BIOCHEMICAL ADAPTATION

BIOCHEMICAL ADAPTATION

Mechanism and Process
in Physiological Evolution

Peter W. Hochachka
George N. Somero

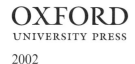

UNIVERSITY PRESS

2002

OXFORD
UNIVERSITY PRESS

Oxford   New York
Athens   Auckland   Bangkok   Bogotá   Buenos Aires   Cape Town
Chennai   Dar es Salaam   Dehli   Florence   Hong Kong   Istanbul   Karachi
Kolkata   Kuala Lumpur   Madrid   Melbourne   Mexico City   Mumbai   Nairobi
Paris   São Paulo   Shanghai   Singapore   Taipei   Tokyo   Toronto   Warsaw

and associated companies in
Berlin   Ibadan

Published by Oxford University Press, Inc.
198 Madison Avenue, New York, New York 10016

Oxford is a registered trademark of Oxford University Press.

Library of Congress Cataloging-in-Publication Data

Hochachka, Peter W.
  Biochemical adaptation: mechanism and process in physiological evolution / Peter W.
  Hochachka, George N. Somero.
    p. cm.
  Includes bibliographical references and index
  ISBN 0-19-511702-6; 0-19-511703-4 (pbk.)
  1. Adaptation (Physiology) 2. Physiology, Comparative. 3. Molecular evolution. I.
  Somero, George N. II. Title.

QP82.H632 2001
572.8'38-–dc21   2001032142

9 8 7 6 5 4 3 2
Printed in the United States of America
on acid-free paper

Dedicated

to C. Ladd Prosser and Knut Schmidt-Nielsen

teachers, researchers,

pathfinders, and role models

Preface

The eighteen years that have elapsed since we last attempted to fit the broad field of "biochemical adaptation" between two covers have witnessed an explosive growth of information in virtually every area of study encompassed by our field. This statement holds whether the topic in question is metabolic regulation, protein structure–function relationships, the control of gene expression, the physics of intracellular water, or the evolutionary origin of new classes of proteins. The information explosion that students of biochemical adaptation have experienced during this period has of course been matched by equally and often more explosive growth in other biological disciplines. At the time we wrote our last volume, even optimists like ourselves would have underestimated the amount of progress that would take place in the biological sciences during the closing decades of the past century. In particular, we probably would not have foreseen that many of the questions that served as focal points of our previous volume would receive detailed answers by the time we set out on our next writing effort.

Yet, as we are all aware, such progress comes with both positive and negative aspects, a kind of good news/bad news situation. Thus, the excitement that accompanies discovery of the wealth of new knowledge in biology is sometimes paired with a sense of desperation: How are we to assimilate all of this new detail (the proverbial "trees" of information) while retaining within our scientific field of vision a clear overview of the "forest," that is, of the major integrative theories of our discipline? How must our existing theories be modified in the face of new data? Can entirely new conceptual syntheses now be developed on the basis of recent discoveries? How are we to deal with cross-disciplinary challenges that also abound? How do the discoveries and theories of one field impact the status of sister disciplines, ones that may lie close to the periphery of our scientific field of vision? The challenges faced in dealing with "informational" issues of these sorts are heightened by the fact that new experimental approaches, important new theoretical developments, and a great deal of new jargon have entered biology. These manifestations of progress frequently have the unfortunate consequence of making much of the literature seem as though it is penned in a foreign language. Can a biologist any longer read the table of contents in widely focused journals like *Science* and *Nature* and hope to comprehend what all of the articles related to "biology" are about? An unfortunate trend linked to progress in biology is increased specialization: Investigators find themselves feeling most comfortable and secure (and most apt to be funded) when dealing with a limited suite of phenomena and techniques. Biologists more and more frequently seem to be speaking to a restricted set of their peers, those specialists to whom they can talk their particular language.

Despite the trend toward increased specialization, many biologists strive to carry out and to communicate integrative analyses that represent synthetic, cross-disciplinary contributions. In these analyses, data from many types of experimentation, performed at different levels of complexity in the hierarchy of biology phenomena, are incorporated into investigations of broad-scale questions. The present volume is an attempt to reach this very goal. We approached this project with the desire to integrate a wide range of information from studies of topics like the regulation of gene expression, metabolic biochemistry, protein structure–function relationships, genomics, and proteomics into a framework that would allow the reader to gain deeper understanding of broadly important issues in evolution, ecology, biodiversity, and biogeography. As the subtitle of this volume is meant to suggest, we have taken an integrative approach in two different senses of the term. First, we have attempted in each topic covered to traverse as many rungs on the reductionist ladder as was possible with available information. Through these exercises we have tried to place a fundamental mechanistic foundation under higher level phenomena such as biogeographic patterning. Second, we have sought to integrate analyses of mechanisms with accounts of how these mechanisms came to be through evolutionary change in the genetic repertoire of organisms. We provide examples of how mutations finely tune gene products for dealing with particular environmental challenges, and we show how entirely new biochemical potentials arise through the development of new classes of genes. Mechanism and process thus serve as integrating themes in the chapters to follow. We hope that our focus on integrative approaches to the study of biochemical adaptation will provide for readers a mode of analysis that will become a routine way of viewing many biological issues. The success of this volume will be measured in part by the degree to which we have summarized important facts and concepts—"trees" and "forests"—as they were known near the beginning of the 21st century, and more importantly, by whether we have taught our readers what we view to be the most effective ways of addressing questions about the mechanisms and processes of biochemical adaptation.

The coming decades in this so-called "Century of Biology" will offer enormous opportunities and challenges. New technological approaches (such as those used for obtaining detailed information in genomics, proteomics, magnetic resonance and other imaging modalities, and remote-sensing field physiology, to mention a few topical areas) will vastly increase the amount of information we have before us. And, paired with new means for acquiring information, we can expect equally rapid growth in the suite of algorithms used to analyze the torrent of new data. Students of biochemical adaptation must be prepared for these advances and be ready to exploit them, at least when these new advances are relevant for our purposes. If recent history is an indication of what the following decades will bring, progress in biochemical adaptation will often depend on successful incorporation of methods and theories developed for "model" organisms like humans, fruit flies, or zebra fish into investigations of organisms of interest to the comparative biologist. However, novel technologies per se do not necessarily and inevitably lead to creativity and advancement of a field. Comparative biologists interested in biochemical adaptation must not lose sight of the important questions and principles of their field, even as they incorporate new theories and methods from sister disciplines in biology. To the degree that we are able to adapt new approaches when applicable to long-standing questions about adaptation, our field will enjoy an even brighter future. We hope that this volume serves in some small way as a stimulus to these endeavors.

Completing this volume would not have been possible without the support of many of our colleagues. First and perhaps foremost, PWH wishes to thank a group of graduate and postdoctoral research students: Chris Moyes, Les Buck, Chris Doll, Tim West, Steve Land, Jim Staples, Mark Mossey, Petra Motishaw, Mark Trump, Gary Burness, Grant McClelland, Sheila Thornton, Gunna Weingartner, Jim Rupert, Charles Darveau, Cheryl Beatty, Peter Arthur, Kevin Campbell, and Yan Burrelle. Many of PWH's insights are really products of their creativity, enthusiasm, and hard labor. Additionally, several colleagues have been hugely instrumental in "pulling reptilian scales" off of PWH's eyeballs so that he could "see" better. Space will not permit mentioning all of these, but will allow especial thanks to Raul Suarez, Michael Guppy, Gordon Matheson, Carlos Monge, Peter Allen, Bob Boutilier, Dave Jones, Bill Driedzic, Dan Costa, Barbara Block, Brian Murphy, Michael Hogan, Peter Lutz, and Keith Webster. Each in their own way made PWH aware of aspects of adaptation that he otherwise would have overlooked or under emphasized. Warren Zapol, an ever-fussing deeply committed friend and colleague, has been aware (and, along with Mont Liggins, has kept PWH as aware as possible) of clinical implications of many aspects of adaptational biochemistry. Dick Taylor (until his premature death) and Ewald Weibel were continuous sources of inspiration and their questions at physiological levels of organization often created intellectual fun and fermentation for those of us working at molecular and metabolic levels of organization.

GNS, too, wishes to thank his current and former students and postdoctoral associates, all of whom have provided inspiration and encouragement, not to mention loads of interesting data, many of which will be found in this volume. Several of these colleagues have been generous with their time and energy in helping develop the ideas and exposition of the present volume. In particular, gratitude is owed to Dr. Peter Fields, who did yeoman service as a critic and editor throughout the writing of chapters 1, 6 and 7, and Drs. Glenn Johns, Dietmar Kültz, Jason Podrabsky, Jonathon Stillman, and Lars Tomanek, who played important roles in critiquing chapters 6 and 7. Development of many of the ideas found in the book benefited from discussions with Drs. Barb Block, D. Wayne Bolen, John Carpenter, Jim Childress, Mary Clark, Andy Cossins, Elizabeth Dahlhoff, Mark Denny, Dave Epel, Allen Gibbs, Andy Gracey, Steve Hand, Gretchen Hofmann, Linda Holland, Jen-Jen Lin, Philip Low, Donal Manahan, Eric Sanford, Serge Timasheff, Patrick Walsh, Paul Yancey, and Tzung-Horng Yang, and with current doctoral students, Rachael Ream and Caren Braby. Students in Stanford University's course in Ecological and Evolutionary Physiology also played important editorial roles, through critiquing handouts that were based on embryonic versions of book chapters.

One of the special joys of our profession sometimes arises from following the experimental organism under study to its natural habitat; or, as Per Scholander would have put it, great joy arises from taking the laboratory to the study organism rather than vice versa. In this context, we both would like to acknowledge our numerous colleagues around the world who have made, and in most cases continue to make, the entire endeavor more interesting by combining the adventures of intellect with the adventures of scientific expedition.

In addition, we wish to express our deepest sense of gratitude to Brenda and Amy, who have accepted with comforting humor that Peter and George (respectively) are fundamentally "workaholic" husbands, who year after year are almost certain to find excuses for shorter-than-planned holidays so that they can pursue varied academic projects. Claire, Gail, Gareth, and (until lately) Panda supplied comic relief, encouragement and support to PWH even at the lowest moments in life—when his cranial nerves were trashed by a nasty virus and death was at his door. GNS' spirits enjoyed continual buoyancy from Gabe, whom he thanks along with Patty and Bud, who made Gabe's entry into the family possible. GNS would not have been able to complete his part of the bargain without substantial support from the faculty and staff at the Hopkins Marine Station; they established a working environment in which it was possible to juggle teaching, research, and administrative duties while retaining sufficient ATP to complete this volume.

Lastly, we thank Ms. Diana McPhail, Mr. Chris Patton and Ms. Freya Sommer for their work on illustrations, and our editor, Kirk Jensen, for unrivalled if unrequited patience. Ms. Lissa Herschleb designed for us a cover creature that aptly portrays, at an anatomical level, the concept of "unity in diversity," which serves as a unifying theme in our treatment of biochemical adaptation. The smile on the imaginary creature's face may be taken as a reflection of the pleasure we have had in reviewing the fascinating topics that constitute the literature of our field. We hope that the book brings our readers a comparable sense of enjoyment.

Peter W. Hochachka
Vancouver, British Colombia

George N. Somero
Pacific Grove, California

Contents

BIOCHEMICAL ADAPTATION

1

The Goals and Scope of This Volume

THE CHALLENGES OF ADAPTATION

The central question to be addressed in this volume is, How have living systems, which are based on a common set of biochemical structures and processes and subject to a common set of physical–chemical laws, been able to adapt to the enormously wide spectrum of environmental conditions found in the biosphere? The biosphere comprises habitats having a remarkably varied set of physical, chemical, and biotic characteristics, many of which seem "extreme" or "highly stressful" from our human perspective as a 37°C species living on the planet's surface and exposed to an oxygen-rich atmosphere. The diversity of life forms found in the varied habitats of the biosphere indicates how successful adaptation has been in allowing exploitation of virtually all regions of the earth's land and waters. Yet we can ask whether the diversity we find in morphology and other highly visible attributes of organisms is paired with a high degree of adaptive diversification at the biochemical level. Are all organisms relatively alike "under the skin," that is to say, biochemically, despite their vast differences in habitat preferences, body plan, and mode of life? As we will learn, the answer to this question represents a fascinating combination of "yes" and "no." To develop this answer, we will first characterize the adaptational challenges facing biochemical systems and then examine how these systems have been modified through evolution to permit the same fundamental types of structures and processes to be sustained in all organisms, in all environments. We will show how an underlying unity in biochemical design persists in the face of a remarkable degree of adaptive diversification in biochemical structures and processes.

The challenges to biochemical systems that are imposed by the environment, challenges that would seem to be tremendously diverse because of the wide range of habitat conditions encountered by organisms, ultimately arise from only *two* principal sources. First, the core biochemical constituents of all organisms—enzymatic and structural proteins, nucleic acids, and lipoprotein structures like cellular membranes—and the interactions among them are susceptible to direct perturbation from several environmental factors. Specifically, temperature, hydrostatic pressure, radiation, water availability, O_2-derived free radicals, and the solute composition and concentration of the medium may exert profound effects on the biochemical structures on which life depends. This sensitivity to the environment often is a manifestation of a critical feature of the design of biochemical systems. Each of the above essential biochemical constituents of cells must retain a *delicate balance between stability and instability* in order to maintain its functional properties. This *marginal stability of structure* that is so essential for function renders biochemical systems highly vulnerable to physical and chemical forces. One challenge of adaptation, then, is to ensure that the appropriate structural states of the biochemical constituents on which life depends are sustained in the face of environmental conditions that threaten their integrity.

A second fundamental source of sensitivity to the environment and, therefore, a second major challenge for adaptation, derives from the fact that, in order to sustain life, cells must be capable of maintaining an *adequate level of energy turnover*—the synthesis of adenosine triphosphate (ATP) and reducing power and use of these "energy currencies" in biological work. The Second Law of Thermodynamics states that disorder increases with time, so all systems, living or not, tend to move toward a state of maximal entropy. One of the hallmarks of living systems is their ability to channel energy through metabolic processes in manners that allow maintenance of the high degree of order that is characteristic of life. For example, turnover of large quantities of ATP is required to maintain transmembrane gradients in ion concentrations. These gradients are critical for a wide range of physiological activities in all types of cells. Large amounts of energy must be expended to replace denatured proteins and to add sufficient new quantities of proteins to support growth and reproduction. All of these processes require synthesis of ATP, which is used to perform the work that is required to circumvent the threats posed by the Second Law. In addition, reducing power, as supplied by reduced nicotinamide adenine dinucleotide phosphate (NADPH), is needed to power reductive steps in biosynthetic processes such as those involved in lipid synthesis. Many environmental changes, even if they do not directly damage the structures of biochemical systems, threaten the cell by affecting its ability to sustain adequate rates of energy turnover. We will see how these threats arise from the chemical environment, notably from reduced availability of molecular oxygen or water, and from the physical environment, for instance, from the effects of reduced temperature.

To summarize, the central challenges faced by all organisms in adaptation to the environment comprise (i) offsetting the direct perturbation of marginally stable biochemical structures by physical and chemical factors, and (ii) coping with the effects of environmental change on rates of metabolic processes. Structure and process must be defended if life is to persist, and the manners in which diverse taxa have responded to these two fundamental challenges under a host of environmental conditions form the focus of this volume.

To see how these adaptive biochemical feats are accomplished, we first must develop an analytical frame of reference that will enable us to study adaptive change in a logical and rigorous manner. The "challenges of adaptation" involve philosophical issues for the scientist as well as environmental challenges for organisms.

CONCEPTUAL APPROACHES TO BIOCHEMICAL ADAPTATION STUDIES

The philosophical "challenge of adaptation" arises from difficult conundrums that are linked to the concept of "adaptation." In recent decades these conceptual issues have led to substantial debate about the nature of adaptation and the appropriate means for studying it. These deliberations have served as a strong "selective force" that has driven an evolutionary change (perhaps even a *revolutionary* change, in the Kuhnian sense of the word "revolution") in our perspective on adaptive processes. If we are to answer satisfactorily the question that opens this chapter, we must understand what this intellectual ferment is all about.

To fulfill the goals of this volume, then, we must first construct a conceptual foundation that will provide a solid base on which we can develop our analyses of diverse types of adaptive change. This foundation must provide *logical definitions* of the vocabulary we will employ when we discuss adaptation, and it must delineate *how the process of adaptation needs to be studied* in order to allow meaningful conclusions to be drawn about the interactions between environment and organism. Building this foundation also will entail developing a historical perspective on the broad field of physiology. This historical viewpoint can help us to understand how the study of adaptation arose and how it has evolved, as the field of physiology has differentiated into a number of distinct subdisciplines.

What Do We Study When We Examine Biochemical Adaptation: What Is a "Biochemical Trait"?

It seems logical to begin our foundation-building effort with a most basic question: What do we study when we examine biochemical adaptations? What may seem like the obvious answer to this question, namely "biochemical traits," is by no means a simple or unambiguous answer, for it immediately should draw our attention to the difficulty entailed in defining just what a "trait" of an organism is. The difficulty a physiologist or biochemist faces in defining what a trait is arises from a common and fundamental challenge that *every* experimental biologist faces. One of the primary requirements for doing experimental biology is this: the investigator must "dissect out" from nature a study system that is (i) simple enough to be experimentally tractable, yet (ii) is not so overly simplified that it fails to teach us about the properties of the ecosystem, organism, cell, or macromolecule as it actually exists in its natural condition. Delineating the appropriate study system is a problem that faces all biologists, whatever the spatial or temporal scale of their investigations. As we show throughout this volume, making decisions about the right study system is a tall order for both technical and philosophical reasons.

The mandatory "dissection" process involved in studying biochemical traits creates two primary types of problem. One problem is a general one that obtains whether or not the biochemist is interested in examining the adaptive value of a biochemical trait. This common problem relates to the difficulties that arise when data from studies of simplified systems are used to extrapolate back to the much more complex reality of the living organism in its natural habitat. Let us try to delineate this problem in some detail, so we can better appreciate the challenges we face in studying biochemical adaptation.

A biochemist typically must "dissect" an organism into separate biochemical constituents in order to carry out the intended studies. For instance, through isolating and purifying one protein from among tens of thousands in the cell, detailed, closely controlled in vitro experiments can be done on this particular study system (or "biochemical trait," if you will). This requirement for simplification is absolutely necessary for controlled experimentation, yet is also the source of a major philosophical problem: How do we know that the properties we measure in an isolated system resemble those

of the system in situ? Can the isolated object even be called a "trait" if, through our efforts at isolating the object for controlled study, we alter it in ways that cause its properties in vitro to differ from those present in vivo? For instance, is an individual protein a "trait"? Although one may tend to think that this question can be answered affirmatively, we will see that problems arise with this answer because the functional characteristics of proteins are so strongly influenced by the local milieu in which they carry out their roles. Thus, to adequately describe a protein's status in vivo we may need to understand how the protein of interest is influenced by (i) its hydration state, (ii) the pH of the medium, (iii) the concentrations of regulatory molecules in solution, (iv) interactions with the abundant low-molecular-mass osmotic solutes (osmolytes) of the cell, and (v) interactions with other proteins and other types of macromolecular components of the cell. The observations obtained through in vitro study may fall short of telling us what the protein—the so-called "trait" under study—is like in vivo. A key point arising from this conclusion is that the assignment of "adaptive significance" to a trait may be strongly influenced by the set of study conditions used to examine the trait.

Similar concerns about the effects of studying systems in isolation arise at all levels of biological organization, not only in the context of biochemistry. For example, can we meaningfully study the adaptive importance of a single organ to the diving response of a seal—or must we adopt a more integrative perspective and determine how the function of the organ of interest is affected by, and integrated with, the activities of other organs? Just how do we draw boundaries around "traits" so as to perform biologically realistic experiments and deduce how the characteristic of interest is adaptive to the organism?

In addition to this basic challenge that affects all experimental biologists faced with the need to "dissect out" a tractable study system, there is a further problem linked to the concept of "trait" that arises for the biochemist interested in elucidating mechanisms of adaptation and describing these adaptations in a logically consistent manner. To appreciate the nature of this complex problem, it is necessary to examine in some detail the concept that lies at the very core of our analysis: *adaptation*.

What Is "Adaptation"?

Adaptation is a concept that enjoys widespread use—and suffers from widespread misuse. To develop a firm conceptual foundation for the analyses of adaptation presented in subsequent chapters, it is essential to define carefully the way in which this intellectually charged word is to be used. This is a considerable challenge, for a number of reasons. First, "adaptation" is used both in the context of process and in reference to specific traits (or character states) of existing organisms. Therefore, in discussing adaptation it is critical to clarify whether we are referring to the historical process by which attributes of organisms change to enhance fitness, or whether we are restricting our discussion entirely to the characteristics and current utility of the trait of interest.

A second major challenge arises from the difficulty of demonstrating rigorously that a particular trait in fact has adaptive properties. As Gould and Lewontin (1979) illustrated in their landmark article, "The spandrels of San Marco and the panglossian paradigm: a critique of the adaptionist programme," the study of adaptation is fraught with the danger of lulling ourselves into believing that, if a trait *seems* adaptive for some particular purpose, it *must be so*—and it must have arisen for just this purpose. It is easy to pen "just-so" stories that, while intuitively appealing, may turn out to be in error. For instance, when we examine the diving response it will be shown how traits that seem to be critical adaptations for diving are in fact ancestral traits that arose in the non-diving ancestors of contemporary seals and their relatives and have persisted in this lineage, in some cases without any diving-adaptive alterations in the trait (chapter 4). These traits may contribute to breath-hold diving, but their origin had little or nothing to do with the diving response per se. If we adopt the terminology associated with "adaptation" that has been introduced by Gould, Lewontin, Vrba, and others, such "phylogenetic baggage" should

not be referred to as adaptations at all (Gould and Lewontin, 1979; Gould and Vrba, 1982; for a comprehensive analysis of "adaptation," see Rose and Lauder, 1996).

Let us examine this terminology to learn how it can clarify the discussion of adaptation. In the rigorous analysis of Gould, Lewontin, and Vrba, definitions of "adaptation" and related terms take into account the two aspects of adaptation emphasized at the beginning of this section: the *process* through which a trait arose (original selective advantage; the raison d'être for the trait) and the *current utility* of the trait. The concept "adaptation" is defined in a restrictive sense to refer to a trait (i) that enhances the fitness of an organism, and (ii) whose current beneficial characteristics reflect the selective advantage of the trait at its time of origin. Clearly, to analyze adaptation in this rigorous manner, one must know a great deal about the evolutionary history of traits and the phylogenies of the organisms being studied. We return to the issue of phylogeny later on, and discuss methods that may help us distinguish between "phylogenetic baggage" and true adaptive variation.

Despite the problems pointed out by Gould and others, making well-grounded evaluations of adaptive significance can be straightforward. For many traits, their current benefits seem very likely to reflect the selective advantage that favored their origins. For example, the benefits obtained by contemporary organisms through using molecular oxygen as a terminal electron acceptor, and thus acquiring a high yield of ATP per mole of substrate catabolized, are most likely the same as the benefits that originally favored selection for aerobically poised catabolic pathways and the electron transport chain. The roles played by molecular chaperones in protein maturation and repair of denatured proteins in contemporary organisms are very likely the benefits that initially favored the evolutionary development of these ubiquitous proteins. Chaperones are present in all organisms, and their occurrence and common physiological function in all species argue strongly that their original functions were the same as the functions we see today. Traits such as the respiratory chain and molecular chaperones thus can be viewed as "adaptations" in the restrictive sense of the word defined by Gould, Lewontin, and Vrba, because it seems highly probable that each trait continues to benefit contemporary organisms in the same fundamental way it benefited the first organisms to acquire the trait.

The life of a student of biochemical adaptation is not always this easy, however. In many cases, a trait that is currently beneficial (adaptive) would not be termed an "adaptation" in the narrow historically determined sense of Gould et al. We can point to numerous instances in which the current benefit or adaptive significance of a trait is not the same as the benefit of the trait at the time of its time of origin. The varied functions of the polyhydric, three-carbon alcohol glycerol provide a good case study of this issue. This study of glycerol's roles in physiology will lead us to seriously re-examine what we mean by a "trait" and how we must "dissect" organisms for studying adaptation.

Glycerol plays a broad range of adaptive roles in contemporary organisms. For example, glycerol is used by certain freeze-resistant invertebrates (e.g., Arctic beetles) and fishes (e.g., smelt and greenling) to lower the colligative freezing points and enhance the supercooling abilities of body fluids (see chapter 7). Was this the original adaptive value of glycerol at the time that the biochemical pathways for its synthesis arose? This seems highly unlikely. Glycerol plays essential structural roles in lipid chemistry, forming a key backbone element in depot lipids (triacylglycerides) and phospholipids (phosphoglycerides). Its importance in this context is almost universal. Glycerol also is a substrate for energy metabolism, where it plays an important role in ATP-generating pathways. Glycerol also stabilizes proteins and membranes under conditions of cellular dehydration, when it may function as a "water substitute," among other roles (chapter 6). Which benefit of glycerol accounts for the initial evolution of its biosynthetic pathway? Although in the absence of a time machine we cannot answer this question definitively, it seems very probable that glycerol's initial selective advantage related to one of its presently most widely occurring functions: lipid structures or energy metabolism. Both of these uses of glycerol almost certainly predated its uses as an anti-freeze and supercooling agent or as a mechanism for tolerance of desiccation. However, which of these two widely occurring "primitive" uses of glycerol came first remains an open question. More to the point of our analysis, however, is the question of what terminology to use when we describe one of the "nonprimitive" uses of glycerol.

To follow the terminology of Gould and Vrba (1982), it is appropriate to view glycerol's roles in resistance to freezing and in tolerance of desiccation as *exaptations*, which are defined as the exploitation of a trait (in this case a chemical) for an entirely new function, one unrelated to the original selective value of the trait. Older terminology for this type of phenomenon would refer to glycerol as being "preadapted" to assume a role in resistance to freezing and desiccation—an adaptation "waiting to happen."

As should be evident from this discussion of the multiple functions of even a simple molecule like glycerol, it is often difficult, if not impossible, to discern exactly what adaptive role the trait in question initially played. We will return to this conundrum at many junctures in this volume. In similar quandaries, some authors employ the term *aptation*, which refers to beneficial values of traits in a *nonhistorical* manner. Use of the term aptation is an honest confession of ignorance on the part of the investigator. Data may strongly support the conjecture that a trait is currently beneficial, but there may be no data that provide a historical perspective concerning the origin and original utility of the trait. Thus, aptation is probably the most legitimate term to use in the discussion of many currently beneficial traits. In other words, many of the traits that are commonly viewed as adaptations should logically be regarded as aptations, because of our lack of historical insight into the original selective advantage of the trait. In fact, some currently beneficial traits may have arisen as *nonadaptations*, traits that arose as a necessary consequence of some evolutionary process, but which conferred no selective advantage to the organism.

What Do We Mean by "Origin of a Trait"?

The definitions given above of "adaptation" and its verbal congeners reemphasize the importance of treating adaptive change in the dual context of the current value of the trait in question and the evolutionary process that led to the trait's origin. To deal adequately with this two-fold nature of adaptation, however, a closer look at the concept of "trait" is mandated at this juncture. This reexamination of just what we choose to define as a trait will force us to reexamine the seemingly clear-cut distinction between adaptation and exaptation. How we choose to "dissect" an organism biochemically will help to determine which of these two terms is the appropriate one to use in examining adaptive change at the biochemical level.

Let us again consider the glycerol molecule. Just what trait are we really studying when we examine adaptation in contexts like freezing resistance and tolerance to desiccation? If we answer by saying "the three-carbon polyhydric alcohol glycerol," we may be giving an answer that is naïve and simplistic in terms of providing a context for discussing adaptation. To discuss the role of glycerol in a biologically realistic manner, the trait we define as "glycerol" may need to encompasses not only the chemical itself, but also the physiological systems in which it is embedded. At a minimum, these systems would include a number of different proteins that are involved in the synthesis and further metabolism of glycerol and in the regulation of its intracellular concentration. The latter types of proteins may include membrane-localized transporters and gene regulatory proteins whose activities are influenced by the concentration of glycerol or by environmentally imposed stresses that determine the cell's needs for this molecule (chapter 6). The context in which we should analyze the adaptive importance of glycerol, in any of its many roles, thus comprises two distinct factors: (i) the intrinsic properties of the molecule itself, for instance its stabilizing effects on proteins and membranes and its infinite miscibility with water; and (ii) the abilities of the cell's metabolic pathways, membrane-localized transporters, and gene

regulatory systems to closely control the concentration of glycerol in the body fluids as a function of environmental stress.

The nature of the trait "glycerol" described in this broader sense forces us to reexamine our earlier decision to regard the benefits of glycerol in freezing resistance and tolerance of desiccation as exaptations. Although it is true that glycerol is unlikely to have been selected originally for either of these functions, it is also true that substantial amounts of selective fine-tuning of metabolic regulatory systems, membrane transporter functions, and gene regulatory mechanisms have been required to support the use of glycerol in some of its derived functions, for instance, in resistance to freezing. Therefore, if we elect to offer a more inclusive definition of the trait "glycerol," and include in our definition the mechanisms or functional systems responsible for controlling glycerol's concentration, then the benefits of glycerol in freezing resistance, tolerance of desiccation, and other functions different from its original role can be properly referred to as adaptations. Perhaps a rigorous analysis of glycerol's adaptive roles in freezing resistance and tolerance to desiccation would restrict use of the term "adaptation" to the alterations in the regulatory systems used to control glycerol's concentration. The molecule itself might still be viewed as an exaptation, one whose new benefits arose through refinements of the regulatory mechanisms used by the cell to mediate adaptive shifts in concentration. Although we agree with the inherent logic of the latter argument, namely that the glycerol molecule functions in several *exaptive* roles as a result of *adaptive* changes in the systems controlling its concentration, we prefer to group together the molecule and the processes involved in its synthesis, degradation, and transmembrane movements as a single trait, "glycerol." We view "glycerol" in this way because in so doing we believe we are defining the trait of interest in a more biologically meaningful manner, one that encompasses the complexity of the selectively important features in question. Therefore, when we refer to glycerol as an adaptation for withstanding desiccation or subfreezing temperatures, we are employing the term adaptation in the historical sense of Gould et al., even though a restrictive definition of glycerol as the molecule per se would require use of the term exaptation to refer correctly to these secondary benefits of the three-carbon polyol.

The analysis given to the trait "glycerol" reflects a general issue that will appear throughout this volume: adaptive variation commonly involves adjusting the production of a type of constituent (a chemical, a metabolic pathway, an organelle) in ways that enhance the organism's fitness. The constituent per se may have arisen for the same benefit for which it is now used, or the constituent may be an example of exaptation. In either case, it is justified to use the term adaptation to describe how changes in the mechanisms that alter the constituent's concentration or functional properties help to make the organism more fit.

One additional example of how biochemical traits may be recruited for new functions may be helpful in clarifying further our use of the word "adaptation." This example concerns the origin of the Krebs citric acid cycle as a mechanism for facilitating catabolism of diverse substrates for ATP generation. Many of the reactions we associate with this cycle are thought to have had as their original function the biosynthesis of carboxylic acid skeletons for incorporation into amino acids. When these synthetic reactions were linked to the oxidation of acetate, a complete cycle was generated that is capable of funneling large quantities of reducing equivalents to the electron transport chain for aerobic production of ATP. Melendez-Hevia et al. (1996) demonstrate that although there are several different chemical ways for achieving this goal, the design of the Krebs citric acid cycle is the best chemical solution: it has the least possible number of steps and it achieves the greatest yield of ATP. The key point, however, is not the remarkable efficiency of this pathway, but rather the fact that a preexisting set of metabolic reactions needed for synthesis of carboxylic acid intermediates for amino acid biosynthesis was recruited (exapted) for an important new function: the supply of reducing equivalents to the electron transport chain. The changes in enzymatic potential that led to this new use for "old" biosynthetic reac-

tions would certainly seem to warrant use of the concept of "adaptation."

We hope that our use of the term "adaptation" will strike the reader as being logical and, of equal importance, biologically realistic in the sense that descriptions of the evolution of complex physiological systems mandate an integrative perspective. It may prove helpful to our understanding of how physiological traits should be delineated and studied if we take a brief look at the evolution of the discipline of physiology itself—its origins and its subsequent diversification into numerous specialties.

A HISTORICAL PERSPECTIVE: WHAT IS "PHYSIOLOGY"?

As the subtitle of this volume suggests, this book has a strong focus on "physiology," a discipline that the dictionary defines quite simply as "the study of biological function." But *what* physiology is to serve as the focus of our treatment? Even a cursory look at the suite of current biological journals or the rows of physiology texts in any science library will reveal a host of different adjectives lying before the noun physiology. In many cases, these adjectives merely denote the particular level of biological organization or the type of organism that serves as the focus of the journal or book, for instance, *cellular, molecular*, and *neural* or *plant, microbial*, and *vertebrate*. More germane for our purposes in the present discussion, however, are some of the adjectives that denote different conceptual approaches to physiology. Among these conceptual adjectives are *comparative, environmental, ecological, evolutionary, adaptational*, and *integrative*. These conceptual approaches to the study of physiology will be central recurring themes throughout this volume, as we analyze diverse functional traits of organisms in the contexts of (i) how a particular trait helps "fit" (adapt) the organism to its particular environment, (ii) how and why these traits originated during evolution, (iii) how a given trait may assume new adaptational significance when environmental conditions change or when the lineage itself evolves to have new characteristics, and (iv) how the function of one trait is integrated into the web of physiological processes of the whole organism. Our study of physiology, then, will present the mechanisms of diverse functional systems in a way that elucidates each system's current utilities, its origin, and its interactions with the environment and with other physiological components of the organism.

When and Why Did Different "Physiologies" Arise?

To understand the different conceptual approaches to physiology, it is helpful to have an historical perspective. The earliest physiology (which probably would be recognized today as an early form of medical physiology because of its emphasis on human physiology) focused on *mechanism*—on how organisms "work." Knut Schmidt-Nielsen's 1972 text on animal physiology is aptly entitled How Animals Work, a title that serves as a concise shorthand statement of the primary objective of *mechanistic physiology*. Mechanistic physiology, at least the modern experimental version of this discipline, has roots that can be traced into the seventeenth century, for instance in the work of Harvey on the circulation of the blood. The field grew significantly during the eighteenth century, for instance through the development by Lavoisier and Priestly of the theory of oxygen and its role in respiration. Mechanistic physiology flourished in the nineteenth century, as exemplified by the investigations of great physiologists like Bernard, who emphasized the critical importance of conserving the status of the internal milieu; Helmholtz, who established many of the basic principles of vision and hearing (as well as developing major physical theories such as the conservation of energy); and Pasteur, whose genius led to spectacular advances in physiology on several fronts (fermentation, nature of disease, and disproving the spontaneous generation of life). These giants of mechanistic physiology not only helped develop momentum for one of the core disciplines in the biological sciences, but they also established a rich tradition that characterizes most, if not all, branches of physiology: the borrowing from physics and chemistry of critical concepts and techniques

that facilitate a rapid advancement of the physiological sciences, broadly defined. The current exploitation by physiologists of the techniques of imaging (e.g., magnetic resonance imaging) and molecular biology represents an intellectual continuum in this regard.

Not too many decades after the beginnings of mechanistic physiology, which initially focused strongly on humans and other mammals, the breadth of species coming under the scrutiny of physiologists grew, a pattern perhaps driven by a mixture of natural curiosity about diversity and "unusual" organisms, and the realization that some questions are best addressed with a particular type of organism (Somero, 2000). This latter point of view, which is commonly termed the *August Krogh Principle* (Krogh, 1929; see Krebs, 1975) states that, for any question that a physiologist chooses to address, nature provides an ideal study organism (or, as we shall see in later chapters, the ideal gene, the ideal protein, and so forth). The utility of this principle is not restricted to physiology, of course. For instance, much of the progress of the field of genetics is based on the insightful choice of organisms such as *Drosophila*, bacteriophages, and *Escherichia coli*, species that provide study systems that exemplify the August Krogh Principle.

The search for optimal study systems has been one of the driving forces in what is commonly termed *comparative* physiology, the examination of a common type of physiological system in diverse species. This search for good experimental systems has led to the development of powerful research programs that exploit diverse organisms that offer unique experimental benefits. The giant axon of the squid is one classic example of the August Krogh Principle at work. However, the use of diverse organisms because of their utility as good "model systems" is only one of two major benefits that accrue from comparative physiology. As we will demonstrate in numerous contexts in this volume, a second great strength of the comparative approach (whether used by a physiologist, an anatomist, or a biochemist) is that it allows fundamental principles to be deduced from the comparative examination of naturally occurring variation among species (or conspecifics). For instance, if we examine a particular physiological process in organisms adapted to widely different environmental conditions, conditions that strongly perturb the process in question, and find that selection has favored strong conservation of some aspects of the process in all species, in all environments, we may learn a clear lesson about "what really matters" about the physiological system in question. Comparative study at the molecular level may reveal how conservation in critical functional traits is achieved by structural modification; explaining function in terms of structure is a key goal of physiology. If one creatively combines the comparative approach, in the sense just described, with the August Krogh Principle for selecting the optimal study system, then research in elucidating basic aspects of physiology may be especially productive.

Comparative physiologists examining species adapted to widely different environments quickly learned that there often is a strong correlation between the characteristics of the physiological system under study and the environmental conditions faced by the species. Thus, a third adjective, *environmental*, enters the picture. Much comparative physiology can be described as "environmental" or "ecological" or "adaptational" physiology because of the attempt made to elucidate how traits, or modifications thereof, fit the organism to the particular suite of environmental or ecological conditions it faces. This major current in physiology has revealed a multitude of fascinating examples of evolutionary change in response to a variety of abiotic environmental factors, including oxygen availability, temperature, salinity, and hydrostatic pressure, and biotic interactions, for instance, intensity of predator–prey interactions. These responses of organisms to the abiotic and biotic characteristics of their world are the primary subject matter of this volume.

Consideration of how traits have been acquired initially and, then, transmitted through lineages has become an increasingly exciting and important discipline within physiology. There are two distinct reasons for the ferment in this field, which is called *evolutionary physiology*. One catalyst for the development of this field has been a reexamination of the logic that must be used in exploring the evolution of traits, especially traits for which adaptive interpretations are given. Above, we discussed some of the logical issues involved in employing the concept of adaptation. In elucidating the evolution and adaptive significance of traits, a major challenge is to remove from the analysis as fully as possible the influences of phylogeny per se, so that we can more definitely establish if the trait found in the species under study is truly an adaptation in the sense of the terminology developed by Gould and others. Thus, one needs to show that a particular trait, a putative adaptation, is truly something that has been selected to enhance the organism's survival, and is not merely some type of "phylogenetic baggage" that just happens to be a characteristic of the organism because it is a fish, a crab, a seal, a member of the Archaea, and so forth. (Note: Phylogeny is defined as the *actual* evolutionary history of a group of organisms. A *phylogenetic tree* represents a *hypothesis about* a phylogeny.)

Felsenstein (1985) and others (see, e.g., Garland and Carter, 1994) have developed and exploited methods such as Phylogentically Independent Contrasts (PIC) analysis, which attempts to remove from comparative analysis as much as possible the effects of "phylogenetic baggage," in order to allow more rigorous testing of hypotheses about adaptation. These and other methods for distinguishing adaptive change from the mere effects of phylogeny are by no means foolproof. These approaches introduce assumptions that may or may not mesh with reality (for instance, PIC analysis assumes that evolution occurs by a Brownian model). Despite their limitations, the combination of these methods with the August Krogh Principle has led to a much more rigorous analysis of physiological adaptation. This being said, it is reassuring that PIC analysis has not led to a wholesale discard of the conclusions and conjectures of prior efforts in *adaptational* physiology. As Garland and others have pointed out, use of these new algorithms typically leads to the (comforting) conclusion that a less rigorously established adaptive explanation is likely to be correct, especially in cases involving comparisons of distantly related species, for which "phylogenetic baggage" may not create problems for interpreting the significance of variation. Nonetheless, as we will show in various contexts in this volume, PIC analyses have often provided a strong corrective influence in studies of adaptation. At times these analyses (which often are reanalyses of earlier data to which a strong taxonomic foundation has now been appended) have upset intuitively plausible, long-held explanations for the function and origins of traits (Garland and Carter, 1994).

A second major pillar supporting evolutionary physiology is molecular biology. The theories and techniques of molecular biology have expanded and refined the generation of phylogenetic trees, because molecular characters are (i) available in all organisms, and (ii) evolve by well-understood mechanisms. While classical morphology-based phylogenies have been available for many decades—and, it should be emphasized, their accuracy is often supported by subsequent molecular phylogenies for the group in question—the advent of molecular phylogenetics has provided a plethora of easily obtainable orthologous characters for any new group one wishes to study, characters that are often entirely independent of the adaptational hypotheses being examined.

Molecular biology's contributions to evolutionary physiology extend well beyond the generation of phylogenetic trees, however. Elucidation of mechanism and of structure–function relationships has been vastly enhanced by adoption of molecular approaches. For instance, site-directed mutagenesis can be used to modify specific sites in a protein's sequence to test rigorously the conjectured role of an amino acid residue in adaptation to environment. More complex genetic manipulations of organisms have been used for such purposes as testing the importance of enzyme compartmentation in flight muscle metabolism (see Maughan and Vigoreaux, 1999). Studies in which specific genes are deleted may demonstrate the importance of a given gene product, and may also reveal how the absence of this gene product is compensated through modifica-

tions of other physiological systems. Molecular approaches thus not only may allow a clearer picture to be developed of the evolution of a trait through an extended lineage, but also may permit definitive tests to be conducted concerning the putative adaptive importance of a trait. We will see repeatedly in this volume how the exploitation of molecular approaches for these two purposes has allowed evolutionary physiologists to elucidate process and mechanism in biochemical adaptation.

Our exploration of physiological terminology has now taken us to the last adjective in our list: *integrative*. What is integrative physiology, and why is this field gaining an increasing relevance within biology? One way to begin to answer this question is to remind the reader of a viewpoint expressed by certain leaders in genomic research, including principals of the Human Genome Project: "the future is physiology" (see "A Focus on Function," *Nature Genetics* 250: 243–244 (2000)). Once genomes have been sequenced, the challenge becomes one of discovering what all of these genes actually do and what all of the functional roles of proteins are. In other words, once we have learned the set of "words" in the dictionary, we can begin to look in great detail at all of the "sentences," "paragraphs," and "texts" involved in biological function. In essence, we need to be antireductionist in our approaches: begin with the information encoded in DNA, see what proteins result and how their expression is modulated, learn what metabolic transformations occur as a result of possessing this battery of proteins, and, eventually, learn how the organism functions in the real world to which it is more or less well adapted. Integrative physiology can be seen as perhaps the most inclusive discipline within biology, for it attempts to integrate across all levels of biological organization, from the molecular to the ecological and biogeographical.

There is also an experimental design facet to integrative physiology. For example, integrative analysis performed at the biochemical level may allow an investigator to avoid many of the pitfalls that derive from the need of the experimentalist to "dissect" from the organism a biochemical system that can be studied in a closely controlled manner. Integrating the protein or other molecule under study into the fabric of its natural environment can, in effect, put the "bio" back into biochemistry. Integrative biochemistry stresses the critical nature of interactions among large and small constituents of the cell. One major theme of this volume is that, to appreciate as deeply as possible how a physiological system "works," it generally is necessary to understand the types of complementary roles played by large molecules—macromolecules like proteins, DNA, and RNA plus ensembles of macromolecules and lipids in membranes—and small molecules (which we frequently refer to as *micromolecules*, to distinguish them from macromolecules). Despite the fact that physiology (whatever the adjective that precedes it) has come to focus more and more on macromolecules, the milieu in which macromolecular structure and function are supported is a critical element in any physiological investigation. Integrating information involving macro- and micromolecules is key for understanding both mechanistic and evolutionary aspects of physiology. We touched on this issue when we discussed the difficulties entailed in defining a biochemical trait. Integrative physiology is, in many ways, a philosophical perspective in biology that will be needed increasingly as genomic information is exploited, as a first step, to develop a comprehensive—an integrated—view of life.

THE ELEMENT OF TIME IN ADAPTATION

Another theme that runs through this volume concerns the importance of the element of time in processes of adaptation. Numerous examples in the following six chapters will show that, as a general rule, the complexity of an adaptive response is positively correlated with the time that is available to fabricate the response. This statement refers not only to the obvious fact that evolutionary change founded on new or rearranged genetic information is apt to allow the most elaborate forms of adaptation, but also to phenotypic change occurring during the lifetime of an individual. Often the initial cellular response to an environmental change

is modulation of activities of biochemical systems currently operative in the cell. Such "immediate" adaptations may be highly effective in redirecting metabolic flux in manners that compensate for an environmental insult. For instance, a decrease in availability of oxygen may shift ATP generation from aerobic to anaerobic pathways.

Following these short-term modulations of *preexisting* biochemical systems, the cell commonly alters the expressions of genes to provide new types of biochemical potentials or to change the quantity of a particular type of protein already present in the cell. These intermediate time scale adaptations are commonly referred to as either *acclimations* or *acclimatizations*. The distinction between these two terms relates to whether the response is occurring under controlled laboratory conditions, in which only a single variable of interest (e.g., temperature or oxygen availability) is being altered—acclimations, or in natural habitat conditions, where several variables in addition to the variable of interest may change—acclimatizations. Acclimations and acclimatizations are often discussed as instances of *phenotypic plasticity*, the ability to alter the phenotype in response to environmental change. The evolution of phenotypic plasticity requires development of a complex set of tightly integrated environmental sensing and gene regulation mechanisms that allow the organism to sense and then respond appropriately to an environmental change. At many junctures in this volume we will focus on these regulatory systems and their kinetics, to reveal how organisms sense environmental change and how the layers of regulatory control in species with different complexities—for instance, prokaryotes, single-celled eukaryotes and metazoans—help to determine how rapidly adaptive responses can be made. In fact, one of the key distinctions found among different types of organisms is the speed with which adaptive changes can be fabricated. For example, alterations in gene expression tend to occur far more rapidly in prokaryotes than in eukaryotes, whereas alterations in the activities of preexisting biochemical pathways may occur at similar rates in both groups. Generation times differ by several orders of magnitude among species, so evolutionary adaptation is apt to occur at strikingly different rates in different species.

UNITY AND DIVERSITY IN BIOCHEMISTRY

Perhaps the most fundamental theme that will emerge from the discussions contained in the following six chapters is that life manifests a remarkable pairing of *unity* and *diversity*. This "yin–yang" aspect of life will be seen in virtually all of the contexts in which we discuss adaptive change. Perhaps the French expression says it best, "Plus ça change, plus c'est la même chose." The more things change—the more diverse or extreme are the conditions to which organisms adapt—the more we find that a consistent set of biochemical properties is rigorously conserved. Much of the diversity found at the biochemical level represents, in the most fundamental way, the conservation of key traits that form the biochemical architecture of all species. Even the most radical adaptations found in so-called extremophiles reflect the conservative nature of biochemical adaptation.

The conservative trends we will highlight in our analysis of biochemical adaptation may come as something of a surprise. The diversity of life is perhaps more obvious than its unity, at least when organisms are examined with the naked eye or even with sophisticated microscopes. The variety of taxa that are found in the biosphere and their remarkable diversities in form, function, and habitats are phenomena obvious to all observers of nature. However, the underlying unity of biochemical design that one finds among organisms is a phenomenon that is equally remarkable. The ability of diverse life forms to thrive in such a wide spectrum of habitats is largely a result of adaptive processes that allow retention within all types of organisms of a core set of structures and processes. Underlying biochemical unity is preserved at the same time that diversity is generated.

It is probably not an overstatement to say that one of the major triumphs of twentieth-century biochemistry was discovering the unity of life at the level of cellular function. Thus,

today it is almost axiomatic that the genes specifying the "core" components of cellular function and structure are highly conserved in most if not all lineages. Included in this list are: (i) genes for enzymes involved in DNA replication, DNA repair, transcription, translation, protein synthesis, and proteolysis; (ii) genes for mainstream metabolic pathways such as glycolysis, the Krebs citric acid cycle and the electron transfer system, gluconeogenesis, amino acid, fatty acid, and nucleotide synthesis and catabolism, and waste nitrogen (ammonia, urea, and uric acid) metabolism; (iii) genes for membrane-localized ion channels, ion or metabolite transporters or exchangers, and ion or metabolite pumps; (iv) genes for biogenesis and degradation of intracellular motors, microfilaments, sarcoplasmic reticulum, and mitochondria and other organelles; and finally (v) genes for directly sensing changes in the extracellular environment and for transducing that information to appropriate intracellular targets. All of the above genes, except category (v), which we shall discuss further below, usually occur either as single copies or at most are duplicated one to several times. Thus, whereas protein isoforms for these core components of biochemistry are common, typically no more than several variants on a given protein theme are found.

How many genes, then, are required to encode proteins needed for core biochemical functions? If we consider the yeast as a representative single-celled eukaryote, then about 6,000 genes (Goffeau, 2000) appear to be required to generate the suite of functions allowing a single-celled eukaryote to survive. As emphasized already, most of these genes are highly conserved not only in single-celled organisms, but also in cells of multicellular eukaryotic organisms. This conservation is a key underpinning of the biochemical unity found at the cellular level in all living systems. But what types of genetic change can explain the diversity found in nature?

Origins of Physiological Diversity of Cells

Given the core unity of structure and function of cells, we are faced with a key issue: What types of genetic change underlie the physiological diversity of advanced multicellular organisms? One clue to an answer to this question comes from comparisons of genomes of yeast to those of multicellular organisms. Consider genomes of the nematode *Caenorhabditis elegans* (Wilson, 1999) and the insect *Drosophila melanogaster* (Adams et al., 2000; Wixon and O'Kane, 2000). The genome of the former contains about 19,000 genes and the genome of the latter comprises about 14,000 genes. Assuming that about 6,000 of these genes are the same as in yeasts (albeit we pair this assumption with the caveat that the biology of yeast obviously involves an unknown number of yeast-specific genes) we can ask what the additional approximately 8,000–13,000 genes are used for. In a context closer to home, the current Human Genome Project (Bentley, 2000; Kornberg and Krasnow, 2000; Venter et al., 2001) is estimating that our species requires even more genes: somewhere near 35,000 to 40,000. Again, if we assume that some 6,000 of these genes are homologous with genes of yeast involved in supporting core biochemical functions, the question arises: What are the rest (some 30,000 genes) used for?

A first hint about the answer to this question actually is already evident in the gene and protein composition of single-celled eukaryotes like yeast, especially the category (v) genes mentioned above. Category (v) genes are those specifying proteins that interface the inside functions of single cells with their environment, either the external world or the extracellular fluids. They are involved in sensing and signal transduction. Interestingly enough, these types of genes are more highly duplicated than most other families of genes, and, therefore, the number of protein isoforms encoded by category (v) genes are typically much higher than for other types of proteins. This condition can be well illustrated by protein kinases. Protein kinases, as we shall see in various places in this book, are critically involved in many signal transduction pathways. Instead of two to several isoforms, over 1,000 protein kinase isoforms may be present in eukaryotic cells (Hunter, 2000). The number of isoforms of protein kinases varies among species: yeast

(*Saccharomyces cerevisiae*) has 114 protein kinase genes, *C. elegans* has approximately 400, and the human genome is predicted to contain greater than 1,100 protein kinase genes. Of course, not all protein kinase isoforms are expressed under any given condition and the types of protein kinases encoded in the genome differ among eukaryotes. The differential expression and differential evolution of these kinds of genes—the category (v) group of genes above—supply raw material for evolutionary change and species specificity. That this is one key point of departure for physiological diversity in multicellular organisms is strongly supported by studies showing that genes involved in such functions are the most differentiated of all, that is, they are expressed in most numerous isoforms of all. We shall see later in this book (see the discussion of osmosensing in chapter 6, for example) that the complexity of physiological systems in multicellular organisms requires ever more complex sensing, signal transduction, and communication, as body plans attain higher levels of complexity. The control networks that have evolved are hugely complex by comparison with single-celled eukaryotes such as yeasts. We hypothesize that the need for these kinds of functions in metazoans explains in part why these species possess so many more genes than are found in unicellular eukaryotes. More formally, the hypothesis is that genes whose products are involved in such processes as interorgan communication, in cell–cell communication, in development and differentation, in general sensing and signal transduction, in immune defense systems, and in host defense against pathogens and parasites, are fundamental to the evolution of physiological diversity. We believe that this is a key element in resolving one major aspect of the unity—diversity duality of biological systems. Several thousand or so genes in unicellular and multicellular organisms seem to be involved in so-called "core processes" central to cell-level survival and representative of the "unity" of biochemical design. So-called "none-core" functions, such as those listed immediately above, are what a substantial fraction of the remainder of the protein-encoding regions of the large genomes of complex eukaryotes represents—these are the genes that account for physiological diversity.

The Problem of Evolving Physiological Systems

Although the above analysis supplies us with some general guidelines as to the basis of unity and the origins of diversity in biological systems, it does not give a good indication of the size of the problem: How big are the differences between single cell function and function involving interactions among multiple cells? To get a feel for this issue, consider the physiology of wound healing. This physiological function in vivo is in part orchestrated by fibroblasts, which fortunately can be studied in cultured form. When fibroblasts in culture are deprived of nutrient for several hours and then are reintroduced to serum as a culture medium, they begin to divide and proliferate; at a cellular level, the fibroblasts are doing most (if not all) of the things they would do in normal wound-healing physiology. Analyzing shifts in expression among approximately 8,600 genes using DNA microarrays, Iyer et al. (1999) showed that a huge (517-gene) transcription program is regulated in this complex physiology. On the order of 10 different time courses of expression were found for the hundreds of genes required to orchestrate the appropriate functional response. Of course, wound healing is just one kind of physiological system that is required in multicellular organisms, but it is not required in single-cell eukaryotes like yeast. Indeed, most physiologists would admit that, in the total scheme of things, wound healing represents a relatively simple physiological system. All the more informative, therefore, is the insight of how many new genes, compared to the total number of genes possessed by single cell eukaryotes, would have to be found to perform this function. If over 500 genes are required for evolving and regulating a simple physiological system, would 9,000, 35,000, or more be required for the complex, integrated physiologies of mammals, birds, or other metazoans? Until at least most of the genes in fully sequenced genomes are identified, the

answer to this question remains unknown. However, the indications are that as the complexity of physiological systems increases, the recruitment of new genes will be mainly for those in category (v) above—not for those that are involved in "core" cell function and structure.

The Problem of Evolving Organ Systems

The evolution of physiological systems in multicellular animals is often associated with the evolution of organ systems, which also often occur in lineage-specific patterns and thus contribute to observed physiological diversity. What are the dimensions of the problem of organ making? How many genes are involved in going from a single cell condition to an organ with species-specific functions? For most organs and tissues, we do not have enough data for any serious insight into this problem. However, a study of the mammalian pancreas may supply us with some guidelines. When Zhang and colleagues (1997) analyzed the expression of 45,000 genes in normal and cancerous pancreatic cells, they found that only 268 transcripts (or less than 1%) were pancreas-specific. However, many more pancreas specific genes may be involved in the initial development of the organ per se. While we have no information on this for the pancreas, John Steeves of the University of British Columbia has some insight on this question for the development of the advanced nervous systems. According to Steeves (personal communication), it is commonly assumed in today's neuroscience disciplines that up to one half of the genome may be involved in the development and differentiation of mammalian or avian central nervous systems (CNSs). Thus, organ-specific physiology in some cases may be achieved with a modest number of genes (as percentage of the whole genome), but organogenesis may well represent another huge reservoir of genes that are required for metazoans but that would be of no use in prokaryotic systems. And again, those genes that are recruited in this process specify protein products (i) that define organ-specific structures and functions (endocrine functions in the case of the pancreas; neuronal functions, in the case of the CNS), (ii) that interface the organ-specific cell with its extracellular environment or integrate its function with the rest of the organism's physiology, and (iii) that are involved in development and differention of the organ; i.e. proteins that are involved in organogenesis. In short, organ-specific genes specify proteins that are involved in sensing, signal transduction, organogenesis, and physiological communication.

Species Diversity

To reiterate, the implications of these new studies are: (i) that unity of biological systems derives mainly from the conservation of "core" genetic programs (involving perhaps several thousand genes) for "core" cellular-level functions and structures; (ii) that the complexity and diversity of physiological systems arise in large part from genes that are involved in internal communication and in interfacing the organism with its environment; (iii) that going from single cell eukaryote function to complex physiological function in multicellular organisms requires huge numbers (probably tens of thousands) of genes; and, finally, (iv) that tissue and organ specific development and differentation in multicellular organisms may require a large fraction of the genome of metazoans, even if tissue-specific physiology per se may not require an inordinate number of additional genes (268 in the case of the pancreas). The final question of biological diversity that arises concerns the species level: How much new or different genetic machinery is required to make a new species, the ultimate threshold indicator of biodiversity?

Interestingly, there is a huge data base relating to this question, which we will not have the time or space to explore here in any detail. Suffice it to say that many molecular biologists have tried to evaluate this very question in many settings—in the rapid evolution of fishes in east African rift valley lakes, in the postglacial evolution of fishes in north temperature regions of the world, in nematodes, in insects, and in primates—to mention a few well-studied groups. The same general conclusion arises from all of these exceptional examples, and this result can be illustrated by well-known studies in primate evolution involving the separation of chimpanzees from the human lineage. The problem (and in some senses the paradox) is that protein and gene sequences in the common chimpanzee and in humans are remarkably similar. In fact, human and chimpanzee proteins appear to be nearly 99% identical at the amino acid level (King and Wilson, 1975), and it is widely assumed that the same percentage similarity prevails at the DNA level (Normile, 2001). Yet no one could mistake the two species as one. What these examples suggest is that only exceedingly minimal changes in genome sequences may be necessary to specify separate species, possibly with larger percentage changes in gene expression patterns (Normile, 2001). Of course, the longer any two such related lineages evolve separately from each other, the greater the genetic differences between them may become. However, in terms of the origins of unity and diversity, it is humbling as it is surprising to realize how very small the differences in the overall genome may be between two lineages as they separate from each other and thus extend our planet's biodiversity.

Despite what appears to be a minimal requirement for genetic change in the origin of species, it is important to remind ourselves that populations within a species, especially species that occur over wide geographic ranges and comprise populations that do not frequently interbreed, may show high degrees of genetic divergence, even though the disparate populations retain the ability to interbreed (an excellent example is populations of salamanders in the *Ensatina eschscholtzii* complex [Wake, 1997]). Genetic variation within species obviously provides important "raw material" for adaptation to localized conditions throughout a species' biogeographic range. The classic work of Dennis Powers and his colleagues on latitudinal variation in populations of the killifish *Fundulus heteroclitus* illustrates the critical role of this type of intraspecific genetic variation in adaptation to local habitat conditions (Powers et al., 1993). These studies have documented adaptive variation in (i) the kinetic properties of allelic variants of lactate dehydrogenase-B (LDH-B), (ii) the quantities of LDH-B expressed in different populations, and (iii) the structures of the gene regulatory regions governing transcription of the *ldh-b* gene (Schulte et al., 2000). The studies of *Colias* butterflies by Ward Watt and colleagues also have provided fascinating accounts of the roles played by allelic variants of enzymes in adaptation to local environmental conditions (Watt, 1995; Watt et al., 1985). A review of the role of adaptive allelic variation is found in Watt and Dean (2001).

CONCLUSIONS AND CHALLENGES FOR THE FUTURE

We hope that this introductory chapter helps to prepare the reader for the varied analyses of biochemical adaptation presented throughout this book. We have tried to construct a conceptual framework to use in the analysis of adaptation, a framework whose elements include concepts and issues of a complex philosophical nature. To assist the reader in obtaining an overview of this field, we have also tried to "give away the plot" of the story, by indicating the major conclusions that arise from this analysis of biochemical adaptation. These overarching conclusions include the highly conservative nature of adaptive change—the preservation of biochemical unity in the face of diversity of adaptive challenges. Achieving this conservative goal requires not only the appropriate gene products, for instance, enzymes whose thermal characteristics fit them to their particular thermal niche, but also gene regulatory mechanisms that ensure that appropriate types of genes are activated to effect adaptive change. In this context we have tried to outline the hierarchical nature of adaptation, in two different senses. One is a temporal hierarchy in which the time available to the organism to fabricate its adaptive response will govern strongly the types of "raw material" it can exploit in dealing with an environmental challenge. The other hierarchy reflects the organizational complexity of the organism. Here, we emphasized that the requirements for intercellular and interorgan coordination in complex metazoans create regulatory challenges not faced by unicellular species. These requirements

for complex integration and coordination of biochemical adaptations appear to have played major selective roles in the proliferation of genes encoding proteins that play regulatory roles, for instance, protein kinases and phosphatases. The question, "Why do complex organisms contain so much DNA?" may be answered in part by the complexity entailed in regulating the adaptive responses found in metazoans.

Reviewing and analyzing the literature on biochemical adaptation that has appeared during the last 10–15 years of the twentieth century is something of a heady experience: the mixture of good questions, new theoretical frameworks for studying physiological evolution, and powerful new experimental approaches that have come to characterize this field has allowed a remarkable degree of growth in our understanding of the nature of adaptive change in diverse biochemical systems. However, in each chapter we will try to illustrate both the achievements and the current shortfalls that exist in this discipline. On the one hand, many central questions about adaptation remain at best partially resolved. On the other hand, the advent of new conceptual and technical approaches appears to ensure continued rapid growth of knowledge about the fundamental ways in which genes and gene products become attuned to diverse environmental conditions. One of the primary goals of this volume is to generate enthusiasm in the reader for tackling the tough problems that remain in this field. Application of comparative and evolutionary approaches to these questions will yield the two types of important dividends we illustrate throughout this volume: insights into the fundamental nature of biochemical design in all species and a deeper understanding of the sources and significance of biochemical diversity.

REFERENCES

Adams, M.D., S.E Celniker, R.A. Holt, C.A. Evans, J.D. Gocayne, P.G. Amanatides, S.E. Scherer, P.W. Li, R.A. Hoskins, R.F. Galle, R.A. George, S.E. Lewis, S. Richards, M. Ashburner, S.N. Henderson, G.G. Sutton, J.R. Wortman,

M.D.Yandell, Q. Zhang, L.X. Chen, R.C. Brandon, Y.H.C. Rogers, R.G. Blazej, M. Champe, B.D. Pfeiffer, et al. (2000). The genome sequence of *Drosophila melanogaster*. *Science* 287: 2185–2195.

Bentley, D.R. (2000). The human genome project—An overview. *Med. Res. Rev.* 20: 189–196.

Felsenstein, J. (1985). Phylogenies and the comparative method. *Am. Nat.* 125: 1–15.

Garland, T.J., and P.A. Carter (1994). Evolutionary physiology. *Annu. Rev. Physiol.* 56: 579–621.

Goffeau, A. (2000). Four years of post-genomic life with 6000 yeast genes. *FEBS Lett.* 480: 37–41.

Gould, S.J., and R.C. Lewontin (1979). The spandrels of San Marco and the panglossian paradigm: a critique of the adaptationist programme. *Proc. Roy. Soc. Lond. Ser. B*. 205: 581–598.

Gould, S.J., and E.S. Vrba (1982). Exaptation—a missing term in the science of form. *Paleobiology* 8: 4–15.

Hunter, T. (2000). Signaling—2000 and beyond. *Cell* 100: 113–127.

Iyer, V.R., M.B. Eisen, D.T. Ross, G. Schuler, T. Moore, J.C.F. Lee, J.M. Trent, L.M. Staudt, J. Hudson, M.S. Boguski, D. Lashkari, D. Shalon, D. Botstein, and P.O. Brown (1999) The transcriptional program in the response of human fibroblasts to serum. *Science* 283: 83–87.

King, M.C., and A.C. Wilson (1975). Evolution at two levels in humans and chimpanzees. *Science* 188: 107–116.

Kornberg, T.B., and M.S. Krasnow (2000) The *Drosophila* genome sequence: Implications for biology and medicine. *Science* 287: 2218–2220.

Krebs, H.A. (1975). The August Krogh Principle: "For many problems there is an animal on which it can be most conveniently studied." *J. Exp. Zool.* 194: 221–226.

Krogh, A. (1929). Progress in physiology. *Am. J. Physiol.* 90: 243–251.

Maughan, D.W., and J.O. Vigoreaux (1999). An integrated view of insect flight muscle: genes, motor molecules, and motion. *News Physiol. Sci.* 14: 87–92.

Melendez-Hevia, E., T.G. Waddell, and M. Cascante (1996). The puzzle of the Krebs citric acid cycle: Assembling the pieces of chemically feasible reactions and opportunism in the design of metabolic pathways during evolution. *J. Mol. Evol.* 43: 293–303.

Normile, D. (2001). Comparative genomics: Gene expression differs in human and chimp brains. *Science* 292: 44–45.

Powers, D.A., M. Smith, I. Gonzalez-Villasenor, L. DiMichelle, D. Crawford, et al. (1993). In: *Oxford Surveys in Evolutionary Biology*, ed. D. Futuyma and J. Antonovics, 9: 43–107. Oxford: Oxford University Press.

Rose, M.R., and G.B. Lauder (1996). *Adaptation*. San Diego: Academic Press, 511 pp.

Schmidt-Nielsen, K. (1972). *How Animals Work*. Cambridge: Cambridge University Press, 114 pp.

Schulte, P.M., H.C. Glemet, A.A. Fiebig, and D.A. Powers (2000). Adaptive variation in lactate dehydrogenase-B gene expression: Role of a stress-responsive regulatory element. *Proc. Natl. Acad. Sci. USA* 97: 6597–6602.

Somero, G.N. (2000). Unity in diversity: a perspective on the methods, contributions, and future of comparative physiology. *Annu. Rev. Physiol.* 62: 927–937.

Venter, J.C., et al. (2001). The sequence of the human genome. *Science* 291: 1304–1351.

Wake, D.B. (1997). Incipient species formation in salamanders of the *Ensatina* complex. *Proc. Natl. Acad. Sci. USA* 94: 7761–7767.

Watt, W.B. (1995). Allozymes in evolutionary genetics: beyond the twin pitfalls of "neutralism" and "selectionism." *Rev. Suisse de Zool.* 102: 869–882.

Watt, W.B., and A.M. Dean (2001). Molecular-functional studies of adaptive genetic variation in prokaryotes and eukaryotes *Annu. Rev. Genet.* 34: 593–622.

Watt, W.B., P.A. Carter, and S.M. Blower (1985). Adaptation at specific loci. IV. Differential mating success among glycolytic allozyme genotypes of *Colias* butterflies. *Genetics* 109: 157–175.

Wilson, R.K. (1999). How the worm was won—the *C. elegans* genome sequencing project. *Trends Genet.* 15: 51–58.

Wixon, J., and C. O'Kane (2000). Featured organism: *Drosophila melanogaster*. *Yeast* 17: 146–153.

Zhang, L., W. Zhou, V.E. Velculescu, J.E. Kern, R.H. Hruban, S.R. Hamilton, B. Vogelstein, and K.W. Kinzler (1997). Gene expression profiles in normal and cancer cells. *Science* 276: 1268–1272.

2

Cellular Metabolism, Regulation, and Homeostasis

ENERGETIC HUB OF LIVING CELLS

One of the great insights arising from biochemical research, starting in the 1930s and extending to present times, is that almost all cell work functions—biosynthetic work, ion pumping work, mechanical work—are coupled to the hydrolysis of adenosine triphosphate or ATP (Atkinson, 1977). When coupled with the requirement that at steady state cells, tissues, organs, and organisms must be in energy balance, this means that at steady state ATP demand pathways must be balanced with ATP supply pathways both at low and at high work rates. The energetic hub of living cells thus can be described as an ATP cycle with steady-state requirements for flux through the ATP demand pathways of the cycle to be balanced by flux through the ATP supply pathways. Before proceeding to the issue of how this regulation is achieved, we need to digress and describe the pathways cells use to regenerate ATP.

THREE BASIC ATP-SYNTHESIZING PATHWAYS

The simplest mechanism for generating ATP is phosphagen mobilization. In vertebrate tissues such as muscle containing creatine phosphate (PCr) this mobilization is catalyzed by creatine phosphokinase (CPK), a process which requires no O_2 and can be written as follows:

$$PCr + ADP + H^+ \rightarrow ATP + creatine$$

Other phosphagens (such as arginine phosphate, lombrocine phosphate, tauromyocine phosphate) are found in many invertebrate muscles.

Fermentation, or the partial (O_2 independent) catabolism of substrates to anaerobic end products, is a second means of forming ATP. In animals, the commonest fermentative pathway is that of anaerobic glycolysis (figure 2.1). At high pH (> 8.0), the summed reaction can be written as follows:

$$glucose + 2ADP^{3-} + 2HPO_4^{2-}$$
$$\rightarrow 2 \, lactate^{1-} + HATP$$

At low pH (< 6.0), the adenylates are more protonated and the reaction can be written:

$$glucose + 2HADP^{2-} + 2H_2PO_4^{1-}$$
$$\rightarrow 2 \, lactate^{1-} + 2H^+ + 2HATP^{3-}$$

The pathway of glycolysis is phylogenetically ancient and many of its features are strongly conserved. However, the terminal dehydrogenases are subject to adaptive change; in many invertebrate organisms, lactate dehydrogenase is replaced by functionally analogous imino acid dehydrogenases. In such event, an imino acid (octopine, alanopine, strombine, tauropine, or nopaline) replaces lactate as the anaerobic glycolytic end product. However, neither the proton stoichiometries nor the ATP yields are changed (Hochachka and Mommsen, 1983). If glycogen is the substrate fermented instead of glucose, the yield of ATP is 3 moles ATP formed per mole glucosyl unit. If glucose is the starting substrate, $2 \, \mu mol$ ATP per μmol glucose are conserved. In goldfish and carp, prolonged anaerobiosis can lead to ethanol fermentation, but this pathway is not known to be utilized to a significant extent in any other vertebrate species.

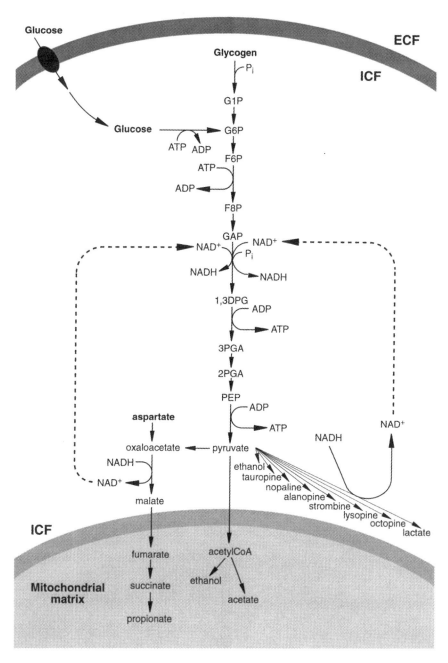

Figure 2.1. Common fermentation pathways in animal tissues. The dominant pathways are glycolysis (glucose as carbon source) or glycogenolysis (glycogen as carbon source); often both pathways are referred to generically as glycolysis. In vertebrate tissues glycogen or glucose are typically fermented to lactate as the major anaerobic end product; carp and goldfish, however, can form lactate or ethanol. Many hypoxia tolerant invertebrate species utilize imino acid dehydrogenases: these reactions involve the reductive condensation of pyruvate and an amino acid to form imino acid end products. With taurine, proline, alanine, glycine, lysine, or arginine as cosubstrates, the end products formed are tauropine, nopaline, alanopine, strombine, lysopine, and octopine, respectively. The energy yields are the same as in the more familiar glycogen (glucose) fermentation to lactate. (Modified from Hochachka, 1994.)

In addition to carbohydrates, some amino acids can also be fermented. Aspartate, for example, can be fermented to succinate or propionate, a process that in molluscs is stoichiometrically coupled to glucose (or glycogen) fermentation. Another major category of potential fuel, the fats, are so reduced that they are not fermented by animal cells (presumably, unlike dioxygen, there is not enough oxidizing "power," or not a high enough electron affinity, in organic electron acceptors such as pyruvate to ferment fats).

The third means for generating ATP requires O_2. In animal fermentations, an organic molecule (e.g., pyruvate) serves as a terminal proton and electron acceptor, forming an organic end product (e.g., lactate). In contrast, O_2 is required as a terminal acceptor for the complete oxidation of substrates such as glucose, glycogen, fatty acids, or amino acids. As discussed in chapter 3, O_2 was not always available as one of the substrates for oxidative metabolism and organisms in primordial times had to rely on anaerobic metabolic processes.

AEROBIC PATHWAYS OF METABOLISM

The pathways by which such complete oxidations are achieved are much more complex than most fermentation pathways. In the case of glucose, the first phase of complete oxidation (namely, the conversion of glucose to pyruvate) is the same as in glycolysis. However, instead of being reduced to lactate, pyruvate is converted to acetylCoA, which serves as the entry substrate into the Krebs cycle, a process occurring in the mitochondrial matrix. The two carbons of acetylCoA appear as CO_2 with the simultaneous formation of reducing equivalents in the form of NADH. Under anaerobic conditions, NADH is reoxidized to NAD^+ by an organic substrate that is reduced in the process (pyruvate, for example, being reduced to lactate; fumarate similarly can be reduced to succinate). Under aerobic conditions, NADH is reoxidized to NAD^+ via the electron transport system (ETS) located in the mitochondrial inner membrane or cristae (figure 2.2). During the electron transfer process, H^+ ions are pumped out of the mitochondria across the inner mitochondrial membrane.

The developed H^+ concentration gradient plus an electric potential across the membrane supply the driving force for ATP synthesis from ADP and Pi, a thermodynamically unfavorable reaction catalyzed by ATP synthase (Karrasch and Walker, 1999). The latter is a mitochondrial enzyme located on, and spanning, the inner mitochondrial membrane. At least when in submitochondrial particles, ATP synthase saturation kinetics involve ADP positive site–site interactions in catalysis. One group has proposed that ADP saturation in vivo also shows site–site interactions (n, the interaction or Hill coefficient increasing from 1, meaning no interaction, to 2); however, others have not found this, so this issue at this time must be considered to remain unresolved.

The net reaction for glucose oxidation (via glycolysis, the Krebs cycle, the ETS, and ATP synthase) can be written as follows:

$$glucose + 36(ADP + Pi) + 6O_2 \rightarrow 36ATP$$
$$+ 6CO_2 + 42H_2O$$

When fatty acids are the fuel being combusted, the pathway of oxidation is termed the β-oxidation spiral, which, following fatty acylCoA formation, involves four basic steps:

1. acylCoA + FAD^+ $\rightarrow$ α-β-unsaturated acylCoA + $FADH_2$
2. α-β-unsaturated acylCoA + H_2O $\rightarrow$ β-hydroxyacylCoA
3. β-hydroxyacylCoA + NAD^+ $\rightarrow$ β-ketoacylCoA + NADH + H^+
4. β-ketoacylCoA + CoASH $\rightarrow$ acylCoA (−2 carbons) + acetylCoA

This pathway, also located in the mitochondria, generates acetylCoA which is then completely metabolized by the Krebs cycle, the ETS, and ATP synthase. The overall equation for fatty acid oxidation, using palmitate as an example, can be written as:

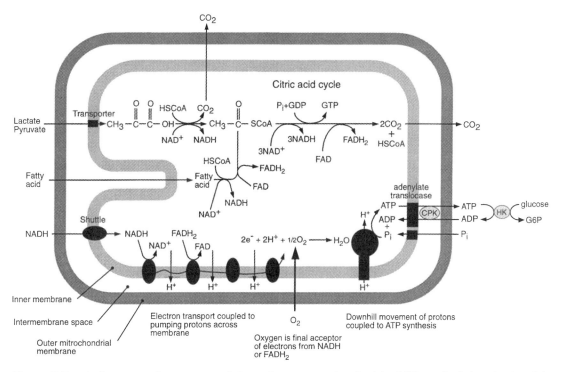

Figure 2.2. A diagrammatic summary of the main processes involved in ATP synthesis in mitochondria. Key substrates of oxidative metabolism (pyruvate, FFA, ADP, Pi, etc.) are transported into the matrix through specific transport proteins (these are termed specific transporters or exchangers in the physiological literature; often they are termed permeases in the biochemical literature). O_2 is thought to simply diffuse through the mitochondrial membranes into the matrix. NADH generated glycolytically in the cytosol is not transported directly into the matrix because the inner mitochondrial membrane is impermeable to NAD^+ and to NADH. Instead a so-called shuttle system is used to transport the reducing equivalents in NADH to the electron transfer system (ETS). ATP as a product of metabolism is transported out of the matrix via the adenylate translocase; then high energy equivalents are transferred via creatine phosphate shuttles to cytosolic sites of ATP utilization (see figure 2.14 for further discussion of this process). (Modified from Hochachka, 1994.)

$$palmitate + 23O_2 + 129(ADP + Pi) \rightarrow 129ATP$$
$$+ 16CO_2 + 145H_2O$$

In most mammalian muscles, amino acids are not a major fuel for oxidative metabolism, although they may be in numerous other animals. When amino acids are the fuels being combusted, they are metabolized by pathways that all ultimately feed into the Krebs cycle, where the intermediates can be fully metabolized (figure 2.3). Being at about the same oxidation state as carbohydrates, the ATP yields of amino acids during oxidation are also similar. For example, alanine oxidation

yields 15 ATP/alanine, exactly the same value as for pyruvate. Oxidation of glutamate yields 27 ATPs, while the oxidation of proline could in theory be coupled to the synthesis of 30 ATPs (Hochachka and Somero, 1984).

While the complete oxidations of fats and carbohydrates yield $CO_2 + H_2O$, the complete oxidation of amino acids yields $CO_2 + H_2O$ and as well as ammonia. Three fates of this so-called nitrogen waste product are common in animals: it can be excreted into the outside medium (ammonotelism, which is common in many aquatic animals); it can be excreted as uric acid (uricotely, common in reptiles and birds); or, it can be excreted as urea (common

(A)

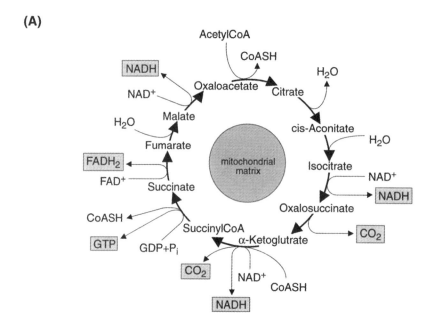

Figure 2.3(A). The Krebs cycle is initiated with the condensation of oxaloacetate and acetylCoA and ends with the formation of oxaloacetate from malate. Two carbons enter the cycle and two carbons are released as CO_2 in one turn of the cycle; in steady state, the cycle is therefore a catalytic system (intermediates are neither accumulated nor depleted) analogous to a super-enzyme. The cycle is considered the hub of cell metabolism, the final and common pathway for the complete catabolism of most carbon fuels.

(B)

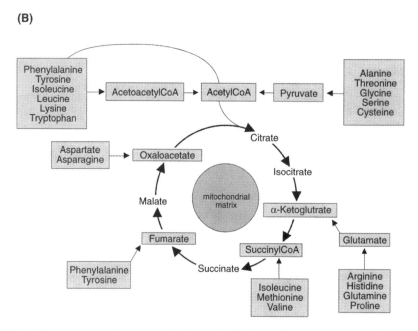

Figure 2.3(B). Sites of entry of amino acids into the Krebs cycle; these are requisite steps for the complete catabolism of amino acids and proteins. (Modified from Hochachka, 1994.)

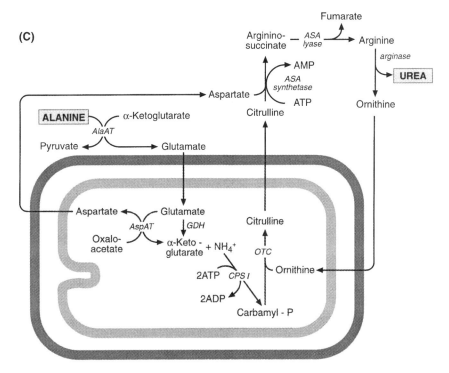

Figure 2.3(C). Ureagenesis via the urea cycle during alanine catabolism in the mammaliam liver. The urea cycle (highlighted) comprises (1) arginase, (2) ornithine-carbamoyl transferase, (3) argininosuccinate synthetase and (4) argininosuccinate lyase. In mammals, CPS I (carbamoylphosphate synthetase I) serves as a feeder enzyme to the urea cycle, leading to the incorporation of amino-acid-derived ammonia and bicarbonate into citrulline. In fishes, CPS III plays the same role; instead of NH_4^+, it preferentially utilizes glutamine as a nitrogen donor; thus in fishes, glutamine synthase also serves as a feeder enzyme to the urea cycle. Amino acid nitrogen can also be funnelled into aspartate and the urea cycle via glutamate dehydrogenase and aspartate aminotransferase reactions. Fumarate from the urea cycle is recovered via parts of the Krebs cycle plus aspartate aminotransferase. Additional abbreviations used: AlaAT, alanine aminotransferase; ASA, argininosuccinate; AspAT, aspartate aminotransferase; GDH, glutamate dehydrogenase; OTC, ornithine transcarbamylase. (Modified from Campbell, 1991, and Walsh and Mommsen, 2000.)

in some fishes, amphibans, and mammals). While earlier studies focused mainly on the pathways to urea and urate (figures 2.3(C) and 2.3(D)), recent studies have also addressed evolutionary and adaptational aspects of waste nitrogen metabolism (e.g., see Walsh and Mommsen, 2000, for an interesting essay on evolutionary aspects of ammonia and urea production in fishes).

For practical purposes, then, the above relatively small numbers of metabolic pathways are the main means by which cells can balance energy production with energy utilization rate. Our ability today to summarize so complex a set of processes so easily and so simply is a resounding endorsement of the research achievements of workers in this area during the second half of the twentieth century. While a great deal of detail remains to be filled in, for our purposes here it is the functional properties of these metabolic pathways and processes which are of greater inherent interest. So let us begin with the most usual metabolic state of all—that of the basal or resting state. Surprisingly, at least at first glance, animals use a considerable amount of energy in the basal or standard state, when no net work is done and all the free energy is dissipated. Why should this be so? What is basal or standard metabolism all about?

(D)

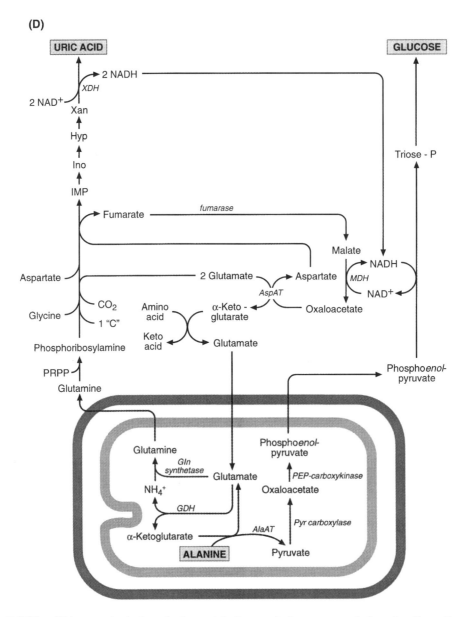

Figure 2.3(D). Uricogenesis during alanine catabolism and gluconeogenesis in avian liver. Some abbreviations are as in figure 2.3(C). 1 "C" refers to one-carbon units; MDH, malate dehydrogenase; XDH, xanthine dehydrogenase; PRPP, phosphoribosylpyrophosphate; IMP, inosoine monophosphate; ino, inosine; hyp, hypoxanthine; xan, xanthine.

BASAL OR STANDARD METABOLIC RATE

Basal or standard metabolic rate (BMR or SMR) is the steady-state rate of heat production by a whole organism under a set of of basal or or "standard" conditions, respectively.

Because the literature on mammals usually uses BMR, while the comparative literature tends to prefer SMR, we shall use these terms interchangeably, although we share a slight preference for SMR. In mammals the conditions under which SMR can be validly estimated are as follows: first, the subject must be in the adult stage of development; second, the subject must be postabsorptive (for humans, an overnight fast is the usual requirement), normothermic, and unstressed in any other way; and third, the subject must be "at rest" but not asleep (in humans, the subject is traditionally supine). Standard metabolic rate can be measured either directly as heat production or indirectly by measuring oxygen consumption or $\dot{V}O_2$ (the volume of O_2 consumed per kg per min). Resting metabolic rate, or RMR, is a similar measurement, but in this case the organism is not postabsorptive. The traditional interpretation of SMR (or BMR) is that it defines "maintenance"—the lowest metabolic rate or level commensurate with life (of course, as we shall see later, there are lots of exceptions to this general statement).

CONTRIBUTIONS TO SMR

An important insight is that the contribution to SMR is tissue specific (see Rolfe and Brown, 1997). Thus in humans, the relative *sizes* of liver, gastrointenstial (GI) tract, kidney, lung, central nervous system (CNS), heart, and muscle are 2, 2, 0.5, 0.9, 2, 0.4, and 42%, respectively, and these together add up to about 50% of total body mass. However, the *contributions* of these same tissues to SMR are 17, 10, 6, 4, 20, 11, and 25% respectively, equivalent to over 90% of SMR; all the remaining tissues (about 50% of the body) contribute only about 5% to SMR. What is more, this breakdown is also species specific. For the rat, for example, these same tissues contribute 20, 5, 7, 1, 3, 3, and about 25% to SMR, or about 75% of the total; metabolism of the rest of the body accounts for the remaining 25% of SMR.

PROCESSES CONTRIBUTING TO SMR

One of the reasons that different tissues/organs contribute differently to SMR is because they are specialized for different kinds of energy-demanding functions. As a rough approximation for mammals, the dominant ATP "sinks" or ATP-consuming processes are protein turn-over, the Na^+ pump, the Ca^{2+} pump, myosin ATPases, gluconeogenesis, ureagenesis, mRNA synthesis, and substrate cycling, contributing 20, 7.5, 6, 5, 8, 3, < 2, and < 2% respectively to whole body SMR (figure 2.4). A detailed breakdown on a tissue-by-tissue basis is unavailable for most species, but for humans these data are available for the two dominant sinks: protein turnover and Na^+ pumping. They show that the contribution of protein turnover to SMR varies from 74% in the case of the gut (this clearly is the main energy sink for the rapidly turning over cells of the GI tract) to as low as 3% in the case of the heart (a tissue which turns over relatively slowly).

O_2 UPTAKE NOT COUPLED TO ATP SYNTHESIS

All of the above ATP consuming processes contributing to SMR are those that would be expected by most comparative physiologists and biochemists. Two additional energy sinks might not be, because they are much less frequently mentioned in the literature. One of these includes nonmitochondrial reactions that consume molecular O_2—there are many of these that in total account for about 10% of SMR (and these too, of course, are tissue/organ specific). This means that only 90% of the O_2 consumption of SMR is mitochondrial. What is more, apparently another 20% of the mitochondrially located O_2 consumption of SMR is due to proton leak (Brookes et al., 1998) through a nonspecific cation channel in the inner mitochondrial membrane (figure 2.4).

STATE 4 VERSUS STATE 3 IN VITRO PROTON LEAK

A first key fact (see Brand, 1995, 1997; Rolfe and Brown, 1997) is that in isolated mitochondria, this proton leak is readily demonstrable in state 4 (all requirements for mitochondrial metabolism present except ADP) but the leak is mainly abolished, or at least, becomes harder to demonstrate on transition to state 3 (ADP-

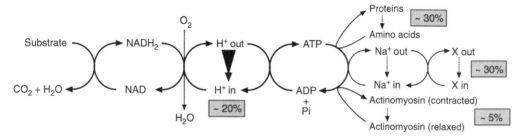

Figure 2.4(A). Various ATP-demanding processes that are assessed as major contributors to mammalian aerobic energy metabolism under basal or standard conditions; this rate of metabolism is called the standard metabolic rate or SMR. Basal and resting metabolic rates (BMR and RMR, respectively), are defined in the text. Current estimates indicate that about 90% of the O_2 consumed in the SMR state is due to mitochondrial metabolism; about 10% is due to various reactions consuming dioxygen. In mammals, about 80% of the mitochondrial associated O_2 consumption is coupled to ATP synthesis, while about 20% is uncoupled by the mitochondrial proton leak. Of the O_2 consumption associated with ATP synthesis in the standard state, about 25–30% is used for protein synthesis; about 19–28% is used by Na^+-K^+-ATPase; and about 5% by contractile work of various kinds of muscles (in the SMR state, energy demands due to muscle work arise largely from the heart, from postural muscles, and from smooth muscles, with only a modest contribution from essentially inactive skeletal muscles). ATP required for proteolysis is unclear, but could approach about 5%. Another 7% of O_2 consumption may go toward sustaining substrate cycling in glycolysis, triglyceride turnover, and the Cori cycle. Whole body RNA turnover in humans is estimated to contribute 2% to SMR, while DNA synthesis contributes even less. Gluconeogenesis contributes about 3–8%, ureagenesis, about 2%, and other ATP-consuming processes presumably account for the remainder. This diagrammatic summary, based on Rolfe and Brown (1997), indicates that over 10% of the O_2 consumed in the SMR state is unaccounted for. As discussed in the text, the contributions of different intracellular processes to SMR display tissue/organ specificity and species specificity. Indeed, the contributions of different tissues and organs to the SMR show species (including size) specificity.

saturated respiration). The corollary is that the P/O or the ATP/O_2 ratios are state dependent and the prediction would be that in any given tissue in vivo, the P/O ratio should be lower in the resting state than in activated states (because with proton leak H^+ flux is to some degree dissociated from ATP-linked O_2 consumption). This prediction has not been systematically examined on a tissue-by-tissue basis, so far at least. A new noninvasive technology, magnetic resonance spectroscopy (MRS), allowing in vivo interrogation of ATP and other metabolites in living tissues, is being applied to evaluate the physiological in vivo P/O values (see further discussion below on P/O ratios in working muscle).

LIPID COMPOSITION AFFECTS PROTON LEAK

A second important feature worth emphasizing is that the proton leak is affected by the lipid composition of the inner mitochondrial membrane. In general, the fatty acyl chains of phospholipid components of membranes can vary in their degree of unsaturation. The proton leak increases with the incorporation of polyunsaturated fatty acids (FAs); the greater the number of double bonds, the greater the proton leak (Hulbert and Else, 2000). As we shall note in the chapter on temperature relations, fatty acyl composition of membranes, including the inner mitochondrial membranes, changes in various physiological states (during cold acclimation in ectotherms, during preferential dietary intake of polyunsaturated FAs, and so forth). The corollary of these observations is that the proton leak and therefore the P/O ratios in tissues may be influenced by physiological or environmental conditions.

PROTON LEAK IN ECTOTHERMS VERSUS ENDOTHERMS

For many years, comparative physiologists and biochemists have known that plasma and mitochondrial membranes of ectotherms differ in the phospholipid composition from the homologous membranes in endotherms: the latter typically have more polyunsaturated phospholipids forming the bilayers of their membranes. These observations set the stage for another provocative result; namely, that proton leak is greater in endotherm than in homologous ectotherm tissues, when compared at constant body temperature (Hulbert and Else, 2000). The corollary of these results is that in SMR states, P/O ratios in homologous tissues in ectotherms are potentially higher than in endotherms; i.e., mitochondria in state 4 in endotherms should be more leaky than state 4 mitochondria in ectotherms at the same body temperature. As further discussed in chapter 7, this may be one of the costs endotherms pay for a high and constant body temperature.

Na^+ AND K^+ LEAKS OF PLASMA MEMBRANES

Interestingly, in addition to mitochondrial membrane differences, the properties of the plasma membranes in ectotherms compared to endotherms show similar differences in degrees of unsaturation of the phospholipid constituents. The higher proportion of polyunsaturated fatty acyl chains in endotherms in turn correlates with three- to four-fold higher Na^+ and K^+ background conductance and hence-higher

Na^+ pump (or Na^+-K^+-ATPase) activities in endotherms than in ectotherms (see Hulbert and Else, 2000).

EVALUATING THE PROTON LEAK IN VIVO

All of the above studies of proton leak under specific in vitro conditions in theory might add up to quite an impact on SMR in the in vivo state. Is this observed? Unfortunately, the data are not entirely clear. Rolfe and Brown (1997) estimate that up to 20% of the mitochondrially based O_2 consumption observed in vivo under standard conditions might be due to proton leak; on a tissue-specific basis (for the two tissues for which data were available), their estimate for proton leak is 26% of liver SMR and more than 50% for skeletal muscle SMR under in vivo standard conditions. However, in vivo, liver metabolic rates are normally impressively high (about 3–4 μmol O_2 consumed per g tissue per min) and one would expect most mitochondria at these high O_2 consumption rates to be in state 3 (i.e., reduced proton leak). Most of the data reviewed by Rolfe and Brown (1997) referred to isolated mitochondria or to isolated hepatocytes in the resting state; however, in vivo one never finds hepatocytes in the resting state. They are perpetually working very hard, turning over proteins, making glucose and glycogen, making urea, and biosynthesizing many other macromolecular components required for normal function. Hence it is likely that proton leak estimates in the range of 20% of liver SMR are higher than might occur in vivo.

The same argument may be used for the brain and CNS. Plasma and mitochondrial membrane bilayers in the CNS in mammals are notably rich in long-chain polyunsaturated FAs, so one might expect brain mitochondria to be more leaky with unusually low P/O ratios. This probably does not occur in vivo because the CNS normally displays very high metabolic rates (under BMR conditions in humans, brain metabolic rates are in the range of 3 μmol O_2

per g per min, comparable to above values for the liver in vivo). And, as in the liver, such high ATP synthase activity would presumably out-compete the nonspecific proton leak for the common intermediate, H^+, and would thus keep this uncoupled respiration to a minimum.

In muscle the situation is different. Here rest-ing metabolic rates are indeed low, about 0.15 μmol O_2 per g per min, which may be low enough for significant amounts of proton leak. In vivo this could mean lower P/O ratios during SMR than during activated metabolism. Again there is evidence that in vivo, this problem may be avoided. Using ^{31}P magnetic resonance spec-trosocopy (MRS), Myers and his coworkers (see chapter 3) estimated the ATP cost per con-traction under the same in vivo conditions in which they were also able to estimate O_2 con-sumption per contraction. The ratio of the two of course is an in vivo estimate of the ATP/O_2 ratio, which under working conditions is essen-tially 6 (or close to theoretical maximum). Equally important, plots of $\dot{V}O_2$ (on the vertical axis) versus work intensity (on the horizontal axis) extrapolate through SMR for muscle in the resting state, or at zero work. This would not be expected if the resting muscle sustained a proton leak as large as 50% of SMR; in fact, the simplest interpretation of these data is that the ATP/O_2 ratio at rest is also not far below 6, implying a lower proton leak than currently estimated (Rolfe and Brown, 1997). However, the mechanism for slowing down the proton leak in resting muscle remains unknown. Further work is clearly required to clarify the situation in this tissue, since perfused muscle apparently displays quite a large and easily measurable proton leak (Rolfe et al., 1999). Be that as it may, proton leak appears to represent a significant, if modest, fraction of metabolism under some conditions but it seems to be reduced as metabolic rates move above the SMR.

ALLOMETRY AND PROTON LEAK

One final instructive observation is that the phospholipid composition of membranes also varies with body size. Systematic comparisons of homologous tissues in large-to-small animals shows increasingly polyunsaturated FAs in the phospholipid bilayers of plasma and inner mito-chondrial membranes. Predictably it is found that state 4 mitochondria prepared from tissues of small animals display more proton leak than do similar preparations from large animals (Hulbert and Else, 2000). The implications again are that P/O ratios in small animals may be lower than in homologous tissues of large animals—compared under basal (standard) conditions. Like the tissue specific differences noted above, these predictions are yet to be fully explored (see chapter 7).

ALLOMETRY AND BMR OR SMR

Despite the uniformity of structure and func-tion at the cellular level, living things are pack-aged into what at first glance may seem to be an amazing diversity of sizes: the largest and most complex of animals and plants weigh some 21 or more orders of magnitude more than the simplest of microorganisms. Biologists recog-nize that from these observations two funda-mental features of life arise. The first is that the huge variety of sizes is central to the ability of organisms to diversify so extensively that they have literally covered our planet, with mil-lions of species exploiting nearly all of its envir-onments to a terrestrial plus aquatic biomass of about 1×10^{19} g wet weight (Kump et al., 1999) and an near-equivalent intraterrestrial micro-bial biomass (Pedersen, 2000). The second fea-ture is that organisms adjust their structure and function to allow for the consequences of their size through allometric scaling relationships. These are usually expressed in the form

$$Y = Y_0 W^b$$

where Y is a process rate (such as resting or standard metabolic rate, SMR), Y_0 is a normal-ization constant, W is the weight of the organ-ism in grams, and b is a scaling exponent. In plots of log SMR versus log body weight, b is the slope of the line, and Y_0 is the intercept.

In one of the first extensive analyses of this problem, Kleiber (1932) showed that for a

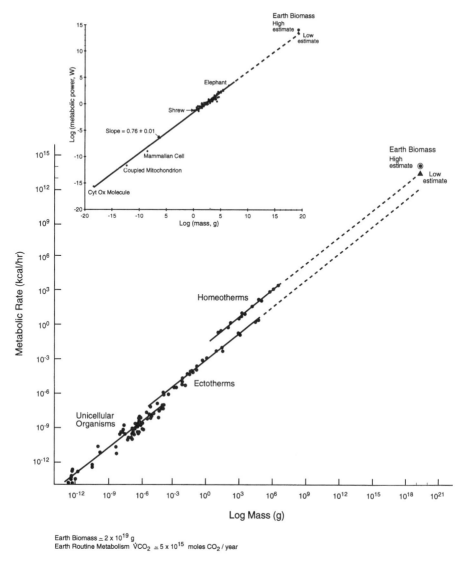

Figure 2.4(B). A plot of log of body weight in grams versus log of metabolic rate is shown for unicellular organisms, ectotherms, and homeotherms, modified from Hemmingsen (1960). In the Hemmingsen (1960) review, the data for unicellular and ectothermic organisms are corrected to $20°C$, while the data for birds and mammals (endotherms) is corrected to $39°C$. The routine global "metabolic rate" of the earth's biomass is added to the original data. The earth's biomass and a low estimate of $\dot{V}CO_2$ is from Kump et al. (1999); a higher estimate of CO_2 flux for the earth's biosphere comes from Des Marais (2000). Intraterrestrial microbial biomass estimates are from Pedersen (2000). The total biomass (terrestrial + aquatic + microbial) adds up to about 2×10^{19} g wet weight; while the total CO_2 flux is about 5×10^{15} moles CO_2 per year. The data for the earth's biomass are remarkably close to a simple extrapolation of the data from Hemmingsen (1960). The inset shows a similar plot of standard O_2 consumption rates from cytochrome oxidase to the largest mammals, modified from West et al. (2000). Again, these data are extrapolated to the high and low estimates of the earth's metabolic rate. West et al. (2000) calculated the in vivo cytochrome oxidase, mitochondrial, and cell-level metabolic rates for cardiac myocytes. As noted in the text, similar data for these components from other tissues may not yield fits that are as good as shown in this figure. Nevertheless, the impressive conclusion that arises from both of these plots is that a scaling coefficient of 0.75 fits the available data on O_2 consumption rates for organisms varying in size by over 20 log cycles (30 log cycles when we include the earth's biomass).

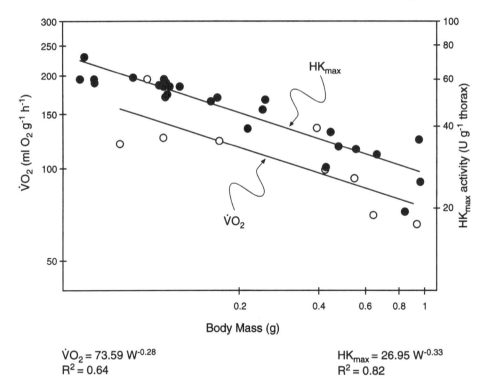

$\dot{V}O_2 = 73.59 \ W^{-0.28}$
$R^2 = 0.64$

$HK_{max} = 26.95 \ W^{-0.33}$
$R^2 = 0.82$

Figure 2.4(C). Allometric scaling of flight metabolism in Euglossine bees (Euglossa, Exaerete, Eulaema, Eufriesea) plotted on the same log–log scale as the maximum flight muscle hexokinase HK_{max} activity. Each point corresponds to the average value of a single species. Open circles represents $\dot{V}O_2$ data measured in nine species by Casey et al. (1985). Filled circles represents hexokinase maximal activity measured in 28 species by Darveau, Suarez, and Hochachka (unpublished data). Note that no difference in slopes between the two data sets could be detected. (Unpublished data are courtesy of R.K. Suarez and C.A. Darveau.)

group of endotherms spanning six orders of magnitude in body weight SMR increased with body mass with $b = 0.75$. This scaling relationship (with $b = 0.75$) has been found over and over again since these seminal studies, not only for endotherms, but for most organisms so far examined. Figure 2.4(B) illustrates the data reviewed by Hemmingsen (1960) for unicellular organisms, for ectotherms, and for endotherms. Whereas Y_0 varies, the slope b is usually close to 0.75. A review by West et al. (2000) has extended these data to include 389 mammals, mammalian cardiac myocytes, coupled heart mitochondria, and even heart cytochrome oxidase, the terminal O_2 uptake site in mitochondrial metabolism (figure 2.4(B), inset). According to Lovelock (1979), the biosphere of the earth itself may be viewed as a single

organism, Gaia, with steady-state CO_2 and O_2 flux rates that can be viewed as the routine metabolic rates of the earth. Using published data on earth biomass and using high (Des Marais, 2000) and low (Kump et al., 1999) estimates of total global CO_2 flux, as $\dot{V}CO_2$ (equivalent, at steady state, to the earth's $\dot{V}O_2$, or volume of O_2 consumed), we have added the earth's metabolic rate to the data set in figure 2.4(B). Given the admitted uncertainties in our knowledge of the biomass of the biosphere, the two estimates for the earth's metabolic rate fall impressively close to the average line for endotherms and only slightly above the line for ectotherms. Since ectotherms form a huge fraction of the earth's biomass, it is important to emphasize that these estimates of the earth's metabolic rate are not equivalent to organism-level SMRs in figure 2.4(B). Instead the data represent global routine or sustained metabolism. For most organisms so far studied, sustained metabolic rates are usually about two- to four-fold higher than SMRs (Peterson et al. 1990), and this may explain why the value for $\dot{V}CO_2$ for the earth's biosphere is somewhat higher than might be expected, given that much of the biosphere is formed of ectothermic, not endothermic, organisms. Still, the conclusions are quite dramatic: there is a surprising uniformity for the value for *b* for living material varying in weight over some 30 log cycles. To put this into perspective for those readers unfamiliar with log cycles, this represents a span of mass of living material of $\sim 1,000,000,000,000,000,000,000,000,000,000$ fold—from prokaryotes to planet earth, from microbes to Gaia!

For a metabolic biochemist, there are two most striking features of figure 2.4(B). First, a single exponent, *b* in the 0.75 range, seems to apply to all the data so far collected; and second, the metabolic rate of a gram of cells declines as body size increases. We shall first examine the latter because, from a metabolic biochemistry viewpoint, this is the most fundamental consequence of the scaling relationships summarized in figure 2.4(B). (Note: for systems obeying the 0.75 "rule," when SMR per gram is on the vertical axis, the slope is negative and $b = -0.25$; either of these slopes refers to the so-called 0.75 "rule"). To illustrate the magnitude of this scaling effect, if we consider a small rodent compared to an elephant, the ATP turnover rate per gram in the former is some nine times higher than the ATP turnover of a gram of elephant (West et al., 2000). Most of the metabolic regulation literature has completely overlooked this most basic of data sets, so it remains a mystery why a tissue in a large animal should have a lower in-vivo metabolic rate than the same homologous tissue in small animals. Since the intracellular structural and functional organization of homologous cells is the same irrespective of organism size, it is not intuitively obvious why cell metabolism should monotonically decline as organism body size increases.

Our discussion of contributors to SMR may be helpful in resolving this problem. Thus if we incorporate all the above information into the allometric scaling relationships (figure 2.4(B)), we can make the following summary statements: at a minimum, as body size increases adjustments are made (i) in organ/tissue level contributions to SMR, (ii) in the relative contributions of plasma membrane ion leaks and consequent needs for Na^+-K^+-ATPase (a dominant ATP sink in most organs/tissues in most organisms), and (iii) in the relative contributions of proton leak in mitochondrial inner membranes. Additionally, it appears (iv) that all steps in the path of O_2 from air to mitochondria to variable degrees are coadjusted for body size (Weibel, 2000) and (v) that several key positive modulators of mitochondrial metabolism (such as [ADP] levels and phosphorylation potentials) are also adjusted to body mass, the smaller the organism, the higher the potential activating signal available for turning on O_2 consumption (Dobson and Headrick, 1995; more on metabolic regulation below). A common denominator for all of these processes under SMR conditions appears to be the degree of saturation of plasma and mitochondrial membrane phospholipids (for that reason, the cell membrane is termed a metabolic pace maker [Hulbert and Else, 2000]): the larger the organism, the greater the percent saturation of plasma and mitochondrial membranes, the lower the ion leak-related O_2 demands, the lower the phosphorylation potential, and thus finally the lower the per gram tissue O_2 consumption rates.

WHY $b = 0.75$ HAS PERPLEXED BIOLOGISTS

Given these multiple adjustments to change in body size, from mitochondrial, to cellular, to tissue, and to organ levels of organization, the uniformity of the data in figure 2.4(B) remains impressive to biologists; in fact, given these known and complex adjustments, it is striking that *b* so often equals 0.75 and is an applicable scaling parameter covering nearly 30 orders of magnitude in biomass weight. Many biologists have pondered this problem. Why should $b = 0.75$ rather than a more simple surface-to-volume ratio ($b = 0.67$) or rather than the simplest direct relationship ($b = 1$), or indeed rather than any other relationship? So far there has been no satisfactory explanation. While numerous earlier hypotheses have been presented, until recently, none have been fully encompassing and complete (see Schmidt-Nielsen, 1984, for earlier literature in this area). A model proposed by West and Brown and their colleagues (West et al., 2000), however, purports to have at last found the answer to this perplexing question and their model has received lots of attention by the biological community. It is notable that so far metabolic biochemists have not examined their ideas, which is why it may have been overlooked that their underlying assumptions appear to contain a flaw so fundamental that in our opinion it is fatal to the model.

In developing their model, West et al. (2000) have emphasized three fundamental assumptions: (i) a fractal-like branching system is required for delivery of carbon and energy sources (fractal branching is a pattern which is self-similar at any level in the system from beginning to end); (ii) the final branch is a size-invariant unit (the alveolus in the lung; the capillary in the circulatory system; the cytochrome oxidase molecule in cell metabolism); and (iii) the energy required to distribute carbon and energy sources is minimized. A key insight of the West et al. analysis is that the surface-exchange areas of fractal systems scale with species weight according to the 0.75 relationship, not the 0.67 surface area/volume "rule." So far, so good. However, in developing their scaling model their most fundamental assumption (not overtly stated) is the fourth: namely, that because the above fractal structures obey the 0.75 scaling "law," the flow rates or O_2 delivery rates through these fractal systems determine the SMRs of organisms. Their model argues that this dependence (of metabolism on flow through a system whose structure obeys the 0.75 power "law") causes the 0.75 power dependence observed when SMRs are compared across a wide range of body sizes. Many biologists like this interpretation because of its simplicity (one single structural explanation for why $b = 0.75$) and because it is intuitively easy to appreciate.

If life were so simple, metabolic biochemists trying to figure out how metabolism is regulated would have long ago solved the problem. In reality, as we shall see later in this chapter, what metabolic biochemists and molecular physiologists have found is that SMR is rarely determined simply by flow of carbon and energy into the system. In reality, control of metabolism is vested in, and shared by, many steps in the overall flux of substrates (including O_2) from entrance points to terminal points. Metabolic biochemists over and over again have shown that when the correlation between metabolism and delivery occurs, especially in hypometabolic and in SMR states and to a lesser degree in hypermetabolic states, the cause–effect relationship is the reverse of that assumed and required by the West et al. model; that is, energy demand has major determining effects on flow (O_2 and carbon fluxes), not vice versa. (e.g., Arthur et al., 1992a; Korzeniewski, 2000; Thomas and Fell, 1996). Thus the assumption that flow or O_2 delivery determines SMR is probably fatal to the West et al. fractal model of scaling. Our assessment is that their recent flurry of papers on the topic (see symposium series in West et al., 2000) are no more successful in sorting out the SMR scaling problem than any other earlier attempts.

METABOLIC SCOPE FOR ACTIVITY

Fry (1947) first introduced the concept of scope for metabolic activity, defined as the difference in an organism's maximum metabolic rate under any given environmental conditions and its basal or resting metabolic rate (RMR) under the same conditions. In a penetrating analysis whose heuristic influences continue to this day, Fry emphasized that biological (behavioral and physiological) options available to ectotherms in any given environment were often a direct function of their scope for activity in that environment. Fry's model starts with RMR and moves upwards to the point of maximum sustainable ATP turnover rates (figure 2.5). Whereas Fry's concept was restricted to aerobic metabolism (or the $\dot{V}O_2$ max), it is obvious that the scope for activity depends upon the time

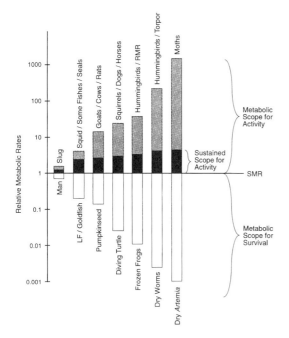

Figure 2.5. Metabolic scope for activity (defined as the difference between maximum metabolic rate and the SMR) and the metabolic scope for survival (defined as the difference between the SMR and maximally suppressed metabolic rates). Hummingbird estimates shown for normothermic conditions and for torpor metabolic rates (the latter gives the full biological scope for activity). Suppressed metabolic rates for the aquatic organisms assume temperatures of about $20°C$ (except for the pumpkinseed, where suppressed metabolism occurs during overwintering hibernation at about $4°C$). (Modified from Hochachka (1990.)

(and therefore metabolic pathways) available for the response. Anaerobic pathways can generate very high power outputs for short time periods; aerobic pathways can sustain highest rates for somewhat longer time periods; and finally, there is another ceiling for aerobic pathways that Diamond and his coworkers (Petterson et al., 1990; Diamond and Hammond, 1992) refer to as the sustained scope for activity: this is the level at which the organism can sustain activity essentially indefinitely.

METABOLIC SCOPE FOR SURVIVAL

In an alternative pattern of metabolic response to environmental stressors, the organism controllably reduces metabolism—usually in defense against a lack of heat, oxygen, or water—to levels that are well below SMR or RMR. Some capacity for the use of this metabolic arrest or controlled metabolic suppression strategy is seemingly universal, although it appears to be more commonly used in ectothermic animals (Hochachka and Guppy, 1987; Guppy et al., 1994). The great comparative physiologist, Kjell Johansen, referred to this strategy as "turning down to the pilot light"—which indeed captures the flavor of this metabolic defense response. Because survival in these cases may depend upon just how low the pilot light can be set and the minimal metabolic rate commensurate with maintenance of the living state, elsewhere one of us (Hochachka, 1990) has referred to the difference between SMR and the minimum in any given environment as the metabolic scope for survival. As instantly evident in figure 2.5, the scope for survival is a conceptual mirror image of Fry's original concept of scope for activity.

DIFFERENCE BETWEEN SMR AND $\dot{V}O_2$ max EQUALS SCOPE

Animals vary a lot in their metabolic scopes for activity and this variability arises largely from differences in anaerobic and aerobic metabolic potentials. Phosphagen-driven scopes can be very large indeed, the first few seconds of phosphagen mobilization possibly achieving several-thousand-fold increases in rates of ATP utilization. The "scope for activity ceiling" powered by anaerobic glycolysis is generally considered to be lower than that achievable with phosphagen hydrolysis, but it can be sustained for somewhat longer. Studies on the scope for $\dot{V}O_2$max are most numerous and they show that most species have a scope for this kind of aerobic metabolism of 5–20 times SMR. However, some species are remarkably lethargic (by aerobic standards); the slug, for example, displays an almost immeasurable aerobic scope for activity. Species such as the hummingbird are able to depress their metabolism by nightly torpor. The difference in metabolism of these birds as they start off the day and their hovering metabolic rates can exceed two orders of magnitude. Similarly, by taking advantage of a hypothermic effect on metabolic rates, some insects, such as moths, are able to sustain a scope for activity extending to three orders of magnitude. However, the latter two examples are exceptional in the animal kingdom and as a rule of thumb it is found that the scope for $\dot{V}O_2$max normally is in the range of five- to 20-fold above SMR (figure 2.5). However, these highest rates of aerobic metabolism are sustainable for only short time periods (e.g., in many studies of mammals it takes about 6 min to make an accurate measurement of $\dot{V}O_2$max and this is often the cutoff point for the estimate of maximum scope). For humans, by arbitrary definition $\dot{V}O_2$max is reached when any further (usually stepwise) increase in work rate occurs with no further increase in O_2 consumption—this rate of ATP turnover can only be maintained for a short time period (for only a few minutes even in well-trained individuals). As mentioned, the latter limitation led Diamond and his colleagues to propose the concept of sustained scope for activity: this metabolic rate is about two to seven times above SMR for most animals that have been studied to date (Peterson et al., 1990).

EFFECT OF BODY SIZE ON $\dot{V}O_2$ max

As might be expected from the discussion of the scaling of SMR, body size also affects $\dot{V}O_2$max. Perhaps the best data available on this parameter for evaluating scaling relationships are from the studies on a range of mammals by Weibel and Taylor's group. Over a range of approximately three orders of magnitude, these studies found that the $\dot{V}O_2$max for mammals scales with an exponent of between 0.81 and 0.86 (see Weibel, 2000). At face value, since SMR scales with a lower exponent, this means

that the bigger the mammal, the larger the metabolic scope for activity. In our analysis of SMR above, we noted that the phospholipid composition of mitochondrial and plasma membranes, as well as ion leak properties of both, changed systematically in comparisons of small and large animals. Many of these changes, such as mitochondrial proton leak, might well put small animals at a disadvantage compared to large animals. For these reasons, and perhaps in part, because larger animals have a greater proportion of proximal leg muscle mass relative to body mass (Nevill, 1994), the slightly higher value for the scaling exponent for $\dot{V}O_2$max than for SMR might well be anticipated and is consistent with the basic biochemical differences between small and large mammals.

Even if the fractal scaling model of West et al. (2000) does not seem to apply to SMR, the question arises as to whether or not it may be more appropriately applied to $\dot{V}O_2$max; this is because when O_2 fluxes approach maximum sustainable values, the relative importance of O_2 delivery to overall control of flux may increase (Jeneson et al., 2000). In the case of a super-athletic species such as the thoroughbred horse, as found in an interesting analysis by Jones (1998), the lung comes closest to representing the classical "rate-limiting" step in the path of O_2 from air to mitochondria, but even in such species, control is shared by other steps in the overall flux pathway. (To sort out the varied contributions to control of net flux, experimenters determine the fractional change in overall O_2 flux caused by a fractional change in flux through any given step or process; such fractions for different steps in the overall flux are termed control coefficients. Qualitatively, if the O_2 flux capacity of the pulmonary gas-exchange surface area, for example, is increased by 50% but only a 25% change in overall net O_2 flux is observed, the control coefficient for pulmonary O_2 diffusion is 0.5, equal to the fractional change in overall O_2 flux/fractional change in lung diffusion capacity. In these models, all the control coefficients in the pathway by definition add up to 1. In a system with a classical single rate limiting step, say O_2 delivery, the control coefficient for that step would be essentially 1; i.e., all control vested in this process.)

Just as in super-athletic animal species, for a small subset of elite human athletes, at $\dot{V}O_2$max the functional capacity of the lung is reached and a condition termed "desaturation" is observed (blood passing through the lung cannot become fully-saturated [Sheel and McKenzie, 2000]). Despite this apparent limitation, outstanding $\dot{V}O_2$max values achieved are possible because of compensatory increases in cardiac output and thus O_2 delivery to working tissues. These small subsets of elite endurance human athletes, like elite animal performers such as thoroughbred horses, are unique in that they come close to fulfilling one of the fundamental requirements of the West et al. scaling model: strong dependence of metabolism on O_2 delivery through the fractal structure of their lungs. As in the case above, however, in these elite human performers at $\dot{V}O_2$max, control of O_2 flux still is shared with other steps, especially with muscle energy demand pathways (Wagner, 2000).

In the West et al. scaling model, the lung is the first fractal system, while the heart and circulation together represent a secondary fractal system that is coupled to that of the lung; perhaps this secondary fractal system supplies the key rate-limiting function required by the model? Unfortunately, this possibility is also not realized. As in the case of the lung, in exercising humans, even at $\dot{V}O_2$max, this fractal system is not the only controller of O_2 flux. Instead, experimental studies indicate that energy demand (set by skeletal muscle workload) is probably the major contributor to control of this fractal system; that is, workload is the dominant controller of cardiac output and circulatory O_2 delivery to working tissue mitochondria, rather than vice versa (Wagner, 2000). Thus, under $\dot{V}O_2$max conditions, O_2 delivery through the fractal structure of the circulation system does not appear to be a major determinant of O_2 consumption rates, as is required by the West et al. model.

Finally, in the West et al. scaling model, a "virtual" intracellular circulation system represents a third fractal system coupled to the fractal systems of the lung and the circulation

systems. Although one of our own analyses indicates possible roles for intracellular convection systems (Hochachka, 1999), their main metabolic consequences are to stabilize substrate and product concentrations as fluxes increase in energy-yielding pathways during exercise. Moreover, at the cellular level, perhaps more so than at either the lung or the circulation, energy demand pathways (such as actomyosin ATPases, Ca^{2+}-ATPases, and Na^+-K^+-ATPases) make large contributions to control of respiration and of ATP synthesis rates (Hochachka, 1994; Korseniewski, 2000; Thomas and Fell, 1996). Thus, just as under SMR conditions, under $\dot{V}O_2$max exercise, for all three fractal systems in the West et al. model of scaling of metabolism to body size, the key condition that O_2 delivery rates determine O_2 consumption rates cannot be met. Instead of a physiological delivery system serving as a single rate-limiting process, in vivo the operational rule of thumb seems to involve sharing of control, with regulatory contributions arising at all the major steps in carbon flux, in O_2 consumption and in ATP turnover.

MULTIPLE CONTRIBUTORS, MULTIPLE CONTROLLERS

Realizing the roles of multisite contributions to control of metabolism allows us to take a completely different tact in accounting for observed b values. In this view, the multiple-causes model of allometry, there are multiple contributors to control, each with their own characteristic b values, that in sum determine the value of the b scaling coefficient for overall energy metabolism. In traditional single-cause models of allometry, the scaling coefficient for the master rate-limiting step must be -0.25; it is assumed to determine the b value for overall metabolism. In models assuming a global b value of -0.25 with shared control, the value of the scaling coefficient for any given controller could deviate from -0.25, so long as this deviation is compensated for by other controllers. The situation can be illustrated by considering the simplest case of control being shared by two steps. The first scales as -0.1, while the second scales as

−0.4; if both contribute 50% to overall control of SMR (both control coefficients equal to 0.5), then the scaling coefficient for SMR equals −0.25. Real systems are much more complex than this and theoreticians working in this area devote huge effort to quantify control contributions of different processes. For energy metabolism in mammals operating at varying rates between basal and maximum levels, major contributors to control include the lung (Jones, 1998), the heart and circulation (Wagner, 2000), cellular level energy supply pathways, which themselves have steps with low and high control contributions (Thomas and Fell, 1996), and finally the ATP demand pathways (Hochachka, 1994). For example, during high work rates, muscle actomyosin ATPase constitutes a major energy demand pathway that may contribute up to about 50% of control of overall metabolic rates (Korzeniewski, 2000). Actomyosin ATPase activity is hard to quantify in vitro, but those studies that are available show that its specific activity decreases with increasing body size in mammals and that $b = -0.23$ (Lindstedt et al., 1985). Like this enzyme, many components in the complex pathways of energy supply and energy demand display b scaling coefficients close to −0.25, but many do not. For example, in mammals, citrate synthase scales with the value of b equal to about−0.1; several other enzymes show their own unique scaling coefficients (Emmett and Hochachka, 1981). When coupled or integrated together into a unitary functional system, one could well expect on chance grounds alone that the b values for the dominant control sites would add up to global b values for metabolism that varied significantly from −0.25. Exhaustive analyses of SMR in 487 mammal species, arranged in zoogeographical clusters, show that this variation in b values is indeed observed (Lovegrove, 2000). One can think of this as an allometric cascade, with the b value for overall energy metabolism being determined by the control coefficients and the b values for all steps in the complex pathways of energy demand and energy supply.

In addition to scaling studies of $\dot{V}O_2$max in mammals, good data are available on the scaling of flight metabolism in insects. The Euglossine bees (Casey et al., 1985) supply a case in point. For this group, plots of mass-specific metabolic rate during flight versus log body mass yield a slope = −0.28, which is similar to the scaling coefficient for wing beat frequency (an index of the main energy demand pathways used during flight). Perhaps because of a higher signal/noise ratio for this smaller number of species studied, $b = -0.28$ is not significantly higher than the expected average value for animal SMR of −0.25. From various kinds of studies, it is evident that bee flight is largely powered by carbohydrate metabolism, in which hexokinase (HK) plays a key regulatory role (Hochachka and Somero, 1984). Hence, it is particularly instructive that the amounts of this enzyme, or the maximally available catalytic HK activity per gram of flight muscle, also scales with bee body mass with a b exponent (−0.33) similar to that for flight metabolism. While the correlation is interesting, the authors of these studies, Charles Darveau and Raul Suarez (personal communication) emphasize that correlation is not necessarily the same as cause. They caution that in studies such as theirs, factors or functions that correlate with scaling of whole body metabolism (with SMR or with $\dot{V}O_2$max) are not necessarily the causal agents of the scaling relationships observed. Readers will probably realize that causes and correlations in science are often confused by researchers, especially when disciplinary boundaries are crossed.

SOME FINAL THOUGHTS ON ALLOMETRY

Because of the intense interest in allometry, we should end this discussion with a final question: Is there a universal biologically important principle underlying the 0.75 power "law"? West et al. (2000) certainly believed there was such a principle when they initiated their search for an explanation for why $b = 0.75$ for SMR in so many organisms and so many functions. After reviewing current information on this question, however, we suspect that they answer may be no. In fact, from our analysis the thought arises that biologists and physiologists may have been making too much of the 0.75 power of scaling of SMR with body mass. Nature "had to choose" some sort of scaling relationship; for O_2 consumption under standard conditions, the value is often close to 0.75 but the reader must realize that this value is a composite outcome of numerous (organ level down to subcellular level) adjustments in processes contributing to SMR, and that this value is often violated in nature. The reason the relationship looks as good as it does in transformations such as figure 2.1 is because the data are plotted on log scales. When we are dealing with some 30 log cycles (there are 30 zeroes in this number!), a three- to ten-fold violation is hardly noticed. There are numerous species whose SMRs are either much lower than the statistical average for the data so far generated and many whose SMRs are three or more fold higher. What is more, the slopes obtained for the scaling of SMR varies within different mammalian groups according to ecological and environmental situations (polar, neotropical, Afrotropical, Australasian, or Indomalayan) and according to physiological parameters (such as nutrition, short-term mobility and long-term endurance), leading Lovegrove (2000) to argue that, when found, the "expected" slopes of 0.67 or 0.75 are merely statistical interspecies averages with little predictive value.

The same is true for $\dot{V}O_2$max: the mass-specific O_2 consumption rates of running antelope at maximum sustained speeds (Weibel, 2000) are essentially the same as for shrews or wood-mice, despite over 1000-fold differences in body sizes! Similarly, we have already noted that bee flight metabolism scales to −0.28, similar to, but perhaps not exactly the same as, −0.25, and these studies have the advantage of using species within a common phylogenetic group, thus avoiding phylogeny-related artifacts. So the 0.75 power "law" is a law only in name: it is frequently seriously violated with no functional consequences that cannot be readily circumvented. What's more, most of the additional (and numerous) physiological characters that also conform to the 0.75 power law (Lindstedt and Calder, 1981; West et al., 2000) co-correlate with each other and with O_2 consumption rates. Thus once nature "chose" a scaling relationship for one of these functions (and we believe perhaps the most critical one would be the value of b for major ATP demand pathways, such as muscle work, and thus for $\dot{V}O_2$max), much of the rest had to follow. Meanwhile, there is a huge amount of metabolic biochemistry that does not conform to the 0.75 power law at all. As more molecular physiologists also begin to look at this problem there probably will be more and more such biochemical processes uncovered. To choose one random example, it is already evident that specific gene expression rates need not scale with body mass (Yang and Somero, 1996; Burness et al., 1999), just as brain lactate dehydrogenase catalytic capacity, compared within a fish species over a 1000-fold size range (!), was found to be independent of body mass (for more literature in this area, see Hochachka and Somero, 1984). Given these complexities, one wonders if the search for a single explanation for the 0.75 power relationship between SMR and body mass is like the search for the Holy Grail: it may be fun, but do not expect us to believe it when you claim you have found it!

SIZE OF METABOLIC SCOPES FOR SURVIVAL

Animals also vary widely in their scope for survival. Species that can effectively use this strategy of defense against environmental stress generally display a maximally suppressed metabolism that is 5–20% of the RMR (in ectotherms, RMR is often hard to measure and the literature often uses the term routine metabolic rate as the reference point for defining either scope for activity or for survival). Species such as the African lungfish or the common goldfish under environmental hypoxia stress sustain metabolic rates that are typically about 20% of standard rates at any given environmental temperature. Suppression of metabolism during fall and winter in a temperate zone fish, the pumpkinseed, reduces metabolism to less than 10% of summer rates, a metabolic energy saving comparable to that found in overwintering hibernation in mammals. Aquatic turtles in overwintering submergence sustain metabolic rates that are only 2–5% of normoxic, normothermic rates, while frozen frogs suppress metabolism even further, down to about 1% of normothermic. Dry biological systems (desiccated *Artemia* cysts, helminths, and rotifers have been well studied) sustain metabolic rates that can be suppresed by at least three orders of magnitude (figure 2.5). In some of these examples, such as the lungfish and pumpkinseed, this strategy relies only on suppression of aerobic metabolism. In many cases (such as aquatic turtles) the environmental stress includes O_2 lack and in such cases metabolic suppression includes down-regulation of anaerobic pathways (this field is so large and has immense practical implications; hence the use of this strategy for surviving O_2 limitation stresses will be discussed in detail in chapter 3).

SIGNIFICANCE OF SCOPE
FOR SURVIVAL

One of the main benefits of metabolic suppression in response to deficiencies in oxygen, heat, or water is that the strategy in effect slows down biological time. Recall that unlike clock time, biological time is always a function of metabolic rate. If we consider a particular physiological, metabolic, or catalytic activity, each homologous process takes 40, 20, and 7 times longer in whales, elephants, and humans than in mice; this is because of the scaling of metabolism with body size, small animals being much more metabolically active per gram of tissue than large animals. This means that a second to a mouse is equivalent to 7, 20, and 40 seconds to a human, an elephant, and a whale. Elsewhere (Hochachka and Guppy, 1987) this relationship has been examined closely and found to be universal. Because aquatic turtles in northern ponds use metabolic arrest mechanisms during underwater hibernation, an overwintering (180-day) "dive" is metabolically equivalent to about a 1-day episode at 20°C and normoxic ATP turnover rates. In the case of a diving elephant seal or Weddell seal operating at a core body temperature of 37°C, a 60

min period of ischemia/hypoxia sustained by a hypoperfused kidney, because of metabolic suppression, may be equivalent to about a 1 min ischemic stress for the kidney at normoxic ATP turnover rates. Because larvae of the gall fly remain frozen for perhaps 120 days during harsh winters (and are thus severely hypometabolic), this time is equivalent to about 1 day of hypophagia at normal metabolic rates. In all these kinds of cases, the size of metabolic problems arising due to oxygen, heat, or water lack—and the ease with which they can be resolved—are proportional to the degree of metabolic arrest possible. At the limit, expressed by entrance into an ametabolic state, anhydrobiotic cells of organisms such as the *Artemia* cyst or of dry helminths come close to escaping from time altogether. A wonderful illustration of this very phenomenon (which appeared in the literature while this book was in preparation) was the discovery of microbial cysts which were collected in salt deposits where they had been trapped in salt crystals for a period of 250 million years! Of course no chemical system can escape the Second Law of Thermodynamics, but these dry biological systems clearly are pushing the envelope towards its extreme.

Environmental stressors under these conditions are of little consequence, which is why metabolic suppression strategies are so widely used as effective adaptations against harsh and extended environmental conditions. This leads directly to the second major advantage of the arrested state: enhanced resistance to external physical and chemical hazards (Hochachka and Guppy, 1987). Enhanced resistance in part may be a direct consequence of the arresting mechanisms used. For example, cold torpor in the common carp involves a classic segregation of nucleolar components of hepatocytes, which is a coarse control mechanism for turning down DNA-dependent RNA synthesis beyond the level expected simply by the decrease in temperature. Metabolic suppression also may provide means for stabilizing or protecting otherwise relatively labile components in cell structure and function (enzymes, mRNA, and membranes). Cytochrome oxidase in preencistment *Artemia*

(Hand and Hardewig, 1996) normally displays a half-life of hours to days, as in most other organisms; in metabolically arrested *Artemia* cysts, however, cytochrome oxidase is stabilized and protected from normal degradation events and its half-life is extended to minimally 80 days (actually the experimental techniques used were unable to accurately assess this and the half-life could be many-fold greater). Similar stabilization of other macromolecules such as mRNA also is observed (Van Breukelen et al., 2000). Anhydrobiotic systems are so well protected in this state that they are able to tolerate remarkable stressors. *Artemia* cysts have been shown to survive greater than 330°C temperature oscillations, vacuum conditions, and exposure to high doses of X-rays, gamma rays, fast neutrons, high-energy electrons, proton beams, and ultraviolet radiation. Although the protective mechanisms being utilized are still very much under investigation, it appears that the impressive resistance to harsh physical environments arises from the loss and redistribution of cell water by "water substitutes" such as trehalose, sorbitol, and glycerol. These polyols favor conditions which stabilize macromolecular structures like proteins, membranes, and intracellular organelles (see chapters 6 and 7).

FUEL UTILIZATION DURING METABOLIC SUPPRESSION

In systems that use metabolic arrest as a defense against O_2 lack, anaerobic metabolic pathways almost always necessarily come into play. As indicated above, carbohydrate (as glycogen) or amino acids are the main fuels available for fermentations in animals. In many hypometabolic systems, oxygen is not necessarily limiting and in these fuel selection during the environmental stress period is of major concern. In early phases of estivation in the lungfish, the major fuel used appears to be lipid. When lipid reserves become depleted, proteins are mobilized and amino acids serve as precursors for gluconeogenesis and for catabolic substrates. Interestingly, glycogen especially in muscles seems to be conserved, presumably because arousal and escape from the cocoon in which estivation occurs require muscle work fueled by glycogen (Dunn et al., 1983).

Fuel selection during hibernation in mammals is also pretty well worked out (see Hochachka and Somero, 1984). Hibernation in mammals is defined as a state of metabolic and physiological down-regulation, usually with hypophagia and concomitant drop in body temperature (T_b). In small mammal hibernators, T_b during hibernation usually is close to that of the environment; in large mammal hibernators (bears), T_b during hibernation (30–32°C) is more modestly suppressed. Fat is seasonally stored in preparation for hibernation and it is the main fuel utilized during early stages of hibernation. Interestingly, many hibernators, such as ground squirrels, store more fat than needed prior to entrance into hibernation; often there is enough fat "on board" to sustain the organism—probably never necessary—through two complete hibernation seasons. Why they incorporate such a large "margin of safety" is unclear.

Fat is generally considered an ideal fuel for this kind of hypometabolic state because it supplies glycerol as a precursor for glucogenesis (glucose usually remains the main fuel for cells of the CNS, for RBCs, and for some cells in the kidney, to mention three well-known examples). Additionally, fat catabolism yields metabolic end products no more noxious than CO_2 and H_2O.

Amino acids (and precursor proteins) also are frequently used to variable degree under hypometabolic states, such as starvation, estivation, or hibernation, as sources of glucose precursors and as direct energy sources. In addition to CO_2 and H_2O, amino acid catabolism of course releases ammonia, which in hibernation or in estivation creates added metabolic problems. The amount of regulatory and metabolic machinery that organisms have invested in order to deal with ammonia indicates how serious ammonia-associated problems actually are; thus it is important to examine this metabolic end product in some detail.

NH$_4^+$ VERSUS NH$_3$

The balance between NH$_4^+$ versus NH$_3$ and the resultant physiological consequences depend upon key features of biochemical reactions involved in animal nitrogen metabolism. Three themes can be found running through this literature (Walsh and Mommsen, 2000).

(i) The amount of free ammonia generated in the tissues is generally limited by reliance on amino acid transaminase enzymes for nitrogen metabolism.

(ii) A second physiologically highly relevant feature is that nearly all ammonia-producing reactions yield NH$_4^+$, rather than NH$_3$. The explanation for this is straightforward: already protonated amine groups of amino acids are in large measure the source of liberated NH$_4^+$. These reactions often do not consume a proton directly from solution, but add hydrogen from a reduced source (H$_2$O, NADH, etc.) to an already charged $-$NH$_3^+$ moiety. Since one aspect of ammonia toxicity arises from its protonation (NH$_3$ + H$^+$ → NH$_4^+$) being strongly favored at physiological pHi and thus its tendency to raise intracellular pH, metabolism seems in a sense "preadapted" for minimizing these effects by releasing mostly NH$_4^+$.

(iii) Un-ionized ammonia (NH$_3$) is released by only a limited number of reactions, specifically when unprotonated $-$NH$_2$ groups (as in the amide of glutamine or asparagine, or the nitrogens of purine rings) are removed. Generally, fish do not rely heavily on purine degradation to uric acid for excretion of nitrogen; therefore, generation of large quantities of NH$_3$ by these means would not appear to present a problem in fish. However, formation of muscle NH$_3$ by these pathways, for example by AMP deaminase, has been implicated as an adaptation for postexercise pHi stabilization (Hochachka and Mommsen, 1983).

AMMONIA/AMMONIUM TRANSPORT METABOLITES

Because of the risk of ammonia intoxication, neither NH$_4^+$ nor NH$_3$ are the main means by which this form of nitrogen is moved around

the body. Instead, amino acids are the usual means for distributing NH$_4^+$/NH$_3$ among the various tissues. In mammals, glutamine and alanine are usually considered to be the dominant internal transport molecules, shuttling NH$_4^+$/NH$_3$ nitrogen to and from tissues (Campbell, 1991; Walsh and Mommsen, 2000). Glutamine assumes a key role as detoxification product in the brain and other tissues and as general nitrogen currency. This amino acid is also the prerequisite nitrogen donor for the synthesis of carbamoylphosphate via CPSase I (in mammals) and CPS III (in fish) en route to urea and via CPSase II en route to pyrimidines. Additionally, glutamine contributes two of the four nitrogen atoms of nascent purine rings. Two kinds of evidence (high amounts of glutamine synthetase and substantial increases in glutamine concomitant with depletion of glutamate and ATP in the brain of ammonia-exposed fishes) have been presented in support of glutamine's role in ammonia detoxification in fish brain. Similarly, glutamine appears to be a general intertissue nitrogen carrier, above and beyond its specific role as a detoxification molecule specific to the CNS. Considering the abundance and activity of glutamine synthetase along the digestive tract, glutamine may also constitute an important export product of the gastrointestinal tract.

In mammals, alanine is considered to be the main carrier of excess muscle nitrogen to the liver, as part of the glucose–alanine cycle, and indeed, this abundant plasma amino acid has been identified as a key carrier of nitrogen from muscle, at least during starvation. The presence of a glucose–alanine cycle is unlikely for fishes, however, because of the generally slow turnover of glucose and sparing release of alanine from muscle following exhaustive exercise.

Many organisms, including mammals and fishes, tie up (and transport) relatively large amounts of nitrogen in the form of creatine and creatine phosphate in their muscles. In fact, the total muscle creatine pools tend to be larger in fish muscle than in mammalian muscle, although the reasons for the higher retention (or higher flux?) are not obvious and deserve some experimental attention. In the mammals, creatine synthesis and turnover extend over several organs: (i) the kidney for production of the arginine-derived precursor guanidino-acetate; as a common principle in metabolic pathways, it is this first step, the activity of the arginine:-glycine amidinotransferase in kidney, that controls arginine flux into this pathway and thus the rate of overall creatine synthesis. The enzyme is down regulated by dietary creatine and its expression is enhanced by growth hormone. And (ii), the liver is the site of methylation to yield creatine. Once made, other organs are then involved in the final disposition of the creatine formed in liver and kidney: muscles (smooth, cardiac, and skeletal forms), the CNS, and sperm are three such key tissue sites which are utilized for transporting, metabolizing and turning over creatine. Thus one, often underemphasized, consequence of creatine physiology is its role in minimizing the pool of free NH_4^+/NH_3 that the organism would otherwise have to deal with.

In summary, then, the above short overview indicates that organisms from very early on probably minimized the threat of ammonia intoxication by metabolic mechanisms which serve to limit the amount of free ammonia in cell/body fluids formed in the first place. However, some formation and accumulation are inevitable. In mammals, and other animals that depend upon the urea cycle, this excess NH_4^+/NH_3 together forms the precursor pool for urea synthesis.

UREA CYCLE—COSTS AND PROPERTIES

While the expression and regulation of the urea cycle are widely appreciated (Campbell, 1991, 1995; Walsh and Mommsen, 2000), a few general functional properties of this pathway of nitrogen metabolism need to be mentioned here.

(i) First and foremost, urea production by the urea cycle is an expensive proposition, requiring 5 moles ATP for each mole of urea produced; that is why ureagenesis makes a significant contribution to BMR, as noted above.

(ii) The pathway provides for entry points of nitrogen from a variety of amino acid sources, notably from the glutamate dehydrogenase reaction feeding into both glutamine and aspartate (figure 2.3(C)).

(iii) The isoform of carbamoyl phosphate synthetase (CPS) in fish used for urea synthesis is typically CPSase III. CPSase III uses glutamine (in preference to ammonia) as a nitrogen donor, is activated allosterically by the compound N-acetyl glutamate, is localized mitochondrially, and is not inhibited by UTP. The use of CPSase III by most piscine systems requires that the enzyme glutamine synthetase (GSase) be intimately involved with the urea cycle. The ubiquitous CPSase II isozyme also utilizes glutamine preferentially, but functions primarily in pyrimidine biosynthesis. It is cytosolic, it is not activated by N-acetyl glutamate, and it is substantially inhibited by UTP. Finally, the mitochondrial CPSase I isozyme that forms the entry step into the urea cycle in mammals, utilizes ammonia preferentially to glutamine, is activated by N-acetylglutamate, and is not inhibited by UTP. All isoforms of CPS are catalytically relatively inefficient enzymes whereever they are found and thus they must be retained at high concentrations to maintain reasonable fluxes of nitrogen towards urea; in liver of hibernators, for example, CPS I constitutes nearly 20% of mitochondrial protein. While the finer details of CPSase isozyme expression throughout phylogeny appear to still be unfolding, the general pattern is that CPSase II is a characteristic of most organisms, CPSase III is expressed in some fish and invertebrates, and CPSase I is expressed in the lungfish, amphibians, and mammals. Thus, in modern-day organisms it is safe to say that CPSase I or III is required for full urea cycle function. Indeed, in phylogenetic studies, if the correct CPSase isozyme type can be determined and if substantial ornithine-carbamoyl transferase activities are expressed, the two characteristics together can be assumed to be diagnostic for the presence of a functional urea cycle in the organism under study (Walsh and Mommsen, 2000, supply literature in this area).

MULTIPLE ROLES OF UREA

Perhaps because urea is energetically costly to make, organisms have found ways of getting the most out of its production (a kind of maximization of bang for buck!). A minimal list of roles which are not purely excretory, so-called "alternative" roles for urea in animals, includes the following: (i) urea as a major balancing osmolyte in selected fishes; (ii) urea as a contributor to buoyancy in marine cartilaginous fishes; (iii) urea as a nontoxic nitrogen transport form in ruminant and pseudo-ruminant mammals; (iv) urea as a major part of the urine concentration mechanism of the mammalian kidney; and (v) urea in the maintenance of acid–base balance by the stoichiometric removal of HCO_3^- and NH_4^+ ions. In addition, (vi) although under normal circumstances urea is not the dominant nitrogen product excreted by most teleosts, urea production appears as a backup and preferred pathway in some teleosts experiencing restrictions on ammonia excretion caused either by an inappropriate aquatic medium or by air breathing (see Walsh and Mommsen, 2000).

UREA AND NITROGEN CYCLING

Again, perhaps because urea is expensive in terms of moles of ATP required per mole synthesized, in nitrogen- or energy-limiting situations, organisms have worked out ways to minimize its loss by recycling it through their bodies. The quintessential mammalian examples of this are ruminants. In the physiological conditions encountered by these organisms, nitrogen is at a premium and as one adaptive solution to this problem urea is transferred into the gut where it is hydrolyzed by bacterial ureases to release its carbon and nitrogen. Indeed, it is hypothesized that gut bacteria in these organisms are able to produce additional amino acids that can be subsequently utilized by the host organism. This kind of urea and nitrogen recycling may also occur in fishes under unique nitrogen-limited conditions (Walsh and Mommsen, 2000).

In mammalian hibernators, the reduced amount of urea that is formed also is cycled through to the gut, where it is hydrolyzed by intestinal bacteria and the released ammonia is re-utilized. In bears, which Nelson et al. (1998) argue have developed hibernation to its epitome among mammals, these metabolic processes are fine tuned to perfection: the animal becomes a self-sustained closed metabolic support system with no carbon or water intake, no urine or digestive waste, and only a modest drop in body temperature (down to about 32°C).

FUEL SELECTION DURING WORK: THE SPAWNING SALMON

We have already emphasized that the choice of metabolic (anaerobic vs aerobic) pathways used to supply ATP for tissue work functions dictates the fuel selected. In addition, even under purely aerobic metabolic conditions, however, the fuel selected to sustain the imposed work may vary and may depend upon conditions. The spawning migration of salmon strikingly illustrates the problem (Mommsen et al., 1980). In the case of some of these species, such as the sockeye salmon of the Northwest coast of North America, spawning migrations can exceed 1,100 km and must represent one of the most awesome biological achievements in nature worldwide. These migrations involve steady continuous upstream swimming and the animals remain hypophagic right through spawning. With no feeding, the migrating salmon, a kind of closed self-sustaining life support system, initially mobilizes lipids to fuel the spawning migration. Mostly this kind of swimming is powered only by slow-twitch or red muscles, which compared to white muscles characteristically have higher fat oxidative capacities (more mitochondria and higher activities of enzymes in fat catabolism pathways). If the migration is relatively short, it can be completed utilizing only fat metabolism pathways. However, in the case of an 1,100 km sockeye migration in the Fraser River of British Columbia, most fat is utilized during the first third of the journey and at this time the salmon begin to mobilize

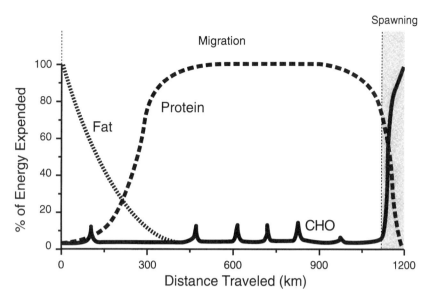

Figure 2.6. Qualitative patterns of fuel selection during spawning migration in Pacific salmon. These particular patterns are from studies summarized from Mommsen et al. (1980). They indicate that during early stages of migration, fats are the preferred fuels; as they are depleted, protein catabolism kicks in and gradually becomes the dominant carbon and energy source. Carbohydrates (CHO) are presumably utilized periodically during migration (e.g., during bursts of swimming probably most commonly encountered while swimming against or jumping rapids). These are shown as blips in an otherwise low steady-state utilization rate. Muscle and liver glycogen reserves are conserved until the end of the migration, when they are thought to power the energetically expensive swimming behaviors associated with spawning.

body protein reserves (figure 2.6). One of the fundamental insights arising from these studies is that not all tissues serve as potential protein reserves: the gut and fast-twitch (or white) muscles are the primary protein sources fueling this metabolism. Another insight is that even within these tissues, not all proteins are "targets" for degradation; some (for example, bound but not soluble, HKs) are preferentially protected. One such subset of proteins are those involved in the metabolic pathways required for interconversion of the free amino acids being formed from protein breakdown so that only a few amino acids (alanine, glutamine, leucine, isoleucine, and valine) are directly fed into ATP-yielding catabolic pathways (see figure 2.4). Whether these amino acids are used directly as a fuel for muscle metabolism during swimming, or whether they are first converted to carbohydrate (through gluconeogenesis in the liver) is an aspect of this system that remains uncertain. In

any event, these protein and amino acid reserves then fuel the salmon migration all the rest of the way to the spawning grounds.

Having arrived at destination, the spawning behavior itself is very energetically demanding. To this point, carbohydrate (as liver, white muscle, and general tissue glycogen) reserves have been conserved throughout most of the migration (we imagine that the only reliance upon muscle glycogen may occur during the scaling of rapids and falls periodically encountered in upstream migration, but of course there are no direct data on this point [see blips in figure 2.6!]). Now in the final throes of reproductive behavior, the salmon taps into its liver and glycogen reserves which fuel the energetically expensive, white-muscle-dominated, activities of nest building, territorial defense, and sexual interactions with spawning females. When these fuels are gone, the salmon is ready to die.

PRINCIPLES EMERGING FROM THE SALMON MODEL

Five clear-cut principles emerge from the salmon migration studies. First, different fuels (lipids, proteins, carbohydrates) are mobilized in sequential order. Second, the order of recruitment is based in part on availability and in part on function. Third, carbohydrates (as glycogen) are conserved for emergency functions. Fourth, internal proteins are used only under extreme conditions; for most purposes, only two fuels are used: lipids and carbohydrates (in the absence of protein mobilization, the free amino acid pool is too minute to form a significant fuel). Fifth, muscle fuel preference displays some fiber type specificity (fats mostly catabolized by red muscles; carbohydrates and proteins are mobilized mainly in white muscles). Interestingly, this model turns out to be surprisingly appropriate for exercise performance in mammals, including humans.

LIPID MOBILIZATION, DELIVERY, AND FATES ARE RELATED TO FFA PROPERTIES

Before exploring the selection of fuels per se during activated metabolism in mammals, it is important to point out that during exercise work, lipid catabolism can tap into two storage sources: muscle intracellular triglyercide pools or fat reserves in the adipose. During long-term sustained performance, the latter is critical, but of course requires delivery of the fuel from adipose to working muscle. Triglycerides are transferred in the blood in a complex form, packaged as VLDLs (very-low-density lipoproteins) or as HDLs (high density lipoproteins), which enter the capillaries and serve as substrates for endothelial lipoprotein (LP) lipase. By this means (figure 2.7) fat is transferred from adipose and is delivered to muscle in the form of free fatty acids (FFAs).

In addition, FFAs can be delivered to working muscles in the free form in solution. However, their extreme hydrophobicity limits their solubility in plasma water and the bulk of the plasma FFA pool is bound to albumin and circulated to target tissues in the complexed form. There are several functional consequences. First, being lipid soluble, FFAs are membrane permeable and no specific membrane-located transporters are required for uptake into the tissue. Second, the concentrations of most FFAs are low, in the 0.1–0.2 mM range. Third, FFAs are probably never saturating to mitochondrial metabolism. Fourth, reduced availability may in fact limit the maximum rate at which exogenous FFAs can be utilized by working muscles.

Once in the cell, the above properties of FFAs further determine the way they are handled. In the first place, their low solubilities explain why nature evolved a fatty acid binding protein (FABP) and the initial fate of FFAs entering the cytosol is FABP–FFA complexing to facilitate diffusion through the cytosol. FABP is found in both heart and skeletal muscles, the amount varying with the oxidative capacity of the tissue (see figure 2.8). FABP–FFA complexes supply the FFA required for the first key step in their catabolism: conversion to their acyl form. Partial oxidation can occur in the peroxisomes but 8-C or shorter acylCoA chains are completely oxidized in the mitochondria. Additionally (van der Lee et al., 2000), FABP can enter the nucleus where FFA are bound by fatty acid receptors (FARs), which interact with fatty acid response elements (FAREs) responsible for the regulation of gene expression (figure 2.7).

GLUCOSE UTILIZATION, DELIVERY, AND FATES ARE RELATED TO ITS SOLUTION PROPERTIES

The above complex means by which fats are mobilized contrast strikingly with the way carbohydrates are mobilized in large part due to the different chemical properties of glucose versus FFAs. As in the case of FFAs, carbohydrates often need to be mobilized from a central depot (in this case, the liver) to sites of utilization at working tissues and the transported metabolite in animals is almost always glucose (there are some invertebrates which use trehalose or galactose). Glucose is a very water

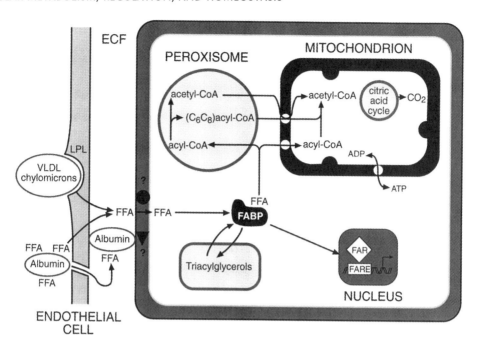

Figure 2.7. The complex pathways and processes involved in fat catabolism in vertebrate tissues such as cardiac and skeletal muscles. FFAs arrive at the cell boundary either via VLDL or albumin-associated and enter the cell either by simple diffusion or through transporters. In the cytosol, FFAs are bound by FABPs, which increase the rate and amount of FFA that can be transferred to sites of utilization. Shorter chain FFAs are converted to acetylCoA in peroxisomes; longer chain FFAs are directly transferred to mitochondria (via a complex system involving acylcarnitines) as long-chain acylCoA derivatives; these enter the β-oxidation spiral and are released as acetylCoA for entrance into the Krebs or citric acid cycle in the mitochondrial matrix. Fatty acid receptors (FARs) in the nucleus bind to fatty acid response elements (FAREs) and in turn regulate the production of enzymes in their own metabolism. (Modified from Veerkamp and Maatman, 1995.)

soluble, highly hydrophilic molecule, which as a result is membrane impermeable. To get it across plasma membranes into cells, nature relies upon glucose transporters. These membrane proteins are part of a gene family specifying five or more glucose transporters (Bastard et al., 1998; Wieczorke et al., 1999). Muscles express two isoforms, glucose transporter (GLUT) 4, which is insulin response, and GLUT 1, which is insulin nonresponsive. Even though glucose transporters are near-equilibrium and fully reversible (net inward flux depends purely on concentration gradients), they may play an important regulatory function in exogenous glucose metabolism. Overexpression of muscle glucose transporters for example quite strongly influences muscle carbohydrate metabolism. On a moment-to-moment basis, the regulation occurs in part by translocation of GLUT from membrane bound intracellular, to plasma membrane locations, properly oriented and hence accessible to exogenous glucose.

One of the consequences of the properties of glucose is that it can and does occur at relatively high concentrations (in the 5 mM range and higher in most mammals). Glucose is usually saturating to glucose transporters in target tissues such as muscle and heart. And finally, limitations to glucose utilization occur at the level of the glucose transporter or further downstream, but not at the level of availability per se.

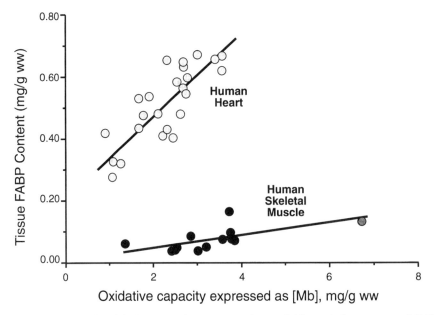

Figure 2.8 Empirical relationship between the content of myoglobin and the content of FABP in different areas of the human heart and in various types of skeletal muscles. Both protein concentrations are expressed in terms of mg protein/g wet weight (ww) of tissue. (Modified from Van Nieuwenhoven et al., 1995.)

CARBOHYDRATE AND FAT: FUELS FOR PROLONGED EXERCISE IN MAMMALS

For practical purposes, in rats and in humans, the picture emerging from a lot of research in exercise physiology is that two fuels, carbohydrate and fat, are available for prolonged exercise. Two factors, length of exercise and intensity of exercise, determine the details of the energetic contribution of these different fuels to muscle work (figure 2.9 (A–E)). In controlled submaximal exercise tests of up to 4 hours duration in humans, for example, intracellular stores of glycogen and triglyceride dominate fuel use in early stages of exercise (50% of the required ATP coming from glycogen oxidation, about 25% coming from triglyceride oxidation, the rest from plasma-borne fuels). However, after 4 hours, muscle glycogen reserves are pretty well exhausted and muscle glycogen contribution to ATP demand falls to near zero. Triglyceride stores are substantially larger than are glycogen stores, so even after 4 hours, the oxidation of this intracellular fuel contributes over 10% of the required ATP. Mostly, however, the required energy is now derived from the oxidation of plasma-borne glucose and FFAs (Brooks, 1998; Coyle, 1995).

CARBOHYDRATE OXIDATION IN HIGH-INTENSITY EXERCISE

Exercise physiologists working with human athletes for years have realized that exercise intensity is another important determinant of fuel preferences, the second parameter mentioned above. At exercise intensities in the range of 25% of $\dot{V}O_2$max, the two dominant fuels being oxidized are plasma FFAs and intracellular triglyceride, but the pattern changes as exercise intensity rises. At about 50% of $\dot{V}O_2$max,

A

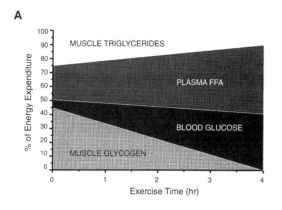

B

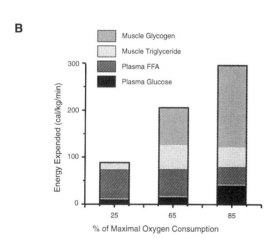

C

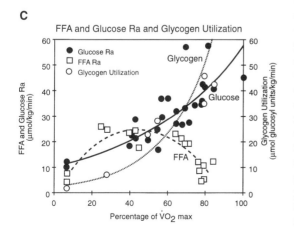

D

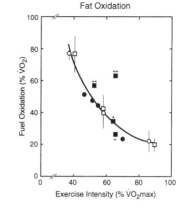

E

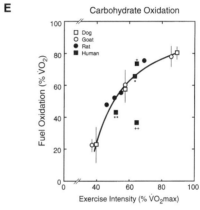

Figure 2.9 (A) Relationship between submaximal exercise duration and the percent contribution of blood borne fuels versus endogenous glycogen in humans. (Modified from Coyle, 1995.) (B) The absolute exercise intensity (expressed here in terms of percent of maximum oxygen consumption rates in humans) is a key determinant of the relative contributions of exogenous blood borne versus endogenous fuels to the energy demands of working tissues (Modified from Coyle, 1995.) (C) The influence of exercise intensity on fuel selection here is indicated by turnover rates for exogenous fuels (Ra actually expresses rates of appearance in the blood during glucose and FFA utilization) and in terms of direct rates of utilization of endogenous muscle glycogen. (Modified from Brooks, 1998.) (D) The influence of exercise intensity on fat contribution to energy demand, as percent of maximum metabolic rate ($\dot{V}O_2$max) in four species of mammals. (Modified from Weibel et al. (1996) and McClelland et al., 1998.) (E) The influence of exercise intensity on glycogen and glucose contribution to energy demand, expressed as percent of maximum metabolic rate ($\dot{V}O_2$max) in four species of mammals. (Modified from Weibel et al. (1996) and McClelland et al., 1998.)

intracellular glycogen and triglycerides are the dominant fuels. Finally, as exercise intensity increases towards the maximum sustainable ($\dot{V}O_2$max), there is a monotonic decline in fat contribution to the ATP demand with a concomitant increase in the contribution of intracellular glycogen (figure 2.9 (C–E)). This effect is so striking that Brooks refers to the phenomenon as a crossover and the conceptual framework describing it as the crossover theorem (Brooks, 1998).

WHY CROSSOVER FROM FAT TO CARBOHYDRATE OCCURS

To figure out the biological meaning of the crossover (Figure 2.9 (C–E)), we need to know why this occurs. In mammals the answer seems to be a simple conseqence of power obtainable from different metabolic pathways: maximum ATP turnover rates supported by fat oxidation in mammals are only about two-thirds the maximum ATP turnover rates supportable by glycogen oxidation (figure 2.10). The reasons for

these features in mammals are unclear but the difference is definitely not a necessary consequence of burning fat versus glycogen during muscle work. We know this because many insects are able to fly at very high flight muscle ATP turnover rates burning fat or carbohydrate. What is more, hummingbirds can hover burning either fat or glycogen and this form of flight is considered the most energy demanding of all activities this animal is likely ever to encounter. In fact, hummingbirds frequently start off the day on arousal from torpor with fat as the only fuel. Following feeding (which of course requires hovering flight), they switch toward a carbohydrate-dominated fuel (figure 2.11), but this is probably due to their glucose-rich food, rather than to biochemical necessity. Be that as it may, the data so far make it clear that in mammals, but not birds or insects, the power input sustainable on glycogen oxidation is substantially higher than on fat oxidation. That is probably why mammals rely more and more upon glycogen the closer they come to $\dot{V}O_2$max. It turns out they get an added advantage from this metabolic organization.

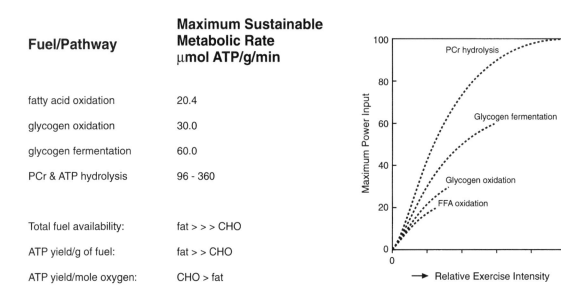

Fuel/Pathway	Maximum Sustainable Metabolic Rate µmol ATP/g/min
fatty acid oxidation	20.4
glycogen oxidation	30.0
glycogen fermentation	60.0
PCr & ATP hydrolysis	96 - 360
Total fuel availability:	fat > > > CHO
ATP yield/g of fuel:	fat > > CHO
ATP yield/mole oxygen:	CHO > fat

Figure 2.10. Relationship between fuels, pathways, and maximum metabolic rates. (Modified from Hochachka and Somero, 1984, and McGilvery, 1973.)

A

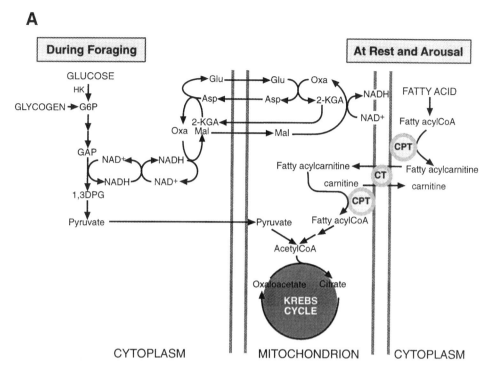

Figure 2.11(A). Pathways and fuels utilized during foraging compared to during rest and early arousal from torpor in hummingbirds.

B

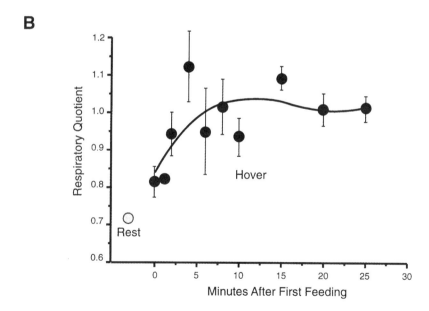

Figure 2.11(B). The RQ or respiratory quotient (μmol CO_2 produced/μmol O_2 utilized) during rest and during feeding. At rest (in hummingbirds, this means before foraging begins) this species primarily utilizes lipid as fuel for metabolism, indicted by an RQ of close to 0.7. During hovering flight (measured during feeding), the RQ is about 1, indicating that this very high intensity of exercise is primarily fueled by carbohydrate (either by blood borne glucose per se or by endogenous glycogen or by both). (Modified from Suarez, 1992.)

HIGH ATP YIELD/OXYGEN: ANOTHER BIOLOGICAL REASON FOR THE CROSSOVER

There is another biochemical explanation for using glycogen when a mammal approaches its $\dot{V}O_2$max, and this relates to the ATP yield. Again, it has been well known that fat oxidation uses oxygen less efficiently than glycogen catabolism does. This is in part because fat oxidation reduces FAD^+ to FADH as well as NAD^+ to NADH; subsequent FADH oxidation misses one of the ATP-conserving sites in the electron transfer system (ETS). By itself, this would lead to an 11% greater yield of ATP per oxygen (11% more mmol ATP per mmol oxygen). However, in experimental tests, the difference between carbohydrate and FFAs is always found to be substantially greater; values of 30–50% are commonly reported as the size of the FFA oxygen-wasting effect. For a mammal operating at or near to $\dot{V}O_2$max, where O_2 availability might well be limiting, there may be a huge advantage to get "the most bang for the buck" and thus to oxidize glycogen rather than fat. In birds with a more effective lung (cross-current-based unidirectional air flow) O_2 is less likely to be limiting and this is even more true of insects, where tracheoles deliver molecular O_2 in the gaseous form directly to individual mitochondria in the working flight muscle cells. In this context, it is not surprising that in humans and other mammals that have been studied to date, intracellular glycogen is the main fuel for muscle work at exercise intensities approaching $\dot{V}O_2$max. By this fuel preference, the exercising skeletal and cardiac muscles get 30–50% more ATP per oxygen (mmole for mmole), when O_2 may be limiting (see Hochachka, 1994, for literature in this area).

CARBOHYDRATE PREFERENCE CAN BE DETECTED NONINVASIVELY

Interestingly, studies of hypobaric hypoxia defense adaptations in the human heart have shown that the above metabolic organization can be visualized noninvasively and in vivo using ^{31}P MRS. To put this into perspective,

it should be recalled that the mammalian (including the human) heart normally displays a distinct opportunistic metabolism: it uses whatever is most available, all else being equal. In the postabsorptive state, when glucose is not super-abundant, this means that the heart is normally fueled by FFAs delivered by the circulation. Under these conditions, FFA derived acetylCoA feeds directly into the Krebs cycle and the adenylates are largely equilibrating with mitochondrial metabolism. Under these conditions, free ADP concentrations are considered to be low, in the $10–30\,\mu$M range; when these pools of ADP equilibrate with creatine phosphokinase (CPK), phosphocreatine (PCr) concentrations are necessarily high, as are [PCr]/[ATP] ratios. The reason for emphasizing the latter ratio is because it can be monitored by ^{31}P MRS, while the ratio [PCr]/[ADP] cannot be monitored because [ADP] is always well below detection limits.

When the above picture is evaluated in the heart of humans indigenous to high-altitude (hypoxic) environments, a striking result is obtained: the [PCr]/[ATP] ratio is on average only half the value found in lowlanders under normoxic conditions. The explanation for this intriguing finding (see chapter 5) is that heart metabolism in Himalayan Sherpas (and presumably other high-altitude lineages) has an elevated preference for carbohydrate (probably plasma glucose) compared to lowlanders. The complete oxidation of glucose of course requires an aerobic glycolytic pathway, which displays high enzyme catalytic capacities and much higher K_m values for ADP (in the $300\,\mu$M range for phosphoglycerate and pyruvate kinases). When this high K_m and high activity pathway interacts with the high activity near-equilibrum enzyme, CPK, the steady-state concentrations obtained include ADP high enough to satisfy glycolysis. CPK thus equilibrates at lower [PCr]/[ATP] ratios, which is why the paper describing the phenomenon (Hochachka et al., 1996b) referred to this ratio as a "signature" of a carbohyrate fuel preference in the heart. This metabolic organization of course is rationalized the same way we rationalize the crossover theorem: on a mole for mole basis, the yield of ATP/O_2 is 30–50% higher than it would be if the heart maintained a low-lander normoxic preference for fat as a fuel for its metabolism.

FUEL PREFERENCE AND ACCLIMATION TO HYPOBARIC HYPOXIA

Given the above discussion it is not surprising to find that reserachers have looked for an effect of hypobaric hypoxia acclimation on the crossover phenomenon in humans and in animals. In humans, Brooks and his colleagues found that glucose contribution to exercise ATP demands goes up on acute exposure to hypobaric hypoxia (equivalent to about 4000 m altitude). After acclimation and at the same absolute exercise intensity, the glucose contribution to ATP demand substantially increases—consistent with the above energetic advantages. However, an independent study comparing athletic versus nonathletic animal species (dog versus goat was the comparison used) noted that when the data are plotted as a function of relative metabolic rate (percent of each species' $\dot{V}O_2$max), then the percent contribution of carbohydrate to ATP demand during exercise is the same for the two species. To McClelland et al. (1998) this suggested that the main determinant of the crossover from fat to carbohydrate was exercise intensity, not hypoxia acclimation per se, a concept which they subsequently proved. Their work suggests that the main reason humans show an increased glucose preference after acclimation to high altitude is because they are tested at the same absolute (but substantially high percent of $\dot{V}O_2$max) exercise intensity as at sea level. In either event, the biological significance of the empirical fuel preference observed is that this metabolism gains more ATP per oxygen, which would be advantageous under potentially O_2-limiting work conditions.

SPECIAL ROLE OF LACTATE IN FISH

Fish are one of the favorite models for comparative physiologists working in this area because the white muscle (WM) and red muscle

(RM) are anatomically separated; in most species, the WM mass, which can constitute over two-thirds of the animal's body mass, greatly exceeds the RM mass, but the arrangement nevertheless allows particularly clear identification of some fiber type specific properties. At the same time that this arrangement is advantageous to the experimenter, it raises a serious problem for the fish; namely, the potentially huge pool size of lactate that may form in WM during bursts of swimming. The problem is that the WM mass (about 70% of total body size) exceeds the plasma volume (about 5% of body mass) by a very large factor indeed. During burst swimming many fish accumulate lactate to levels exceeding 20 mM and some, the tuna for example, sustain over 100 mM concentrations after particularly strenuous bursts of swimming. If all of this lactate were to spill out into the circulation, the plasma lactate concentrations would rise into molar ranges! We believe that is why fish WM is particularly good at retaining lactate in situ during periods of burst work, then is also particularly good at recharging that pool of lactate back to muscle glycogen, again in situ (Moyes et al., 1992). Workers in this area often refer to this metabolic organization as a "metabolic spring" which is discharged during bursts of swimming and is recharged during recovery, with minimal loss of lactate to the circulation.

ROLE OF LACTATE IN SUSTAINED EXERCISE IN MAMMALS

The traditional view of lactate in mammals during high-intensity exercise used to be rather similar to the extreme picture described above for fish; the main difference was that a larger fraction of lactate was thought to be released into the circulation, then recycled to the liver for reconversion to glucose via gluconeogenesis (lactate carbon could then be either stored as liver glycogen or returned as glucose to muscle where it could be stored as muscle glycogen). Over the last 10–15 years, Brooks and his colleagues have been especially active in modifying this old-fashioned picture of lactate metabolism and lactate cycling during and following exercise (Brooks, 1998; Brooks et al., 1996). According to their data, lactate is a far more dynamic metabolite. When formed, it is efficiently released into the circulation and is rapidly distributed to all parts of the body, especially to other actively working muscles and to the heart, where it serves as a perfectly good substrate. Special biochemical adaptations allowing this more dynamic function include monocarboxylate transporters (MCTs) for speeding up release and uptake of lactate at sites of production and at sites of utilization. MCTs, like GLUT isoforms, are part of a gene family (at least seven isoforms of MCT are now known) and specific isoforms seem to be kinetically specialized for particular lactate fluxes (the evidence here so far is largely circumstantial and such putative specialized function probably is better described as our expectation based on tissue-specificity of MCTs). Additionally, some provocative evidence confirms what many people in this field have been observing from time to time over the last two decades: the occurrence of intramitochondrial LDH isoforms. Localizing LDH in the cytosol and in the mitochondrial matrix is also known to occur in spermatozoa and in both settings this raises the possibility of pyruvate–lactate hydrogen shuttles to augment traditional mechanisms (such as the aspartate–malate and α-glycerophosphate shuttles) for moving reducing equivalents into and out of the matrix (Brooks et al., 1999a,b). Be that as it may, this work suggests that the probable main function of muscle glycogen-derived lactate during high-intensity exercise is to rapidly and efficiently distribute carbohydrate carbon throughout the body and especially to other sites of high ATP turnover. Although this model does not change the overall balance between carbohydrate versus fat contributions to overall energy demand during exercise, it certainly adds critical details about the complex intra- and inter-tissue pathways by which that carbohydrate is fluxed in vivo from glycogen to CO_2 and water! Such lactate cycling is not restricted to working muscles.

LACTATE CYCLING IN THE MAMMALIAN CNS

The metabolism of the mammalian brain is usually considered to display three key characteristics: (i) it displays an almost absolute requirement for glucose as a carbon and energy source (the glucose being plasma derived); (ii) glucose uptake, oxygen uptake, and oxygen delivery (i.e. perfusion) are closely coupled, the ratio between these processes being the same in steady states at low and high tissue work rates; and (iii) the absolute ATP turnover rate of the brain on a per gram basis is surprisingly high (in humans, the brain accounts for 15–20% of the oxygen consumed during RMR or, gram for gram, a metabolic rate equivalent to that of heavily working muscle!). These are empirical observations that are found to hold under normoxic and hypobaric hypoxic conditions, and they are fine as far as they go. However, when the CNS is examined at a cellular level, it appears that this seemingly simple metabolic picture is actually far more complex. To understand the complexity the reader should recall the cellular organization of the brain: neurons do not receive carbon substrates and oxygen directly from the capillaries because they are separated from the capillaries by astrocytes (figure 2.12). Indeed astrocytes account for a high percentage of the routine metabolism of the brain and they regulate the flow of fuels to the neuron. Just as in the case of the above interactions between muscle fiber types, there are fascinating metabolic interactions between astrocytes and neurons: glucose taken up by astrocytes from the plasma circulating through capillaries is partially metabolized to lactate, which in turn is shuttled to the neurons for further oxidation in the neurons. The coupled astrocyte plus neuron metabolism of glucose represents its complete oxidation, so these details do not violate the overall description of CNS metabolism that has been well appreciated by neuroscientists for decades.

Interestingly, this lactate shuttling is not the only important metabolite exchange between these two cell types: they also exchange glutamate and glutamine. Glutamate in small quantities is released at neuronal synapses as an

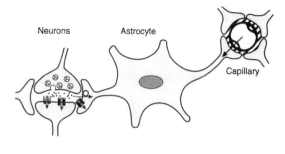

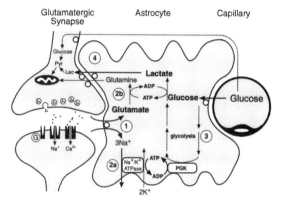

Figure 2.12. Upper diagram illustrates cytological relationships between neurons, astrocytes, and blood vessels. Astrocytes are ideally situated for sensing synaptic activity, since one of their main functions is to eliminate glutamate and K$^+$ ions accumulating in the extracellular fluids after neuronal activation. Astrocytes also form the first cellular barrier to glucose transfer from blood to the brain and are likely a major glucose uptake site. Astrocytes can also provide intermediates such as lactate to neurons. The lower diagram is a model for coupling of synaptic function to glucose energy metabolism. Key functions are numbered. (1) At glutamatergic synapses, the action of glutamate is terminated by an efficient glutamate uptake system located in astrocytes. (2a) Glutamate is cotransported with Na$^+$ resulting in an increase in cytosolic Na$^+$ and thus in Na$^+$-K$^+$-ATPase activation. (2b) Glutamate is converted to glutamine by glutamine synthase. (3) Activation of Na$^+$-K$^+$-ATPase supplies ADP for aerobic glycolysis. (4) The net effect (of glutamate stimulation of glycolysis) is formation of lactate that is released from astrocytes as a fuel for neurons. Whereas the figure indicates glucose uptake by astrocytes as the dominant process, the lower diagram also indicates that some glucose may diffuse directly to neurons. Abbreviations: pyr, pyruvate; lac, lactate; PGK, phosphoglycerate kinase. (Modified from Magistretti and Pellerin, 1999.)

excitatory signal; it is important that such synaptic transmitters have a short lifetime and one means for assuring this is rapid glutamate uptake by the astrocytes. The glutamate is then converted to glutamine, which is then returned to neurons for reconversion to glutamate. This forms an intertissue metabolite cycle that salvages glutamate and assures its efficient use as a tightly regulated excitatory neurotransmitter (figure 2.12).

AMINO ACID USE DURING EXERCISE IN INVERTEBRATES

To complete this brief survey of fuel preferences in activated metabolic states such as exercise, it is worth recalling that in many invertebrates the free amino acid pool may be an important energy source for the exercising organism. This is the case, for example, in cephalopods (which may have an unusually active proline catabolism) and in some insect species that are absolutely dependent upon proline catabolism. Many invertebrates use arginine phosphate as a phosphagen and these species by definition have an active arginine metabolism during exercise involving either anaerobic or aerobic muscle metabolism. As mentioned above, these species also have lost lactate dehydrogenase (LDH) in their phylogeny. The glycolytic function of LDH is typically replaced by imino acid dehydrogenases (Hochachka and Mommsen, 1983): octopine, strombine, alanopine, tauropine, and nopaline dehydrogenases utilizing arginine, glycine, alanine, taurine, and proline, respectively as cosubstrates with pyruvate in NADH-dependent reductive condensations, reforming NAD in the process (see figure 2.1).

AMINO ACID USE DURING EXERCISE IN MAMMALS

Unlike the salmon and invertebrate models above, in which amino acids can be utilized (especially if and when lipids become depleted), in most situations in mammals, muscle work displays a minimal dependence upon proteins and amino acids. For most species, this has not been quantified, but in humans, where data are available, the contributions of amino acids to overall energy demands of exercise are modest and fall as exercise continues. However, their anapleurotic (literally "filling up") roles remain of course, and the amino acid pool is crucial for augmenting the Krebs cycle intermediates and for preventing depletion of them during work (Brooks et al., 1996).

PRINCIPLES EMERGING FROM MAMMALIAN AND COMPARATIVE STUDIES

Six clear-cut principles emerge from the above studies. First, different fuels (lipids, proteins, carbohydrates) are mobilized in sequential order, but the order may be species specific and not all species effectively utilize all three categories of fuel. Mammals, for example, seem to rely almost exclusively on carbohydrate and fat as fuels for high-performance exercise. Cephalopods, also capable of very high exercise intensities and high ATP turnover rates, preferentially utilize carbohydrates and amino acids, but do not use lipids very effectively in support of exercise costs. Second, the order of fuel recruitment, as in the salmon model above, usually is based in part on availability and in part on function. Third, in mammals, fuel preference depends on duration and especially on intensity of exercise. At exercise intensities close to $\dot{V}O_2$max, carbohydrate (as glycogen) is preferred over fat and in fact is the main fuel utilized in mammals, presumably because its metabolism conserves more ATP per oxygen than does fat oxidation, which should be advantageous when O_2 supplies become limiting. This relationship does not seem to change during exercise in humans following hypoxia acclimation. In the heart, this strategy also appears to be part of a hypoxia defense arsenal in humans indigenous to hypobaric environments. Fourth, in mammals, lactate is more than just a dead-end metabolite in anaerobic glycolysis. Instead it is an efficient means for rapidly distributing carbohydrate carbon around the body and especially to muscle sites of high ATP turnover. For these functions, a family of moncarboxy-

late transporters have evolved that speed up the movement of lactate into and out of cells. Additionally, muscle cells seem to retain mitochondrial isoforms of LDH that may well be crucial to vigorous lactate contributions to high-intensity exercise. Fifth, muscle fuel preference displays some fiber type specificity (fats mostly catabolized by red muscles; carbohydrates and proteins are mobilized mainly in white muscles). And sixth, there is no "best" fuel; for each individual species, it all depends upon the kind of performance required and the fuels available.

Up to this point in the discussion, the metabolic rate adjustments (down-regulation in metabolic scope for survival; up-regulation in metabolic scope for activity) as well as the adjustments in fuel preferences were assumed to be regulated. Now it is time to address this issue in greater detail. Although this problem can be addressed in a variety of ways, to biologists the most intuitively obvious problem is how to maintain cellular homeostasis in the face of large changes in metabolic rate in different physiological (or work) states.

CONTRASTING DEMANDS OF HOMEOSTASIS AND TISSUE WORK

As traditionally defined, the term homeostasis refers to the constancy of the internal milieu in the face of external perturbations; the latter in principle may be caused by extracellular factors, or in the case we shall consider, by change in intracelluar biological function (Hochachka and Somero, 1984). Of all tissues in the vertebrate body, skeletal muscle displays the special quality of being able to routinely sustain very large changes in work and metabolic rates. Compared to 1.5- to 2-fold differences in metabolic rates between resting metabolic rates (RMRs) and activated states, which is common to many tissues (liver and brain, to mention two), skeletal muscles in most animals must be able to sustain up to, or even over, 100-fold changes in ATP turnover rates. Among vertebrate endotherms, the highest muscle metabolic rate (in the range of $600 \, \mu$mol ATP $\times \, g^{-1} \times \, min^{-1}$) appears to be that of hummingbird breast muscle during hovering flight—a rate over 500 times muscle RMR (Suarez, 1992). During muscle ischemia, hypoxemia, or hypoxia, the metabolism of muscle, like that of many other tissues under conditions of oxygen lack, may need to sustain a suppression of metabolism even below resting rates (Hochachka and Guppy, 1987), thus even further extending the enormous range between lowest and highest sustainable ATP turnover rates of this remarkable tissue.

THE STANDARD METABOLIC CONTROL MODEL

Current popular interpretations of how these kinds of large-scale differences in steady-state energy turnover are regulated assume cybernetic feedback control circuitry. The standard theory is summarized in figure 2.13 (see Balaban, 1990; Chance et al., 1986; From et al., 1990; Kushermick ct al., 1992). Following activation signals arriving at the muscle cell, an increase in ATP demand "turns on" cell ATPases whose catalytic function leads to increased product (ADP, Pi, H^+) concentrations; the latter then serve as substrates and as positive feedback signals for accelerating ATP supply pathways (figure 2.13). Metabolites such as ADP and Pi are thought to be pivotal in mitochondrial metabolic control, but powerful activation of cell work also demands a proportional activation of catalytic function at essentially every enzyme step involved in ATP supply and ATP demand pathways. Hence, if substrate, product, and modulator concentration changes are to be the main mediators of large (100-fold or more) change in ATP turnover rate, one would anticipate equally large perturbations in pool sizes of numerous intermediates. This would be especially true for regulation processes based on Michaelis–Menten kinetics, where the kinetic order cannot exceed 1 (Atkinson, 1977, 1990; that is, percent change in catalytic rate (ATP turnover rate) cannot exceed the percent change in substrate concentration driving the metabolic rate change (Hochachka, 1994; Hochachka and Matheson, 1992). Whereas "homeostasis" demands "con-

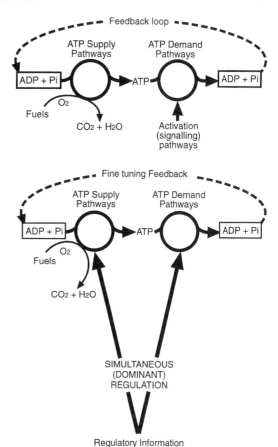

Figure 2.13. Upper panel is a summary diagram of the standard model of metabolic regulation; in this conceptualization, accelerating tissue ATP utilization leads to increasing concentrations of ADP and Pi, which serve as substrates for oxidative phosphorylation, to activate ATP production. Lower panel summarizes an alternate model of metabolic regulation in which ATP demand and ATP supply pathways are simultaneously activated during large-scale change in tissue work rates. See text for further details.

stancy of the internal milieu," muscle work would thus appear to require drastic changes in intracellular conditions, the degree of perturbation being somehow related to the intensity of work. The problem (and paradox) is how the conflicting demands of homeostasis versus metabolic regulation are resolved in muscle during different work and metabolic states; that is, how muscles sustain both metabolic homeostasis and metabolic regulation.

TWO THEORETICAL FRAMEWORKS FOR PROBING METABOLIC REGULATION

Since about the 1960s, two general frameworks (we shall term them models I and II) accounting for metabolic regulation have dominated thinking in the field. These two views can be nicely illustrated by considering the vertebrate phosphagen system (figure 2.14). Model I assumes (i) that the total acid-extractable pool of Cr + PCr (termed tCr) occurs in aqueous solution and is fully accessible to creatine phosphokinase (CPK), (ii) that solution chemistry rules apply globally in muscle cells in vivo, and (iii) that the main CPK-phosphagen function is to "buffer" ATP concentrations during large-scale changes in muscle work and in ATP turnover rates (figure 2.14(A)). Model II hypotheses consider (i) that the structural organization of phosphagen containing cells physically constrains tCr, (ii) that solution chemistry rules may apply in vivo mainly to localized PCr/Cr pools, and (iii) that intracellularly localized CPK isoforms in vivo create complex and possibly directional pathways of PCr and Cr metabolism—forming so-called creatine shuttles in metabolism (figure 2.14(B)). Model I considers the cell essentially as a bag of enzymes in which simple solution chemistry rules apply; Model II sees the cell as a highly structured system with intracellular ultrastructure incorporating constraints on metabolic processes and in the extreme impos-

ing 3D order on metabolic function. The polarization illustrated by these two views extends throughout the metabolic regulation field and has caused the field to progress along two surprisingly independent paths with minimal communication between them. Both views, however, must accommodate the empirical observations on how real biological systems work in differing metabolic states. A good place to start our analysis is with a reappraisal of pathway fluxes and pathway intermediates under different metabolic states to sense the size and nature of the problem we are facing.

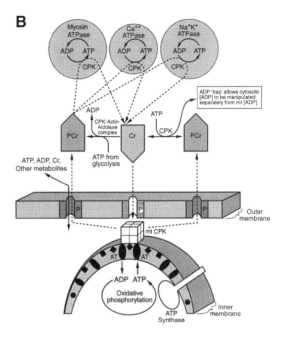

Figure 2.14(B). A summary of a large amount of information gained over many years of research that suggests that cell structure and isoform-specific CPK localizations powerfully influence the behavior of the CPK system. Studies by Wallimann and his coworkers used an ADP trapping system to manipulate the cytosolic ADP separately from the mitochondrial ADP pool. These data showed that ADP formed by mitochondrial CPK (mt CPK) is required for maintaining high rates of ATP turnover; they are consistent with the concept of the CPK system as a shuttle of high-energy phosphate groups from sites of ATP production to sites of ATP utilization. This figure is a composite summary of several studies from the Wallimann group (see Kay et al., 2000).

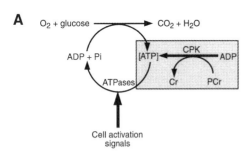

Figure 2.14(A). A summary of the classical role of creatine phosphokinase (CPK) in "buffering" ATP concentrations during change in tissue energy demand. This view of creatine function assumes that the cytosol is analogous to a simple aqueous solution and it assumes that CPK has access to the complete intracellular pool of phosphocreatine (PCr) and creatine (Cr) at all times.

KEY REGULATORY PROPERTIES OF REAL METABOLIC SYSTEMS

It is a rule of thumb in biology that many physiological and molecular functions are the sum of individual processes linked in sequence; in isolation many such individual processes have no clear functions at all. For metabolic pathways, integrated function often is evaluated by comparing changes in flux through the pathway per se with changes in concentrations of substrates and products of individual enzyme reactions within the pathway. Such approaches very early on indicated that enzymes in multistep pathways are surprisingly well integrated. Examples of this are shown for ^{31}P MRS visible phosphate metabolites for human muscle work in essence monitoring the path of ^{31}P during ATP turnover (figure 2.15). These data show that [PCr] and [Pi] both change with muscle work, that the change is an accurate reflection of the change in ATP demand, and that the quantitative response differs in slow- versus fast-twitch fibers. It is less marked in the former than the latter, and these metabolites are even less (actually immeasurably) perturbed during work transitions in the heart. What is more, ATP concentrations are perfectly protected through these kinds of work transitions in all of the three (slow, fast, and cardiac) muscle types. Similar data are shown for the path of glycolysis in figure 2.16 in rat fast-twitch fibers, fish fast-twitch fibers, and rat heart. Again, even if change in flux demanded by change in work perturbs the concentrations of pathway intermediates, what is most striking is how small these changes are compared to the huge changes in pathway flux (figure 2.16). Even in extreme cases (Wegener et al., 1991; Blum et al., 1990, 1991), such as in very high capacity metabolic pathways in insect flight muscles or in the electric organ of electric fishes, greater than 100-fold flux changes in pathways of ATP demand and ATP supply can be achieved with only minor perturbation in concentrations of pathway intermediates.

To explain this precision and integration of linked sequences of enzyme function, several regulatory models are currently being evaluated by workers in this field (Hochachka et al.,

1998). These include (i) simple feedback and mass action controls, the standard model above, (ii) allosteric controls, (iii) models involving the regulation of e_o (the concentration of functional catalytic sites) by means of alteration in protein interactions (as in actomyosin ATPase), by change in phosphorylation state (as in pyruvate dehydrogenase), by change in redox state (as in V-type ATPases), by Ca^{2+} activation, or by translocation from inactive to an active intracellular location (as in glucose transporters), and (iv) various versions of metabolic control analysis (Fell and Thomas, 1995; Thomas and Fell, 1996) originally introduced over a decade ago (these make minimal assumptions at the level of enzyme mechanism). The diversity of mechanisms and models of enzyme regulation arise in part from the differing requirements at different loci in metabolism (figure 2.17).

CONTROL REQUIREMENTS DEPEND ON TYPE OF ENZYME

Many and perhaps most enzymes in metabolic pathways obey Michaelis–Menten kinetics and operate under near-equilibrium conditions (at equilibrium, of course, forward and reverse fluxes for such enzyme reactions are the same and there can be no net forward or reverse flux). During pathway and enzyme activation (Staples and Suarez, 1997; Suarez et al., 1997), net forward flux for such enzymes is achieved by modest adjustments in substrate(s)/product(s) concentration ratios (figure 2.17(A)). Several requirements arise for such enzymes in vivo. First of all, since the chemical potential driving the net forward reaction is usually modest, large amounts of enzyme are the rule in order to be able to match the flux rates required in vivo. This is achieved by high enzyme content or by high k_{cat} (turnover number per active site on the enzyme), or by both mechanisms at once. Traditionally, for most metabolic biochemists, this is the explanation for "near equilibrium" enzymes occurring at relatively enormous concentrations—the higher the enzyme concentration, the closer to equilibrium is in vivo function—and for "near equilibrium" enzymes

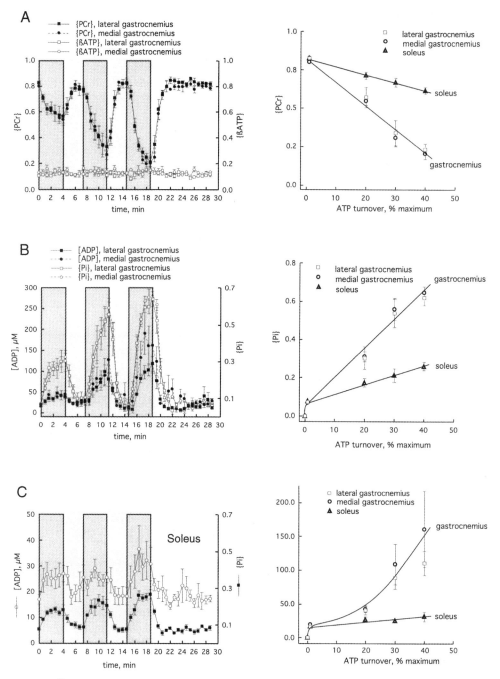

Figure 2.15. ^{31}P magnetic resonance spectroscopic (MRS) analysis of changes in PCr, ATP, Pi, and ADP monitored simultaneously in human gastrocnemius and soleus during three different exercise intensities, 20%, 30%, and 40% of maximum (bars), with rest periods in between and recovery at the end of the protocol. To standardize the data, {PCr} and {ATP} are expressed as the ratios of each to the sum of easily MRS-measurable phosphate metabolites: [PCr] + [ATP] + [Pi], while ADP is given in molar units, since it is calculated from the CPK equilibrium. Left panels in A, B, and C indicate representative MRS data. Right panels show plots of work intensity (% maximum ATP turnover rate) as the independent parameter and metabolite concentrations at the end of each work bout are plotted as dependent parameters (on the vertical axes). (Modified from Allen et al., 1997.)

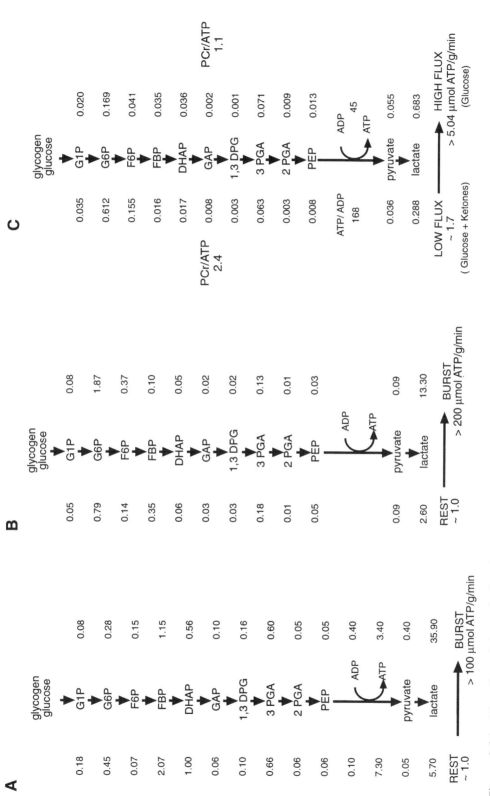

Figure 2.16. The effect of change in flux through the glycolytic path (low vs high work rates) for two (A: trout muscle; B: rat gastrocnemius) skeletal muscle systems in vivo (modified from Hochachka, 1994) and (C) for perfused rat heart preparations in vitro (modified from Kashiwaya et al., 1994). One of the instructive insights arising from these kinds of studies is the so-called [s] stability paradox: remarkably stable concentrations of pathway intermediates during changes in pathway fluxes that can approach or exceed 100-fold. See text for other details.

A

Near Equilibrium Enzymes

e.g. PEP + ADP ⟷ ATP + pyruvate

- net flux occurs with only minimal changes in substrate or product concentrations
- 'driving force' is modest
- high enzyme concentration required to drive a given change in velocity

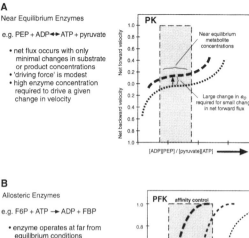

B

Allosteric Enzymes

e.g. F6P + ATP → ADP + FBP

- enzyme operates at far from equilibrium conditions
- 'driving force' is high (modulators drastically alter the *s* vs *v* relations)
- lower concentration of enzyme required to drive a given change in velocity

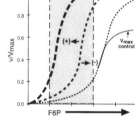

C

Phosphorylation (or Redox) Controlled Enzymes

e.g. pyruvate + NAD + CoA → acetylCoA + CO_2 + NADH

- enzyme operates at far from equilibrium conditions (enzyme in extreme cases operates as fully ON or fully OFF)
- change in flux varies with e_O, not with change in [substrates] or [products]
- lowest concentration of enzyme needed for a given change in velocity of the reaction

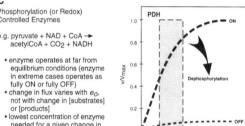

Figure 2.17. How matching of flux of substrate to product at each step in a complex metabolic pathway such as glycolysis with the overall maximum flux through the pathway (J_{max}) is achieved may depend upon the kind of enzyme functioning at any specified locus. Traditional explanations for three kinds of enzymes are summarized above. Panels (A), (B), and (C) summarize processes thought to allow for large changes in flux with more moderate changes in substrate and product concentrations for three different kinds of enzymes. See Hochachka et al. (1998) and text for further details.

being catalytically especially efficient. Triose phosphate isomerase (TPI) is one such example. In tissues with a high (aerobic or anaerobic) glycolytic potential (such as various fast-twitch

muscles) the enzyme occurs at almost millimolar concentrations and its high k_{cat} means that its in vivo activity (in terms of μmol substrate to product per g per min) is enormous. In fact, studies carried out over two decades (see Hochachka, 1980, 1994; Fersht, 1985) showed that selection for high efficiency has pushed this enzyme towards a state of catalytic "perfection": any further improvement in the enzyme's efficiency would not be expressed in higher reaction rates because it would be limited by diffusion-based enzyme–substrate encounter.

Most metabolic pathways also contain allosteric enzymes that function under quite different conditions and that are much more subject to regulation. Allosteric regulation (Fersht, 1985; Hochachka and Somero, 1984) is based on positive or negative modulators binding at sites other than the active site (hence the term "allosteric" rather than isosteric, which would apply to modulators competing with substrate at the active site). Phosphofructokinase (PFK) in glycolysis is a quintessential example of an allosteric enzyme (figure 2.17(B)). PFK in vivo operates far from equilibrium, it tends to work largely in the forward direction, catalyzing the reaction

$$F6P + ATP \rightarrow ADP + F1,6P$$

The enzyme is product activated by both ADP and F1,6P (also termed FBP), by F2,6P, AMP, ammonia, and high pH. F6P saturation curves are sigmoidal with an interaction coefficient, n, of 2 or more. This means that when one F6P is bound, the affinity of the next site for F6P rises; in this sense, F6P is a substrate and an activator of the enzyme acting upon it. Most modulators affect PFK by shifts in substrate affinities, rather than in V_{max}, except for the cosubstrate ATP: at high concentrations ATP becomes a substrate inhibitor of the reaction. Taken together, these regulators add up to a pattern in which energy-rich conditions down-regulate PFK activity, while energy-depleted conditions up-regulate PFK. These properties mean that the chemical potential driving the forward reaction tends to be very high and high fluxes can therefore be sustained with lower enzyme activities (i.e., lower enzyme concentrations are required and lower k_{cat} values are quite tolerable).

Still other enzymes are regulated essentially in on–off fashion. Pyruvate dehydrogenase (PDH), for example, is regulated by phosphorylation–dephosphorylation mechanisms (by protein kinases and protein phosphatases, respectively). The ATP-dependent PDH kinase-catalyzed reaction converts PDH to the low-activity (off) form, which is favored under energy-saturated conditions, while a phosphatase hydrolyzes this bond, releasing Pi and converting PDH back to its high-activity (on) form (figure 2.17(C)). This may be viewed as a kind of coarse control system; fine control of PDH catalytic activity is achieved by NADH and acetylCoA product inhibition. As in the case of PFK, PDH functions far from equilibrium and the chemical potential driving the forward reaction is high. This means that the same maximum in-vivo flux capacities can be matched by lower enzyme concentrations and lower catalytic efficiencies than in the case of near-equilibrium enzymes such as TPI. Similar phosphorylation-based on–off type controls of enzyme activities were first discovered for glycogen phosphorylase in the 1960s and have been shown for numerous other enzymes. Although protein kinase and phosphatase couplets are the most common, they are not the only means by which enzymes can be held in either on or off states. Two other mechanisms we will briefly mention are those based on protein–protein interactions and on redox change in –SH residues. Actomyosin ATPase is an example of the former (Grabarek et al., 1992), V type ATPase, of the latter (Harvey and Wieczorek et al., 1997). At rest, actomyosin ATPase in skeletal muscle is catalytically inert, held that way by troponin c; Ca^{2+} activation (during excitation–contraction or EC coupling) relieves troponin c binding and unleashes this enzyme's huge catalytic activity. Low- and high-activity forms of V-type ATPases are similarly regulated by hypoxia or other parameters that change local redox (reducing the S–S bridge to –SH). Because the concentration of catalytically active sites (e_o) is effectively low in the off state and high in the on state, this category of mechanisms is referred to as e_o reg-

ulation of enzyme activity (Hochachka and Matheson, 1992). The exceptionally huge metabolic flare-up associated with electric organ discharge in electric fishes may supply a particularly clear example of this kind of regulatory mechanism (Blum et al., 1990, 1991).

HOW TO EXPLAIN HOMEOSTASIS OF PATHWAY INTERMEDIATES

Given this diversity in the nature of enzymes that in vivo are linked together to form single metabolic or physiological functions, it is all the more perplexing to find, and challenging to account for, the empirical observation: that enzymes linked in linear series to form metabolic pathways are so exquisitely integrated that large changes in pathway flux are sustained with minimal perturbation of pathway substrates and products. [ATP] is almost perfectly homeostatic under most conditions (except under very extreme O_2 limited or fatigue conditions) and other intermediates in pathways of ATP supply or ATP demand are stabilized within less rigorously controlled concentration ranges (where these changes may reflect change in ATP turnover rates, but clearly cannot cause them (see figures 2.15 and 2.16). A cursory count shows that the percent changes in concentrations of more than 60 substrates and intermediates (in glucose, fat, and amino acid catabolic pathways) quantified to date are far less than the percent changes in flux rates with which they correlate. This is observed over and over again, for low-capacity and high-capacity pathways. The only metabolite that seems to be an exception is oxygen. Even this turns out not to be a real exception, but the story here is so fascinating and so complex that we need to reason our way through the empirical evidence.

OXYGEN DELIVERY ($\dot{Q}O_2$) IS KEY TO REGULATION OF $\dot{V}O_2$

There is a huge literature on how O_2 functions both as a substrate and as a potential regulator of tissue metabolism over varying times of exposure and we shall not review this comprehensively at this time. There are both physiological and biochemical aspects to controlling the relationship between O_2 delivery and O_2 consumption. As energy demand changes, physiological mechanisms must be harnessed for appropriate perfusion changes. Multiple metabolite signals (adenosine, K^+, H^+, endothelins, nitric oxide) are utilized for coordinating perfusion with cell-level energy demands. Nitric oxide (NO) has received particular attention over the last decade. NO is formed from arginine in a reaction catalyzed by nitric oxide synthase (NOS), which in mammals occurs as three different isoforms (Forstermann and Hartmut, 1999). NOS I or ncNOS was originally discovered in neurons, NOS II or iNOS was originally discovered in cytokine-induced macrophages, and NOS III or ecNOS was originally discovered in endothelial cells. This field of research is far too large to explore in detail here. It should suffice to point out that NO released by NOS catalytic activity serves in perfusion regulation by direct vasodilation and indirectly through Hb binding. The latter mechanism is only now being worked out in detail, but it already appears that NO binding to Hb occurs at the lungs, while its release is favored at the tissues; the lower the oxygen tension, the greater the need for NO-mediated vasodilation, and the greater the NO release from Hb (Gow et al., 1999). These kinds of studies go a long way towards explaining why numerous studies have found essentially 1:1 relationships between $\dot{Q}O_2$ and tissue (especially muscle) work. For example, studies using dog gastrocnemius (Arthur et al., 1992a), found such a relationship over an 18-fold change in ATP turnover rate. Later, Hogan et al. (1992) used the same preparation to analyze subtle submaximal work changes; these transitions were sustained with no change at all in [PCr], [ATP] and other [metabolites]. Yet through these transitions a 1:1 relationship between $\dot{V}O_2$ and $\dot{Q}O_2$ was maintained—results similar to many other data from other laboratories on different tissues and organs. The conclusion arising is that this is the only metabolite signal so far identified that varies 1:1 with work over realistic biological rate changes. That is why we and many others in the field accept

that O_2 plays a key role in regulating up or down change in ATP turnover. But how is the O_2 signal transduced within the cell?

OXYGEN SIGNAL TRANSDUCTION IS NOT BASED ON INTRACELLULAR [O_2]

Interestingly, the answer to this question remains unclear. So far the only mechanisms proposed by traditional studies in this area assume simple diffusion paths from capillaries and calculate smooth diffusion gradients within the cell ending in mitochondrial O_2 sinks. However, this approach has been less than satisfactory for, to unravel the puzzle of how O_2 delivery translates into effects on metabolism within the cell, we require hard data on intracellular O_2 concentration. The difficulty is that for most tissues this key parameter remains elusive and unknown; only in muscle is the situation more favorable. In this tissue, myoglobin (Mb) represents a direct intracellular detector of [O_2]. Mb is a relatively small, monomeric respiratory pigment occurring in heart and mitochondria-rich skeletal muscles at concentrations of less than 0.5 mM; in muscles of marine mammals such as seals, Mb concentrations reach into the 4–5 mM range. Gene knockout experiments (Garry et al., 1999; Goedecke et al., 1999) show that even if mice can survive without Mb they can do so only by activating compensating mechanisms such as increasing capillary densities and blood O_2-carrying capacity. It is therefore usually assumed that Mb is functionally important under usual physiological conditions. At 37°C, O_2 solubility in physiological solutions is about 1 μM/torr. Because the reaction $Mb + O_2 \leftrightarrow MbO_2$ is always in equilibrium, with a P_{50} of 3 torr (K_d of about 3 μM), whenever [O_2] is less than saturating for Mb, %MbO_2 directly estimates intracellular [O_2].

Earlier attempts to make such estimates with working muscle preparations almost exclusively relied upon near-infrared spectroscopy. More recently, MRS is being used to take advantage of a histidine-H being ^{1}H MRS "visible" in deoxyMb but being MRS "invisible" in oxyMb (figure 2.18). For the first time, this

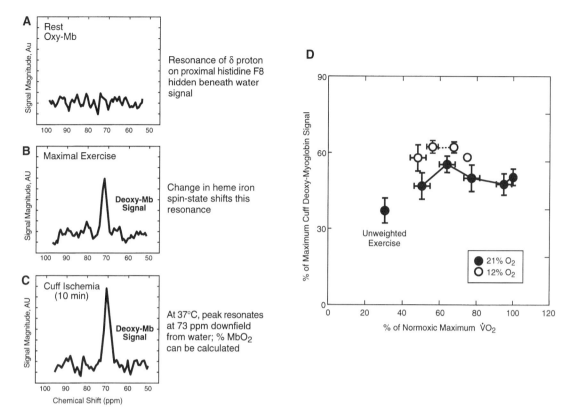

Figure 2.18. (A)–(C) How ^{1}H MRS can be used to estimate the %MbO$_2$ in muscles that contain a high enough concentration of myoglobin to make an F8 histidine 1H MRS visible. (D) A study using this technology to evaluate the %MbO$_2$ in human working thigh muscle going from unweighted exercise to maximum exercise. Under these kinds of conditions, where most of cardiac output can be directed to a small working muscle mass, very high rates of O$_2$ delivery and thus of aerobic metabolism and work are possible (equivalent to about 100μmol ATP/g muscle/min). Despite these very high metabolic rates and associated very high O$_2$ fluxes, %MbO$_2$ remains almost constant at about 50–60%. (Modified from Richardson et al., 1996.)

new technology supplies workers in the field with a noninvasive window on the oxygenation state of muscles in different work and metabolic states, at least for muscles with a high enough [Mb] to be ^{1}H MRS "detectable." When first applied to both working human skeletal muscles (Richardson et al., 1996) and to heart (Jelicks and Wittenberg, 1995) the same instructive results were found: essentially stable %MbO$_2$ through large changes in work rate. In such studies, as soon as a workload is imposed (even very-low-intensity exercise, such as unloaded pedaling), %MbO$_2$ quickly establishes a new steady state, usually between 40% and 70% saturation, both as a function of time

and as a function of tissue work intensity. Along with gold-labeling studies showing a random Mb distribution in rat heart and skeletal muscles (figure 2.19), the MRS data imply that %MbO$_2$ and intracellular [O$_2$] both remain relatively constant up to the maximum sustainable aerobic metabolic rate of the tissue. Just as CPK serves to "buffer" ATP concentrations during changes in muscle work so Mb apparently serves to "buffer" intracellular [O$_2$] in different metabolic states.

Parenthetically, it should be acknowledged that the volumes of interest in these kinds of MRS studies are large and the MRS data necessarily are averages of large numbers of fibers.

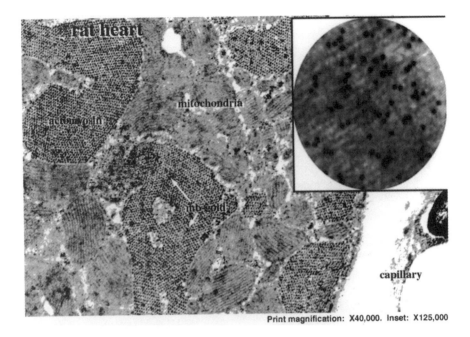

Print magnification: X40,000. Inset: X125,000

Figure 2.19. Distribution of gold-labeled Mb in rat heart electron micrographs: Two magnification levels are shown. At all magnification levels analyzed, Mb distribution showed no specific localizations. Knowing that Mb is randomly distributed in the cytosol of muscle cells constrains models of its in-vivo functions. See text for further details. Electron micrographs are courtesy of S. Shinn and P.W. Hochachka, University of British Columbia.

Human muscles like muscles in other mammals are formed from mixtures of fiber types and as work intensity rises for a given muscle mass, there may be changes in recruitment and in the percent contribution of different fiber types. This problem does not arise in studies of heart muscle, which is biochemically rather homogenous. While Richardson et al. (1996) apparently avoided this artifact, this does not seem to be the case in the Mole et al. (1999) study on an unknown mix of fibers in human calf muscle. Evidence of the problem initially arises from their ^{31}P MRS data, which showed an expected linear decrease in [PCr] as work increased; at maximum aerobic work, [PCr] changed by maximally about threefold. Since the same [PCr] change occurs when gastrocnemius work rate reaches only 40% of sustained aerobic maximum, but much smaller changes in [PCr] occur in (the mainly slow fibers of) soleus during the same work transition (Allen et al., 1997), it is probable that the regions of interest

in the Mole et al study may have overlapped into muscles rich in slow-twitch fibers, where the change in [PCr] is less for a given level of work than in fast-twitch fibers. Otherwise it would be difficult to understand why their preparation had to be pushed to its maximum work level to achieve the same percent [phosphagen] shifts that Allen et al. (1997) observed at only 40% of aerobic maximum. For these reasons, the %MbO$_2$ values recorded at different work intensities almost certainly represent different combinations of fiber types. Nevertheless, these studies found that at about 50% and 80% of sustained aerobic maximum work rate (representing huge ATP turnover rates, equivalent to about 50–80 μmol ATP $\times$ g^{-1} $\times$ min^{-1}), %MbO$_2$ did not change significantly (stabilized at about 65–70% MbO$_2$), in agreement with earlier studies; however, at the maximum work rate, a further modest desaturation to about 50% MbO$_2$ occurred, which is not in full agreement with the data of

Richardson et al. (1996). Because of the mixed fiber and recruitment problems, readers should not be surprised by these modestly different results; and, at least tentatively we consider that the small discrepancies probably arise from artifacts caused by differing metabolic states in different fiber types. Thus they do not strongly influence our main conclusion that $[O_2]$ is largely homeostatic.

In fact, even if most workers probably would accept that Mb should function to buffer intracellular $[O_2]$, the significance of this has not been fully appreciated. As Carl Honig explained to one of us (PWH) in a discussion in 1987, this may be because of a too enthusiastic acceptance of traditional diffusion models assuming smooth gradients across the capillary-muscle cell threshold all the way to the mitochondrial sinks. Such models, which assume complete homogeneity and necessarily ignore the issues of fiber type and recruitment heterogeneity, are not accepted by the Honig group. According to Honig et al. (1992), the structure of the capillary-muscle system develops steep gradients (and localized high O_2 fluxes) only at the capillary-muscle interface but very shallow gradients within the muscle cell per se, as indeed found by the more recent MRS data on %MbO_2 in vivo. That is why Hochachka and McClelland (1997) accepted the MRS data on %MbO_2 at face value and emphasized that, under normoxic conditions, O_2 is perfectly homeostatic in the sense that its concentration is stable even while its flux to cytochrome oxidase can change by two or more orders of magnitude. In the examples above, the concentration of O_2 ranged between $2-4\,\mu M$ during pathway flux changes from about 1 to over $80\,\mu mol\ ATP \times g^{-1} \times min^{-1}$ (these high mass-specific metabolic rates are achieved because most of the cardiac output during these protocols is available for supporting the work of relatively small muscle masses).

To recapitulate, the situation arising from these studies of oxygen and metabolic regulation can be summarized as follows. First, because of the buffering role of Mb, oxygen concentrations are low (in the P_{50} or K_d range) and intracellular $[O_2]$ gradients must be quite shallow. Second, it is emphasized by the

Honig, Gayeski, and Connett group (see Honig et al., 1992) that the capillary–muscle contact surface area is only a fraction of the surface area of inner mitochondrial membranes and cristae; by definition this means that the highest gradients and highest O_2 fluxes are at the capillary–muscle cell threshold and that these gradients are necessarily much shallower in the cytosol. Thirdly, the low intracellular [oxygen] remains essentially stable (i.e., remains effectively buffered by the $MbO_2 \leftrightarrow Mb + O_2$ equilibrium, throughout large changes in work and metabolic rates. Nevertheless, $\dot{V}O_2$ and O_2 delivery are closely related, suggesting a key role for O_2 in metabolic regulation.

MECHANISMS ACCOUNTING FOR O_2 FLUX TO CELLS

Given that it is $\dot{Q}O_2$—not intracellular $[O_2]$—that correlates with work rate, the problem we still are left with is how the O_2 signal is transmitted to the machinery of cell metabolism. At this time, we admit that there is no widely accepted resolution of this problem. The traditional answer, of course, assumes oxygen diffusion down smooth concentration gradients from capillary plasma to tissue mitochondria. A second mechanism assumes accelerated intracellular O_2 transfer by Mb-facilited diffusion in Mb-containing cells (in this case two species are diffusing to the mitochondrial targets at once: molecular O_2 and MbO_2). A third mechanism assumes that lipids (either phospholipid bilayers or triglyceride droplets) form the preferred path of O_2 diffusion because of the greater O_2 solubility in lipids than in aqueous phase. A final mechanism is that of O_2 sensing. When we first recognized this puzzling problem of O_2 transmission and realized the limitations of the classical diffusion model to explain the observations, we postulated an O_2-sensing system presumably located in the cell membrane (or even more distally) and signal transduction pathways or mechanisms for "telling" the cell metabolic machinery when and how potently to respond to changing availability of O_2 (Hochachka, 1994). Whereas each of the above explanations of O_2 transfer can claim to be able to account for observed O_2 fluxes under some conditions, none of the above mechanisms is able to easily explain why the flux rates vary with O_2 delivery rather than with intracellular O_2 concentrations.

All of the above mechanisms represent so-called traditional explanations and, as briefly mentioned above, they are formulated within the Model I framework of cell function: this is the view of cells as watery bags in which solution chemistry rules basically dominate the functional behavior of the system. Model II views of the cell are very different and assume that intracellular conditions are so complex that solution behavior is not necessarily the rule. The Model II view (of metabolic ragulation in general and of O_2 regulation in particular) takes an entirely different tack and postulates that intracellular circulation, not diffusion, is the main means for bringing ligands and their binding sites together during upwards or downwards transitions in metabolic and tissue work rates. Let us review how this picture differs from the more classical or traditional framework discussed above.

MODEL II: CELL STRUCTURE DEMANDS AN INTRACELLULAR PERFUSION SYSTEM

Conceptually, the major difference between the above traditional approach to metabolic regulation and Model II is the emphasis placed upon intracellular order and structure. The points of departure for the latter view are three different lines of evidence favoring intracellular perfusion but not favoring diffusion as the dominant means for regulating enzyme–substrate encounter (including cytochrome oxidase–O_2 encounter). First and most fundamental is the structural argument: ultrastructural, histochemical, and cytochemical studies do not indicate the cell as a static bag of substrates and enzymes, but rather a 3D membrane-bound microcosm housing an internal milieu filled with complex organelles, motors, membranes, cables, trabeculae, and channels. Rather than a dead-still solution (as would be required for formal application of laws of diffusion), the

internal medium is very much "alive" in the sense that movement is the rule of thumb—movement of organelles, of particles, and of cytosol (so-called cytoplasmic streaming at rates from less than 1 to $80\,\mu m\ sec^{-1}$). This intracellular convection is metabolically controlled, it varies with metabolic state, it is based on ATP-dependent and ATP-utilizing myosin motors (so-called unconventional myosin isoforms) which can be activated to run on actin filaments, and it behaves for practical purposes like an intracellular circulation system. What is more, because of the conservative nature of macromolecular structures and functions, we have good reasons for thinking that this, and comparable systems based on kinesin and dynein motors running on microtubules, are widespread and probably characteristic of all cells (see Hochachka, 1999a,b, for literature in this area).

In contrast to what might be expected of a bag of enzymes and substrates, over a half-century of research has clearly concluded that many metabolic pathways and their component enzymes are restricted to specific cell compartments and numerous so-called soluble enzymes show intracellular binding to specific intracellular sites. Order and structure is the name of the game, as far as the literature on cell ultrastructure is concerned, and it is not a diffusion-dominated game. Take away the order and the system behavior falls apart; sometimes function is lost completely. A good example of this comes from genetic studies of *Drosophila* flight muscle metabolism. While earlier studies had shown that ALD, GAPDH, and GPDH colocalize mainly at Z-disks, Wojtas et al. (1997) used clever genetic manipulations (that influenced binding but not overall catalytic activities) to show that mislocating these enzyme activities in the cytosol rather than correctly bound to Z-disks would render *Drosophila* flightless—a dramatic demonstration that even if all three enzymes are expressed at high activities, their 3D organization is part and parcel of in-vivo regulated function of the pathway (figure 2.20).

Second is the argument on macromolecular functional constraints. As we might expect from the above (and indeed find), the intracellular

(a)

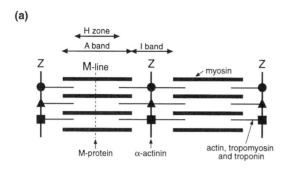

(b)

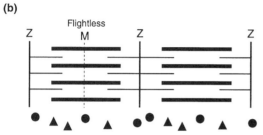

(c)

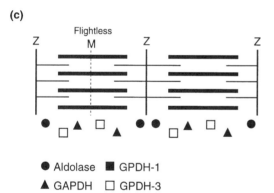

● Aldolase   ■ GPDH-1

▲ GAPDH   □ GPDH-3

Figure 2.20. In normal *Drosophila* muscle (a), three key glycolytic enzymes (aldolase, glyceraldehyde-3-phosphate dehydrogenase (GAPDH), and glycerol-3-phosphate dehydrogenase isoform 1 (GPDH-1) are all known to be colocalized on the Z-line of myofilaments. Genetic manipulations which prevent binding of these enzymes to the Z-line (b) make *Drosophila* unable to fly, even if transfected (c) with glycerol-3-phosphate dehydrogenase (GPDH) acvitity (in this case, a different isoform, GPDH-3, was transfected). These clever genetic studies show that structural localization of glycolytic enzymes, not only overall catalytic activity, is critical to normal muscle function. See text for further details. (Modified from Wojtas et al., 1997.)

mobilities of enzymes and of carrier proteins such as Mb are not equivalent to those in simple aqueous solutions. For example, intracellular diffusibility estimates for Mb in the cytosol range from as low as one fiftieth that found in simple solutions (Juergens et al., 1994; Papadopoulos et al. 2000) to values of about half that in simple solution (Wang, D. et al., 1998). Interestingly, the latter MRS study estimated rotational diffusion, while the former study estimated translational diffusion; as indicated below, these may change independently. Just as Mb appears to be less mobile within the cytosol than previosuly believed, so also are cytosolic enzymes apparently rather restricted in their intracellular mobility (the larger the protein, the greater the mobility restriction)—again this picture is not easily compatible with the concept of the cell as a bag of enzymes whose functions are determined mainly by self-diffusion and substrate diffusion at appropriate rates. With enzyme and myoglobin translational mobilities reduced to only a fraction of that expected in aqueous solutiion, diffusion of macromolecules becomes a highly inefficient means for assisting in enzyme–substrate encounter (or in the case of myoglobin, for assisting O_2 flux through the cytosol).

Third is the argument on metabolite mobility: because of the complexity of the internal milieu, the translational mobility even of simple molecules may be restricted compared to simple solutions and this is especially true in the mitochondrial matrix (Scalettar et al., 1991). To illustrate the problem, let us consider a small metabolite, creatine, that is found in cytosol and in mitochondria. Studies with ^{14}C-labeled Cr (Hochachka and Mossey, 1998) show that CPK is unable to readily equilibrate the entire pool of PCr + Cr in fish white muscle (fast-twitch fibers) over hour-long time periods. At the same time, parallel ^{1}H MRS studies (Trump et al., 2001) show that in human muscle in vivo the intracellular behavior of Cr is highly constrained. One set of studies, focusing on the methyl hydrogens show that Cr mobility is metabolic state dependent: three- to four-fold less mobile in ischemic fatigue than in muscle at rest. Another set of studies focusing on the methylene protons found that the methylene protons only in PCr were MRS visible; on PCr conversion to Cr during muscle work, the methylene protons become MRS invisible (in simple solutions MRS cannot distinguish these in PCr and Cr). Taken together these data supply powerful evidence that the behavior of metabolites in vivo may be much more precisely regulated (and certainly much more constrained) than previously expected (for literature in this area, see Hanstock et al, 1999; Trump et al., 2001). Another study showed that three factors (viscosity, binding, and interference from cell solids) could account for translational diffusion of a metabolite-sized analogue in cytosol being decreased to only 27% that observed in water. As in the MRS studies, these workers (Kao et al, 1993) also demonstrated mobilites that were state dependent: during osmotic stress (twofold cell volume increase), when metabolism is known to be increased, there is a correlated (if unexplained) sixfold increase in the apparent translational diffusion coefficient, while rotational diffusion remains constant. The complex and metabolic state-dependent diffusion behavior of metabolite-sized molecules would not readily facilitate enzyme–substrate encounters as required for simple solution models of regulated cell function.

Given these constraints, several workers (Coulson, 1993; Wheatley and Clegg, 1994; Hochachka, 1999a,b; Wheatley, 1998, 1999) consider diffusion by itself to be an inadequate, inefficient, and minimally regulatable means of delivering carbon substrates and oxygen to appropriate enzyme targets in the cell under the variable conditions and rates that are required in vivo. Instead, we favor an hypothesis—almost demanded by the rules imposed by a structured and ordered internal milieu—of an intracellular convection or perfusion system as an elegantly simple resolution of the problem of how substrates (including O_2) and enzymes are brought together. From our present point of view (Hochachka, 1999a,b), the key advantage of this model is that it easily explains how enzymes and substrates can be brought together and how reaction rates can occur at widely varying rates with minimal change in substrate concentrations—this is the empirical starting point of the paradox in this whole field which,

to our minds, has never been satisfactorily explained (for O_2 or for any other intermediate in mainline metabolism). As in the perfusion of organs/tissues such as muscle mentioned above, rates of intracellular metabolic reactions by this model are simple products of intracellular perfusion rates: the greater the perfusion rates the greater the metabolic rates with no concomitant changes in substrate concentrations required. In this view, during osmotic activation of metabolic rate, the sixfold increase in metabolite mobility observed (but not explained) could well represent a similarly large increase in intracellular convection. In the case of the MRS data, a fourfold change in Cr mobility in hypometabolic ischemic muscle may well represent a similar change in intracellular convection (this is viewed as a coarse but dominant control, which to be sure need not rule out other fine tuning control mechanisms, the kinds that have so far absorbed much of metabolic research).

For O_2 transport, this view places the function of a half-O_2-saturated, randomly distributed Mb into an entirely different perspective where the fundamental purpose of an intracellular Mb may be to equalize $[O_2]$ everywhere in the cytosol—this would assure that intracellular convection would always be delivering similar amounts of O_2 per unit volume of cytosol to cytochrome oxidases (and would simultaneously minimize or even destroy intracellular O_2 gradients). While this model is consistent with the minimal intracellular O_2 gradients in muscle cells proposed by the Honig, Connett, and Gayeski work (Gayeski and Honig, 1991; Honig et al., 1992), it takes on a quite different meaning. Finally, the concept of an intracellular perfusion system supplies purpose and meaning to intracellular movements (motor driven or otherwise induced cytoplasmic streaming) which have been mainly ignored by traditional metabolic biochemists to this time. If accepted, the concept of intracellular convection modifies our overall view to include an intracellular component to the chain of convective and diffusive steps in the overall path of O_2 from air to mitochondria.

In considering the concept of intracellular convection, early pioneers in this field may have been prone to over-enthusiastic pressing of their case; this is understandable, since it seems to explain much previously puzzling data so easily (Coulson, 1993; Wheatley and Clegg, 1994). Nevertheless, there clearly remain critical functions that are largely or solely diffusion based, so the understandable over-enthusiasm with which Model II proponents minimize the importance of diffusion in energy metabolism puts them at risk of throwing the baby out with the bathwater. To finally assemble a model that can realistically explain a realistic working range of metabolic systems, what seems to be required for the future is an opening up of channels of communication between the above two very differing views of metabolic regulation.

All of the above discussion on the functional properties of metabolic pathways has focused on short-term responses. The question arises of the effects of adjustments over acclimation or intermediate time courses; because studies with humans and mammals dominate this field, we will refer to these as "training effects" rather than acclimations (the term that is used elsewhere throughout this book).

TRAINING FOR ANAEROBIC EXERCISE: POTENTIAL ADAPTATION SITES

A minimal list (see Hochachka, 1994; Brooks et al., 1996, for additional literature) of theoretically adjustable aspects of anaerobic metabolism, primarily in muscle, must include:

1. increasing size of muscles utilized for the exercise (i.e., hypertrophy),
2. fiber-type replacement,
3. increasing levels of endogenous substrates (CrP and glycogen),
4. increasing levels of key enzymes in anaerobic metabolism and its control,
5. adjustments in isozyme type at specific loci in metabolism, and
6. improving buffering capacity of working muscles.

WORK-INDUCED MUSCLE HYPERTROPHY

The simplest adaptive response to prolonged, if periodic, burst-work demands on muscle, simply to make more of what is already present, i.e., hypertrophy, is in fact so obviously utilized that it has become a fad in many modern societies. All of us will be familiar with the image of a frail weakling reading with avid interest appealing advertisements on body-building, and the social advantages that go with same. This popular lore seems to have a scientific basis because the widely desired hypertrophy of muscle cells and their concomitant increase in strength in fact is an *adaptational response mainly to repeated bouts of anaerobic work* and is either not elicited or is more modestly expressed in endurance training. Although widely recognized, hypertrophy is poorly understood and underlying mechanisms are still largely unclear with only a few general features being well established (Duncan et al., 1998):

(a) Hypertrophy is assumed to be stimulated by exercise per se, for exercise can act independently of anabolic hormones (growth hormone, insulin, glucocorticoids) and even takes precedence over endocrine signals for muscle depletion (e.g., during starvation).

(b) The process involves RNA and protein biosynthesis, although it is still unclear if any cell division per se is involved. Inhibition of RNA or protein synthesis predictably blocks hypertrophy.

(c) The muscle mass increase represents mainly an increase in tissue protein, as a result of increased rates of synthesis and decreased rates of degradation. Increase in muscle weight, for example, is directly proportional to the increase in ^{3}H-labeled amino acid incorporation into proteins. Interestingly, even before increased RNA and protein synthesis can be demonstrated, stimulated muscle shows an increased ability to accumulate specific amino acids from the blood, and actually this is one of the earliest biochemical events signaling that the tissue will hypertrophy.

(d) Several lines of evidence indicate that some biochemical consequences of exercise per se or of the contractile process per se depend on amino acid uptake. (For example, muscle contracting isometrically takes up amino acids more rapidly than muscle shortening against no load.)

(e) The muscle mass increase during such work-stimulated growth represents mainly an increase in fiber size.

(f) The muscle mass increase represents an increase in soluble and myofibrillar proteins, as well as in collagen. However, the soluble proteins tend to be augmented disproportionately, which may reflect changes in contractile properties (reduced contractile speed, for example) as well as changes in metabolic capacities. Such changes could also be mediated by interconversions between slow-twitch oxidative and fast-twitch glycolytic fibers, so it is important to assess this possibility as well.

REGULATING % FAST-TWITCH FIBERS

Since there are major biochemical differences between red, intermediate, and white fiber types, increasing the percentage of white fibers may represent another possible way of adjusting the anaerobic power of a muscle. This theoretical possibility is raised by electrical stimulation and cross-innervation studies in animals which show that fibers *can* be converted one into the other. What is more, when one considers a longer (phylogenetic) time scale, one of the commonest adaptations for performance style is in the type and amount of muscle fiber retained in working muscles. This is best illustrated in teleosts, where species that rely mainly or solely upon burst-type swimming maintain a large white muscle mass but reduced red muscle; furthermore, the red muscle that is present takes on many of the biochemical properties of white muscle (reduced capillarity, reduced mitochondrial abundance, reduced levels of oxidative enzymes, and so forth). Similar differences are also well illustrated in the muscles of burst-flying birds, such as grouse and partridges. Even in humans there is

evidence for such genetically fixed differences between individuals. In athletes that are particularly good at anaerobic exercises (weightlifters, for example), the proportion of white fibers is typically higher than in individuals particularly good at sustained, aerobic work.

Earlier studies assessing fiber-type plasticity in training programs had difficulty in demonstrating that such effects might actually occur during, or in response to, the exercise regime, although there was some evidence for the interconversion of intermediate and white fiber types. However, the use of immunohistochemical techniques for distinguishing fast myosin (FM) and slow myosin (SM) have shown that intermediate fiber types contain both myosin isozymes, and moreover that the proportions of these can change with physical training. However, no such changes can be measured for the SM and FM isozymes in red and white fiber types. Thus, as repeatedly observed, the potential for adjusting the percentage fiber composition of mammalian muscle by exercise training programs is limited (probably to conversion of type IIx to type IIa during anaerobic training). Electrical stimulation, however, is another matter (Pette and Vrbova, 1999). The model of chronic low-frequency stimulation for the study of muscle plasticity was developed over a three-decade period. The protocol leads to a transformation of fast-twitch, fatigable muscles toward slower, fatigue-resistant ones. It involves qualitative and quantitative changes of all elements of the muscle fiber studied so far. Both functional and structural alterations are caused by coordinated replacement of fast protein isoforms with their slow counterparts, as well as by altered levels of expression. This remodeling of the muscle fiber encompasses the major, myofibrillar proteins, membrane-bound and soluble proteins involved in Ca^{2+} dynamics, as well as mitochondrial and cytosolic enzymes of energy metabolism (Simoneau and Pette, 1998). Most transitions occur in a coordinated, time-dependent manner and result from altered gene expression, including transcriptional and posttranscriptional mechanisms. Mechanistic insights arising from these kinds of electrical stimulation models are now being further developed with newer techniques, including the use of transgenic mice (Carlson et al., 1999).

GLYCOGEN AND tCr (PHOSPHOCREATINE + CREATINE) POOL SIZES

If the proportion of white fibers in working muscle is not increased during training for anaerobic work, to what extent might the anaerobic potential of muscle be improved simply by elevating the stored supplies of PCr and glycogen? Again, this mechanism appears to be utilized in long-term phylogenetic adaptation, particularly in the case of glycogen. It turns out that it also is utilized to some extent during training programs. In sprint-trained rats, for example, muscle PCr levels are higher than in controls particularly when the training is coupled with altitude stress (see Hochachka, 1994). Such an elevation in creatine phosphate level does not typically occur in humans, but even if the concentration does not rise, the hypertrophy of skeletal muscle that accompanies anaerobic training in effect increases the total *amount* of phosphagen available during burst work; what this means is that the *total amount of energy extractable from phosphagen is proportionately elevated.* Exactly the same considerations apply for glycogen, which also occurs in higher concentrations in muscles of athletes trained for anaerobic exercises.

Parenthetically, we should mention that various social pressures in human athletics have led to a huge interest in the use of creatine supplementation in an attempt to nudge the tCr upwards. The word "nudge" is the appropriate one, because, interestingly enough, even high Cr supplementation doses lead to barely statistically significant increases in the tCr pool; recent ^{1}H MRS studies (Trump et al., 2001) for example, could show no effect on the MRS visible pool size in soleus muscle at rest and only modest increases in the gastrocnemius. In mammals, including humans, tCr seems to be regulated at about $30 \mu M$ levels; however, in fish fast-twitch muscle, tCr pools can reach the $50 \mu M$ range (Parkhouse et al., 1988). It remains a mystery why the tCr pool in humans or in other mammals cannot be increased with Cr supplementation by a much larger factor than is actually observed experimentally.

TRAINING EFFECTS ON ENZYME LEVELS

In animals that are specialized for burst-type locomotion, not only is the proportion of white type fibers high, so also are the levels of enzymes in adenylate, creatine phosphate, and glycogen metabolism. In tuna white muscle, for example, which can sustain one of the highest rates of burst swimming thus far analyzed by biologists, the activities of myokinase, CPK, and various glycolytic enzymes are unusually high; lactate dehydrogenase, for example, occurs at over 5,000 units per gram (assayed at $25°C$), which contributes to potentially very high rates of glycolysis (Guppy et al., 1979). Thus, it is not surprising to find the same mechanism being utilized during anaerobic exercise regimes in animals and humans; particularly good data are available for CPK, myokinase, and LDH. The effects are presumably quite general, and indicate that enzyme concentrations stabilize after training at about 120–150% of pretraining levels (Holloszy and Booth, 1976). In addition, it must be remembered that the total content (total catalytic power) of enzymes of anaerobic metabolism is also elevated by simple hypertrophy of muscle during training. Thus the power output of muscle following such training will be elevated by an amount determined by a combination of (a) the degree of hypertrophy, and (b) the percentage change in concentration of enzymes in anaerobic metabolism.

ANAEROBIC EXERCISE TRAINING AND ISOZYME EXPRESSION

The properties of anaerobic metabolism are also strongly determined by the isozyme arrays present at each step in the anaerobic glycolysis of vertebrate muscle, so the question arises as to whether or not training can lead to adjustments in isozyme arrays utilized. The answer appears to be affirmative, but it must be cautioned that only a few studies are available. One of the best involves LDH, which is composed of five isozyme types; these are tetramers formed from the random association of A (muscle type) and B (heart type) subunits to generate A_4, A_3B_1, A_2B_2, A_1B_3, and B_4-type LDH. In humans, during sprint training, both the total LDH activity and the proportion of A_4 LDH increase and this appears to be the case in horses as well (Guy and Snow, 1977). Whether or not such isozyme adjustments during anaerobic exercise regimes turns out to be general remains uncertain and in need of further study.

ANAEROBIC EXERCISE TRAINING AND MUSCLE BUFFERING CAPACITY

The production of large amounts of lactate plus protons during burst work indicates the need for intracellular buffers. In vertebrate muscles, intracellular buffering is dominated by histidine imidazole groups. These may either occur as free histidine (in some teleosts), as histidine-containing dipeptides, or as protein-bound histidine residues. In teleosts, for example, the concentration of free histidine is highest in powerful burst-swimmers; tuna white muscle contains nearly 100μmol free histidine per gram of tissue and can accumulate lactate during intense anaerobic glycogenolysis to about the same levels. In mammals, about half the total histidine in muscle is protein-bound; the rest is present in the form of dipeptides, carnosine, anserine, and ophidine; concentrations can get up to about 50μmol g^{-1}, making these the dominant solutes in the cytosol. In general, the buffering capacity of muscle is proportional to its glycolytic activity, and so it is reasonable that during training for anaerobic exercises the buffering capacity of muscle is appropriately adjusted (Abe et al.. 1985).

AEROBIC EXERCISE TRAINING: POTENTIAL ADAPTATION SITES

Just as in our analysis of anaerobic training, it also is useful to begin our discussion of aerobic

training by considering possible sites and functions in aerobic work which theoretically may be adjustable (see Brooks et al., 1996; Hochachka, 1994). These then will supply us with a framework for analyzing aerobic training effects that are actually demonstrable in practice. A list of such theoretically adjustable determinants of aerobic performance must include:

1. increasing size of muscles utilized (i.e., hypertrophy),
2. adjusting proportions of red, intermediate, and white fiber types,
3. increasing levels of endogenous substrates (triglyceride and glycogen),
4. increasing levels of key enzymes in pathways contributing to aerobic oxidation of substrates,
5. increasing number (and possibly enzyme organization) of mitochondria, and
6. reducing activity levels of enzymes in anaerobic metabolism in concert with elevating aerobic metabolic potential.

In addition, because aerobically working muscles remain open systems, we may expect important adaptations occurring at higher levels of organization: in cooperative metabolic interactions between liver and muscle and between adipose tissue and muscle, in particular. These adaptations may involve:

1. simple adjustments in glycogen and triglyceride storage depots,
2. adjustments in the capacity of liver and adipose tissue to release glucose and fatty acids, respectively, during aerobic work,
3. adjustments in the capacity of muscle to take up blood glucose and blood free fatty acids, either for immediate catabolism or for deposition as endogenous storage (as muscle glycogen or muscle triglyceride), and
4. adjustments in the capacity to deliver O_2 to working muscle and in its capacity to take up O_2 from blood.

These are the kinds of adjustments that would appear to be theoretically possible, given what we have learned above about metabolic support for aerobic work. How do such theoretical expectations match up with fact? It turns out not as well as in our analysis of anaerobic training effects, since the first two possibilities actually appear not to be utilized.

HYPERTROPHY IS NOT SEEN IN AEROBIC TRAINING

One of the most striking differences between aerobic and anaerobic training is that two key characteristics of the latter (*hypertrophy* plus an increase in *strength*) are not evident in the former. In rodents, for example, training on motor-driven exercise treadmills for several weeks leads to large increases in endurance and in respiratory capacity, but no indication of muscle hypertrophy. Nor under such training regimes is there any increase in muscle strength (Holloszy and Booth, 1976). Thus this potentially useful adaptive response does not seem to be a part of the arsenal of training adaptations utilized by mammals.

WHITE FIBERS ARE NOT CONVERTED TO RED DURING AEROBIC TRAINING

Because between-species comparisons in teleosts, birds, and mammals consistently show a correlation between the proportion of red fibers in working muscles and aerobic performance preferences, it is surprising that again this obvious theoretical possibility is not typically utilized during aerobic training in mammals. On the contrary, some of the differences between red and white muscle fibers are accentuated (see below) in aerobic training, implying that there are advantages to retaining different fiber types. These advantages may arise from the way in which substrates are utilized (by working red and white muscles) and from enzymatic adjustments occurring in each.

AEROBIC TRAINING AND ENDOGENOUS SUBSTRATE SUPPLIES

Since the power output of muscle is highest when it utilizes either glycogen or glycogen plus fat in combination, it is instructive that endogenous depots of *both* these substrate sources are elevated following aerobic training regimes (Holloszy and Booth, 1976). This means the total amount of energy that can be extracted from endogenous sources is elevated by an exactly proportionate amount. Similarly, high levels of endogenous substrates in red muscles are observed in species well adapted for sustained aerobic performance.

AEROBIC TRAINING AND ENZYMES IN AEROBIC METABOLISM

As we emphasized above, the aerobic metabolic potential of muscle depends upon the integrated activities of several metabolic pathways (unlike the single pathway of glycolysis that is used in anaerobic work). So it is to be expected and is indeed observed (Holloszy and Booth, 1976) that increased respiratory capacity of muscle depends upon elevated activities of enzymes:

1. in the activation, transport, and oxidation of long-chain fatty acids,
2. in the oxidation of ketone bodies,
3. in the Krebs cycle,
4. in the mitochondrial electron transfer system,
5. in Krebs cycle augmentation pathways,
6. in hydrogen-shuttling pathways,
7. in the initiation of blood glucose metabolism, catalyzed by hexokinase, and
8. in the uptake of blood glucose, facilitated by glucose transporter (GLUT 1 and 4) isoforms.

Typically, these elevations occur in all three fiber types, but they are most pronounced in red muscle, least in white muscle. Whereas the total amount of power that a muscle can generate is determined by the substrate that is available to it (from endogenous or exogenous sources), the rate of energy generation of course depends upon the catalytic power of its catabolic machinery; the observed training effects on levels of key enzymes in aerobic metabolism and upon substrate supply therefore imply that both the total power output *and* its rate of generation are elevated during aerobic training. Again, similar adjustments are apparently genetically fixed in phylogenetic adaptations for sustained performance.

AEROBIC TRAINING AND MITOCHONDRIAL ABUNDANCE

The above changes in enzyme levels in training appear to result from an increase in enzyme protein concentration (rather than from other possible mechanisms such as altered catalytic efficiency). For those enzymes in aerobic metabolism that are mitochondrially located, ultrastructural studies of muscle in humans and rodents indicate elevations in *both size and number* of mitochondria, leading to an increase in total mitochondrial protein. In addition to making more of what is already present, adaptation at this level also leads to alterations in enzymatic composition and organization of mitochondria. An expression of such reorganization of the mitochondria is gained by comparing quantitatively the degree of training-induced change (Holloszy and Booth, 1976). Thus, some enzymes increase in activity a lot, some a little, while still others are essentially unchanged in activity, when expressed on a muscle weight basis. The signal transduction pathways and the activity-specific gene expression controls are gradually being unravelled (Leary and Moyes, 2000; Pette and Vrbova, 1999). Analogous but genetically fixed elevations in mitochondrial abundance are observed in between-species comparisons of animals varying greatly in endurance performance capacities (Hochachka, 1994).

AEROBIC TRAINING AND GLYCOLYTIC ENZYME LEVELS

Since essentially the same pathway may be utilized in both aerobic and anaerobic glycolysis, it is interesting to inquire into the effects of aerobic training on glycolytic enzyme levels in muscles (Baldwin et al., 1973). For one enzyme, hexokinase, the situation is quite clear; it displays an elevation in activity in all muscle fiber types following aerobic training. Levels nearly double in intermediate fibers, increase by about 1.5-fold in red muscles, and increase by about 30% in white muscle. The data on other glycolytic enzymes are less clear. Red muscles show a slight increase in levels of glycogen phosphorylase, pyruvate kinase, and lactate dehydrogenase, while in intermediate muscles these same enzymes decrease in activity by about 20%. Similarly, there are adjustments in the ratios of A_4 (muscle type) and B_4 (heart type) LDHs. In white muscle, there occurs a small (15%) decrease in lactate dehydrogenase activity following aerobic training.

In our view such modest changes in glycolytic potential are consistent with the idea that these enzyme levels are conserved largely for emergency (i.e., anaerobic) needs periodically imposed on the system. Since flux through anaerobic glycolysis is much higher than through aerobic glycolysis, enzyme levels must be tailored to the former, not the latter. As a result, under aerobic conditions, the catalytic potential of glycolytic enzymes should be well in excess of needs. The one exception to this, understandably enough, is hexokinase. During anaerobic conditions, the main carbon source being fermented is glycogen, but during sustained aerobic work, the importance of glucose rises as a function of duration of performance. In performance intense and long enough to fully deplete glycogen in working muscle in an hour, liver-derived glucose accounts initially for about 10% of the total energy being utilized but for about 20% by the end of the work bout. Since hexokinase acts as a control site in aerobic glycolysis, its elevation would facilitate such utilization of glucose, so it is not surprising that aerobic training leads to higher activity levels in muscle. Indeed, it would be more surprising if this did not occur.

EXERCISE TRAINING EFFECTS ON PDH

Pyruvate dehydrogenase (PDH), which catalyzes the conversion of pyruvate to acetylCoA for entry into the Krebs cycle, is positioned at a key interchange site between anaerobic and aerobic pathways of energy metabolism. Interestingly, it responds both to acute exercise as well as to exercise training. Following submaximal endurance training, the interplay between these pathways is altered so as to favor pyruvate flux into the PDH reaction, not into the LDH reaction; at least in part because of this mechanism, muscle in the post-training state displays less lactate production at the same workload. Interestingly, the active form (PDHa) of this enzyme complex is not different between conditions (Putman et al., 1998) but the steady-state %PDHa is lower after training, so that the response potential is higher (Nakai et al., 1999). Before training, glycolytic fluxes associated with high work rates exceed the PDH response capacities; possibly because of a higher phosphorylation potential, training thus improves the matching of glycolytic to PDHa fluxes, favoring lower muscle lactate production than found before training (Heigenhauser and Parolin, 1999).

AEROBIC TRAINING EFFECTS ON LIVER GLYCOGEN AND GLUCOSE

The increasing dependence of muscle metabolism upon liver-derived glucose during sustained performance emphasizes the importance of intertissue metabolic interactions during exercise. The increased glucose production from the liver (with increasing workload or work duration) is initially due primarily to activated liver glycogenolysis. At later stages, as liver glycogen becomes depleted, the continued release of glucose depends upon activated gluconeogenesis (mediated by insulin and glucagon). About two- to tenfold gluconeogenic activation can occur during exercise, but to our knowledge the effect of training on this process has not been ascertained. Although several precursors for de novo glucose formation in the liver under these conditions are utilized (including alanine, glycerol, pyruvate, and lactate), of these lactate is quantitatively by far the most important. This critical and provocative observation begs the question of the origin of such lactate, which again seems to remain unanswered by researchers in this field. Be that as it may, it is when this process becomes critical that fat becomes the main carbon and energy source for continued aerobic exercise. It is important to ask if the mobilization of fat is similarly influenced by aerobic training regimes.

AEROBIC TRAINING EFFECTS ON TRIGLYCERIDE METABOLISM

In both rodents and humans at least, several aspects of triglyceride metabolism are now known to be influenced by training. Capacities in muscles for fatty acid oxidation, for triglyceride formation by esterification of α-glycerophosphate, and for triglyceride deposition are all elevated following training (Holloszy and Booth, 1976). Interestingly, even the capacity to take up triglyceride from the blood is elevated. This capacity is represented biochemically by the membrane-bound enzyme lipoprotein lipase, which hydrolyzes triglyceride in chylomicrons in the blood. Lipoprotein lipase activity is increased threefold in intermediate muscle fibers, twofold in red and white fibers of rats following a long aerobic training program. A metabolically critical consequence of triglyceride and fatty acid uptake and metabolism by muscle following aerobic training is that it may cause a reduction in rates of glucose oxidation. This indeed is considered an important reason why trained animals deplete their liver glycogen reserves more slowly than untrained animals during extended, submaximal exercise. Although there are no direct measurements on rates of fatty acid release from adipose tissue to blood, the slight elevation in blood free fatty acids during extended exercise (when fatty acid oxidation rates are also elevated) is clearly consistent with increased flux from adipocytes to muscle.

AEROBIC TRAINING EFFECTS ON O_2 DELIVERY AND O_2 EXTRACTION

For completion of the discussion it is useful to remind the reader that the delivery of O_2 to working muscles, and the extraction of O_2 by working muscles, must be closely integrated with the metabolic adjustments described above. That indeed is the case, and it is of course well known that aerobic training induces an adaptive increase in the maximum cardiac output and thus in the total amount and total rate of O_2 delivered to muscle. Although in theory the delivery of O_2 to muscles could also be increased by preferential perfusion (i.e., redistribution of cardiac output), this mechanism does not appear to be utilized. So the question arises: Does the increase in cardiac output during aerobic exercise proceed in step with the overall increase in maximum O_2 uptake rates? The answer turns out to be negative.

Although there is a great deal of individual variation, on average the increase in maximum cardiac output appears to account for only about 50% of the rise in maximum O_2 uptake rates occurring in response to training (see Brooks et al., 1996). The other 50% or so of the increase is accounted for by improved extraction of O_2 by the working muscles, which is reflected in larger AV PO_2 differences and lower O_2 tensions in venous blood. How improved O_2 extraction is achieved, however, is a problem area in need of further research.

EVOLUTION-DRIVEN SCOPES FOR ACTIVITY

To this point in our discussion, we have focused mainly on two time courses over which the activities of metabolic pathways can be modulated: the acute and the acclimation (or training) responses. When we turn to the problem of how these response pathways are fine tuned through evolutionary time, good physiological

data sets do exist (Bishop, 1999) but good biochemical data sets are rare. Some of the best studies, interestingly enough, are to be found in the literature on fish muscle biochemistry and performance. In this area, biologists have long realized that fishes differ greatly in their locomotory patterns and capacities, ranging from the fast-start, burst-swim specialists, to species that can swim steadily but slowly for intermediate or long time periods, and finally to species that can swim steadily and rapidly for long time periods and long distances. Just as in the athletic spectrum considered above for mammalian and human athletes, adjustments can occur:

- in the phosphagen and CPK content of red muscle (RM) and white muscle (WM)
- in the glycolytic enzyme amounts in RM and WM
- in the mitochondrial volume densities and capillary densities in RM and WM
- in the contractile properties (muscle protein isoforms) in RM and WM
- in the EC coupling properties (Ca^{2+} ATPase, Ca^{2+} channel, and ryanodine channel isoforms)
- in the relative amount of RM versuss WM
- in the myoglobin (Mb) content of RM and WM
- in the blood volume as percentage of body mass
- in the red blood cell (RBC) mass
- in the hemoglobin concentration per RBC, and
- in the heart size as % of body mass.

Extensive studies carried out since the 1980s, make it clear that up- or down-regulation of the biochemical machinery of red and white muscle (i) goes hand in hand with coordinate physiological adjustments (affecting fuel and oxygen supply capacities) and (ii) can be so extensive that it exceeds the WM–RM distinctness normally expected. For example, mitochondrial enzyme concentrations per gram of WM in scombroids can be higher than the homologous enzyme levels in RM of some sluggish Amazon fishes. Or, in the RM of some Amazon fishes the concentrations of enzymes in anaerobic metabolism may be higher than in the WM of more hypoxia-sensitive fishes from more oxygen-rich, usually colder, waters. The up- or down-regulation of metabolic pathway capacities raises important questions about what is involved in such processes and about how they are regulated (Hochachka, 1980, 1994).

ENZYMES ARE PROPORTIONATELY UP- OR DOWN-REGULATED

The first problem that we must consider is that the catalytic and regulatory properties of enzymes in a given pathway are not the same. The pathway of glycolysis, for which there are good data available, is composed of some enzymes which are reversible and operate near equilibrium, while others are allosteric and still others are phorphorylation controlled, often essentially irreversible in vivo. Similarly, the turnover numbers of enzymes in the sequence vary substantially. Since enzymes with such different catalytic and regulatory properties are linked in sequence to form metabolic pathways, it is not surprising that the amount of enzyme required at any step for sustaining in vivo functions may be reaction specific—a problem already alluded to above. Probably the two key parameters determining how much enzyme is required at each step for matching in vivo pathway fluxes are (i) the catalytic efficiency or turnover number of the enzyme (μmol substrate converted to product per μmol enzyme per min) and (ii) the distance from equilibrium at which the enzyme operates in vivo (Suarez, 1992; Suarez et al., 1996). These two factors need not be related, but a generalization often found in the literature is that highest turnover numbers are found for equilibrium enzymes. For a given flux in vivo, enzymes with low turnover numbers functioning near equilibrium are at one extreme and by definition are required at relatively high concentrations; for convenience, we shall refer to enzymes within a pathway that occur at high concentrations for a variety of reasons as hE. At the other extreme, much lower concentrations of enzymes with high

turnover number functioning far from equilibrium are required to sustain a given in vivo flux; we shall refer to enzymes that occur at low concentration relative to hE as lE. If catalytic efficiency and distance from equilibrium were the only two factors determining the amount of enzyme required, then comparable enzyme concentration profiles for a pathway such as glycolysis would occur in all tissues examined. While similar patterns of hE and lE enzymes in glycolysis may be seen when comparing homologous tissues (Baldwin et al., 1973; Betts and Srivastava, 1991; Srivastava and Bernard, 1986), this is not always observed (Fersht, 1985), so other regulatory factors (such as the need for bidirectional or glycolytic vs glucogenic function) may be important as well. For example, along with a regulatory cascade of protein kinases and phosphatases, glycogen phosphorylase is well known to be "plated out" on glycogen granules and this structural feature may influence the required amount of enzyme. In any event, what we would expect and find is that component enzymes vary in a spectrum from lE to hE depending upon tissue specific metabolic conditions. Traditionally, metabolic biochemists refer to hE enzymes as "equilibrium enzymes," while lE enzymes are "regulatory enzymes," either allosteric or phosphorylation controlled. It is recognized that there is a gradation between these in terms of in-vivo concentration, distance from equilibrium for in-vivo function and quantitative contribution to control in varying metabolic states. So-called "equilibrium" enzymes, such as enolase (ENOL) for example, can sometimes operate quite far from equilibrium and display surprisingly high control coefficients.

With this background, a key question arises: during upwards or downwards scaling of the glycolytic capacity of a tissue, how are enzymes with such different properties scaled to match each other and the maximum flux capacity (J_{max}) of the pathway? A good way to examine the questions is to compare how these different kinds of enzymes are adjusted during large-scale upwards or downwards scaling of glycolysis in evolutionary time.

EVOLUTIONARY REGULATION OF GLYCOLYTIC PATH CAPACITY

The differentiation of WM and RM in fishes provides an interesting system for probing these issues. Qualitatively, the patterns of hE and lE enzymes in the glycolytic pathway are similar in both muscle types. Through evolution within specific lineages and through ontogeny within species like the tuna, the capacity of the glycolytic pathway in white muscle is drastically up-regulated compared to the pathway in red muscle (Guppy et al., 1979; Hochachka, 1980). To achieve this large-scale up-regulation, the enzymes for each individual step are changed to variable degree: hexokinase (HK) and phosphofructokinase (PFK) concentrations change the least, while triose phosphate isomerase (TPI) and lactate dehydrogenase

(LDH) concentrations increase the most. Phosphorylase, phosphoglucomutase, phosphoglucoisomerase, aldolase, phosphoglycerate kinase, enolase, and pyruvate kinase (PHOS, PGM, PGI, ALD, PGK, ENOL, and PK, respectively), in tuna WM are elevated by an intermediate amount and are expressed at about three- to five-fold higher levels than in RM (figure 2.21(A)). Analyses of low-capacity to high-capacity glycolytic pathways in different combinations (low-capacity RM → high-capacity RM; low-capacity RM → high-capacity WM; low-capacity WM → high-capacity WM) always show the same result: the largest relative changes are for hE type enzymes. Similar conclusions arise from comparisons of mammalian slow and fast muscles: the activities of PHOS, PFK, GPDH, PK, and LDH, in rat quadriceps (mainly fast-twitch) muscle exceed

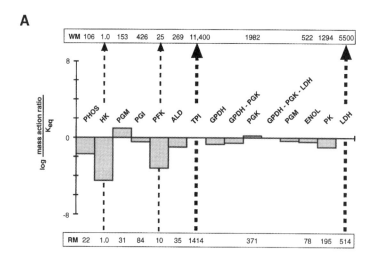

Figure 2.21(A). Summary diagram illustrating the distance from equilibrium (log of the observed mass action ratio/K_{eq}) for glycolytic enzymes in muscle during steady-state performance. These particular data were obtained from swimming rainbow trout (Dobson and Hochachka, 1987; Parkhouse et al., 1988), but the pattern is similar for the pathway in most muscles (Kashiwaya et al., 1994), and probably most tissues. Equilibrium enzymes operate relatively close to equilibrium (hence the nomenclature). Regulatory enzymes, such as PFK, operate far from equilibrium. Enzyme activities for the pathway in tuna red muscle (RM) and white muscle (WM) are given below and above, respectively. Enzyme activities (in μmol substrate converted per g tissue per min) are from Guppy et al. (1979) and Hochachka (1980). Within each pathway, equilibrium enzymes typically occur at high levels compared to regulatory enzymes, a feature that may be influenced by enzyme turnover numbers. Up-regulating glycolytic capacity from RM to WM levels shows that equilibrium enzymes are increased the most (TPI and LDH, shown with large arrows); regulatory enzymes are increased the least (HK and PFK, shown with smaller arrows). These patterns are seen for the glycolytic path in many other biological settings and are observed for other metabolic pathways. See text for further details. (Modified from Hochachka et al. (1998).

B

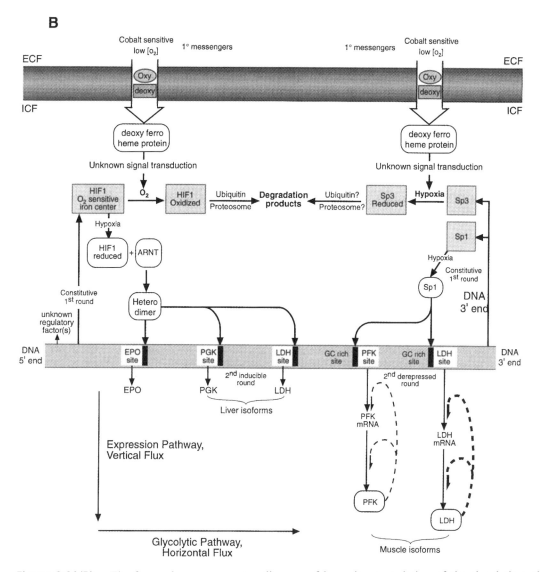

Figure 2.21(B). The figure shows a summary diagram of hypoxia upregulation of the glycolytic path in hypoxia responsive tissues. A poorly understood oxygen sensing and signal transduction pathway integrates the constitutive synthesis of two transcription factors, HIF1 and Sp3 (first round of gene function). These transcription factors are thought to coordinate hypoxic induction of the pathway by mechanisms discussed in detail in chapter 3. During hypoxic induction of the pathway, each enzyme seems to modulate its own expression pathway (shown as dotted feedback loops; dark arrows indicating large positive modulation for LDH muscle isoforms, lighter arrows indicating less potent activation for PFK). Control mechanisms could act on transcription, at translation through mRNA effects, or post-translationally (Bachurski et al, 1994; Beelman et al., 1996; Kollia et al., 1996; Williams and Neufer, 1996). Degree of induction (absolute amount of protein synthesis) appears greater for hE than for lE type enzymes. In terms of functional integration, vertical expression pathways are fine-tuned during hypoxic up-regulation to match the new horizontal pathway flux capacity. The differing response patterns of hE and lE enzymes apply to other—and possibly to all—metabolic pathways. See text for further details and references. The diagram is based on an analysis of hypoxia defense mechanisms (Hochachka et al., 1996) and on studies of hypoxia responsive genes discussed in chapter 3.

those in soleus (mainly slow-twitch) muscle by three- to six-fold. In this case, the RM versus WM relative differences between hE and lE type enzymes are not as striking as in fishes, probably in part because fiber types are mixed in mammalian muscles (Baldwin et al., 1973).

In these studies, and others discussed below, the parameters usually measured are enzyme catalytic activities per gram of tissue. However, the activities of isoforms of most of the WM and RM glycolytic enzymes overlap and the turnover number for each enzyme-catalyzed reaction step is similar in the two tissues. Since measured maximum activities per gram are linear functions of enzyme concentrations, fish RM versus WM enzyme activities per gram are probably reasonable reflections of enzyme concentration profiles. Actually the enzymes of glycolysis are so extensively studied that it is commonly assumed that their catalytic activities are a good reflection of enzyme concentration per se; exhaustive analyses of mammalian data, for example, shows that ratios of catalytic activities per gram of tissue are similar to ratios of molar concentrations of catalytic sites (Srivastava and Bernard, 1986). Because of the hE–lE structure of the glycolytic path in fish muscles, this means that up-regulating overall pathway capacity requires differential (enzyme-specific) amounts of synthesis: more absolute amounts of synthesis of hE than of lE type enzymes.

Since the turnover numbers for homologous (WM and RM) glycolytic enzymes are similar, at any given step another determinant of location on the hE–lE spectrum is the distance from equilibrium for in-vivo function. That is why we would expect, and indeed find, a general relationship between the degree of up-regulation of different enzymes and the degree of disequilibrium of in-vivo function. To illustrate the situation, the amounts of each enzyme in tuna RM and WM are compared on a plot of each enzyme's distance from equilibrium during steady-state muscle work (figure 2.21(A)). The degree of disequilibrium at each enzyme reaction is similar in fish muscles to that observed in the heart (Kashiwaya et al., 1994); however, even if this pattern may well be common to the glycolytic path in all tissues, fine details

vary in different tissues or in different metabolic states. Nevertheless, in the fish muscle example, enzymes such as TPI and LDH seem to function the closest to equilibrium and the activities of these are increased the most in the up-regulation of RM to WM glycolytic capacity. This is similar to the situation in mammalian muscles and explains why TPI, a quintessential equilibrium enzyme driven by evolution to catalytic perfection (i.e., a state where the turnover number is so high that maximum catalytic velocity is limited by diffusion-based enzyme–substrate interaction [Fersht, 1985]), nevertheless is required at higher concentrations (approaching the mM range) than any other enzyme in the glycolytic sequence. With in-vivo substrate and product mass action ratios almost at thermodynamic equilibrium, TPI at any lower concentrations would be unable to match required fluxes during activated glycolysis (Staples and Suarez, 1997; Suarez et al., 1997).

Regulatory enzymes, which under physiological conditions are considered to be largely irreversible, are seen to function far from equilibrium (figure 2.17(B)), as in the heart. The driving force for such enzymes when activated, for example, by allosteric positive modulators, is high and presumably for this reason, up-regulating glycolytic capacities from RM to WM levels requires modest increases in enzyme concentrations. Any remaining shortfall in catalytic capacity of such enzymes could be easily compensated for by positive modulators. (The similar HK levels in tuna RM and WM, despite much higher glycolytic capacity of the latter, probably reflect the observation that WM relies mostly on glycogen, not glucose, as fuel for the pathway.) Other enzymes, such as PHOS, PGM, PGI, ALD, GPDH, PGlM, ENOL, and PK, operate at intermediate distances from equilibrium, again as in the heart, and intermediate increases in enzyme concentrations occur in WM compared to RM.

Apparently what this means is that through evolutionary time the genetic program for glycolysis has been set so that for a high-capacity pathway hE type enzymes are up-regulated the most, while lE enzymes are increased the least. If this same situation applied to short-term regulation of the glycolytic path, it would require separate genetic controls for each enzyme in the pathway. The paradox is that in short-term adjustments (such as in hypoxic induction of the glycolytic path and in muscle electrical stimulation where repression of glycolytic enzymes is observed) the genes for the pathway of glycolysis are coordinately regulated as a single unit.

REGULATING THE GLYCOLYTIC PATH AS A UNIT

Initial insights into this problem come from studies showing that on exposure to hypoxia, cells in culture increase expression of enzymes in glycolysis, while simultaneously decreasing the expression of enzymes in aerobic metabolic pathways (Murphy et al., 1984; Robin et al., 1984). On average, all glycolytic enzyme expression in L8 myoblasts increased by about 2.4-fold in hypoxia; these are modest changes compared to the long-term evolutionary adjustments noted above. Subsequent studies (Webster and Murphy, 1987; Webster et al., 1990) showed that the reciprocal coordination (of genes for glycolytic versus oxidative enzymes) occurs at the transcription level, and more recently still (Ebert et al., 1996; Firth et al., 1995; Jiang et al., 1996; Semenza, 1999; Semenza et al., 1994; Wang and Semenza, 1995; Wang G. L. et al., 1995), molecular studies revealed that glycolytic up regulation during hypoxia is preceded by induction of a transcription factor (Hypoxia Inducible Factor 1 or HIF1). Hypoxia Inducible Factor 1, a basic helix–loop–helix (BHLH) heterodimeric inducer, along with Sp3, a transcription factor acting as a repressor (Webster et al., 2000) appear to be part of a universal oxygen-sensing and signal transduction system (figure 2.21(B)) involved in the hypoxia-dependent regulation of genes for proteins as different as EPO, VEGF1, GLUT1, and GLUT3, and glycolytic enzymes, including PFK L, ALD A, GPDH, ENOL1, PGK1, and LDH A. This control system will be further analyzed in our chapter on hypoxia tolerance. Suffice here to mention that it was the search for hypoxia-mediated regulation of

EPO expression that led to the discovery of additional roles for HIF1 in control of glycolytic expression (Bunn and Poyton, 1996). The picture of coordinated hypoxia control of the glycolytic path that is emerging is that of each gene having its own promoter and enhancer sequences, although not all the glycolytic genes have so far been analyzed (Webster et al., 2000).

An important and largely overlooked feature of these data is that conditions for induction of the pathway are different for hE versus lE type enzymes. As in the examples given above for skeletal muscle glycolysis, tissue culture L8 cells in normoxia express large amounts of some enzymes and small amounts of others. In hypoxia, the same percentage induction of an hE enzyme such as LDH and an allosteric lE enzyme such as PFK requires that quite differing amounts of absolute enzyme product be made in the two cases—a lot of the former, a little of the latter—a theme identical to the above comparisons of the glycolytic path in fish red and white muscles. Although this pattern has not been systematically explored, at least some control appears to lie at transcription. In Hela cells, for example, normoxic expression rates require a lot more mRNA for LDH than for PFK; furthermore, hypoxia induces a lot more mRNA for LDH than for PFK. A qualitatively similar picture emerges when we analyze the data for glycolytic enzyme activities (i) in transformed cells compared to quiescent cells or in cells stimulated by mitogenic agents to proliferate compared to quiescent cells (Darville et al., 1995), and (ii) in electrically stimulated muscles which typically sustain a large induction of enzymes in aerobic metabolic pathways, but a repression of glycolytic enzymes (Simoneau and Pette, 1998). Parenthetically, we might add that analogous differences between hE and lE enzymes are observed during induction or repression of enzymes in aerobic metabolism, although the genetic controls here are complicated by participation of nuclear and mitochondrial genes and hypoxic repression is not HIF1 mediated (see chapter 3 for further discussion of this area).

TRANSCRIPTION AND TRANSLATION RATES FOR hE AND lE STEPS IN METABOLIC PATHWAYS

Taken together, these data uncover two features in the genetic regulation of metabolic pathways like glycolysis. First of all, genes for glycolytic enzymes are coordinately expressed, even if they do not appear to be regulated as operons. Operons in eukaryotic systems have only recently been identified (Zorio et al., 1994) and do not seem to be widespread (Goodridge, 1987). Instead, coordinate control is achieved by connecting each gene to common inducing signals (such as hypoxia).

This feature of coordinate control perhaps is to be expected (Semenza, 1999). The second control feature of the pathway is not; namely, that the flux from each gene to each enzyme in the pathway seems to depend on the kind of enzyme being synthesized. High amounts of expression or high rates of expression, required for hE enzymes often operating close to equilibrium, are scaled down to lowered amount or rate of expression for lE enzymes usually operating further from equilibrium. To our knowledge, mechanisms are not yet known by which the different genes of the glycolytic sequence can be differentially activated (unique gene → product expression for each enzyme in the pathway). However, there are several control or amplification mechanisms possible at various stages between transcription and completion of protein synthesis. Thus, indications of differential mRNA synthesis for equilibrium versus regulatory enzymes, observed but not systematically researched, suggest at least some gene-specific control at transcription (Gallie et al., 1991). Recent studies also raise the possibility of control of mRNA stability and function ((Czyzyk-Kreska et al. (1994). A major pathway of mRNA degradation in yeast cells involves the shortening of the poly(A) tail which triggers a decapping reaction and so exposes mRNA to $5' \rightarrow 3'$ degradation; mRNA-specific rates of decapping and decay could result from differences in interactions between the decapping enzyme and gene-specific transcripts (Beelman et al., 1996). Finally, it is possible that during hypoxic induction flux rates from genes to enzymes for all steps in glycolysis are the same, and that differing amounts of products are maintained by differential proteolysis. However, this would be wasteful of carbon and energy (a kind of futile cycle or energy short circuit) and would still confront the same specificity problem as above (knowing which enzymes to degrade and at what rate). Besides, despite a large data base on protein synthesis and proteolysis, none suggests that degradation rates vary with the hE versus lE nature of the enzyme target (Argiles et al., 1996; Hochstrasser, 1996; Nair and Schwenk, 1994).

The problem with the above kinds of control concepts is that they beg the question: How does each gene "know" the functional (hE or lE) state of the enzyme it specifies? In other words, how does it "know" how much enzyme product to make? Analagous control problems in other areas of cell function are often solved by negative feedback modulation by the product of the pathway; in our case, this would require feedback by the protein being expressed. A good example of just such a negative feedback control involves α-tubulin autoregulation of its own synthesis rate by means of an unique amino-terminal tetrapeptide mediating transcript specific-mRNA decay (Bachurski et al., 1994). The α-tubulin isoform also modulates its own synthesis rate through mRNA stability, but the decay pathway for this mRNA is not currently understood. Similarly, one class of cold shock proteins involved in protecting against cold-induced unfolding of particularly sensitive enzymes or other polypeptides, interact with their mRNAs in such a way as to automatically self-regulate their own synthesis (see chapter 7).

In summary, then, we are left with an interesting situation (figure 2.21(B)): either (i) we assume a feedback loop from enzyme product synthesized to the gene or mRNA being activated, a unique feedback loop for each gene in the glycolytic sequence (this would explain why enzyme levels are reflected in mRNA levels for hE versus lE enzymes), or (ii) we assume that each gene → enzyme pathway is genetically programmed and uniquely primed for unique amounts or rates of transcription, translation, and protein assembly. While both may be intellectually appealing, available studies do not allow clear resolution of the issue at this time.

FINE TUNING hE AND lE REQUIRES GENE → ENZYME → GENE INFORMATION FLOW

The discussion so far leads to the conclusion that an interesting information flow circuit is required: genes → enzymes → genes. The first arm of this has been generally understood for decades; a special version is the well-known induction of energy-yielding pathways by increase in energy demand of working muscles—the training effect noted above (Simoneau et al., 1990; Viru, 1994; Williams and Neufer, 1996). However, the second arm of the circuit (enzymes → genes), to this point has been under-emphasized and it differs from the kinds of concepts that are pervasive in studies of muscle training and use–disuse transitions. In muscle, this control loop (i.e., feedback from metabolism to genes) is an important mechanism underlying tissue plasticity; it is traditionally considered to be initiated by altered activity or energy demand (use, disuse, denervation, or electrical stimulation) but to be mediated (i) by low-molecular-weight metabolites (such as creatine, spermidine, or spermine), or (ii) by hormones (Viru, 1994; Williams and Neufer, 1996). The possibility of a direct enzyme → gene control loop so far remains unexamined in muscle, but such regulation is known in other systems. In proline metabolism in bacteria, for example, one protein has two activities: proline dehydrogenase and pyrroline-5-carboxylate dehydrogenase that together catalyze oxidation of proline to glutamate. When exogenous proline is available, this complex enzyme is attached to the cell membrane and plays its normal metabolic function. In the absence of proline, it detaches, binds to DNA, and represses expression of both proline dehydrogenase and a proline transport protein, the switch from membrane-bound enzyme to DNA-binding transcription factor being mediated by a change in the redox state of the enzyme (Brown and Wood, 1993; Muro-

Pastor and Maloy, 1995). Some glycolytic enzymes such as PGK have specific DNA binding sites (Bryant et al., 1997) and this also raises the possibility for direct enzyme → gene control circuitry.

Whatever the mechanism, this feedback, an acknowledged basis of muscle plasticity, shares certain features with muscle differentiation. Current studies indicate that muscle differentiation depends upon four myogenic BHLH transcription factors (termed MyoD, myogenin, myf5, and MRF4 in the literature), whose function is potentiated by myocyte enhancer factors, especially MEF2 (Molkentin et al., 1995). The genes for these BHLH transcription factors are referred to as "master genes" because they in turn regulate batteries of genes further downstream. Interestingly, fiber type specific plasticity also is regulated by BHLH proteins; disuse atrophy, for example, induces MRF4 but not myogenin in slow muscles, whereas myogenin but not MRF4 transcripts rise dramatically in fast-twitch muscle (Loughna and Brownson, 1996). It may be that similar controls also could contribute to the differential up- or down-regulation of specific enzymes in metabolic pathways such as glycolysis, but thus far this has not been evaluated.

For molecular physiologists, the significance of the enzyme → gene feedback loop is especially significant for it may mean that the integration of linked enzyme sequences is occurring simultaneously in two directions (figure 2.21(B)): horizontally (flux through the linked enzyme reactions of the glycolytic path) and vertically (amount or rate of transcription and translation, and thus information flow from genes to enzymes). The former can be a very-high-flux system (moment to moment response time); the latter of course is a much lower flux system (response time of hours to days) and its functional capacity appears to vary with cellular energy demand. That is why biological processes such as exercise training, electrical stimulation of muscle, or hypoxia exposure typically alter the expression rates of genes for enzymes in glycolysis or in oxidative metabolic pathways. Even if gene → enzyme pathways are low flux and each may be a relatively minor energy drain, when all are combined their cost becomes significant for under normoxic conditions protein synthesis contributes about one-third of the maintenance energy demands of the resting cell. If the cost of ATP-dependent proteolysis is included, the overall cost of the control circuit (genes → proteins → genes) accounts for approximately 50% of normoxic ATP turnover rates (see Hochachka et al., 1996a and figure 2.4 above).

For evolutionary physiologists, the fundamental insight is that the above conditions apply "across the board" in the evolution of metabolic scope for activity in any particular phylogeny. That is, the stringent integration (i) of gene expression amounts or rates for hE and lE reaction steps in specific pathways with (ii) flux capacities through the linked enzyme reactions forming those same metabolic pathways sets conditions that apply during long-term phylogenetic up or down adjustments of pathways such as glycolysis or the Krebs-cycle-involved in energy generation. Although it is this coadaptation which determines the metabolic scopes for different kinds of locomotory activities in fishes as well as other organisms, the coadaptation of expression pathway capacities with metabolic pathway properties must ultimately also be integrated with the organism-level physiology. Exactly such coadaptations are the focus of an exhaustive series of studies by the Taylor–Weibel group, in which evidence is generated and evaluated for integration of all steps in the path of oxygen from air to mitochondria and even for integrating these processes with fuel selection during exercise (Taylor et al., 1981, 1987, 1996; Weibel, 2000; Weibel et al., 1991, 1996).

At molecular physiology levels, a striking example of how evolutionary adjustments in WM and RM biochemical composition are integrated with performance capacities is found in the tunas, a group of pelagic fishes that is of commercial importance and thus has been particularly well studied. All members of this group are thought to have much (two- to ten-fold) higher metabolic scopes for activity than is common among other fishes and pretty well all of the biochemical fine-tuning or train-

ing options mentioned above have been utilized in improving performance capacities in tunas.

ANAEROBIC METABOLIC SCOPES IN HIGH-PERFORMANCE TUNAS

For burst swimming, the simplest strategy is to build up WM mass as a percentage of body mass, which at once increases total phosphagen and glycolysis-based anaerobic potential. This simplest strategy is used by scombrids generally (WM mass is about 55–60% of body mass) and is not unique to tunas. In tunas, the concentrations of glycolytic enzymes, of glycogen, and of dipeptide buffers also are increased relative to other fishes (including other scombrids), which is a back-up strategy for up-regulating anaerobic burst-swimming potential. A third fundamental WM adaptation in tunas involves the up-regulation of mitochondrial volume densities and of enzymes associated with aerobic metabolic pathways. And finally, a fourth adaptation, influencing the output of all three above processes, is regional endothermy (discussed in more detail below) which allows both RM, and to a lesser degree WM, to operate at some 5–15°C above ambient. These adaptations go a long way towards explaining why tuna are able to accumulate the highest muscle-work-induced lactate concentrations so far found among all vertebrates—up to and exceeding 100 mM concentrations! Whereas at first sight the unexpectedly high aerobic metabolic potential may appear paradoxical, studies indicate that this metabolic potential, especially when coupled with endothermy, is particularly useful for speeding up recovery processes following high-intensity short-term anaerobic work. For example, clearance of lactate following burst swimming in most fishes (salmonids supply a large data base) usually requires 8–12 hours, and even longer in extreme cases, while in tunas the clearance of even higher lactate loads requires only a matter of an hour or so. In fact, tunas express lactate clearance rates close to, or equal to, rates observed in mammals. In fish WM the fate in recovery of the work-induced lactate pool is largely reconversion to glycogen in situ. As noted above, the recovery of PCr following fatigue in tuna WM is linked to the clearance of H$^+$ accompanying the clearance of lactate—a process shifting the CPK equilibrium towards PCr (Arthur et al., 1992b).

AEROBIC METABOLIC SCOPES IN HIGH-PERFORMANCE TUNAS

Biologists have long realized the biomechanical advantages of the tunniform body design for efficient and sustained swimming performance. To match the biomechanics with appropriate biochemistry and physiology, tunas could in principle rely upon four strategies:

(i) they could increase the amount of RM,
(ii) they could increase the rate at which oxygen can be delivered to the working RM (by coadaptation of heart, blood volume, RBC mass, and [Hb] per RBC),
(iii) they could increase the ATP turnover capacities (i.e., the capacities of RM ATP demand and RM ATP supply pathways) by increasing mitochondrial content and/or myofibrillar composition or efficiency, and
(iv) they could increase the potential output of all of the above globally by increasing RM temperature.

When compared to fishes in general, all of the above are in fact utilized. However, when compared only to other members of the lineage, the striking insight (see review by Graham and Dickson, 2000) is that strategies (i), (ii), and (iii) above seem to have been pushed close to some upper limit in scombroids as a group so that within the lineage *tuna RM is remarkable in being unremarkable*: its mitochondrial volume densities, its sarcoplasmic reticulum (SR) form and abundance, its Krebs cycle enzyme content, and its Mb content all are pretty well in the same range as found in scombrid relatives. The microcirculation does show capillary manifolds helping to serve RM cells that are smaller (lower diameter) than in many other fishes, but in terms of numbers of capillaries per muscle fiber, again tuna RM is not remarkably different from RM in other scombroids. Whereas smaller tuna such as the skipjack show strikingly (more than twofold) higher amounts of RM as a percentage of body mass than do related scombroids, larger tunas such as albacore show no unusual amounts of RM (possibly because of the very large body mass of adults and the associated lower mass specific metabolic rates required).

The impressive aerobic metabolic swimming capacities of tunas could in part also be explained by purely physiological adjustments. Several coupled systems allowing for high O_2 delivery—large hearts and consequently large cardiac outputs during exercise, large blood volume, large RBC mass, and high content of Hb in RBCs—all add up to high oxygen delivery to RM during sustained exercise. Heart mass and RM mass show a 1:1 linear relationship and these parameters also correlate with liver gluconeogenic capacities and fuel supply capabilities. All of these kinds of factors are up-regulated in tunas when compared to fishes in general but when compared to scombrid fishes even these factors by themselves appear to be inadequate to account for the observed higher performance of the tunas. In fact, the conclusion emerging from analyses of this problem (Graham and Dickson, 2000) is that in the scombroids as a group the coadaptations of the biochemical machinery of RM and heart and the associated oxygen and fuel delivery systems have been honed close to an upper limit or threshold beyond which it was not possible to readily evolve. Within the lineage as a whole, these physiological, metabolic, and molecular characters therefore can be described as relatively conservative: or, put another way, in the evolution of the tunas within this lineage there was dreadfully little room left for further up-regulating these performance components. The way tunas were able to circumvent these upper limits—by developing the capacity for regional endothermy—is, among teleosts, unusual to say the least.

ENDOTHERMY: A KEY PHYSIOLOGICAL CHARACTER IN THE TUNAS

The final key to understanding the high-performance nature of tunas is endothermy: this is because all the basic RM biochemical machinery and the physiological systems designed to support it with O_2 and fuel delivery, in tunas can operate at higher temperature than in scombrid relatives. Thus one simple mechanism (elevated temperature) can step up the output of all of the above systems at once. This is perhaps their most fundamental evolutionary invention and their greatest single advantage over their pelagic cousins.

EVOLUTIONARY PATH OF ENDOTHERMY IN TUNAS PARALLELS ENHANCED SCOPE FOR ACTIVITY

Endothermy in tunas is based on a simple physiological principle: the insertion of a heat exchanger (a parallel system of arterioles and venules termed a *rete mirable*) somewhere between muscle and gills. Interestingly, this kind of physiology evolved independently at least three times in the Scombridae (figure 2.22(A)): in the billfishes a brain heater organ evolved independently in each of the major lineages (Xiphidae and Istiphoridae) while the tunas evolved a red-muscle-based thermal physiology. The mechanism and biological advantages of brain heaters are discussed elsewhere (Block, 1995; also, see chapter 7). Our main interest here is the muscle heat exchanger. The exact anatomical position of the *rete mirable* varies: it is centrally located in *Allothunnus, Auxis, Euthynus,* and *Katsuwonus*; in these groups essentially all of the blood flow to red and white muscles arrives from arterioles branching off from the dorsal aorta (DA). The venous return is passed through venules in the central rete and during this passage, venous blood heat derived from RM metabolism is transferred to incoming arterial blood, which is thermally equilibrated at the gill to sea water temperatures. This central countercurrent heat exchanger supplies these species with a mechanism for storing heat internally and

maintaining a higher internal (especially RM) temperature than the outside seawater.

A similar principle, but a different anatomical structure, is used to warm up the body in fishes of the genus *Thunnus*. Here, in all extant species of the genus *Thunnus*, essentially all blood flowing to working muscles (especially RM) arrives via two large lateral arteries. Arterioles branch off the lateral arteries and enter the muscle through a lateral rete or lateral countercurrent heat exchanger; blood warmed by RM metabolism returns via the venules in the heat exchanger, so again allowing for an efficient transfer of heat to the incoming colder blood (thermally equilibrated at the gills). Correlated with the appearance of a well-developed countercurrent heat exchanger is the differentiation of a large amount of RM mostly or fully internalized, in contrast to the primitive lateral and superficial localization of RM in most teleosts. The more internalized the RM presumably the more effective the endothermic mechanism, a process that reaches its zenith in the bluefin family.

TRANSITION FROM A CENTRAL TO A LATERAL HEAT EXCHANGER

Examination of current phylogenies of the scombroids (figure 2.22(B)) identifies several key steps (biological innovations) in the evolutionary pathways of these two kinds of endothermic systems in the tunas. First is the occurrence of a primitive central heat exchanger: with the identification of a complex vascular plexus in the hemal arch of *Allothunnus*, the most parsimonious explanation of the occurrence of circulatory systems modified into central countercurrent heat exchangers is that the feature is ancestral. Such a one-point-of-origin is shown in figure 2.22(B). The second major step is the relocalization or "movement" of the RM mass from a lateral superficial position to an axial, internalized one (especially well developed in the anterior part of the body). This reorganization and internalization of the RM in overall body design of tunas coincided with the appearance of a third major innovation—a lateral circulatory supply—and led to

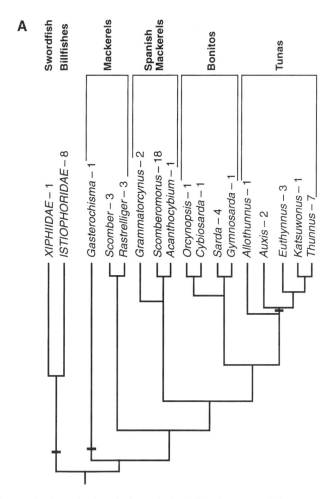

Figure 2.22(A). Phylogenetic hypothesis of the relationships between different groups of scombroid fishes. Endothermic systems evolved three times separately within the scombroids (shown as thick bars): heater organs evolved twice in the billfishes (Xiphiidae and Istiophoridae), while red-muscle-based thermogenic systems evolved in the tunas.

the co-evolution of the lateral heat exchanger. This innovation in the phylogeny of the tunas is shown in figure 2.22(B) as the point where red muscle endothermy is confirmed (at the time of writing, it is not known whether or not *Allothunnus* is capable of some degree of endothermy).

Biologists believe that the main subsequent evolutionary processes (i) incorporated a heat conduction path from RM to the brain (the presumed function of frontoparietal fenestrae in the back of the skull) and a carotid rete or heat exchanger for recycling heat and maintaining a warm brain and retinas; (ii) continued the expansion of the lateral heat exchanger (by establishing hypaxial as well as epaxial lateral circulation); (iii) included the gradual diminution, and, in the advanced *Thunnus*, the complete loss of the central rete; (iv) favored the appearance of visceral retes (a major innovation critical to speeding up kidney, liver, and digestive functions), and (v) favored the complete loss of the postcardinal vein in the most advanced *Thunnus* (not needed once the bulk of the blood supply to and from the RM mass occurred via the lateral circulation and lateral heat exchanger).

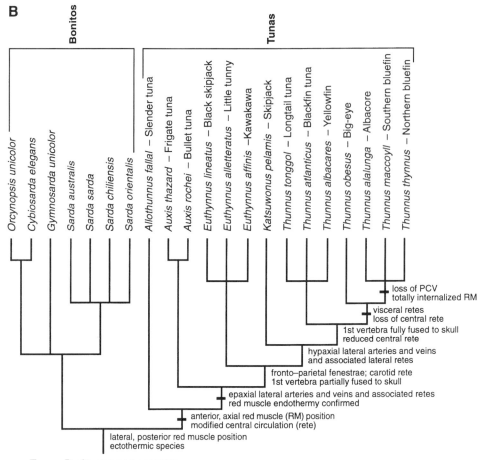

Figure 2.22(B). A phylogeny for all species of the bonito + tuna clade proposed by Graham and Dickson (2000) and based upon both morphological and gene sequence data. Mapped onto this phylogeny are the character states associated with evolution of endothermy and evolution of expanded scope for activity. (Modified from Block, 1995, and Graham and Dickson, 2000.)

RETES EVOLVED SEPARATELY MORE THAN ONCE

Because the differentiation of a countercurrent heat exchanger involves very specific, highly localized, and tightly regulated angiogenesis and tissue differentiation, we consider it most probable that the evolution of each of the above rete systems—the central rete for recycling heat to RM, the carotid rete for recycling heat to the brain, the lateral rete for recycling heat to RM, and the visceral retes for recycling heat to the liver and other viscera—occurred separately and independently. Even the loss of the central rete in the *Thunnus* probably represents a novel evolutionary origin. These key steps in the evolution of tuna endothermy are highlighted on the phylogenetic tree in figure 2.22(B). As far as we know at this time, the last remaining step in this ongoing evolutionary progression was the complete loss of the postcardinal vein (PCV)—a highly precise, highly regulated angiogenesis restricted to the most "advanced" cold water tunas. And finally, the complete internalization of the RM in the temperate zone bluefin tunas, but not the tropical tunas, suggests that this component of endothermy and of metabolic scope may well have arisen more than once in the *Thunnus* lineage as well. Otherwise it is hard to understand why this character is not expressed in the tropical tunas. This model also helps to explain the subtle but real differences in the counter current heat exchanger microcirculatory structures that are observed when comparing Atlantic bluefin and Pacific bluefin tuna, two species that were once thought to be more closely related than modern molecular data indicate (Graham and Dickson, 2000).

The independent evolution of the same solution to a given environmental problem is termed convergent evolution, and within the scombroids this apparently also occurred during the evolution of the brain heater. Recent studies have led Barbara Block and her students to postulate that brain heaters have evolved independently at least three times within the billfish and tuna lineages (figure 2.22(A))—a phenomenon that suggests a significant (and possibly very high) selective advantage to having warm brains and warm bodies in this group of fishes (see chapter 7 for more on this topic).

SUMMARY OF KEY STEPS IN EVOLVING TUNA ENDOTHERMY

Because of the complexity of this system, it may be useful to briefly summarize the key steps thought to be involved in the evolution of endothermy in the tunas:

1. Origin of a primitive central rete in the hemal arch; anterior, axial, internalized relocalization of the RM mass.
2. Some development of lateral arteries and veins, and carotid retes; the development of efficient RM endothermy.
3. Complete (epaxial and hypaxial) lateral retes.
4. A reduced central rete, then a complete loss of central rete; appearance of visceral rete.
5. Complete loss of PCV and complete internalization of RM in cold-water tunas.

The interesting implication is that many of the preconditions for a high metabolic scope were already in place at the phylogenetic origin of the tunas: the proper anatomy (a body form designed for hydrodynamically efficient swimming); the proper physiology (a large amount of RM well supplied with capillaries and capillary manifolds plus an expanded blood volume, RBC mass, Hb O_2 carrying capacity, heart, and cardiac output capacity); and the proper biochemistry (the right kinds of contractile machinery, well supplied with high mitochondrial densities and ample concentrations of enzymes of oxidative metabolism). These key ancestral evolutionary systems within the scombroid lineage were close to an upper threshold and there was little room left for further evolutionary "improvements" here.

The major evolutionary innovation within the tuna lineage was the appearance, first, of central–and then later of—lateral countercurrent heat exchangers coupled with fully internalized RM and additional vascular adjustments (carotid and visceral retes and loss of PCV). With one complex but global mechanism—that allowing for higher operating temperatures—this lineage was thus able to increase the potential output of all of the above biomechanical, physiological, and biochemical components of swimming performance. With one mechanism, we go a long way toward accounting for the higher metabolic scopes for sustained activity that are found elsewhere in this lineage. That is why the evolution of these thermogenic mechanisms (figure 2.22) within the scombroids in essence conveniently describes the evolution of metabolic scope for sustained activity within this group.

CONCLUSIONS EMERGING FROM STUDIES OF SCOMBROID SCOPES

For mechanistic physiologists, two key conclusions arise from these studies of scombroid evolutionary physiology. Firstly, the biomechanical (i.e., anatomical), physiological, and biochemical characters contributing to defining performance capacities were coordinately adjusted toward an upper threshold during the expansion of swimming capacities in scombroids as a group. This means that at the origin, or very soon after the origin, of the scombroid lineage, there already was little room for further improvement of performance by further evolutionary fine tuning any of these kinds of characters. Secondly, that was why a different solution—regional endothermy—had to be found if scombroid lineages like the tunas were going to be able to sustain any further up-regulation of swimming capacity. The ability to maintain a significant part of the physiology and biochemistry of swimming performance at 5–15°C above ambient temperature supplied tunas with a mechanism for increasing the output of all the above performance-linked biochemical and physiological characters. This in turn allowed tunas to override a performance capacity "threshold" or "ceiling'" constraining the evolution of related lineages unable to "fire up" a biological furnace.

For evolutionary physiologists, the take-home messages are different but equally interesting. Firstly, it appears that some characters that are required for the high metabolic scopes of the tunas are conservative and probably ancestral; they appear to be shared with other scombrid lineages. Included in this category are many of the biomechanical (i.e., anatomical) characters for thunniform swimming efficiency, many of the physiological features (high cardiac output and fuel + oxygen delivery systems), and many of the biochemical properties of RM (mitochondrial volume densities, Mb content, capillarity, and even overall RM mass). Whereas these characters are clearly up-regulated when compared to teleosts as a whole, they are not so unusual in tunas compared to other scombrid fishes. This indicates that up-regulation of metabolic scope through these characters has been taken about as far as it can be in the scombrid lineage.

Secondly, it appears that another set of characters that are required for the high metabolic scopes of the tunas are highly adaptable, in the sense that they change during phylogeny and correlate with change in metabolic scope. Included in this category of more adaptable physiological characters are all the components of endothermy: the vascular counter current heat exchangers for warming RM and brain, the internalized red muscle, and the visceral retes for warming the gut and liver. These physiological characters in sum allow the expression of regional endothermy. By allowing higher temperature function, regional endothermy represents an all-pervasive and adaptable means for stepping up the metabolic scope of tunas above and beyond the impressive range already achieved by related (cold-blooded) scombrid cousins.

EXPANDING METABOLIC SCOPE FOR SURVIVAL

In the above example, scope for activity is expanded with one global mechanism (regional hyperthermia); in some animals, under particular stress conditions, there is a need to down-regulate metabolism well below the SMR, and interestingly, regional or whole body hypothermia (i.e., the reverse of the above regional hyperthermia) is the strategy of choice. Extreme examples of this strategy are to found among lineages capable of torpor or hibernation (e.g., overwintering submergence in turtles and overwintering hibernation in mammalian hibernators). In the case of mammalian hibernators, the hypothermia can be so complete and so severe as to represent seasonal energy savings equivalent to nearly 90% of the energy that would otherwise be expended. In overwintering submergence of aquatic turtles, O_2-limitation leads to a powerful hypometabolism, but then the same mechanism (hypothermia) is used to further suppress metabolic processes down to as low as 1% of normothermic basal metabolic rates (see chapter 3).

In still other situations, for example, in deep-diving mammals and birds (see chapter 4), the hypothermia is distinctly regional. In diving animals such as the pinnipeds, the usual hypometabolic mechanisms available for extending submergence time (such as bradycardia, tissue hypoperfusion, reduced O_2 delivery, and thus reduced aerobic metabolic rates) are conservative and seemingly developed about as far as possible. That is why when comparing different species within the pinniped lineage, physiological characters such as bradycardia (with its associated vasoconstriction and hypometabolism of hypoperfused tissues) are *most remarkable by being unremarkable*: they are pretty well the same in all pinnipeds (Mottishaw et al., 1999; Hochachka, 2000). As in the tuna example considered above, where there seems little room left for further up-regulation of performance capacities, in this case there seems to be little room left for further down-regulation of metabolic and physiological processes. To dip down below this threshold (for purposes of extending submergence time), these so-called homeothermic and endothermic organisms activate mechanisms for tissue-specific cooling. In some diving birds, the hypothermia, while regional, can be strikingly large: approaching 10°C, this gains the advantage of a similarly large cold-induced decline in O_2 demand (and hence expansion in submergence time). In seals, the cooling is only a few degrees, but this is nevertheless high enough to lead to a significant (in the 50% range) energetic saving. It is probable that the hypothermic capabilities of pinnipeds correlate with diving duration, like other physiological characters that are adaptable and help to extend diving capacities within this group (Mottishaw et al., 1999).

SUMMARY: EXPANDING SCOPES FOR ACTIVITY OR FOR SURVIVAL

The above analyses are notable and instructive; they indicate that when evolutionary pressures driving biochemical and physiological processes reach some inherent limit, organisms are then required to turn to novel mechanisms (e.g., utilizing global physical parameters such as operating cell temperatures), if they are to achieve either further upward or further downward expansion of metabolic scope. The evolution of high aerobic metabolic scopes so beautifully illustrated in the tunas can be viewed in terms of the assembly of conservative, probably ancestral, characters with more adaptable physiological components (biological innovations including features such as regional tissue-specific endothermy). How these two categories of characters are assembled in any given tuna line-

age specifies the metabolic scope of that lineage. Moving in the other direction, the evolution of expanded hypometabolic capacities, in diving animals such as aquatic turtles (ectothermic example) or pinnipeds (endothermic example) can similarly be viewed in terms of the assembly of conservative, probably ancestral, characters (such as bradycardia and peripheral hypoperfusion with associated metabolic consequences) with more adaptable physiological components (biological innovations such as regional tissue-specific hypothermia). How these two categories of characters are assembled in any given lineage specifies the degree of hypometabolism that is possible and thus the maximum submergence time. Such interplay between conservation and adaptation is a theme that, as we shall see, is repeated over and over again in the evolution of complex physiological systems.

REFERENCES

Abe H., G.P. Dobson, U. Hoeger, and W.S. Parkhouse (1985). Role of histidine-related compounds to intracellular buffering in fish skeletal muscle. *Am. J. Physiol.* 249: R449–R454.

Allen, P.S., G.O. Matheson, G. Zhu, D. Gheorgiu, R.S. Dunlop, T. Falconer, C. Stanley, and P.W. Hochachka (1997). Simultaneous ^{31}P magnetic resource spectroscopy of the soleus and gastrocnemius in sherpas during graded calf muscle exercise and recovery. *Am. J. Physiol.* 273: R999–R1007.

Argiles, J.M., and F.J.Lopez-Soriano (1996). The ubiquitin-dependent proteolytic pathway in skeletal muscle: its role in pathological states. *Trends Pharm. Sci.* 17: 223–226.

Arthur, P.G., M.C. Hogan, P.D. Wagner, and P.W. Hochachka (1992a). Modelling the effects of hypoxia on ATP turnover in exercising muscle. *J. Appl. Physiol.* 73: 737–760.

Arthur, P.G., T.G. West, R.W.Brill, P.M. Schulte, and P.W. Hochachka (1992b). Recovery metabolism in tuna white muscle: rapid and parallel changes of lactate and phosphocreatine after exercise. *Can. J. Zool.* 70: 1230–1239.

Atkinson, D.E. (1977). *Cellular Energy Metabolism and its Regulation.* New York: Academic Press.

Atkinson, D.E. (1990). *Control of Metabolic Processes.* pp. 11–27, ed. A. Cornish-Bowden and M.L. Cardenas. New York: Plenum Press.

Bachurski, C.J., N.G. Theodorakis, R.M.R. Coulson, and D.W.Cleveland (1994). An amino-terminal tetrapeptide specifies cotranslational degradation of b-tubulin but not a-tubulin mRNAs. *Mol. Cellular Biol.* 14: 4076–4086.

Balaban, R.S. (1990). Regulation of oxidative phosphorylation in the mammalian cell. *Am. J. Physiol.* 258: C377-C389.

Baldwin, K.M., W.W. Winder, R.L. Terjung, and J.O. Holloszy (1973). Glycolytic enzymes in different types of skeletal muscle: adaptation to exercise. *Am. J. Physiol.* 225: 962–966.

Bastard J.P., C. Jardel, M.Guerre-Millo, and B.Hainque (1998). Hexose transporters in humans: their role in insulin sensitivity of peripheral tissues. *Revue de Medecine Interne.* 19: 108–118.

Beelman, C.A., A. Stevens, G. Caponigro, T.E. LaGrandeur, L. Hatfield, D.W. Fortner, and R. Parker (1996). An essential component of the decapping enzyme required for normal rates of mRNA turnover. *Nature* 382: 642–646.

Betts, D.F., and D.K. Srivastava (1991). The rationalization of high enzyme concentrations in metabolic pathways such as glycolysis. *J. Theor. Biol.* 151, 155–167.

Bishop, C.M. (1999). The maximum oxygen consumption and aerobic scope of birds and mammals: getting to the heart of the matter. *Proc. Roy. Soc. Lond. Ser.* B 266: 2275–2281.

Block, B.A. (1995). Endothermy in fish: thermogenesis, ecology and evolution. In: *Biochemistry and Molecular Biology of Fishes.* Vol. 1, pp. 269–311, ed. P.W. Hochachka and T.P. Mommsen. New York: Elsevier Press.

Blum, H., J.A. Balschi, and R.G. Johnson, Jr. (1991). Coupled in vivo activity of the membrane band Na^+K^+ ATPase in resting and stimulated electric organ of the electric fish Narcine brasiliensis. *J. Biol. Chem.* 266: 10254–10259.

Blum, H., S. Nioka, and R.G. Johnson, Jr. (1990). Activation of the Na^+K^+ ATPase in Narcine brasiliensis. *Proc. Natl. Acad. Sci. USA* 87: 1247–1251.

Brand, M.D. (1995). Control analysis of energy metabolism in mitochondria. *Biochem. Soc. Trans.* 23: 371–376.

Brand, M.D. (1997). Regulation analysis of energy metabolism. *J. Exp. Biol.* 200: 193–202.

Brookes, P.S., J.A. Buckingham, A.M. Tenreiro, A.J. Hulbert, and M.D. Brand (1998). The proton permeability of the inner membrane of liver mitochondria from ectothermic and endothermic vertebrates and from obese rats: correlations with standard metabolic rate and phospholipid fatty acid composition. *Comp. Biochem. Physiol.* B 119: 325–334.

Brooks, G.A (1998). Mammalian fuel utilization during sustained exercise. *Comp. Biochem. Physiol B* 120: 89–107.

Brooks, G.A., M.A. Brown, C.E. Butz, J.P. Sicurello, and H. Dubouchaud (1999a). Cardiac and skeletal muscle mitochondria have a monocarboxylate transporter MCT1. *J Appl. Physiol.* 87: 1713–718.

Brooks, G.A., H. Dubouchaud, M. Brown, J.P. Sicurello, and C.E Butz (1999b). Role of mitochondrial lactate dehydrogenase and lactate oxidation in the intracellular lactate shuttle. *Proc. Natl. Acad Sci. USA* 96: 1129–1134.

Brooks, G. A., T.D. Fahey, and T.P. White (1996). *Exercise Physiology—Human Bioenergetics and its Applications.* London: Mayfield.

Brown, E.D., and J.M. Wood (1993). Conformational change and membrane association of the PutA protein are coincident with reduction of its FAD cofactor for proline. *J. Biol. Chem.* 268: 8972–8979.

Bryant, J.A., A. Ibrhaim, D.C. Brice, P.N. Fitchet, X.W. Wang, and L.E. Anderson (1997). Does a glycolytic enzyme also participate directly in DNA replication? *SEB Abstr.* C8.6: 107–108.

Bunn, H.F., and R.O. Poyton (1996). Oxygen sensing and molecular adaptation to hypoxia. *Physiol. Rev.* 76: 839–885.

Burness, G.P., S.C. Leary, P.W. Hochachka, and C.D. Moyes (1999). Allometric scaling of DNA, RNA, and enzyme levels: Influence of body size and age. *Am. J. Physiol.* 277: R1164-R1170.

Campbell, J.W. (1991). Excretory nitrogen metabolism. In: *Environmental and Metabolic Animal Physiology*, pp. 277–324, ed. C.L. Prosser. New York: Wiley-Liss.

Campbell, J.W. (1995). Excretory Nitrogen Metabolism in Reptiles and Birds. In: *Nitrogen Metabolism and Excretion*, pp. 147–178, ed. P.J. Walsh and P.A. Wright. Boca Raton, Florida: CRC.

Carlson, C.J., F.W. Booth, and S.E. Gordon (1999). Skeletal muscle myostatin mRNA expression is fiber-type specific and increases during hindlimb unloading. *Am. J. Physiol.* 277: R601–R606.

Casey, T.M., M. L. May, and K. R. Morgan (1985). Flight energetics of Euglossine bees in relation to morphology and wing stroke frequency. *J. Exp. Biol.* 116: 271–289.

Chance, B., J.S. Leigh, Jr., J. Kent, and K. McCully (1986). Metabolic control principles and 31P NMR. *Fed. Proc.* 45: 2915–2920.

Coulson, R.A. (1993). The flow theory of enzyme kinetics: role of solid geometry in the control of reaction velocity in live animals. *Intl. J. Biochem.* 25: 1445–1474.

Coyle, E.F. (1995). Substrate utilization during exercise in active people. *Am. J. Clin. Nutr.* 61: 968S-979S.

Czyzyk-Kreska, M.F., Z. Dominski, R. Kole, and D.E. Millhorn (1994). Hypoxia stimulates binding of a cytoplasmic protein to a pyrimidine-rich sequence in the 3′-untranslated region of rat tyrosine hydroxylase mRNA. *J. Biol. Chem.* 269: 9940–9945.

Darville, M.I., I.V. Antoine, J.R. Martens-Stritjhagen, V.I. Dupriez, and G. Rousseau (1995). An E2F-dependent late-serum-response promoter in a gene that controls glycolysis. *Oncogene* 11: 1509–1517.

Des Marais, D.J. (2000). When did photosynthesis emerge on earth? *Science* 289: 1703–1705.

Diamond, J., and K. Hammond (1992). The matches achieved by natural selection between biological capacities and their natural loads. *Experientia* 48: 551–557.

Dobson G.P., and J.P. Headrick (1995). Bioenergetic scaling: Metabolic design and body-size constraints in mammals. *Proc. Natl. Acad. Sci. USA* 92: 7317–7321.

Dobson, G.P., and P.W. Hochachka (1987). Role of glycolysis in adenylate depletion and repletion during work and recovery in teleost white muscle. *J. exp. Biol.* 129: 125–140.

Duncan, N.D., D.A. Williams, and G.S. Lynch (1998). Adaptations in rat skeletal muscle following long-term resistance exercise training. *Eur. J. Appl. Physiol. Occupat. Physiol.* 77: 372–8.

Dunn, J.F., P.W. Hochachka, W. Davison, and M. Guppy (1983). Metabolic adjustments to diving and recovery in the African lungfish. *Am. J. Physiol.* 245: R651-R657.

Ebert, B.L., J.M. Gleadle, J.F. O'Rourke, S.M. Bartlett, J. Poulton, and P.J. Ratcliffe (1996). Isoenzyme-specific regulation of genes involved in energy metabolism by hypoxia: similarities with the regulation of erythropoietin. *Biochem. J.* 313: 809–814.

Emmett, B., and P.W. Hochachka (1981). Scaling of oxidative and glycolytic enzymes in the shrew. *Resp. Physiol.* 45: 261–267.

Fell D.A., and S. Thomas (1995). Physiological control of metabolic flux: The requirements for multisite regulation. *Biochem. J.* 311: 35–39.

Fersht, A. (1985). *Enzyme Structure and Mechanism.* pp. 1–282. New York: W.H. Freeman.

Firth, J.D., B.L. Ebert, and P.J. Ratcliffe (1995). Hypoxic regulatin of LDH A: interaction betwee hypoxia inducible factor 1 and cAMP response elements. *J. Biol. Chem.* 270: 21021–21027.

Fostermann, U., and K. Hartmut (1999). Nitric oxide synthase: expression and expressional control of the three isoforms. *Naunyn-Schmiedebergs Arch. Pharmacol.* 352: 351–364.

From, A.H.L., S.D. Zimmer, S.P. Michurski, P. Mohanakrishnan, V.K. Ulstad, W.J. Thomas, and K. Ugurbil (1990). Regulation of oxidative phosphorylation in the intact cell. *Biochemistry* 29: 3733–3743.

Fry, F.E.J. (1947). Effects of environment on animal activity. *Publications of the Ontario Fisheries Research Laboratory* 55: 1–62.

Gallie, D.R., J.N. Feder, R.T. Schimke, and V. Walbot (1991). Post-transcriptional regulation in higher eukaryotes: the role of the reporter gene in controlling expression. *Mol. Gen. Genet.* 228: 258–264.

Garry, D.J., G.A. Ordway, J.N. Lorenz, N.B. Radford, E.R. Chin, R.W. Grange, R. Baseel-Duby, and R. Williams (1999). *Nature* 395: 905–908.

Gayeski T.E., and C.R. Honig (1991). Intracellular PO_2 in individual cardiac myocytes in dogs, cats, rabbits, ferrets, and rats. *Am. J. Physiol.* 260: H522–H531.

Godecke, A., U. Flogel, K. Zanger, Z. Ding, J. Hirchenhain, U.K.M. Decking, and J. Schrader (1999). *Proc. Natl. Acad. Sci. USA.* 96: 10495–10500.

Goodridge, A.G. (1987). Dietary regulation of gene expression: enzymes involved in carbohydrate and lipid metabolism. *Ann. Rev. Nutr.* 7: 157–185.

Gow, A.J., B.P. Luchsinger, J.R. Plawloski, D.J. Singel, and J.S. Stamler (1999). The oxyhemoglobin reaction of nitric oxide. *Proc. Natl. Acad. Sci. USA* 96: 9027–9032.

Grabarek, Z, T. Tao, and J. Gergely (1992). Molecular mechanism of troponin-C function. *J. Muscle Res. Cell Motil.* 13: 383–393.

Graham, J. E., and K. A. Dickson (2000). Evolution of thunniform locomotion and heat conservation in scombrid fishes: new insights based on the morphology of *Allothunnus falai.* *Zool. J. Linnean Soc.* 129: 419–466.

Guppy, M., C .J. Fuery, and J.E. Flanigan (1994). Biochemical principles of metabolic depression. *Comp. Biochem. Physiol.* B 109: 175–189.

Guppy, M., W.C. Hulbert, and P.W. Hochachka (1979). Metabolic sources of heat and power in tuna muscles. II. Enzyme and metabolite profiles. *J. Exp. Biol.* 82: 303–320.

Guy, P.S., and D.H. Snow (1977). The effect of training and detraining on lactate dehydrogenase isozymes in the horse. *Biochem. Biophys. Res. Comm.* 75: 863–869.

Hand, S.C., and I. Hardewig (1996). Downregulation of cellular metabolism during environmental stress—mechanisms and implications. *Annu. Rev. Physiol.* 58: 539–563.

Hanstock, C.C., R.B. Thompson, M.E. Trump, D. Gheorghiu, P.W. Hochachka, and P.S. Allen (1999). The residual intra-molecular dipolar coupling of the Cr/PCr methyl resonance in resting human medial gastrocnemius muscle. *Magnet. Reson. Med.* 42: 421–424.

Harvey, W.R., and H. Wieczorek (1997). Animal plasma membrane energization by chemiosmotic H^+ V ATPases control. *J. Exp. Biol.* 200: 203–216.

Heigenhauser, G.J., and M.L. Parolin (1999). Role of pyruvate dehydrogenase in lactate production in exercising human skeletal muscle. *Adv. Exp. Med. Biol.* 474: 205–218.

Hemmingsen, A.M. (1960). Energy metabolism as related to body size and respiratory surfaces and its evolution. *Rep. Steno. Mem. Hosp. (Copenhagen)* 9: 1–110.

Hochachka, P.W. (1980). *Living Without Oxygen*, pp. 1–181, Cambridge, Mass.: Harvard University Press.

Hochachka, P.W. (1990). Scope for survival: A conceptual 'mirror' to Fry's scope for activity. *Trans. Am. Fish. Soc.* 119: 622–628.

Hochachka, P.W. (1994). *Muscles and Molecular and Metabolic Machines.* pp. 1–157, Boca Raton, FL.: CRC Press.

Hochachka, P.W. (1999a). The metabolic implications of intracellular circulation. *Proc. Natl. Acad. Sci. USA* 96: 12233–12239.

Hochachka, P.W. (1999b). Two research paths for probing the roles of oxygen in metabolic regulation. *Brazilian J. Med. Biol. Res.* 32: 661–672.

Hochachka, P.W. (2000). Pinniped diving response mechanism and evolution: A window on the paradigm of comparative biochemistry and physiology. *Comp. Biochem. Physiol.* 126A: 435–458.

Hochachka, P.W. and M. Guppy (1987). *Metabolic Arrest and the Control of Biological Time.* Cambridge, MA: Harvard University Press.

Hochachka, P.W., and G.O. Matheson (1992). Regulation of ATP turnover over broad dynamic muscle work ranges. *J. Appl. Physiol.* 73: 570–575.

Hochachka, P.W. and G.B. McClelland (1997). Cellular metabolic homeostasis during large scale changes in ATP turnover rates in muscles. *J. Exp. Biol.* 200: 381–386.

Hochachka, P.W., and T.P. Mommsen (1983). Protons and anaerobiosis. *Science* 219: 1391–1397.

Hochachka, P.W., and M.K.P. Mossey (1998). Does muscle creatine phosphokinase have access to the total pool of phosphocreatine + creatine. *Am. J. Physiol.* 274: R868-R872.

Hochachka, P.W., and Somero (1984). *Biochemical Adaptation.* Princeton: Princeton University Press.

Hochachka, P.W., L.T. Buck, C. Doll, and S.C. Land (1996a). Unifying theory of hypoxia tolerance: molecular/metabolic defense and rescue mechanisms for surviving oxygen lack. *Proc. Natl. Acad. Sci. USA* 93: 9493–9499.

Hochachka, P.W., C.M. Clark, J.E. Holden, C. Stanley, K. Ugurbil, and R.S. Menon (1996b). ^{31}P Magnetic resonance spectroscopy of the Sherpa heart: A PCr/ATP signature of metabolic defense against hypobaric hypoxia. *Proc. Natl. Acad. Sci. USA* 93: 1215–1220.

Hochachka, P.W., G.B. McClelland, G.P. Burness, J.F. Staples, and R.K. Suarez (1998). Integrating metabolic pathway fluxes with gene-to-enzyme expression rates. *Comp. Biochem. Physiol. B* 120: 17–26.

Hochstrasser, M. (1996). Protein degradation or regulation: Ub the judge. *Cell* 84: 813–815.

Hogan, M C., P.G. Arthur, D.E. Bebout, P.W. Hochachka, and P.D. Wagner (1992). Role of oxygen in regulating tissue respiration in dog muscle working in situ. *J. App. Physiol.* 73: 728–736.

Holloszy, J.O., and F.W. Booth (1976). Biochemical adaptations of endurance exercise in muscle. *Ann. Rev. Physiol.* 38: 273–291.

Honig, C.R., R.J. Connett, and T.E. Gayeski (1992). O_2 transport and its interaction with metabolism, a systems view of aerobic capacity. *Med. Sci. Sports Exer.* 24: 47–53.

Hulbert A.J., and P.L. Else (1999). Membranes as possible pacemakers of metabolism. *J. Theor. Biol.* 199: 257–274.

Hulbert, A.J., and P.L. Else (2000). Mechanisms underlying the cost of living in animals *Annu. Rev. Physiol.* 62: 207–235.

Jeneson, J.A., H.V. Westerhoff, and M.J. Kushmerick (2000). A metabolic control analysis of kinetic controls in ATP free energy metabolism in contracting skeletal muscle. *Amer. J. Physiol.* 279: C813-C832.

Jelicks, L.A., and B.A.Wittenberg (1995). 1H NMR studies of sarcoplasmic oxygenation in the red cell perfused rat heart. *Biophys. J.* 68: 2129–2136.

Jiang, B-H., E. Rue, G.L.Wang, R. Roe, and G.L. Semenza (1996). Dimerization, DNA binding, and transactivation properties of hypoxia-inducible factor 1. *J. Biol. Chem.* 271: 17771–17778.

Jones, J.H. (1998). Optimization of the mammalian respiratory system: symmorphosis versus single species adaptation. *Comp. Biochem. Physiol.* 120B: 125–138.

Juergens, K.D., T. Peters, and G. Gros (1994). Diffusivity of myoglobin in intact. *Proc. Natl. Acad. Sci. USA* 91: 3829–3833.

Kao H.P., J.R. Abney, and A.S. Verkman (1993). Determinants of the translational mobility of a small solute in cell cytoplasm. *J. Cell Biol.* 120: 175–184.

Karrasch S., and J.E. Walker (1999). Novel features in the structure of bovine ATP synthase. *J. Mol. Biol.* 290: 379–384.

Kashiwaya, Y., K. Sato, N. Tshuchiya, S. Thomas, D.A. Fell, R.L. Veech, and J.V. Passonneau (1994). Control of glucose utilization in working perfused rat heart. *J. Biol. Chem.* 269: 25502–25514.

Kay, L., K. Nicolay, B. Wieringa, V. Saks, and T. Wallimann (2000). Direct evidence for the control of mitochondrial respiration by mitochondrial creatine kinase in oxidative muscle cells in situ. *J. Biol. Chem.* 275: 6937–6944.

Kleiber, M. (1932). Body size and metabolism. *Hilgarida* 6: 315–353.

Kollia, P., E. Fibach, S.M. Najjar, A. Schechter, and C.T. Noguchi (1996). Modifications of RNA processing modulate the expression of hemoglobin genes. *Proc. Natl. Acad. Sci. USA* 93: 5693–5698.

Korzeniewski, B. (2000). Regulation of ATP supply in mammalian skeletal muscle during resting state work transition. *Biophys. Chem.* 83: 19–34.

Kump, L.R., J.F. Kasting, and R.G. Crane (1999). *The Earth System*, pp. 1–351. Upper Saddle River, N.J.: Prentice Hall.

Kushmerick, M.J., R.A. Meyer, and T.R. Brown (1992). Regulation of oxygen consumption in fast- and slow-twitch muscle. *Am. J. Physiol.* 263: C598-C606.

Leary, S.C. and C.D. Moyes (2000). The effects of bioenergetic stress- and redox balance on the expression of genes critical to mitochondrial function. In: *Environmental Stressors and Gene Responses* pp. 209–220, ed. K.B. Storey and J.M. Storey. Amsterdam: Elsevier.

Lindstedt, S.L., and Calder W.A. III (1981). Body size, physiological time, and longevity of homeothermic animals. *Quart. Rev. Biol.* 56:1–15.

Lindstedt, S.L., J. Joppeler, K.M. Bard, and H.A. Thronson, Jr. (1985). Estimates of muscle-shortening rate during locomotion. *Am. J. Physiol.* 249: R669-R703.

Loughna, P.T., and C. Brownson (1996). Two myogenic regulatory factor transcripts exhibit muscle-specific responses to disuse and passive stretch in adult rats. *FEBS Lett.* 390: 304–306.

Lovegrove, B.G. (2000). The zoogeography of mammalian basal metabolic rate. *Am. Natur.* 156: 201–219.

Lovelock, J.E. (1979). *Gaia—A New Look at Life on Earth*. Oxford: Oxford University Press.

Magistretti, P.J., and L. Pellerin (1999). Astrocytes couple synaptic activity of glucose utilization in the brain. *News Physiol. Sci.* 14: 177–182.

McClelland, G.B., P.W. Hochachka, and J.-M. Weber (1998). Carbohydrate utilization during exercise after high altitude acclimation: A new perspective. *Proc. Natl. Acad. Sci. USA* 95: 10288–10293.

McGilvery, R.W. (1973). *Biochemistry, a Functional Approach*. Philadelphia: Saunders.

Mole, P.A., Y. Chung, K. Tran, N. Sailasuta, R. Hurd, and T. Jue (1999). Myoglobin desaturation with exercise intensity in human gastrocnemius muscle. *Am. J. Physiol.* 277: R173–R180.

Molkentin, J.D., B.L. Black, J.F. Martin, and E.N. Olson (1995). Cooperative activation of muscle gene expression by MEF2 and myogenic bHLH proteins. *Cell* 83: 1125–1136.

Mommsen, T.P., C.J. French, and P.W. Hochachka (1980). Sites and patterns of protein and amino acid utilization during the spawning migration of salmon. *Can. J. Zool.* 58: 1785–1799.

Mottishaw, P.D., S. Thornton, and P.W. Hochachka (1999). The diving response and its surprising evolutionary path in seals and sea lions. *Am. Zool.* 39: 434–450.

Moyes, C.D., P.M. Schulte, and P.W. Hochachka (1992). Recovery metabolism of trout white muscle: role of the mitochondria. *Amer. J. Physiol.* 262: R295–R304.

Muro-Pastor, A.M., and S. Maloy (1995). Proline dehydrogenase activity of the transcriptional repressor PutA is required for induction of the put operon by proline. *J. Biol. Chem.* 270: 9819–9827.

Murphy, B.J., E.D. Robin, D.P. Tapper, R.J. Wong, and D.A. Clayton (1984). Hypoxic coordinate regulation of mitochondrial enzymes in mammalian cells. *Science* 223: 707–709.

Nair, K.S., and W.F. Schwenk (1994). Factors controlling muscle protein synthesis and degradation. *Curr. Opin. Neurol.* 7: 471–474.

Nakai, N., Y. Sato, Y. Oshida, N. Fujitsuka, A. Yoshimura, and Y. Shimomura (1999). Insulin activation of pyruvate dehydrogenase complex is enhanced by exercise training. *Metabolism: Clin. Exper.* 48: 865–869.

Nelson, D.E., A. Angerbjorn, K. Liden, and I. Turk (1998). Stable isotopes and the metabolism of the European cave bear. *Oecologia* 116: 177–181.

Nevill, A.M. (1994). The need to scale for differences in body size and mass: an explanation of Kleiber's 0.75 mass exponent. *J. Appl. Physiol.* 77: 2870–2873.

Parkhouse, W.S., G.P. Dobson, and P.W. Hochachka (1998). Control of glycogenolysis in rainbow trout muscle during exercise. *Can. J. Zool.* 66: 345–351.

Papadopoulos, S., K.D. Jurgens, and G. Gros (2000). Protein diffusion in living skeletal muscle fibers: dependence on protein size, fiber type, and contraction. *Biophys. J.* 79: 2084–2094.

Pedersen, K. (2000). Exploration of deep intraterrestrial microbial life: current perspectives. *FEMS Microb. Lett.* 85: 9–16.

Peterson, C C., K.A. Nagy, and J. Diamond (1990). Sustained metabolic scope. *Proc. Natl. Acad. Sci. USA* 87: 2324–2328.

Pette, D., and G. Vrbova (1999). What does chronic electrical stimulation teach us about muscle plasticity? *Muscle Nerve* 22: 666–677.

Putman, C.T., N.L. Jones, E. Hultman, M.G. Hollidge-Horvat, A. Bonen, D.R. McConachie, and G.J. Heigenhauser (1998). Effects of short-term submaximal training in humans on muscle metabolism in exercise. *Am. J. Physiol.* 275: E132-E139.

Richardson, R.S., E.A. Noyszewski, K.F. Kendrick, J.S. Leigh, and P.D. Wagner (1996). Myoglobin O_2 desaturation during exercise. Evidence of limited O_2 transport. *J. Clin. Invest.* 96: 1916–1926.

Robin, E.D., B.J. Murphy, and J. Theodore (1984). Coordinate regulation of glycolysis by hypoxia in mammalian cells. *J. Cell. Physiol.* 118: 287–290.

Rolfe, D.F., and G.C. Brown (1997). Cellular energy utilization and molecular origin of standard metabolic rate in mammals. *Physiol. Rev.* 77: 731–758.

Rolfe, D.F., J.M. Newman, J.A. Buckingham, M.G. Clark, and M.D. Brand (1999). Contribution of mitochondrial proton leak to respiration rate in working skeletal muscle and liver and to SMR. *Am. J. Physiol.* 276: C692–699.

Scalettar, B.A., J.R. Abney, and C.R. Hackenbrock (1991). Dynamics, structure, and function are coupled in the mitochondrial matrix. *Proc. Natl. Acad. Sci. USA* 88: 8057–8061.

Schmidt-Nielsen, K. (1984). *Scaling: Why is Animal Size so Important?* Cambridge: Cambridge University Press. 241 pp.

Semenza, G.L (1999). Regulation of mammalian O_2 homeostasis by hypoxia-inducible factor 1. *Annu. Rev. Cell Develop. Biol.* 15: 551–578.

Semenza, G.L., P.H. Roth, H-M. Fang, and G.L. Wang (1994). Transcriptional regulation of genes encoding glycolytic enzymes by hypoxia inducible factor 1. *J. Biol. Chem.* 269: 23757–23763.

Sheel, A.W., and D.C. McKenzie (2000). Hypoxemia during exercise: in health and disease. *Clin. Exer. Physiol.* 2(3): 116–127.

Simoneau, J-A., and D. Pette (1998). Species-specific effects of chronic stimulation upon tibialis anterior muscle in mouse, rat, guinea pig, and rabbit. *Pflugers Arch.* 412: 86–92.

Simoneau, J-A., D.A. Hood, and D. Pette (1990). Species-specific responses in enzyme activities of anaerobic and aerobic energy metabolism to increased contractile activity. *Int. Ser. Sports Sci.* 21: 95–104.

Srivastava, D.K., and S.A. Bernard (1986). Metabolite transfer via enzyme-enzyme complexes. *Science* 234: 1080–1086.

Staples, J.F., and R.K. Suarez (1997). Honeybee flight muscle phosphoglucoseisomerase: matching enzyme capacities to flux requirements at a near-equilibrium reaction. *J. Exp. Biol.* 200: 1247–1254.

Suarez, R.K. (1992). Hummingbird flight: sustaining the highest mass-specific metabolic rates among vertebrates. *Experientia* 48: 565–570.

Suarez, R.K., J.R.B. Lighton, B. Joos, S.P. Roberts, and J.F. Harrison (1996). Energy metabolism, enzymatic flux capacities, and metabolic flux rates in flying honeybees. *Proc. Natl. Acad. Sci. USA* 93: 12616–12620.

Suarez, R.K., J.F. Staples, J.R.B. Lighton, and T.G. West (1997). Relationships between enzymatic flux capacities and metabolic flux rates: nonequilibrium reactions in glycolysis. *Proc. Natl. Acad. Sci. USA* 94: 7065–7069.

Taylor, C.R., E.R. Weibel, J-M. Weber, R. Vock, J. Hoppeler, T.J. Roberts, and G. Brichon (1996). Design of the oxygen and substrate pathways. I. Model and strategy to test symmorphosis in a network structure. *J. Exp. Biol.* 199: 1643–1649.

Taylor, C.R., E.R. Weibel, R.H. Karas, and H. Hoppeler (1987). Adaptive variation in the mammalian respiratory system in relation to energy demand. *Resp. Physiol.* 69: 1–127.

Taylor, C.R., G.M.O. Maloiy, E.R. Weibel, V.A. Langman, J.M.Z. Kamau, H.J. Seeherman, and N.C. Heglund (1981). Design of the mammalian respiratory system. III. Scaling maximum aerobic capacity to body mass: wild and domestic mammals. *Respir. Physiol.* 44: 25–37.

Thomas, S., and D.A. Fell (1996). Design of metabolic control for large flux changes. *J. Theor. Biol.* 182: 285–298.

Trump, M.E., C.C. Hanstock, P.S. Allen, D. Gheorghiu, and P.W. Hochachka (2001). A ^{1}H MRS evaluation of the phosphocreatine(PCr)/creatine (Cr) pool in human muscle. *Amer. J. Physiol.* 280: R889–R896.

Van Breukelen, F., R. Maier, and S.C. Hand (2000). Depression of nuclear transcription and extension of mRNA half-life under anoxia in *Artemia franciscana* embryos. *J. Exp. Biol.* 203: 1123–1130.

Van der Lee, K.A., M.M. Vork, J.E. De Vries, P.H. Willemsen, J.F. Glatz, R.S. Reneman, G.J. Van der Vusse, and M. Van Bilsen (2000). Long-chain fatty acid-induced changes in gene expression in neonatal cardiac myocytes. *J. Lipid Res.* 41: 41–47.

Van Nieuwenhoven, F.A., A.H. Kleine, K.W.H. Wodzig, W.T. Hermens, H.A. Kragten, J.G. Maessen, C.K. Punt, M.P. Van Dieijen, G.J. Van der Vusse, and J.F.C. Glatz (1995). Discrimination between myocardial and skeletal muscle injury by assessment of the plasma ratio of myoglobin over fatty acid binding protein. *Circulation* 92: 2848–2854.

Veerkamp, J.H., and R.G.H.J. Maatman (1995). Cytoplasmic fatty acid binding proteins: their structure and genes. *Prog. Lipid Res.* 34: 17–52.

Viru, A. (1994). Molecular cellular mechanisms of training effects. *J. Sports Med. Phys. Fitness* 34: 309–322.

Wagner, P.D. (2000). Reduced cardiac output at altitude—mechanisms and significance. *Resp. Physiol.* 120: 1–11.

Walsh, P.J., and T.P. Mommsen (2000). Evolutionary considerations of nitrogen metabolism and excretion. In: *Fish Physiology,* Vol. 18, pp. 1–16, ed. P.M. Anderson and P.A. Wright. New York: Academic Press.

Wang, D., U. Kruetzer, Y. Chung, and T. Jue (1998). Myoglobin and hemoglobin rotational diffusion in the cell. *Biophys. J.* 73: 2764–2770.

Wang, G.L., and G.L. Semenza (1995). Purification and characterization of hypoxia-inducible factor-1. *J. Biol. Chem.* 270: 1230–1237.

Wang, G.L., B-H. Jiang, E.A. Rue, and G.L. Semenza (1995). Hypoxia inducible factor 1 is a basic-helix-loop-helix-PAS heterodimer regulated by cellular oxygen tension. *Proc. Natl. Acad. Sci. USA* 92: 5510–5514.

Webster, K.A., and B.J. Murphy (1987). Regulation of tissue-specific glycolytic isozyme genes: coordinate response to oxygen availability in myogenic cells. *Can. J. Zool.* 66: 1046–1058.

Webster, K.A., P. Gunning, E. Hardeman, D.C. Wallace, and L. Kedes (1990). Coordinate reciprocal trends in glycolytic and mitochondrial transcript accumulations during the in vitro differentiation of human myoblasts. *J. Cellular Physiol.* 142: 566–573.

Webster, K.A., D.J. Discher, O.M. Hernandez, K. Yamashita, and N.H. Bishopric (2000). A glycolytic pathway to apoptosis of hypoxic cardiac myocytes. In: *Oxygen Sensing and Molecule to Man. Advances in Exptl. Medicine and Biology* pp. 161–176, 475, ed. S. Lahiri, N.R. Prabhakar, and R.E. Forster, II. New York: Kluwer Academic/Plenum.

Wegener, G., N.M. Bolas, and A.A.G. Thomas (1991). Locust flight metabolism studied in vivo with 31P NMR spectroscopy. *J. Comp. Physiol.* B161: 247–256.

Weibel, E.R. (2000). *Symmorphosis, On Form and Function Shaping Life.* Cambridge, Mass.: Harvard University Press.

Weibel, E.R., C.R. Taylor, and H. Hoppeler (1991). The concept of symmorphosis: A testable hypothesis of structure-function relationships. *Proc. Natl. Acad. Sci. USA* 88: 10357–10361.

Weibel, E.R., C.R. Taylor, J-M. Weber, R. Vock, T.J. Roberts, and H. Hoppeler (1996). Design of the oxgyen and substrate pathways. VII. Different structural limits for oxygen and substrates to muscle and mitochondria. *J. Exp. Biol.* 199: 1699–1709.

West, G.B., J.H. Brown, and B.J. Enquist (2000). The origin of universal scaling laws in biology. In: *Scaling in Biology,* pp. 87–112, ed. J.H. Brown and G.B.West. New York: Oxford University Press.

Wheatley, D.N. (1998). Diffusion theory, the cell, and the synapse. *Biosystems* 45: 151–163.

Wheatley, D.N. (1999). On the vital role of fluid movement in organisms and cells: a brief historical account from Harvey to Coulson, extending the hypothesis of circulation. *Medical Hypotheses* 52: 275–284.

Wheatley D.N., and Clegg, J.S. (1994). What determines the metabolic rate of vertebrate cells. *Biosystems* 32: 83–92.

Wieczorke, R., S. Krampe, T. Weierstall, K. Freidel, C.P. Hollenberg, and E. Boles (1999). Concurrent knock-out of at least 20 transporter genes is required to block uptake of hexoses in *Saccharomyces cerevisiae. FEBS Lett.* 464: 123–128.

Williams, R.S., and P.D. Neufer (1996). Regulation of gene expression in skeletal muscle by contractile activity. *Handbook of Physiology,* Section 12: 1124–1150.

Wojtas, K., N. Slepecky, L. von-Kalm, and D. Sullivan (1997). Flight muscle function in Drosophila requires colocalization of glycolytic enzymes. *Mol. Biol. Cell* 8: 1665–1675.

Yang, T.-H., and G.N. Somero (1996). Activity of lactate dehydrogenase but not its concentration of messenger RNA increases with body size in barred sand bass, *Paralabrax nebulifer* (Teleostei). *Biol. Bull.* 191: 155–158.

Zorio, D.A.R., N.N. Cheng, T. Blumenthal, and J. Spieth (1994). Operons as a common form of chromosomal organization in *C. elegans. Nature* 372: 270–272.

3

Influence of Oxygen Availability

THE FIRST ORGANISMS ON EARTH WERE ANAEROBES

Extracting the maximal amount of chemical bond energy from a reduced organic molecule typically involves degradation to CO_2 and H_2O and to achieve this, molecular O_2 usually must serve as a terminal electron acceptor and thus must be available to the organism. That is why for most present-day organisms, O_2-based combustion of foodstuffs is the sine qua non of metabolic efficiency. Yet biologists today realize that this was not always so. The best available evidence indicates that early stages in the development of life on our planet occurred under highly reducing conditions (Crick, 1981; Gold, 1999). This means that the planet was colonized initially by prokaryotic anaerobes. Genomics, the sequencing and mapping of genomes and analysis of gene and genome function (Hieter and Boguski, 1997), has revolutionized our understanding of this early stage in the biological and, by extension, geological evolution of the planet. The prokaryotic and eukaryotic genomes that have been completely sequenced supply enormous new insights into the coevolution of living systems and of their geological microenvironments. Based on the presence or absence of gene families from 11 such completed genome sequences of free living microorganisms (Hieter and Boguski, 1997), or upon only 16S ribosomal RNA sequences (Woese et al., 1990), molecular biologists arrive at similar summaries of three main roots (Archaea, bacteria, and eukaryotes) to the tree of life (figure 3.1). What is more, these molecular phylogenies place anaerobes close to the root of all of life and corroborate geological arguments favoring a predominantly anaerobic primordial earth.

The introduction and gradual accumulation of O_2 by photosynthesis is considered a major turning point in the development of the geology and life on the planet for two reasons. In the first place, the emission of O_2 after the emergence of complex photosynthetic systems changed the distribution and speciation of numerous redox-sensitive elements (such as iron, uranium, sulfur, copper, and manganese)—this is the basis for the effect on geology and geochemical cycles. Secondly, these geological changes in turn led to new partitioning of living systems between aerobic and anaerobic environments—this is the basis for the biological impact of the emergence of O_2 as a major end product of photosynthesis. Even today the layered microbial communities found in sediments and aquatic biofilms reflect the relatively oxidized conditions at the sediment–water interface progressively down to hypoxic then anoxic conditions in the sediments per se, with electron acceptors being utilized in an order predictable on thermodynamic grounds (increasing electron affinity with increasing severity of environmental hypoxia).

Given initially highly reducing conditions, the photosynthetic release of O_2 as a metabolic end product may well have represented a devastating pollution to the anaerobic world that was already thriving (Lovelock, 1979; Gold, 1999). Hyperoxic conditions can be severely debilitating even to modern-day organisms, probably due to the formation of reactive free radicals. This may be the phylogenetic explanation for the occurrence of enzymes such as lactate dehydrogenase k (LDHk), whose catalytic activity is so O_2 sensitive that it can function as a dehydrogenase only under hypoxic or anoxic conditions. This LDH would have worked well in an anaerobic world, but in an aerobic one it is capable of

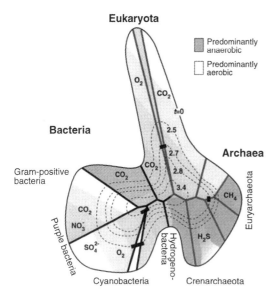

Figure 3.1. An attempt to correlate genomics with the geological record. The tree of life is based on the presence or absence of gene families from the 11 completed genomes of free living microorganisms and is placed in a temporal and evnironmental framework. The genomic framework is similar to the ribosomal RNA tree. Contours, labeled in billions of years, are schematic and are anchored by a few dates from the geological record (indicated by bars). Where the geological record indicates greater than usual diversity, the line depicting the lineage has been expanded. (Predominantly aerobic organisms are coded in white regions, while predominantly anaerobic times and organisms are shaded gray; the darker the gray, the more anaerobic the system.) Several important metabolic byproducts of different lineages are included. (From Banfield and Marshall, 2000.)

function only if protected from O_2 or from reactive oxygen species (ROSs) derived from O_2. The "saturation curve" for O_2 inactivation of LDHk (Reisser et al., 1994), a major anoxic stress protein that like other proteins of this category (see chapter 7), probably involved in facilitating proper folding of newly synthesized proteins (chaperone functions), shows a P_{50} value that is similar to the half-saturation value for hemoglobin, or Hb (Anderson et al., 1983), implying that the latter could to some degree protect the former by O_2 scavenging. Interestingly, it is known that Hb has an extremely ancient origin; homo-

logous genes for Hb are now known in many bacteria, plants, and animals, and almost certainly will also be found in the Archaea. Thus workers in the field assume that Hb origins predate the split between the bacteria and the eukaryotes. While most biologists are familiar with the O_2 transport roles of Hbs typically observed in animal species, in prokaryotes (and possibly in some plants) Hbs may serve in metabolism as electron acceptors, in intracellular O_2 transport, or in O_2 scavenging, the latter presumably representing the primoridal function for organisms in the early anaerobic world (Hardison, 1998) and serving to protect enzymes such as LDHk.

ATMOSPHERIC STEADY STATES ARE NOT FOREVER STABLE

While we normally think of the earth's atmosphere as a given, its composition is not as stable as might be intuitively anticipated. The atmosphere today is composed mainly of nitrogen (almost 79%) and of O_2 (about 20.5%); other gases, such as CO_2 and CH_4 occur at much lower levels (0.035% and 0.0024% respectively). At thermodynamic equilibrium O_2 and CH_4 cannot coexist, so their simultaneous presence means that the condition of our atmosphere is not an equilibrium one. Instead, our atmosphere is in a steady-state condition, with pool sizes of different gases being determined by relative rates of biological and geological processes that produce and that consume different gas components (Lovelock, 1979). Current evidence indicates that since the origin of complex metazoan life (about 0.6 billion years ago) O_2 in our atmosphere has varied from about 15% to as high as 35%, while CO_2 has varied by an even larger (fivefold) factor. Based on well-described responses of present-day organisms to hypoxia and hyperoxic (discussed in detail below), we can with confidence conclude that such huge fluctuations in atmospheric composition had to have equally enormous impact on living systems. Unfortunately, since metabolic and molecular defense mechanisms are not fossilized, we can only surmise what some of these processes may have been, based on the way currently extant species respond to hypoxia or hyperoxia. However, fossils do tell us about the size of different phylogenetic groups and about how size and form changed through geological history. Interestingly, animal gigantism was unusually widespread during the Carboniferous period when the %O_2 in the atmosphere was thought to be at the highest in the planet's history. Dudley (1998), reviewing what is currently known of this topic, points out that Carboniferous animal gigantism was most common among diverse flying insect lineages, but was also expressed in millipedes, arthropleurids (extinct arthropods), and terrestrial labyrinthodont amphibians. For readers unfamiliar with this information, it may be worth mentioning that the wingspans of extinct Protodonata dragonflies were notably large, and in one species exceeded 0.7 m! Millipedes 1 m (!) long, giant arthropleurids, giant Carboniferous wingless hexapods (Diplura and Thysanura), and even giant arachnids round out the Carboniferous caste of terrestrial arthropod giants. Dudley and other workers in this field (see Graham et al., 1995) believe that Carboniferous gigantism occurred in species and lineages relying heavily upon diffusive processes for O_2 transfer from air into the tissues. An elevation of O_2 to the (by today's standards) hyperoxic condition of 35% coupled with a background constant N_2 partial pressure, increases rates of O_2 diffusion by about 67% (Dudley, 1998). For diffusion-limited systems, this situation could represent an enormous advantage and would favor development of gigantism in many invertebrate groups relying upon O_2 diffusion through a tracheal system, through gills, through book lungs or through skin. The same situation is thought to have applied for primitive terrestrial vertebrates. Within this group, large amphibians reached body lengths of up to 2 m in the Carboniferous. That these large amphibians were probably limited by the capacity for cutaneous respiration is supported by studies of contemporary urodeles, in which this physiological function is known to restrict maximum body size through O_2 diffusion limitations (Dudley, 1998).

If the interpretation that Carboniferous hyperoxic conditions favored evolution of animal gigantism is correct, then it might be predicted that the persistence of this feature would also be correlated with the O_2 content of the atmosphere, and this prediction is in fact realized. Thus the relative atmospheric hypoxia that gradually developed in the Permian period also coincided with the disappearance from the fossil record of these diverse animal giants. And again, this is seen in the fossil record of both invertebrate and vertebrate groups. Final confirmation of this overall interpretation arises from studies correlating a secondary peak of hyperoxic conditions in the Cretaceous period with the appearance in the fossil record of the (now predicted and expected) secondary peak of insect gigantism, this time best evident in species within the Ephemeroptera. Equally striking is the subsequent disappearance of such groups with the recurrence of relatively hypoxic conditions (Dudley, 1998).

For most readers there may be no need to further emphasize the global impact of global O_2 availability. However, for the sceptic, we will add one final indication of the importance of O_2 to the well-being and indeed to the biomass of our current world. This example comes from the world fisheries literature, which Pauly (1999) has reviewed and digested. Of the numerous fascinating data that he presented, none is more startling than the observation of a linear relationship between fisheries biomass and O_2 availability. Since Pauly's focus was global in dimension, there can be no more impressive a way to emphasize the critical role of hypoxia in the physiology and biology of present-day organisms: if O_2 is present in abundance, a whole new universe of possibilities is opened up. If O_2 is not present, or only available in limited quantities, life's options are more limited; but, as we shall see below, both microbial and metazoan organisms do manage, and our next goal is to figure out how they do so.

TRUE FERMENTATION VERSUS ANAEROBIC AND AEROBIC RESPIRATION

For aerobic organisms in the oxic world following the appearance of oxygenic (green plant type of) photosynthesis, all strategies for dealing with the problem of O_2 deficiency revolve around replacement functions that in some way compensate for the loss of molecular oxygen. The best of these, at least in energetic terms, are found in denitrifying bacteria. The key metabolic feature of these microorganisms is that when oxygen is absent they are able to respire nitrate instead. The oxidation of substrates such as glucose with either oxygen or nitrate proceeds with a similar, large free energy change and thus both processes are thermodynamically extremely favorable:

$$\text{glucose} + 6O_2 \rightarrow 6CO_2 + 6H_2O$$

$$\Delta G_0' = -686 \, \text{kcal}$$

$$\text{glucose} + 4.8NO_3^- + 4.8H^+ \rightarrow 6CO_2 + 2.4N_2$$
$$+ 8.4H_2O$$

$$\Delta G_0' = -638 \, \text{kcal}$$

Denitrifying bacteria have taken advantage of the similarities between these two processes, developing means to respire nitrate rather than oxygen whenever the latter is unavailable. In this process, nitrate is reduced to N_2, a metabolic end product formally analogous to CO_2 and even less harmful to living cells. Such denitrifiers encompass quite a large group of microorganisms including many bacilli and pseudomonads. In addition, a number of bacteria are able to perform a nitrate–nitrite respiration in which nitrate is reduced to nitrite:

$$\text{glucose} + 12NO_3^- \rightarrow 6CO_2 + 6H_2O + 12NO_2^-$$

$$\Delta G_0' = -422 \, \text{kcal}$$

The nitrite formed is either excreted directly or reduced by non-ATP-yielding reactions to ammonia. The enzyme machinery for both processes, nitrate/nitrite respiration and denitrification, is formed only under anaerobic conditions or conditions of low oxygen tension. In fact, the activities of the enzymes involved in dissimilatory nitrate reduction are strongly inhibited by oxygen. Thus, denitrification and nitrate/nitrite respiration take place only when oxygen is absent or available in insufficient amounts.

Like oxygen respiration, denitrification allows a complete oxidation of the organic substrate to CO_2 and H_2O. For instance, when *Bacillus licheniformis* grows with glucose and nitrate under anaerobic conditions, the substrate is degraded via glycolysis and the Krebs cycle, while $NADH_2$ and $FADH_2$ serve as electron donors for the respiratory chain. Nitrate, however, does not simply replace oxygen; special types of cytochromes and membrane-bound enzyme systems are utilized, which systematically reduce nitrate to nitrite and further to nitrogen in at least four distinguishable steps (figure 3.2).

It is now evident that at least two, and probably more, of the four possible reductive steps are coupled to ATP formation in denitrifying bacteria. As may be expected from thermodynamic consideration, this crucial observation implies an ATP yield per mole of glucose similar to that for normal oxidative metabolism (see Gottschalk, 1979, for literature in this area).

From these considerations, it is clear that the three most fundamental features of oxygen-based respiration are also expressed in nitrate-based respiration:

1. the free energy drop of glucose oxidation is large and negative and the process, therefore, is thermodynamically very favorable;
2. the process leads to the complete degradation of glucose to CO_2 and H_2O without the concomitant accumulation of large amounts of partially catabolized anaerobic end products; and
3. the process is relatively efficient in terms of ATP yield per mole of carbon substrate because of a tight-coupling between electron transfer and phosphorylation.

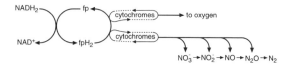

Figure 3.2. Pathways of nitrate and O_2-based respiration; these are mutually exclusive in denitrifying bacteria.

That is why anaerobic respiration, based on nitrate as a terminal electron acceptor, is more similar to oxygen-based (aerobic) respiration than it is to fermentation and is why it must by definition be clearly distinguished from the latter. The great pioneer in this area, Louis Pasteur, first and simply defined fermentation as life in the absence of oxygen. But today, a century after his pathbreaking work, fermentations are more precisely defined as those metabolic processes that occur in the dark and do not involve respiratory chains with either oxygen or nitrate as terminal electron acceptors.

NATURE OF FERMENTATIVE PATHWAYS

In true fermentation, the free energy drop between substrate (say glucose) and anaerobic end products is always modest by comparison with respiration, because fermentation is never based on electron transfer chains coupled to phosphorylation. Rather, true fermentations depend upon a variety of oxidation–reduction reactions involving organic compounds, CO_2, molecular hydrogen, or sulfur compounds. All these reactions are inefficient in terms of energy yield (moles ATP per mole substrate fermented), and, therefore, the mass of cells obtainable per mole of substrate is much smaller than with respiratory-dependent species.

Microbes capable of carrying out fermentations are classified as either facultative or obligate anaerobes. Facultative anaerobes, such as the enterobacteria, utilize O_2 if and when it is present, but if it is absent, they carry out fermentative metabolism. In contrast, obligate anaerobes are unable to synthesize the components of electron transport systems; consequently, they cannot grow as aerobes. Moreover, many of the obligate anaerobes cannot even tolerate oxygen and perish in air; these organisms are referred to as strict anaerobes.

The standard hallmark of fermentation is the accumulation of partially metabolized anaerobic end products. This is an inefficient metabolic strategy because a lot of potential chemical energy is still retained in the end products being formed; moreover, these are often noxious and therefore at high levels may well hinder further microbial growth or metabolism. Anaerobic end products are so distinguishing that true bacterial fermentations are often classified according to the main end product formed: alcohol, lactate, propionate, butyrate, mixed acid, acetate, methane, and sulfide fermentations are commonly found among anaerobic bacteria.

There are two fermentative processes that at first appear to be quite similar to oxygen and nitrate-dependent respirations: the reduction of CO_2 to methane and of sulfate to sulfide. However, on closer examination, it is clear that they bear little resemblance to the process of denitrification. In the first place, the reduction of CO_2 and of sulfate is carried out by strict anaerobes, whereas nitrate reduction is carried out by aerobes only if oxygen is unavailable. Equally important, nitrate respirers contain a true respiratory chain; sulfate and CO_2 reducers do not. Furthermore, the energetics of these processes are very different. Whereas the free energy changes of O_2 and nitrate reduction are about the same, the values are much lower for CO_2 and sulfate reduction. In fact, the values are so low that the formation of one ATP per H_2 or NADH oxidized cannot be expected. Consequently, not all the reduction steps in methane and sulfide formation can be coupled to ATP synthesis. Only the reduction of one or two intermediates may yield ATP by electron transport phosphorylation, and the ATP gain is therefore small, as is typical of fermentative reactions.

DESIGN RULES FOR BACTERIAL FERMENTATIONS

The design rules for fermentative metabolism in bacteria are few in number and are widely expressed in the microbial world. Firstly, the fermentation process always involves the partial oxidation of substrate, although there is a tremendous diversity in choice of substrate. Almost any organic compound can be fermented by some microorganism somewhere. Secondly, the oxidative reaction or reactions must always be balanced by subsequent reductive reactions in order to allow sustained function; organic compounds usually serve as electron and proton acceptors in the reductive reactions leading to the formation of organic anaerobic end products. The end products typically accumulate to some extent and are released to the outside. Thirdly, because the free energy changes associated with substrate conversion to end products are always modest, the ATP yield per mole of substrate fermented is always relatively low. One or two moles ATP per mole substrate fermented is not unusual. Fourthly, some fermentative reactions must be retained not for energy purposes per se but for the generation of key metabolite intermediates which are required for biosyntheses and growth; these may be directly related to anaerobic energy-producing pathways or may be unrelated to them; in the latter case, different substrates may be fermented to satisfy these different needs. Finally, for a unicellular system, it is reasonable and economical not to synthesize all the time all of the enzymes it is able to make but to make only those that are needed under specific and current physiological conditions. That means, the mere presence or absence of specific enzymes in microorganisms is of critical importance and must be very closely regulated. As has been well known in microbiology since the late 1970s, this regulation is achieved by enzyme induction and repression. The former is usually used in regulating levels of catabolic enzymes, while enzyme repression is usually the mechanism exploited for control of anabolic pathways (Gottschalk, 1979).

In the microbiology literature, enzyme induction is so much associated with catabolic enzymes, enzyme repression with anabolic ones, it is useful to emphasize that the levels of enzymes in central metabolic pathways must also be regulated. This is because the requirements for coupling intermediates change with varying O_2 and substrate availability, with varying growth rate, and with varying metabolic rate. In facultatively anaerobic bacteria, for example, a change from aerobic to anaerobic environments removes the need for a complete Krebs cycle; not surprisingly, anaerobic *E. coli* cells stop making 2-ketoglutarate dehydrogenase, KDH, the enzyme connecting the first

and second spans of the Krebs cycle. Other enzymes of the Krebs cycle, in contrast, are still synthesized, and it turns out, for good reasons (figure 3.3). The first span of the Krebs cycle is still required for glutamate synthesis (which in turn is needed for various biosyntheses). Citrate synthase, aconitase, and isocitrate dehydrogenase therefore are maintained even under anaerobic conditions, but their amounts are accordingly reduced. The second span of the Krebs cycle (succinate → oxaloacetate, OXA) under anaerobic conditions works backwards (OXA → succinate) forming ATP at the level of fumarate reduction to succinate, which accumulates as an anaerobic end product. Succinate in turn may be used for other biosyntheses. Thus these enzymes too must be retained under anoxic conditions.

Upon return to well-oxygenated conditions, all of the above processes in microorganisms such as *E. coli* are basically reversed in order to regain the energetic advantages of O_2-based respiration. This transition to greater energy efficiency, however, comes with the cost of dealing with reactive oxygen species (ROSs); namely, superoxide anion radical (O_2^-), hydrogen peroxide, (H_2O_2), and hydroxyl radial (·OH). Reactive oxygen species as by-products of O_2-based metabolism damage many biological molecules, including DNA, proteins, and

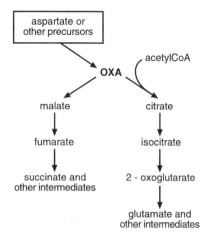

Figure 3.3. Metabolic roles during anoxia of the Krebs cycle reactions in facultatively anaerobic bacteria and yeast.

lipids. To alleviate the toxicity of these compounds, *E. coli* induces the synthesis of protective enzymes such as Mn-dependent superoxide dismutases (SOD-A), and catalase I and this induction in turn is controlled by several now well-defined regulatory proteins. In total, on anaerobic/aerobic transition, *E. coli* employs at least four global gene transcription regulatory systems that monitor the cellular oxidative and metabolic conditions and adjust the expression of more than 70 operons in order to exploit the energetic advantages of O_2 as a terminal electron acceptor in aerobic metabolism (Iuchi and Weiner, 1996).

These design principles are applicable in theory to any cell considered in isolation under anoxic conditions. As such, in their simplest form, they are prerequisite for, and are applicable to, cells in higher organisms. The anoxic microbe, however, is a closed system, and must be entirely self-sustaining and self-sufficient. In contrast, the metazoan in hypoxia remains an open system, in the sense that tissues and organs remain in communication with each other and their metabolic responses to hypoxia may well show significant degrees of tissue specificity and inter-tissue exchanges. Nevertheless, as we shall see below, the availability of cell models for studying hypoxia/anoxia responses of metazoans has hugely accelerated progress in this area.

HYPOXIA TOLERANCE IN THE ANIMAL KINGDOM

For some time now, biologists have known that certain vertebrate species have evolved inordinate capabilities for surviving prolonged periods without oxygen or with greatly reduced supplies of oxygen. Within the invertebrates, the most developed hypoxia tolerance mechanisms appear amongst the Nematodes, the bivalve Molluscs, the Annelids and Platyhelminths. Within the vertebrates, well-known hypoxia-tolerant species are known among the teleosts; included here are many fishes that evolved air breathing as a means of surviving in extremely hypoxic situations. Among the water breathing teleosts, the

Cyprinidae (goldfish and carp being two examples) are particularly hypoxia tolerant. Within the Amphibia, some Apoda species are believed to be extremely tolerant to hypoxia; Anurans are less tolerant, while other groups do not appear to display this feature. Within the reptiles, the Chelonia, especially the aquatic turtles, are known to tolerate hypoxia or even anoxia extremely well; other reptiles all seem to be obligate aerobes. Analysis of the major animal lineages (a simplified tree of animal life, based on Knoll and Carroll, 1999, is given in figure 3.4) shows that hypoxia tolerance probably evolved independently multiple times and that hypoxia tolerant groups are spread throughout the phylogeny.

PHYSIOLOGICAL LINES OF DEFENSE AGAINST LIMITING O_2

Studies of such species shows that the first lines of defense against hypoxia are at physiological levels and are primarily aimed at improving O_2 delivery to compensate for reduced supplies. The most obvious way of improving O_2 delivery to tissues is through adjustments in capillarity, in blood volume or in red blood cell (RBC) mass; these kinds of mechanisms are reviewed in specific contexts in chapters 4 and 5 and will not be further discussed here. However, correlated with these processes are important biochemical adaptations of respiratory pigments such as hemoglobin (Hb) and myoglobin (Mb) in vertebrates and other respiratory pigments such as hemocyanin (Hc) in invertebrates. In the case of Hbs, adaptations to hypoxia may involve (i) increases in Hb content in the blood, (ii) changes in O_2 affinity, (iii) changes in regulatory properties, and/or (iv) changes in regulatory modulators per se—all of which facilitate either O_2 uptake at the gas exchange organs or O_2 release at tissue sites of utilization. Although there are examples of changes in Hb concentration per RBC (in seals, for example, as an adaptation for diving), the first of the above mechanisms is usually realized simply by increasing RBC mass, and will not be further discussed here. The other two mechanisms supply some of the best examples of biochemical

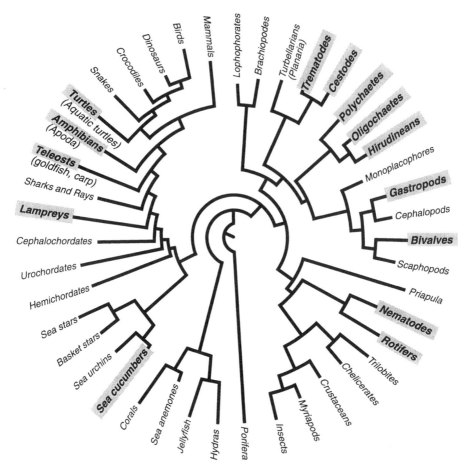

Figure 3.4. A simplified phylogenetic tree of the animal kingdom, modified from Knoll and Carroll (1999), with lineages containing notably hypoxia-tolerant species highlighted (bold type, gray boxes). Even casual analysis suggests that hypoxia tolerance probably arose independently multiple times within the animal kingdom; and, perhaps more signficantly, the figure indicates that hypoxia tolerance is widely distributed.

adaptation to hypoxia currently known and we need to discuss these in some detail. Hb structure is where our analysis must begin, because it forms the basis for Hb functional properties.

MOLECULAR BASIS FOR Hb FUNCTIONAL ADAPTATIONS

Vertebrate hemoglobins are tetrameric proteins made up of four heme-containing subunits, each capable of binding an O_2 molecule. Adult Hbs ($\alpha_2\beta_2$) consist of two kinds of such subunits (termed α and β) that in humans are composed of 141 and 146 amino acid residues,

respectively. Some mammals have fetal Hb (HbF that has γ instead of β chains) and even earlier in development all mammals so far studied express embryonic Hb that contains embryonic α or β chains. Each subunit forms helical segments joined by helical "corners." All Hb subunits display sequence homology that reflects gene duplication during phylogeny. As we shall see below, molecular adaptations involve substitutions at only a few amino acid residues at key positions in the protein moiety. This means that most observed substitutions in different species are conservative replacements (of internal nonpolar or hydrophobic residues and of external polar and nonpolar ones) that have little effect on Hb function. In the deoxygenated state the subunits are braced in a tense or T conformation by salt bridges that are broken upon oxygenation, allowing transition into the relaxed or R conformational state. Effector molecules regulate Hb function mainly by modulating O_2 affinity by strengthening or weakening the T or R states. For example, the Bohr effect (decreased O_2 affinity at low pH, which liberates O_2 in the relatively acidic tissues) is caused by H^+ and CO_2 binding that reduces O_2 affinity by strengthening the T state. Organophosphates such as 2,3-diphosphoglycerate (DPG), found in mammalian RBCs, and inositol pentaphosphate (IPP) found in avian red cells and chloride ions decrease O_2 affinity by homologous interaction between subunits. Within any species, a combination of modula-tors in concert serve to facilitate O_2 loading at the lungs or gills and O_2 unloading at the tissues.

Parenthetically, we should briefly review terminology. Cooperativity between the subunits and thus between the heme groups leads to sigmoidal-shaped O_2 saturation curves (figure 3.5): the first O_2 bound strengthens the R state and thus increases the affinity for the second O_2 bound, and so forth. The strength of subunit–subunit interactions (sigmoidicity of the O_2 saturation curve) is denoted by a coefficient n, which normally varies between 1 (no interactions) and 2–3, but sometimes can even be higher. Another term, the P_{50} or O_2 tension at 50% HbO_2 saturation, is used to describe the O_2 affinity; negative modulators such as DPG or H^+, decrease O_2 affinity (right shift the O_2

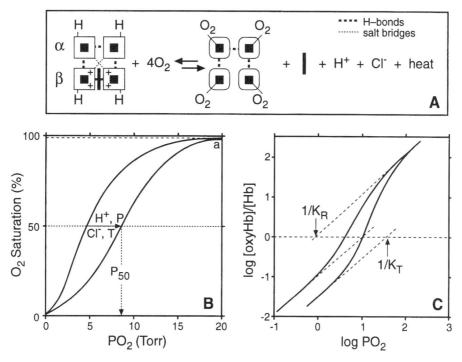

Figure 3.5. (A) Diagrammatic representation of Hb oxygenation, showing the transition from the T(ense) state to the R(elaxed) state with the liberation of protons, organic phosphate modulator (like DPG in mammalian RBCs, or ATP or GTP in fish RBCs, indicated by a bar), chloride ions, and heat. (B) O_2 saturation curves for Hb showing the right shift (decrease in O_2 affinity) with increases in temperature (T) and in concentrations of organic phosphate (shown as P), chloride, or protons. (C) Hill plots for O_2 saturation curves in (B), showing the decreased O_2 affinity in the T state induced by increased temperature or increased concentrations of organic phosphate modulator, chloride, or protons (compare $1/K_T$ vs $1/K_R$ values). Modified from Weber (1995).

equilibrium curve). The Bohr effect refers to H^+-mediated decrease in Hb O_2 affinity (right shifting of the O_2 equilibrium curve); the Root effect also refers to a low pH-mediated decrease in Hb O_2 affinity but in this case, the effect is so pronounced that complete Hb saturation becomes impossible.

The amino acid sequences of large numbers of Hbs are now known and they reveal homologies that reflect phylogenetic relationships between different groups of organisms. Differences in the numbers and identities of amino acids cause variations in molecular weight of Hbs, but all are around 65,000. Each polypepetide subunit has a characteristic secondary structure alternating between α-helical segments (termed A through H, starting from the N terminus). In-between nonhelical segments are named with the letters of adjacent helices (i.e., AB through to GH). The ultimate segments at the N- and C-terminal ends are nonhelical and are labeled NA and HC, respectively. Our preference is not to use this terminology, but, in the literature it is common to refer to individual amino acid residues by their positions in these segments. For example, F8α means the eighth-amino-acid residue in the F helix of the α chain, counting from the amino end of the subunit and F8β means the same thing for the β subunit.

As molecular adaptations involve changes in effector binding, the few sites directly implicated should also be reviewed. In human HbA, DPG binds electrostatically at seven positively charged chain residues; namely, at the N-terminal valine residues (β1Val), β2His, and β143His of both β chains, and at β82lys of one chain. The Bohr protons bind predominantly at the N terminal residues of the α chains and the C termini of β chains (α1Val and β146His); chloride ions bind at α1Val, which interacts with α131Ser and at β82lys (which interacts with β1Val). In bird Hbs, IPP appears to bind at the same site as does DPG in human Hbs, as well as at β135Arg and β139His, while CO_2 binds at the free N-terminal amino groups of α and β chains (Weber, 1995). Regulation of Hb function on a moment-to-moment basis by pH shifts (the Bohr and Root effects), by changes in organic phosphate concentrations,

or by changes in modulators such as chloride ions, is well known to physiologists and will not be explored in detail here. Less well known are studies on the role of nitric oxide (NO) in regulation of Hb transport; we will begin our discussion with this regulation process, since it interfaces between Hb molecular function per se and whole organism physiology.

NITRIC OXIDE AT THE INTERFACE OF ORGANISMAL AND MOLECULAR PHYSIOLOGY

As is well known to most physiologists interested in the control of tissue perfusion, decades of search for the elusive EDRF (endothelial derived relaxation factor) finally culminated in the discovery of a small gaseous molecule, nitric oxide or NO, which is now known to be a kind of universal vasodilator. Three isozymes of nitric oxide synthase (NOS) have been identified and both protein and genomic structures are now known. NOS I (nNOS, originally discovered in neurons) and NOS III (eNOS, generating the classical EDRF, originally discovered in endothelial cells) are low-output, Ca^{2+}-activated enzymes whose physiological function is signal transduction. NOS II (inducible or iNOS originally discovered in cytokine-activated macrophages) is a high-output, largely Ca^{2+}-independent enzyme that produces toxic amounts of NO; this end product represents perhaps the single most important component of the antimicrobial, antiparasitic, and antineoplastic activities of these cells. Interestingly, within species (e.g. humans) the three isozymes show only about 59% identity, while between species comparisons of isozyme homologs show more than 90% sequence conservation for NOS I and III and about 80% conservation for NOS II comparisions. All NOS isoforms produce NO by oxidizing a guanidinium nitrogen of L-arginine utilizing molecular oxygen and NADPH as cosusbtrates; all isoforms contain FAD, FMN, and heme iron as prosthetic groups and require the cofactor BH-4. NOS I function in the central nervous system is highly complex and beyond the scope of our analysis. The classical NOS II functions in defense against bacteria, parasites, or neoplastic cells and NOS III functions in endothelial-derived NO regulation of vascular tone are well described in many modern physiology textbooks and need not concern us further in this context. In 1998, three scientists shared a Nobel Prize for their work on these kinds of NO functions. Since then, another insight of major biological and physiological significance is that arising from Stamler and his coworkers (Stamler et al., 1997) who have demonstrated an important NO transport function of Hb which they postulate serves to facilitate O_2 transport. The workings of this control system are elegant and complex. At the lungs the binding of O_2 to heme irons in Hb promotes the binding of NO to cysteine93 on the β chain, forming nitrosohemoglobin. Deoxygenation is accompanied by an allosteric transition in S-nitrosoHb from the R (oxygenated) to the T (deoxygenated) state that releases NO, making it available for vasodilation at physiologically appropriate times. By thus sensing the physiological O_2 gradient in tissues, Hb exploits conformation-associated changes in the position of cysteineβ93 SNO to bring local blood flow into line with O_2 requirements. In essence, in this regulatory system, Hb serves as an O_2 and a nitric oxide carrier with the latter, on release, serving to vasodilate (to increase flow and thus more O_2 delivery to) the most O_2-needy tissues or most O_2-needy regions of tissues. While a lot remains to be clarified in the details of Hb NO interactions, it is hard to imagine a more refined control system for interfacing whole organism physiology with molecular physiology than this (Gross and Lane, 1999). In view of these interesting findings, the reader will not be surprised to find that so versatile a macromolecule as Hb is adapted for specific functions through phylogenetic times. Interestingly, so far no one has examined interspecies environmental adaptations of NO binding; all of the work in this area to date has focused largely on other, mainly O_2 transport functions of this respiratory pigment.

Indeed, as a carrier of O_2 from lungs to tissues, Hb has long been the subject of intense research by comparative biochemists and evolutionary physiologists. The role of Glu6B → Val replacement in affording heterozygotes at least some defense against malaria, while causing homozygotes to suffer a debilitating anemia, supplies a classic example of microadaptation in the human species. Yet there is more, much more, to the evolution of Hbs than this well-publicized case. In fact the literature on the comparative biochemistry of Hbs is so large that we can only supply a very limited summary of examples which illustrate basic principles of evolution and adaptation of this important physiological system.

HEMOGLOBIN ADAPTATIONS: HIGH-ALTITUDE MAMMALS

It has been known since the 1930s that Hbs in high-altitude animals typically display unusually high O_2 affinities and the camelids of the high Andes supply one of the quintessential examples of this phenomenon. The camelid family comprises six species, two of which are lowland animals (the camels of Asia and Africa) and four of which live at altitudes of 2,000–5,000 m in the Andes (the guanaco, the llama, the alpaca, and the vicuña). The first camelids appeared at the end of the Eocene period in Northern America where they differentiated into separate species, then dispersed either to South America or to central Asia, then more recently to the Middle East and Africa. The P_{50} values for all six species are in the range of 17–22 torr, low compared to other mammals such as humans (26 torr). However, within the camelids per se the high-altitude species display Hbs with higher O_2 affinities than in the Asian or African camels and the molecular basis for this effect is attributed to the β chains. In fact, sequence and Hb functional analyses lead to the following conclusions: (i) Compared to other lowland mammals, all members of the camelid family exhibit a higher than usual O_2 affinity, suggesting they are derived from ancestors with Hbs displaying high O_2 affinities as well. The basis for the high-O_2-affinity ancestral Hb is to be found in the numerous substitutions per dimer between camelids and other lowland species (human HbA is usually used as a reference in these studies). (ii) The high O_2 affinity of the Andean camelids is probably related to a

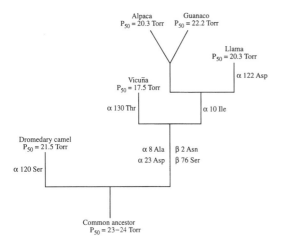

Figure 3.6. A simplified phylogenetic tree for low- and high-altitude camelids based on the α and β chains of Hb. Mutational events postulated to occur at the successive steps are indicated, along with the functional consequences (change in P_{50} value or O_2 affinity). (Modified from Poyart et al., 1992.)

His → Asn substitution in the β chains, which suppresses two DPG binding sites per tetramer. (iii) In this group, the vicuña exhibits the highest O_2 affinity of all these species, which is thought to be due to an Ala → Thr substitution at $\alpha130$ and a His → Asn change at $\beta2$ (Clementi et al., 1994). (iv) The globin chains of the guanaco and the alpaca have identical sequences which may represent the ancestral sequences for the lama, alpaca, and guanaco. (v) Based on these amino acid substitutions, workers in this field generally accept the evolutionary path for Hb within the camelid family shown in figure 3.6. The key insight is that only a few mutations affecting a few key residues are sufficient to adapt the functional properties of Hb to severely hypoxic conditions of the high Andes (Poyart et al., 1992).

HEMOGLOBIN ADAPTATIONS: HIGH-ALTITUDE BIRDS

Because of their super-efficient lungs (one-way air flow), birds are sometimes thought to be in a sense preadapted for hypoxia, but within this group the high-soaring hawks, eagles, and vultures are particularly noteworthy. Anecdotal reports from airline pilots indicate that some African vultures have been observed at altitudes used by modern jets! Rippon's griffon, one such species that can fly at 11.3 km altitudes, contains four Hbs rather than the usual one or two typical of low-altitude birds. These Hbs, termed HbA, HbA′, HbD, and HbD′, exhibit cascaded O_2 affinities, HbA showing the lowest O_2 affinity, HbD′ showing the highest O_2 affinity. This differentiation is consistent with an $\alpha34$ substitution that stabilizes the T structure in HbA, or an $\alpha38$ substitution that stabilizes the R structure in D/D homozygote vultures—molecular adaptations suggesting effective RBC O_2 loading and unloading functions over a broad range of O_2 tensions (Weber, 1995).

High-flying migrating waterfowl represent another interesting source of information on how Hb function can be adapted for high-altitude function. Of these, the bar-headed goose is especially interesting. This species migrates over Mount Everest at altitudes exceeding 9 km where the O_2 partial pressure is only about 30% of that at sea level. The high affinity required for this kind of feat could be achieved by changes in metabolite modulators, but the concentrations of organophosphates (especially of IPP) in the bar-headed goose is in the normal range. Instead the bar-headed goose relies upon a Hb with intrinsically higher O_2 affinities than in sea-level species such as the graylag goose; secondarily and most importantly, these affinity differences are highly exaggerated in the presence of effector molecules such as chloride ions.

Examination of amino acid sequences in bar-headed goose Hb compared to graylag goose Hb indicates three changes in the α chain and only one change in the β chain. Of these, a Pro → Ala at position 119 of the α chain is unique among bird Hb sequences and is thought to be a critical adaptation in the bar-headed goose. The Ala replacement removes an important van der Waals contact between the $\alpha1$ and $\beta1$ subunits, and facilitates shifting the equilibrium from the low-affinity T state toward the high-affinity R state, an interpretation confirmed by X-ray crystallography studies showing elimination of this critical subunit–subunit interaction in the Hb of the bar-headed goose (see Golding and Dean, 1998). The Andean goose (which is actually a duck!) also lives at high altitude (in the 6 km range) and it also has a Hb with a high O_2 affinity. Sequence studies of its Hb indicated that its high affinity arises as a consequence of a Leu → Ser replacement at position 55 of the β chain, which removes the same intersubunit contact as the α chain Pro → Ala substitution at position 119, but this time from the opposite subunit. It is remarkable that single point mutations—obviously representing phylogenetically independent origins (figure 3.7)—occurred affecting the same contact site but on different globin chains in these two geographically widely separated species.

Finally, to test the hypothesis that α chain Pro → Ala or β chain Leu → Ser replacements are singly sufficient to shift the equilibrium

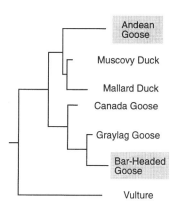

Figure 3.7. A simplified phylogenetic tree showing the distant relationship between the bar-headed goose and the Andean goose, both of which have independently evolved high-affinity Hbs. A mutational event in the evolution of the bar-headed goose led to elimination from the α side of a key interaction between the α and β chains; a high-affinity Hb suitable for high-altitude function was the physiological consequence. In the Andean goose, this key contact between α and β chains was eliminated from the β side; thus a different molecular solution to the problem of requiring a high-affinity Hb was used in the two species. (Modified from Golding and Dean, 1998.)

from the low-affinity T state toward the high-affinity R state, site-directed mutagenesis was used to insert the former into the α chain of human HbA (70% identical to goose globins). Reconstituted tetramers were found to have O_2 affinities that, in the presence of chloride and DPG (the human equivalent of IPP in birds) exceeded normal human Hb by a factor greater than that observed between bar-headed and graylag geese.

In parallel studies, engineering Ser into position 55 of the human Hb β chain also resulted in increased O_2 affinity, notably without measurable disruption of any other functional properties of the novel Hb and without any other X-ray crystallographically measurable effects on Hb structure (see Golding and Dean, 1998).

HEMOGLOBIN ADAPTATIONS: MAMMALIAN FETUS

In the placenta of mammals, a higher O_2 affinity of the fetal blood relative to that of maternal blood favors the transfer of O_2 from mother to fetus. Significantly higher O_2 affinity of the fetal blood is found almost universally among mammals (Poyart et al., 1992), but the combination of mechanisms accounting for this characteristic vary in different species. These mechanisms fall into three distinct categories depending on whether the fetus has a fetal Hb (HbF or $\alpha_2\gamma_2$) or the adult Hb (HbA or $\alpha_2\beta_2$).

In the first group (HbF and DPG present in RBCs), the high O_2 affinity of the fetal blood is based on a partial loss of the regulatory effect of DPG. In human HbF, this results from the replacement of the $\beta143$ (H21) histidine, one of the DPG binding sites, by a serine in the γ chains. Also in this kind of Hb, the N-terminal NA1γ is a glycine, which is partially acetylated and therefore unable to bind DPG well; this further weakens the DPG-HbF complex and also contributes to developing a higher O_2 affinity.

In the second group, illustrated by ruminants, an HbF evolved with a significantly higher O_2 affinity than that of the adult Hb. The bovine fetal subunit differs from the adult bovine β chain at 23 positions and these substitutions are probably responsible for the increase in intrinsic O_2 affinity. As in adult Hb, the residues involved in DPG binding are missing at the N-terminal sequence, indicating that the bovine fetal subunit evolved from the bovine β chain rather than from the γ chain "ancestor" of other HbFs in other species. At birth, calf RBCs contain DPG at relatively high concentrations, which decrease over the first two weeks in parallel with the switch from fetal to adult Hb. Additionally, the transitory high [DPG] coincides with a lowered intracellular pH, which in turn lowers the O_2 affinity in RBCs of the newly born ruminant through the Bohr effect.

Finally, in the third mammlian grouping (dog, horse, rabbit, seal, swine), the fetal Hb is not expressed. In these species, even without HbF, the O_2 affinity of fetal blood is kept higher than that of the adult. This difference is achieved by means of low concentrations of RBC DPG in the fetus and by higher-than-usual concentrations of DPG in the RBCs of adults. In most of these species, this fetal–adult difference in RBC DPG concentration is due to an enhanced catalytic capacity of the terminal part of the glycolytic path (indexed by pyruvate kinase activity, for example), which increases DPG flux towards pyruvate and lactate (see Poyart et al., 1992).

HEMOGLOBIN ADAPTATIONS: HYPOXIA-TOLERANT FISHES

Because of the impressive diversity of fish species, the numbers of Hb studies and hypoxia adaptations in this group are inordinately large. As in the examples above, the most fundamental adaptation level is Hb structure, a primary determinant of Hb function. This is well illustrated by the high O_2 affinity frequently observed in hypoxia-tolerant fishes and low intrinsic O_2 affinity in active fish living in well-aerated water. Within any specific species, the transport of O_2 (and of CO_2 and protons, for that matter) can then be modulated (i) by changes in [Hb] usually by changes in hematocrit, (ii) by changes in concentrations of allosteric regulators, and (iii) by changes in the

expression of Hb isoforms with different functional properties. As in our discussion of this problem area in mammals and birds, we will not further discuss change in RBC mass as a means for improving O_2 delivery capacity, but the other two processes need further evaluation.

FISH Hb: METABOLITE OR ION REGULATORS DURING HYPOXIA

The major metabolite regulators of fish Hbs are probably organic phosphates and protons. The commonest phosphate metabolite regulators are nucleotide triphosphates (NTPs) such as ATP and GTP, but some species (the air-breathing Osteoglossid, *Arapaima gigas*, for example) utilize IPP and still others, DPG. It has been known since the 1960s that hypoxia leads to down-regulation of NTP concentrations in fish (nucleated) RBCs. The response is graded according to severity of hypoxia and new steady-state NTP concentrations may not be established for hours, or even days. Presumably because of frequent exposure to environmental hypoxia, Amazon fishes supply quintessential examples of this kind of Hb functional adaptation (Val, 1996). The decrease in NTP content raises blood O_2 affinity directly through decreased interaction between O_2 binding sites (left shifting the O_2 equilibrium curve and lowering the n coefficient), and indirectly via the Bohr effect (increased pH caused by adjustments to stabilize the membrane electrochemical gradient). The O_2 affinity increase elevates arterial %HbO_2 and blood O_2 capacitance under hypoxia, thus contributing to a reduction in the ventilatory requirements. ATP is the common Hb modulator in some species (trout, plaice, dogfish), while others (such as eel, carp, goldfish, tench, and lungfish) also have high GTP concentrations. When both Hb regulators are present, GTP usually exerts a greater regulatory role than does ATP (expressed as a greater decrease in concentration compared to ATP under hypoxia, as a greater allosteric effect, and as a lesser inhibition of its effect by Mg^{2+} complexing). Interestingly, the decrease in RBC [NTP] is universal among fishes, found even in Antarctic fish species, which are unlikely ever to encounter environmental hypoxia. This observation encourages the view that the hypoxic regulation of [NTP] is a conservative trait acquired early in the evolution of fishes. During early evolution of fishes, atmospheric O_2 and fish RBC [NTP] both may have been low; as environmental O_2 availability increased, natural selection may have favored an increase in RBC [NTP] in order to maintain the P_{50} at appropriate values (Val, 1996; Jensen et al., 1998).

In addition to ATP and GTP, other phosphate metabolites that are found in the RBCs of species such as Amazon fishes include DPG, IP2 (inositol diphosphate), IPP, and IHP. In general the effects of these compounds on fish Hb functions decrease in the following order: IHP, IPP, GTP, ATP, DPG. At this time, unfortunately, there is very little information on details of the evolution of these interesting Hb modulators. Why an air-breathing fish such as *Arapaima* should utilize IPP, while another air breather, a catfish (which uses its stomach as a gas exchange organ), stores DPG in its RBCs and still other species rely only upon NTPs, are issues that remain poorly or not at all understood (Val, 1996).

How or where hypoxia is sensed to allow these adjustments also remains somewhat of a mystery, since the response to environmental O_2 limitation is not the same as for O_2 limitation imposed by strenuous swimming. Whereas regulation of RBC NTP concentration is a universal mechanism for regulating the P_{50} of fish Hbs during hypoxia, the RBC [NTP] remains largely unchanged when the O_2 shortage is due to overexertion. However, it is possible that in the latter case, changes in RBC volume become the dominant mechanism for changing the effective intracellular NTP concentration. The hyperventilation that occurs under these conditions in essence "blows off" CO_2 and thus causes an initial relative alkalosis, with passive redistribution of H^+ and other ions leading to cell swelling. At least at early stages of physical exertion, when O_2 may become limiting, this would lead to an effective decrease in NTP concentration and hence a left shift in the Hb saturation curve (increase in O_2 affinity), as in environmental hypoxia. This phenomenon can be readily shown under controlled experimental conditions (Jensen et al., 1998).

ROLE OF FISH Hb ISOFORMS

Many and perhaps most mammals, including humans, typically express a single main Hb component in their RBCs. Fishes, in contrast, commonly exhibit multiple Hb components, many of which are products of different genes and are termed Hb isoforms, analogous to isozymes in the enzyme field (some Hb isoforms can also be formed during post-transcriptional modification). This field has been well explored (see Jensen et al., 1998). Suffice at this point to emphasize that it is possible to categorize fish according to their Hb isoforms. Class I comprises species that express electrophoretically anodal Hbs that display relatively normal Bohr, Root, phosphate, and temperature effects. Class II includes fish species that express anodal Hbs (properties as in Class I Hbs) and that express cathodal Hbs, exhibiting exceptionally high O_2 affinities and small, even reverse Bohr effects (whereby high O_2 affinity is achieved despite low pH), and exhibiting low thermal sensitivities. Class III refers to fish species that express Hbs that are sensitive to pH (i.e., normal Bohr effect) but relatively insensitive to temperature; a particularly good example of this is found in tuna, which of course display regional heterothermy and in which thermally independent Hb function prevents the unwanted unloading of O_2 on passage through the rete from cold to warm regions of the animal's body (Jensen et al., 1998).

We have known since the 1970s (Powers, 1972) that the occurrence of cathodal Hbs in catfish species appears to be linked with occupation of fast-flowing streams where frequent bouts of activity-induced acidosis and hypoxia would unload anodal Hbs. Fitting this paradigm is the observation of apparently ubiquitous presence of cathodal Hbs in active species such as salmonids and apparently equally ubiquitous absence of cathodal Hbs in relatively inactive or sluggish species such as flatfish (Weber, 1995). Complete sequencing of the eel cathodal Hb has allowed Weber and his associates (Fago et al., 1995) to work out plausible structural explanations for the reverse Bohr effect plus some of its other unique regulatory properties. Parallel studies on eel anodal Hb (Fago et al., 1997) showed that a very large Bohr effect involved the O_2 linked binding of a large number of protons (7–8 H^+ per O_2) in the presence of GTP. What is more these studies go a long way towards a structural explanation for the Root effect in this anodal Hb, which the eel relies upon for O_2 unloading into the swim bladder against exceptionally large O_2 concentration gradients.

LESSONS LEARNED FROM Hb MOLECULAR ADAPTATION STUDIES

The above studies of Hb adaptations assisting survival of fishes, mammals, and birds under sometimes severe hypoxia are highly instructive and lead to several important generalizations: (i) Major shifts in a key physiological function such as loading or unloading can be achieved by one to a few mutations. (ii) Adaptive amino acid replacements may or may not be solely confined to active (i.e., substrate or modulator binding) sites (which means that a common assumption—that amino acid replacements far from active sites must be selectively neutral—is wrong or at least is misleading and incomplete). This is clearly illustrated by the Pro → Ala and the Leu → Ser replacements in the α and β chains of the bar-headed and the graylag geese, respectively, since both of these are remote to the heme O_2 binding site, yet they bring about the required increase in O_2 affinity that is basic to high-altitude operations for these species. (iii) Different solutions (different amino acid substitutions) can be used to achieve the same functional adjustment and to compensate for the same environmental and evolutionary challenge. Again this is well illustrated in the bar-headed and graylag geese studies, showing that the two species solve the problem of improving affinity by different mutations in different genes. The bar-headed goose eliminates the subunit contacts from the α side, while the Andean goose eliminates the same contact from the β side, while a still different suite of replace-

ments at the $\alpha1\beta1$ and $\alpha2\beta2$ Hb subunit interfaces confer high O_2 affinities in vultures that can soar to very high (10–11 km) altitudes (Golding and Dean, 1998). We will see in later chapters that these kinds of evolutionary rules apply widely in animal adaptations to their environment and that these kinds of processes appear over and over again in nature.

RESPIRATORY PIGMENTS AND HYPOXIA ADAPTATIONS IN INVERTEBRATES

Invertebrates use a variety of proteins for the purposes of O_2 storage and transport. As already mentioned above, Hbs are ancient and not surprisingly are found expressed to at least some degree in almost all phyla, where they take on an almost infinite variety of structures. Although the "globin fold" is a common motif, this can be found as individual subunits, as linked subunits, and as extremely large aggregates of globins. Hemoglobins are the primary carriers of O_2 among the annelids; and, while not as common, they are found in other phyla as well. A number of phyla, notably sipunculids, brachiopods, priapulids, and a few annelids bind O_2 via a nonheme iron protein called hemerythrin (Hr). Occurring as single-chain proteins, they are used in associated forms as blood O_2 carriers; when in muscle they are called myoHrs and are used much as Mb is used in vertebrate systems (more on this below). Two phyla, Arthropods and the Molluscs, employ copper proteins called hemocyanins as their principal transport mechanism. Arthropod hemocyanin (Hc) exhibits little sequence homology or structural similarity with Molluscan Hc. However, their O_2 binding sites are similar in the two groups, with O_2 being bound between a pair of copper atoms in both kinds of Hc. Interestingly, Hc occurs free in solution (not in specialized blood cells as the case of Hbs in RBCs of vertebrates) and all Hc forms are very large molecules, consisting of from a few to a dozen or more subunits, all or most of which carry O_2 binding sites. Arthropod Hcs are built up from hexameric aggregates of about 70 kD subunit chains, typically with one O_2 binding site on each sub-unit. Molluscan Hcs, in contrast are constructed from much larger subunits each carrying seven or eight binding sites. Current concepts propose that most invertebrate respiratory proteins (with the exception of Hb) evolved as O_2 carriers after the initial branchings of the major invertebrate phyla, almost certainly in pre-Cambrian times (van Holde, 1998).

Although the above brief summary indicates a rapidly expanding field of invertebrate respiratory pigments, even a cursory examination of the literature makes it clear that much less is known about regulatory details of O_2 transport in these groups. However, it appears that Hc affinities for O_2 are regulated. On a short-term basis, modulators such as pH, lactate, specific cations, and other metabolites alter Hc affinity in such a way as to compensate for variations in O_2 supply on a moment-by-moment basis, both for the Arthropod Hcs (e.g., see Morris and Callaghan, 1998; Reiber, 1995) and Molluscan Hcs (e.g., see Taylor et al., 1995). Similarly, it is well established that Hc affinity for O_2 is fine tuned by evolutionary processes (presumably by sequence adjustments as described above for Hbs); species naturally encountering hypoxic conditions display Hcs that have higher O_2 affinities than found in species living under normoxic conditions (Reiber, 1995). However, unlike the Hb examples given above, the evolution of Hc structures and functions within specific lineages are studies that remain to be completed.

MYOGLOBINS: INTRACELLULAR O_2 STORAGE AND TRANSFER MECHANISMS

Cells and tissues that must sustain very large magnitude swings between basal and maximal metabolism face a serious problem of O_2 delivery from the plasmalemma boundary to the mitochondria. It has long been known that in vertebrates such tissues express and maintain an intracellular respiratory pigment, termed myoglobin or Mb. Mb is a single polypeptide chain, about 16,000 molecular weight, which is analo-gous to a single Hb subunit. As mentioned above, O_2 saturation curves for Hbs are typically sigmoidal, while O_2 saturation curves for Mbs are hyperbolic. As far as we know, Mb O_2 loading and unloading is unregulated and the only means we are aware of for changing Mb function is to increase or decrease the amounts expressed. Mb is thought to play several important physiological functions. First and foremost, it is thought to serve as a bucket brigade for O_2 transfer from the cell boundary to the mitochondria. Secondly, it is thought to speed up the rate of this transfer through faciliated O_2 diffusion; basically, diffusion of MbO_2 supplies an alternate path for, and thus augments, O_2 diffusion to the mitochondria. Thirdly, it has been proposed that MbO_2 serves in the channeling or direct transfer of O_2 to cytochrome oxidase; maximum state 3 rates of mitochondrial O_2 consumption can be shown to be about 30% higher in the presence, than in the absence, of Mb. Fourthly, because Mb O_2 binding is an equilibrium reaction, and because Mb is randomly distributed in muscle cells, it has been proposed that a key function may well be to assure similar O_2 concentrations in all parts of the cell. Because Mb and MbO_2 are both detectable in vivo by modern ^1H magnetic resonance spectroscopy (MRS), it has been possible to show that $\%MbO_2$ and hence $[O_2]$ are both remarkably stable under widely varying work rates, observations leading to renewed interest in the physiological roles of this fascinating molecule (see Hochachka, 1999, for more on this topic).

There are two additional postulated Mb functions that should be mentioned. First, Mb may serve as a simple intracellular O_2 store. In muscles of marine mammals, Mb occurs at 8–12 times higher concentrations than in muscles of most other species, and it is in these kinds of settings that Mb is thought to play an intracellular O_2 storage function (Hochachka and Foreman, 1994). Additionally, there is a linear relationship between the anaerobic capacity of muscles (as indicated by the amounts of lactate dehydrogenase, or LDH, that they contain) and their Mb content. This relationship probably arises because protons generated by anaerobic glycolysis may be buffered by intracellular Mb, an hypothesis first put forth by Castellini, M.A. and Somero, G.N. and which we consider plausible because of a linear relationship between Mb content and empirically measured buffering capacity of muscles (see Hochachka and Somero, 1984 for literature in this area).

PARALLELS IN ORIGINS OF MOLLUSCAN Mbs AND THE ORIGINS OF HEMOCYANINS

While a few invertebrate species have muscles with globin-based Mbs that are homologous with vertebrate Mbs, most invertebrate muscles are not known to contain *any* Mbs. In fact, for most invertebrate phyla, the literature is silent on the question of intracellular respiratory pigments. To many workers in the field (including ourselves) this has been a prickly and perplexing mystery. In at least one group of gastropod molluscs, the problem seems to have been solved as a result of studies probing the origins of respiratory pigments in these invertebrates. The first instructive insight comes from studies

of Hc origins: on the basis of multiple sequence alignments, workers in this field have concluded that arthropod Hc subunits, insect hexamerin subunits, and tyrosinases (O_2-binding enzymes catalyzing the first step in tyrosine catabolism) are all closely related. These studies suggest that the origin of Hc was from ancient tyrosinase-like proteins, while insect hexamerins probably evolved from Hcs (Burmester, 2001; Burmester and Sheller, 1996). A fascinating parallelism is evident in current research into molluscan myoglobins by Suzuki et al. (1998) showing that gastropods display a muscle Mb that is evolutionarily derived from indoleamine 2,3-dioxygenase, an O_2-binding enzyme catalyzing an early step in tryptophan catabolism. Sequence studies have allowed Suzuki et al. (1998) to explore the evolutionary path of this Mb, which appears to have its origins over 200 million years ago within the gastropod lineage (figure 3.8). Additionally, their isolation and characterization studies indicate that this molluscan Mb shows all the functional properties of any typical vertebrate Mb, including reversible O_2 binding and similar P_{50} values. Presumably,

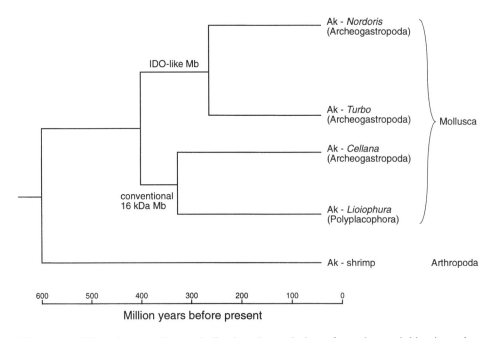

Figure 3.8. A simplified phylogenetic tree indicating the evolution of novel myoglobins in archeogastropod molluscs. Phylogenetic relationships of indoleamine 2,3-dioxygenases or IDOs, IDO-like myglobins, and a shrimp homolog are indicated. (Summary modified from Suzuki et al., 1998.)

therefore, all the functions of vertebrate Mbs mentioned above apply equally well to these molluscan Mbs. Interestingly, these molluscan Mbs all retain a tryptophan binding site, and even express a residual catalytic oxygenase activity from which the Mb reversible O_2 binding function arose.

Whereas these studies solve the problem of intracellular muscle Mbs in this unique phylogenetic group, Suzuki et al. report that this Mb is not present even in relatively closely related cephalopods. Thus the mystery of the missing Mbs in muscles of (especially active) invertebrate groups remains thus far largely unresolved.

WHEN PHYSIOLOGICAL HYPOXIA DEFENSE LINES ARE BREACHED

All of the above respiratory pigment-based mechanisms for adjusting O_2 loading at gas exchange organs, and O_2 unloading at the tissues, serve to calibrate O_2 delivery as a function of O_2 availability. They work well so long as the challenges of O_2 limitation (due to environmental hypoxia, tissue-work-related hypoxia, or tissue ischemia) are not too severe. In other words, these are effective adaptations for aerobic organisms in an aerobic world. However, even within this sphere, systems sometimes become so severely O_2 limited that these physiological lines of defense on their own are simply unable to compensate for the O_2 deficit. To maximize the effectiveness of the above physiological-level hypoxia defense adjustments, all organisms, but especially hypoxia-tolerant species, integrate these processes with back-up biochemical lines of defense against hypoxia. As already mentioned above, some organisms are particularly effective in expressing these back-up mechanisms and thus in surviving extreme O_2-limiting kinds of episodes (or surviving in O_2-limited kinds of environments).

FERMENTABLE FUELS IN HYPOXIA TOLERANCE

Studies of such species (some of which are so anoxia tolerant they are referred to as "facultative" anaerobes [Storey and Hochachka, 1974]) have revealed several molecular and metabolic level strategies of hypoxia adaptation that are widely used. The first of these is a metabolic organization supplying provision for suitable substrates and for their regulated utilization, so that internal stores are not depleted and energy needs of various tissues and organs during O_2 limitation can be matched by substrate availability. In most species the main fermentable fuel is glycogen, which is usually stored in a central depot (liver in vertebrates; mantle and/or hepatopancreas in bivalves), and which supplies the body's bulk needs for glucose. In addition, some amino acids can be fermented to augment the synthesis of ATP in glycogen (glucose) fermentation. Because of the energetic inefficiency of glycolysis, quantitatively large advantages would accrue to those organisms that were able to extend the anoxic survival time on a given amount of glycogen or glucose. To this end, strong selective pressure seems to have led to two main solutions: the first, and conceptually more simple mechanism, involves metabolic suppression. A 10- or 20-fold reduction in ATP turnover during anoxia means a tissue could extend its survival time on glucose or glycogen fermentation by a similar 10- or 20-fold (this obvious strategy is so widely used that workers in this field consider metabolic suppression in anoxia as a sine qua non of a "good" animal anaerobe (more on this below)). In many animals, a second solution for extending the usefulness of glycogen (glucose) stores during anoxia involved the evolution of anaerobic metabolic systems with improved ATP yield.

ENERGETICALLY IMPROVED FERMENTATIONS

It is among the most capable of invertebrate anaerobes, the helminths and the marine bivalves, that we find the best examples of alternative fermentation pathways. Many of these have been reviewed several times elsewhere, so only a brief summary will be considered here. Current concepts view the organization of anaerobic metabolism as a series of linear, and loosely linked, pathways. The most important of these, aside from classical glucose → lactate fermentation (yielding 2 moles ATP per mole glucose) are summarized by Hochachka and Somero (1984) as follows (see chapter 2):

1. glucose → octopine, lysopine, alanopine, or strombine, energy yield 2 moles ATP per mole glucose;
2. glucose → succinate, energy yield 4 moles ATP per mole glucose;
3. glucose → propionate, energy yield 6 moles ATP per mole glucose;
4. aspartate → succinate, energy yield 1 mole ATP per mole aspartate;
5. aspartate → propionate, energy yield 2 moles ATP per mole aspartate;
6. glutamate → succinate, energy yield 1 mole ATP per mole glutamate;
7. glutamate → propionate, energy yield 2 moles ATP per mole glutamate;
8. branched chain amino acids → volatile fatty acids, energy yield 1 mole ATP per mole substrate;
9. glucose → acetate, energy yield 4 moles ATP per mole glucose;
10. $CH_2O + SO_4^{2-} + H^+ \rightarrow H_2S + HS^- + H_2O + CO_2$, energy yield 6 moles ATP per mole glucose.

Pathways 1–4 are known in various bivalve molluscs; 2, 3, 8, and 9 are often utilized by helminths; 5, 6, and 7, while theoretically possible in bivalve molluscs, do not appear to be utilized to any significant extent. Pathway 10, or sulfate oxidation of organic substrates, is well known to occur in the highly reduced layers of benthic silt, but the distribution of this activity between bacteria and lower invertebrate animals is not yet clarified. Since both groups of organisms coexist in what has been termed a "sulfur–sulfide biome" and since both bacteria and at least some invertebrates have the enzymes required for sulfate and sulfide metabolism, we tentatively assume that both contribute to the observed sulfate reduction in benthic sediments (see Hochachka and Somero, 1984).

In this kind of environment, H_2S, which is toxic to most organisms, may accumulate to poisonous concentrations. Interestingly, through evolutionary time numerous aquatic animal species have developed mechanisms for surviving sulfide exposure. One such mechanism involves oxidation of the sulfide, which results mainly in thiosulfate. In a small subset of species, sulfide oxidation is localized in the mitochondria and is coupled to ATP synthesis. The reader must realize, however, that the formation of thiosulfate requires oxygen, which means that these species must be found in regions which contain both O_2 and H_2S (these two gases cannot co-exist at thermodynamic equilibrium, so these organisms rely upon environments that are in a steady state with both O_2 and H_2S present). In such species, if not all sulfide is detoxified, cytochrome c oxidase is inhibited, and a sulfide-dependent anaerobic energy metabolism is turned on (Grieshaber and Volkel, 1998). One of the most successful of organisms capable of thriving in environments containing high concentrations of sulfide is a marine oligochaete, *Tubificoides benedii* (Griere et al., 1999). However, it is dominant invertebrate organisms in hydrothermal vent environments (organisms such as *Riftia*, a giant tube worm or Pogonophoran) that supply the most famous examples of animals whose biology is primed by sulfide oxidation (see Zierenberg et al., 2001), with much of the energy flowing into this large and complex ecosystem being based on intracellular symbionts.

Except for systems using sulfate as an electron acceptor to facilitate the oxidation of organic substrates, the potential for which is not well understood, there is reasonable agreement concerning the pathways by which most of the above end products are formed. For example, in many invertebrates (parasitic helminths, polychaetes, sipunculids, bivalves, cephalopods, gastropods, and probably many other groups as well, PEP functions at a distinct metabolic branchpoint (figure 3.9). PEP carboxykinase (PEPCK) catalyzes carboxylation of PEP to form oxaloacetate, from which ultimately succinate and propionate can be formed. Under other circumstances and in other species (particularly molluscs), PEP is converted to pyruvate, which, depending upon species, or tissue, can be converted into one of several kinds of end products (Schmidt and Kamp, 1996). We should also emphasize that end products such as octopine, alanopine, strombine, and lysopine and the enzymes forming them are formally analogous to, and serve the same functions as, lactate and lactate dehydrogenase in humans: they serve as hydrogen and carbon sinks to maintain redox balance during anaerobic metabolism.

In the reaction path from succinate to propionate in helminths and bivalves, there is still uncertainty as to the way in which CoA is handled and the reaction actually utilized for releasing propionate; in helminths available evidence favors a terminal CoA-transferase step (figure 3.5). Whatever its route, the fermentation of glucose (glycogen) to propionate in bivalves such as *Mytilus* takes on greater importance in long-duration anoxia. The energy yield to the level of succinate is considered maximally at 4 moles ATP per mole glucose, and if the reaction scheme to propionate in figure 3.9 is assumed, the yield rises to a theoretical maximum of 6 moles ATP per mole glucose. The sites of ATP formation involve substrate-level phosphorylations (PGK and PEPCK) to the level of fumarate, plus an electron-transfer-based ATP synthesis at the level of fumarate reductase. The final site of ATP formation in propionate fermentation occurs at the carboxylase reaction (see figure 3.9).

The general pathways for volatile fatty acid (VFA) formation seem to involve three phases:

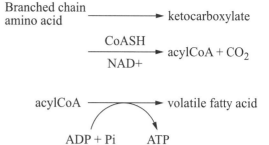

with the last thiokinase step potentially capable of generating 1 mole of ATP per mole of VFA generated. These reactions are not major contributors to ATP yield in most animal anaerobes, but in *Fasciola* they are, probably primarily through being linked to glucose fermentation to propionate. In this situation, overall energy yield in these species can theoretically reach 8 moles ATP per mole glucose plus 2 moles leucine or other branched-chain amino acid utilized.

In oyster heart, in *Mytilus*, and other bivalves as well, aspartate occurs at high (about $15 \, \mu\text{mol g}^{-1}$) concentrations in the normoxic state. In anoxia (figure 3.9) the bulk of the aspartate is fermented to succinate, a process that is particularly important during early states of anoxia. At this time, it is probably redox-coupled to glycolysis. Thus the energy yield increases by 1 mole ATP per mole aspartate fermented to succinate, or by 2 moles ATP per mole aspartate if the fermentation continues to the level of propionate, and the maximum total energy yield becomes 8 moles ATP per mole glucose plus aspartate fermented to propionate.

From the above discussion, it is evident that anaerobic metabolism in many animals can be far more versatile than commonly observed in higher vertebrates and that this raises the possibility of utilizing energetically more efficient fermentations. Estimating how much more efficient than anaerobic glycolysis is complicated by the observation that different combinations of pathways can be utilized at different times in anoxia.

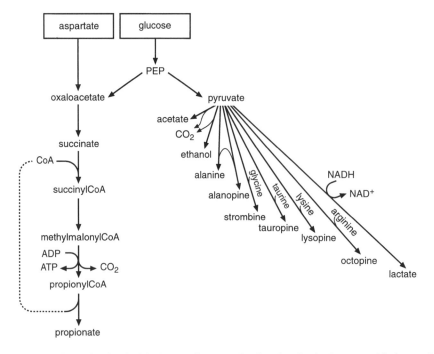

Figure 3.9. The PEP branchpoint in bivalve molluscs and other facultatively anaerobic invertebrates.

But even if a combination of pathways usually is used, the ATP yield can nevertheless be elevated two- to fourfold; any animal anaerobes utilizing such fermentations therefore automatically reduce by a factor of two to four their anaerobic needs for glucose. Although impressive, this factor is still a long way from the order-of-magnitude difference between anaerobic glycolysis and oxidative glucose metabolism.

ANAEROBIC ENERGETIC EFFICIENCIES: ATP/SUBSTRATE OR ATP/H$^+$

In the above discussion, the energy yields of the different anaerobic pathways of metabolism are expressed in terms of moles of ATP per mole of substrate fermented. This is the traditional way to express the energetic efficiency of fermentations and for some purposes it is informative and useful. However, it is important to recall that in vivo these pathways are linked to ATP utilizing pathways (usually ATPases). At steady state, rates of ATP synthesis by these fermentations equal rates of ATP utilization. For classical glycolysis, for example

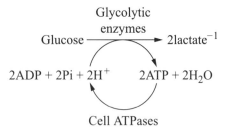

At steady state in vivo, the net reaction is glucose $\rightarrow$ 2lactate^{-1} + 2H$^+$, which is the equation of glycolysis familiar to most students in the field. Unfortunately this way of summarizing the in vivo situation underemphasizes that 2 moles of ATP were cycled through the two metabolic pathways to generate the summed equation. Since H$^+$ accumulation is in fact one of the hazards of anaerobiosis (minimizing acidification is another key defense adaptation against severe O$_2$ deprivation), perhaps a more instructive way of expressing energetic efficiency is in terms of moles ATP/H$^+$ formed. Thus for glucose $\rightarrow$ lactate fermentation, 1 μmol of ATP is turned over per μmol H$^+$ formed, assuming 1:1 coupling with ATPases. For glycogen → lactate fermentation 1.5 μmol of ATP are cycled per μmol H^+ formed. For glucose → succinate fermentation, 2 μmol ATP are cycled per μmol H^+ formed, while for glucose → propionate fermentation the value is 3. This second way of expressing the energetic efficiency of fermentations leads to the important insight; namely, that in adaptational terms, the main advantage gained by utilizing succinate or propionate fermentation in "good" animal anaerobes is being able to turn over up to three times more ATP per H^+ formed and accumulated than in the case of mammalian tissues relying solely upon classical glycolysis.

That is a considerable advantage, yet it does not fully overcome the problem of gradual acidification during anoxia; so other mechanisms must be employed. At least four such additional mechanisms for minimizing the problem of excessive acidification during anoxia are known: (i) The simplest solution is to minimize acidification by large suppressions in ATP turnover rates (more on this below). (ii) Another possibility is to tolerate high production rates by maintaining high buffering capacities of tissues and fluids. (iii) The severity of the problem can be reduced by detoxifying anaerobic end products through their metabolism at sites remote from sites of production; for example, anoxic goldfish and carp during severe hypoxia or anoxia produce lactate in many tissues, but instead of simply accumulating, this lactate is transferred to other sites (mainly white muscle) where it is converted first to pyruvate, then to ethanol, which can be easily released across the gills into the external water. And finally (iv), acidification can also be minimized by utilizing H^+-consuming reaction pathways; for example, under O_2 limitation in muscle AMP is converted to $IMP + NH_3$ and the latter is then protonated to NH_4^- consuming a proton in the process. Since H^+ concentration in these tissues is in the 10^{-7} range, while IMP can increase into the 5 mM range, it is evident that this represents a significant H^+ sink (see Hochachka and Somero, 1984, for literature in this area).

INCREASING YIELD OF ATP/O_2 IS ALSO AN EFFICIENCY ADJUSTMENT UNDER HYPOXIA

In all of the above examples, the activation of fermentation pathways becomes most significant when O_2 is completely lacking (i.e., under totally anoxic conditions). In nature, there are many situations in which the problem faced is not total anoxia, but grades of hypoxia or ischemia. Some examples of these kinds of problems will be discussed in detail below (see chapter 5). Still for the sake of completion we should mention that in this context tissues such as heart and skeletal muscles gain 25–50% more ATP/O_2 by preferentially using glucose instead of free fatty acids as the main carbon and energy source—and this is of considerable advantage when O_2 is in limiting supply.

THE EFFECTIVENESS OF DIFFERENT HYPOXIA DEFENSE MECHANISMS

In overview of the above discussion, we can conclude that two of the most significant hypoxia defense mechanisms found in the animal kingdom include (i) severe down-regulation of energy turnover (Hochachka, 1986, 1998; Storey and Storey, 1990), and (ii) up-regulation of energetic efficiency of ATP-producing pathways (Hochachka, 1993a). The latter involve stoichiometric efficiencies. In hypoxia adaptation, pathways which maximize the yield of ATP per mole oxygen are favored, while in anoxia adaptation, anaerobic pathways are favored which maximize the yield of ATP per mole of H^+ formed in the fermentation (Hochachka, 1993b). In hypoxia or anoxia adaptation, the ratio of anaerobic/aerobic metabolic potentials may well be up-regulated, coincident with up-regulation of glycogen (fermentable substrate) and of buffering capacities. Although all these mechanisms may be useful in surviving hypoxia, evaluation of such hypoxia defense strategies evolved by hypoxia-tolerant animals shows that suppression of energy turnover supplies the greatest protection against, and hence, advantage in, hypoxia. As already mentioned above, the immense advantage of this defense strategy is widely appreciated by many biologists (Guppy, et al., 1994; Hochachka and Guppy 1987; Jackson, 1968, 2000). In one of his last personal communications to one of the authors (PWH), just prior to his premature death, the great comparative physiologist, Kjell Johansen, referred to this strategy as "turning down to the pilot light" and he, like many earlier workers, was acutely aware of its relative importance. Although recognized as a kind of hallmark of reversible entry into and return from states of severe oxygen deprivation, a number of unexplained problems have remained. In particular, it has not been clear (i) how cells/tissues "know" when to turn on their hypoxia defense mechanisms, (ii) which pathways of ATP demand and ATP supply are down-regulated or by how much, (iii) how membrane electrochemical gradients are stabilized and (iv) what gene-expression and protein-expression level adjustments are involved in reorganization of cell structure and function under oxygen-limiting conditions. Studies of cells and tissues from a well-known vertebrate "facultative anaerobe," the aquatic turtle, have used brain cortical slices to probe electrophysiological properties of neurons under anoxia (see Doll, 1993; Doll et al., 1991, 1993, 1994; Lutz, 1992; Sick et al., 1993) and isolated liver hepatocytes (see Buck and Hochachka, 1993; Buck et al., 1993; Land and Bernier, 1995; Land and Hochachka, 1994; Land et al., 1993) to probe cell-level biochemical responses to anoxia. When integrated with independent lines of research at more integrated physiological levels, these studies supply the raw material required for a synthetic cell-level model or general hypothesis of hypoxia tolerance, which goes a long way to answering the above unresolved questions.

HOW CELLS "KNOW" WHEN OXYGEN BECOMES LIMITING

Traditionally, biologists' views of cell-level responses to O_2 limitation are formalized in the concept of the Pasteur effect: as ATP generation by oxidative phosphorylation begins to fall off due to oxygen lack, the energetic deficit is made up by activation of anaerobic ATP supply pathways (Schmidt and Kamp, 1996). In many mammalian cells, aerobic energy metabolism remains constant over wide O_2 concentrations, a metabolic response pattern termed "oxygen regulation." In most and probably all hypoxia-tolerant systems, O_2 consumption rates follow concentrations over equally broad ranges. The apparent $K_m(O_2)$ is low in O_2 regulators and high in O_2 conformers and mitochondrial metabolism in both cases could be viewed as the organism's cell-level O_2-sensing mechanism. In the case of the turtle liver cells, this kind of oxygen sensing would mean activation of anaerobic glycolysis (since this is the only known mechanism for ATP generation without oxygen in these cells). Two observations argue persuasively against this as the means for sensing hypoxia in cells tolerant to oxygen lack. First, hypoxia-tolerant systems rarely activate anaerobic metabolism enough to make up energy deficits; they favor a reduced energy turnover state instead. Secondly, responses to falling oxygen supplies begin at concentrations much higher than the $K_m(O_2)$ for mitochondria, which is typical for O_2-conforming systems. In fact it was the observation of oxygen conformity (see Boutilier and St. Pierre, 2000; Buchner et al., 2000; Hochachka, 1994) that first led workers in this area to postulate the occurrence of a mechanism for sensing molecular oxygen as the cell-level means for detecting hypoxia (discussed further below).

BALANCING ATP DEMAND AND SUPPLY PATHWAYS DURING HYPOXIA

Based on the observation of oxygen conformity and on earlier whole organism studies, it was not surprising to find that when liver hepatocytes encounter oxygen lack, they suppress energy turnover by a factor of almost 10-fold (Buck and Hochachka, 1993; Buck et al., 1993). All else being equal, a mole of ATP could sustain these cells for 10 times longer than under normal conditions. As mentioned, this strategy is frequently observed in hypoxia tolerant cells, but to put the strategy into perspective, it is important to know quantitatively which processes are turned down. To this end the main energy demand functions under normoxia (energetically balanced by the oxygen consumption rates under these conditions) need to be compared to the energy sinks remaining under anoxia. Such studies on turtle hepatocytes show that under *normoxic* conditions, the main energy sinks (table 3.1) are (i) protein synthesis, (ii) protein degradation, (iii) Na^+K^+ pumping, (iv) urea biosynthesis, and (v) glucose biosynthesis. For practical purposes, the ATP demands of these processes account for essentially 100% of the ATP production expected from oxygen consumption (Hochachka et al., 1996; see chapter 2 discussion on fractional contributions to standard metabolic rates).

Most instructive is what happens to the same processes in O_2-limited turtle liver cells. Under conditions of total *anoxia*, the ATP demand of protein turnover drops to less than 10% of normoxic rates; urea biosynthesis drops to essentially zero, as does the biosynthesis of glucose (not unexpectedly, because a major role of the liver under anoxic conditions is to supply glucose for the rest of the body). Although the ATP requirements of the Na^+-K^+-ATPase are also drastically reduced, the suppression in percentage terms is less than for overall ATP turnover. As a result, under anoxic conditions, the Na^+ pump becomes the cell's dominant energy sink, accounting for up to 75% of the ATP demand of the cell (Buck and Hochachka, 1993). In turtle brain these adjustments occur along with a measurable decrease in Na^+-K^+-

ATPase activities per gram of tissue, but in carp brain, the catalytic activities in different brain regions seem to be maintained (Hylland et al., 1997). Although there may well be other more minor energy demand processes remaining under anoxic conditions, the quantitative ATP requirements of the energy demand pathways identified during anoxia account for most of the ATP generated by anaerobic glycolysis (table 3.1).

INTEGRATING METABOLISM AND MEMBRANE FUNCTIONS DURING HYPOXIA

Even if, in percentage terms, ion pumping (as assessed by the activity of Na^+-K^+-ATPase) is the single largest ATP sink during anoxia in turtle hepatocytes, its absolute ATPase or pumping activity is only a small fraction (about 1/4) of normoxic levels. However, direct estimates indicate that the electrochemical potential in anoxic liver cells is essentially the same as in normoxia (Buck and Hochachka, 1993). The only mechanism by which we can account for (i) the large-scale drop in absolute Na^+-K^+-ATPase activity and for (ii) the simultaneous maintenance of normal electrochemical gradients is by means of a similar magnitude decrease in cell membrane permeability (termed generalized "channel arrest" in the literature [Bickler and Buck, 1998; Boutilier and St. Pierre, 2000; Hochachka, 1986]).

Table 3.1. The Main ATP Demand Pathways During Normoxia and Anoxia in Turtle Hepatocytes

Pathway	ATP demand (μmold ATPg^{-1}h^{-1})		
	Normoxia	Anoxia (%)	Suppression
Total	67.0	6.3	94
Na^+ pump	19.1	4.8	75
Protein synthesis	24.4	1.6	93
Protein breakdown	11.1	0.7	94
Urea synthesis	2.0	0.6	70
Gluconeogenesis	11.4	0.0	100

Modified from Buck and Hochachka (1993), Buck et al. (1993), and Land and Hochachka (1994).

In a first attempt at a synthesis of information in this research (Hochachka, 1986), a "channel arrest" component of a hypoxia tolerance theory postulated (i) that hypoxia tolerant cells would have an inherent low permeability (either low channel densities or low channel activities) and (ii) that they would sustain a further suppression of membrane permeability to ions when exposed to oxygen lack (further "channel arrest" by either suppression of channel densities or channel activities). Turtle liver cells display both of these characteristics (especially when compared to mammalian homologs); thus they clearly fit the classical definition of metabolic and channel arrest as two telling signatures of hypoxia tolerance.

In contrast, in turtle cortical cells, only the first criterion is fully met: a background electrical conductivity that is unusually low and when compared at biological temperatures (15 vs 37°C) can be as low as one-twenty-fifth the conductivity of cell membranes of rat cortical cells (Doll et al., 1993). However, when exposed to acute oxygen lack (for up to several hours), there is no further major decrease in background conductivity of these neuronal cells, even though specific ion channels may be down-regulated (Bickler and Buck, 1998). We consider that to be an important reason why the main energy-saving mechanism in turtle brain (Chih et al., 1989) is down-regulation of firing rates or synaptic transmission (involving more localized channel down-regulation and termed "spike arrest" by Sick et al., 1993; Thurman et al., 1993) presumably through adenosine-mediated down-regulation of excitatory amino acid (especially glutamate) release with concomitant increase in release of inhibitory amino acids (Lutz, 1992; Lutz and Manuel, 1999; Nilsson, 1993). This may also explain why the metabolic suppression in brain is substantially less than in liver cells, down to about half rather than one-tenth of normoxic rates (compare Doll et al., 1994 vs Buck et al., 1993). An absence of these kinds of protective mechanisms in hypoxia-sensitive neurons is considered by workers in this field as the main basis for cell damage and ultimately cell death (figure 3.10). The effects of ion channel inactivation extend to key elements of neuronal signaling and are summarized by Bickler and Buck (1998) as follows:

Na^+ Channel inactivation leading to
  Elevated action potential threshold
  Decreased nerve conduction and velocity
  Decreased Na^+ leak and decreased likelihood of Na^+ gradient collapse
  Stabilized Na^+ gradient-linked transporters (glucose, creatine, Ca^{2+}, H^+, transmitters)
K^+ Channel inactivation leading to
  Altered action potential shape
  Altered excitability
Glutamate receptor inactivation leading to
  Decreased excitatory neurotransmission (defense against "excitotoxicity")
  Stabilized intracellular $[Ca^{2+}]$
Voltage-gated Ca^{2+} channel inactivation leading to
  Decreased excitability
  Decreased neurotransmitter release
  Decreased accumulation of intracellular Ca^{2+}
  Decreased likelihood of an autocatalytic Ca^{2+}-mediated cell death cascade
Acetylcholine receptor inactivation leading to
  Decreased excitatory neurotransmission
  Decreased Ca^{2+} influx
  Decreased likelihood of an autocatalytic Ca^{2+}-mediated cell death cascade

A related implication of a lack of change during acute anoxia in global membrane conductivity or a lesser degree of channel arrest in turtle neurons than in hepatocytes is that the ATP turnover rate of anoxic turtle cortical brain cells is higher than in turtle liver cells. Direct microcalorimetric measurements suggest that heat fluxes in anoxic brain cortical tissue are some threefold higher than in anoxic liver cells (Doll et al., 1994). In vivo, of course, anoxic brain survival depends solely upon anaerobic glycolysis (Chih et al., 1989) fueled by plasma glucose derived ultimately from liver glucose. Thus in the turtle brain, hypoxia tolerance equals a more modest metabolic arrest than in liver cells plus the arrest not of "leakage" channels but of channel functions asso-

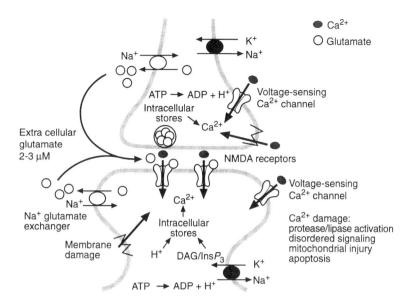

Figure 3.10. A diagrammatic summary of the Ca^{2+}-mediated, self-destruct (excitotoxicity) cascade in hypoxia- or ischemia-sensitive neurons. Key events thought to be occurring are shown for a presynaptic nerve ending (upper diagram) and for a postsynaptic dendritic spine (lower diagram). During anoxic stress (energetic insufficiency), cell membranes depolarize and trigger Ca^{2+} influx through voltage-sensitive Ca^{2+} channels. Anoxic depolarization results in Na^+ influx and the reversal of the Na^+ gradient dependent neurotransmitter re-uptake transporters, flooding the extra cellular fluid (ECF) with excitatory neurotransmitters such as glutamate. Vesicular glutamate release does not contribute significantly to postsynaptic Ca^{2+} influx, since vesicular release fails early on in hypoxia as a result of the loss of ATP; this process does not occur in hypoxia-tolerant neurons in part because ATP concentrations are stabilized during hypoxia or ischemia. Instead of through vesicular release, glutamate directly triggers Ca^{2+} influx via *N*-methyl-D-aspartate (NMDA) receptors. Other contributors to the increase in intracellular Ca^{2+} include membrane damage due to free radical generation, acidification caused by anaerobiosis, and Ca^{2+} triggered Ca^{2+} release from intracellular stores, a process involving diacylglycerol (DAG) and/or inositol triphosphate (InsP3) in intracellular signal transduction. (Modified from Bickler and Buck, 1998.)

ciated with synaptic transmission, in order to remain in energy balance.

The problem of maintaining membrane-linked electrochemical gradients is not unique to the plasma membrane, but extends to other membrane-delineated organelles as well, especially the mitochondria.

REGULATING MITOCHONDRIAL MEMBRANE PROPERTIES

Usually we think of the mitochondrial F_1F_0-ATPase as being the site of ATP production in animal cells. However, when O_2 is absent, this reversible enzyme—the ATP synthase—begins to operate backwards as it actively pumps protons from the matrix in an attempt to maintain the mitochondrial membrane potential (figure 3.11). This means that in anoxia and ischemia, mitochondria change from being ATP producers to potentially important ATP consumers (Lisa et al., 1998). It is obviously advantageous under anoxia to avoid losing a considerable proportion of available energy to hydrolysis, rather than to production, of ATP. Interestingly, this is the strategy that O_2-limited cells actually utilize. An F_1-ATPase inhibitory subunit (IF1) is known to inhibit the hydrolysis of ATP by mitochondria in a pH-dependent manner during anoxia. The IF1 binds to the mitochondrial ATPase at low pH under nonenergizing conditions in a way that reduces its rate of ATP uti-

A

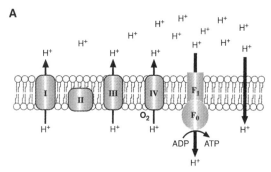

Using the proton-motive force in ATP synthesis

B

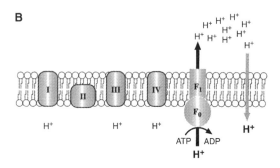

Figure 3.11. Current chemiosmotic concepts of oxidative phosphorylation under normoxic conditions are shown in (A). Protons are pumped across the inner mitochondrial membrane (at Complexes I, III, and IV) thereby generating a proton-motive force that provides the driving force for proton influx through the F_1F_0-ATP synthase. Proton influx is coupled to ATP-synthase-catalyzed phosphorylation of ADP to ATP. At standard metabolic rate (SMR), a significant fraction of the protons pumped out across the electron transfer chain (ETC) leak back into the mitochondrial matrix without synthesizing ATP; i.e., this proton leak effectively uncouples respiration from phosphorylation (see chapter 2 for further discussion of this topic). In the absence of oxygen (B), proton transfer no longer occurs at Complexes I, III, and IV but the reverse operation of the ATP synthase as an ATPase is the cell's attempt to maintain the mitochondrial membrane potential by using ATP hydrolysis to pump protons into the intermembrane space. During oxygen lack in anoxia tolerant organisms such as some frogs, turtles, and fish, the electrochemical gradient across the inner mitochondrial membrane is stabilized at lower values than in normoxia, in this way minimizing the need for, and the activity of, the mitochondrial ATPase in protecting the mitochondrial electrochemical gradient. (Modified from Boutilier and St. Pierre, 2000.)

lization (Rouslin, 1991). Most species exposed to severe hypoxia or anoxia incur an intracellular acidosis, owing to their reliance on glycolysis (see discussion above). Cell acidification then is transmitted to the mitochondrial matrix by way of the Pi/H+ symport, at least in species that possess a functional IF1.

Anoxia-tolerant frogs and turtles belong to the category of species that display a moderate inhibition of their mitochondrial ATPase under anoxic conditions. Since these two species can withstand anoxia for considerable periods of time, they must have a very efficient way to reduce the ATP utilization by their mitochondrial ATPase. If not, almost all the ATP generated by glycolysis could be needed to fuel that process alone. Addressing this problem, St. Pierre et al. (2000) found that during anoxia in frog hearts the mitochondrial electrochemical gradient stabilizes at lower values than in normoxia; this condition then minimizes the need for, and the catalytic activity of, mitochondrial ATPase during anoxia. If this defensive mechanism were not activated, St. Pierre et al. (2000) calculate that the tissue mitochondrial ATPase would become the major ATP sink during anoxia and that its demand for ATP would in fact overwhelm the cell's limited energetic capabilities under these conditions.

HYPOXIC SUPPRESSION OF PROTEIN SYNTHESIS

The only energy-requiring process in normoxic liver cells that is more costly than ion pumping is protein turnover (Buck et al., 1993; Land and Bernier, 1995; Land et al., 1993; Land and Hochachka, 1994), so evaluating this ATP sink under oxygen-limiting conditions is of particular importance. Interestingly, one of the first and most dramatic effects of hypoxia on cell metabolic functions is a rapid and large-magnitude inhibition of protein synthesis. The decline can be so rapid that its time course is difficult to ascertain accurately with currently used techniques for measuring protein biosynthesis (Buc-Calderon et al., 1993; Hand, 1991, 1993; Vayda et al., 1995).

In principle, an hypoxia-induced block could occur at the level of gene transcription or at translation. While in animal models, the mechanism for an initial hypoxia-induced block in protein synthesis is unclear, in plant systems hypoxic suppression of protein synthesis is mediated by a translational block affecting both initiation and elongation. Inhibition of initiation is not well understood, but inhibition of elongation appears to depend upon an accumulation of elongation factor 1α (EF1α), which at low pH appears to form nonfunctional complexes with polysome-associated mRNA (Vayda et al., 1995). Since the role of this elongation factor is to present amino acyl-tRNA to the A site of ribosomes, it is easy to visualize how failure to dissociate from polysomes would prevent peptidyl synthase and translocation. In hypoxia-sensitive systems, such as rat hepatocytes, hypoxia-induced translational arrest and thus blockade of protein synthetic capacity seems to remain general for at least 2 hours (longer term experiments with this preparation are not realistic due to cell damage and cell death—which is also what occurs in natural hypoxia or ischemia stress if O_2 is not again made available to these kinds of cells or tissue).

OXYGEN SENSING AND PREFERENTIAL O_2-SENSITIVE GENE EXPRESSION

While "rescue" of protein synthesis in hypoxia sensitive mammalian cells does not seem feasible without oxygen, exactly such a "rescue" system seems available to hypoxia tolerant cells (Land and Hochachka, 1995). One underlying "rescue" mechanism appears to require the overproduction of key elongation factors such as EF1α; with sustained hypoxia, the latter is overexpressed and accumulates throughout the stress period.

Comparable studies in turtle hepatocytes found (Land and Hochachka, 1995) quite a complex situation. Under conditions of prolonged oxygen lack, the expression of four proteins in turtle hepatocytes was preferentially up-regulated, while the expression of five proteins was preferentially down-regulated. The hypoxia dependence of this system appeared similar to

O_2-sensing and regulatory pathways in erythropoietin (EPO) biosynthesis (Eckardt, 1994; Firth et al. 1994, 1995; Maxwell et al., 1993; Semenza et al., 1994; Wang and Semenza, 1993, 1995). The field of EPO research developed four experimental criteria for discriminating between O_2-sensing and signal transduction pathways versus simple oxygen-dependent metabolic pathways. First, in O_2-sensing pathways, the response should be negated by normoxia even in the presence of metabolic poisons such as cyanide—as observed in the turtle hepatocyte gene expression changes in anoxia. Second, in heme protein O_2-sensing pathways, Co^{2+} or Ni^{2+}, which lock heme proteins in their deoxy conformation, should mimic anoxia effects—as observed in turtle hepatocyte gene expression changes. Third, in heme protein-sensing pathways, carbon monoxide, which locks heme proteins in oxy conformation, should reverse anoxia effects—also observed in the turtle hepatocyte studies. Finally, heme synthesis inhibitors should abrogate the effects of Co^{2+} or Ni^{2+} in heme protein based O_2-sensing pathways—again observed in the turtle hepatocyte gene expression changes in anoxia (Land and Hochachka, 1995). These studies, inspired by developments in EPO research, lead to the conclusion that a putative heme-protein-based O_2-sensing and signal transduction system in turtle hepatocytes serves to activate the expression of a group of several proteins during extended periods of O_2 limitation, but to simultaneously further slow down the expression of another group of several proteins. Molecular details of the O_2 sensor are not known but Bunn et al. (1998) consider that it is likely to involve a heme protein (figure 3.12) in which Co^{2+} or Ni^{2+} can replace Fe^{2+} in the prophyrin ring. Indirect evidence suggests that this kind of sensor is present in all cells and is composed of a multi-subunit assembly containing an NADH or NADPH oxidase capable of generating H_2O_2 and reactive oxygen species (ROSs) which serve in signal transduction to hypoxia response systems in the cell. The O_2 signal transduction pathway in turtle hepatocytes is probably homologous to that found in the liver cells of other vertebrates. In the latter (Keitzmann et al., 1992, 1993), O_2 signal trans-

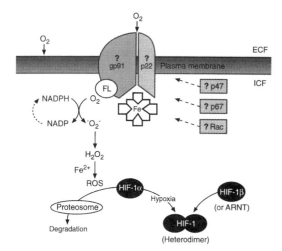

Figure 3.12. The membrane-bound NAD(P)H oxidase model of O_2 sensing proposed by Bunn et al. (1998) is based on neutrophil macrophage enzyme homolog. According to this view, initial sensing is achieved by a heme protein probably formed of two main subunits (gp91 and p22), with a flavin group (FL) participating in the transfer of electrons enabling O_2 to be reduced to superoxide anion via the oxidation of NADPH or NADH (the coenzyme could be NADH; hence the term NAD(P)H used in the literature for this enzyme). In neutrophil/macrophage activation, three additional proteins (p47, p67, and Rac) interact to form a heterooligomeric enzyme complex. The formation of reactive oxygen species (ROSs) from peroxide is catalyzed by iron in a noncatalyzed step (the so-called Fenton reaction). Bunn et al. (1998) propose that under normoxic conditions these oxidizing equivalents mediate the degradation of HIF 1α in the proteosome, thus preventing the formation of the active HIF 1 heterodimer that is required for the induction of hypoxia-sensitive gene expression (see discussion below).

duction seems to include negatively modulating the effects of glucagon on gluconeogenic enzymes such as P-enolpyruvate carboxykinase (PEPCK). The indications are that hypoxia sensitive genes in turtles are not unique; they may be modified versions of similar O_2-sensing and signal transduction control systems in other vertebrates. Mammalian cells and tissues are best understood and we shall use them to illustrate the situation.

COORDINATE INDUCTION OF GLYCOLYTIC ENZYMES GENES IS WIDESPREAD

The glycolytic enzyme pathway consists of 11 separate enzymes that catalyze the fermentation of glycogen or glucose to lactate. Two moles of ATP are generated per mole of glucose, so on a mole-per-mole basis the system is one-eighteenth to one-thirteenth as efficient as oxidative phosphorylation. In 1860, Pasteur observed that the rate of glucose consumption of cells was inversely proportional to the oxygen tension, that is, that glycolysis was positively regulated by hypoxia. More than a century later, Webster and his coworkers reported that the transcription rates of glycolytic enzyme genes were also positively regulated by hypoxia (Webster and Murphy, 1988; Webster et al., 1990; Webster and Bishopric, 1992). Increased transcription rates supported increased steady states of the glycolytic enzyme mRNAs under hypoxia (Webster and Murphy, 1988), as well as increased proteins and enzyme activities (Robin et al., 1984). These earlier reports have been confirmed by a number of later studies in different cells and tissues (Semenza et al., 1996; Firth et al., 1995). Glycolytic enzyme gene regulation by hypoxia appears to be ubiquitous in eukaryotic cells including plants and animals, and induction of the genes varies between about three- and tenfold; there may be some quantitative variability between individual enzyme genes and, as already implied above, between different cells. At least eight of the 11 glycolytic enzymes have been shown to be induced by hypoxia, and the inference is that the complete pathway of genes is hypoxia-responsive (Webster et al., 1990). These inductions probably occur concomitantly with repression of enzymes in aerobic metabolic pathways (Murphy et al., 1984). Most of the enzymes of glycolysis occur as (tissue) specific isoforms; these proteins are either splice variants or, more usually, they are encoded by distinct genes, all of which are considered inducible in muscle and probably in most other tissues as well (Webster et al., 1990). In animal cells at least two pathways have been implicated in the activation of glycolytic enzyme gene expression by hypoxia in different tissues, and these will be discussed below (hypoxia-regulated genes are also well known in plant systems, with some similarities and some differences compared to the picture currently developing for animal cells [see Webster et al., 2000]).

HIF 1 REGULATION OF GENES FOR LIVER-SPECIFIC GLYCOLYTIC ENZYMES

In liver and many other (usually endoderm-derived) tissues, hypoxia induction of genes for glycolytic enzymes is mediated by hypoxia-inducible factor 1, or HIF 1α (figures 3.13 and 3.14). Hypoxia-inducible factor 1 belongs to the family of basic helix–loop–helix transcription factors and in-vivo assembles with another well-known protein (aryl hydrocarbon receptor nuclear transporter, or ARNT; also termed HIF 1β in some of the literature) to form a heterodimer (Wang et al., 1995). Steady-state concentrations of HIF 1α, but not of its mRNA, increase as an inverse function of O_2 tension (see more on this below). Hypoxia-inducible factor 1 has been implicated in the hypoxia-mediated activation of the liver-specific isogenes PFK-L, aldolase-A, PGK-1, enolase-1, and LDH-A (Firth et al., 1994; Semenza et al., 1996). Northern and RNAse protection analyses indicate inductions of five- to tenfold for the endogenous transcripts of these genes in hepatoma L-cells, or HeLa cells exposed to hypoxia for 16 to 20 hours. Other genes that are now known to be regulated by HIF 1 include those encoding glucose transporter 1 (GLUT1) occurring in diverse vertebrate tissues (see Dang and Semenza, 1999); EPO, *in vivo* occurring mostly in kidney cells, but also to a lesser degree, in liver (Maxwell et al., 1993; Wenger and Gassman, 1997); and VEGF1, a growth factor in vascular tissue crucial in vivo to angiogenesis and vascular remolding (Eckardt, 1994; Forsythe et al., 1993; Ladoux and Felin, 1993).

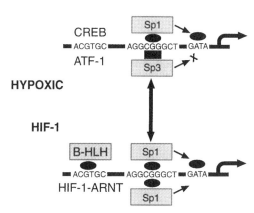

Figure 3.13. Diagrammatic summary of two pathways for hypoxia-mediated regulation of glycolytic enzyme expression proposed by Webster et al. (2000). Under aerobic conditions, HIF 1 is degraded and its binding site is either vacant or is occupied by other transcription factors such as CREB (cyclic AMP responsive binding element) or ATF-1. The site does not contribute to transcriptional activation under these conditions. Under oxygen-rich conditions, members of the Sp1 family of transcription factors compete for binding to the GC-rich site. Of these, Sp1 and Sp3 are the principal factors in muscle, where they appear to be present in approximately equal amounts (and where they bind to the GC-rich site in equal amounts). Sp1 is a transcriptional activator, while Sp3 acts as a repressor, so the transcriptional activation functions of the site are determined by the relative contributions of each factor. Under hypoxic conditions, HIF 1 (represented as a basic helix-loop-helix or B-HLH, above the binding site, and as the heterodimer, below the binding site) is stabilized; as it accumulates it interacts with ARNT to form the active heterodimer that binds at the ACGTGC site and becomes a strong positive transcriptional activator. In parallel, Sp3 is degraded under hypoxia and the GC-box becomes fully occupied by Sp1; repression is relieved, and this site becomes fully active too. (Modified from Webster et al., 2000.)

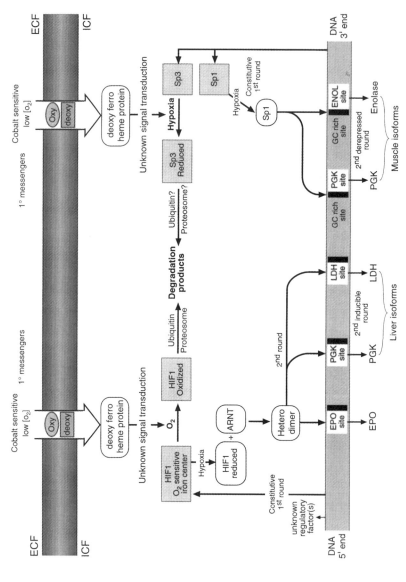

Figure 3.14. A more detailed schematic diagram of oxygen-sensing and signal transduction components involved in regulation of expression of EPO and other hypoxia sensitive proteins in mammalian cells. Direct sensing of molecular oxygen is thought to be mediated by a heme protein, whose activity correlates with a first constitutive round of gene expression leading to production of hypoxia-inducible factor 1 (HIF 1); the concentration of the latter is itself hypoxia stabilized and HIF 1 in turn mediates a second round of hypoxia-sensitive gene expression change leading to enhanced EPO mRNA production and thus to increased EPO expression. Base sequences in the promoter region of the EPO gene (not shown) and the enhancer sequence (located 3′ to the EPO gene) contribute to the hypoxia-sensitive control of transcription rate. Similar and probably homologous enhancer sites are found flanking the PGK gene and may be involved generally in hypoxia (up or down) regulation of genes for enzymes in glycolysis, gluconeogenesis, and the Krebs cycle. In muscle cells hypoxia-sensitive expression is achieved through removal of Sp3 repression; Sp1 binding at GC-rich promoter sites in turn activates genes for muscle isoforms in glycolysis. This summary diagram is based on studies of EPO and of hypoxia-sensitive regulation of glycolytic enzyme expression. (Based on Hochachka et al., 1996; Webster et al., 2000.)

SP3 REGULATION OF GENES FOR MUSCLE-SPECIFIC GLYCOLYTIC ENZYMES

Interestingly, studies show that, in muscle and possibly mesoderm-derived cells in general, there are no HIF 1 binding sites in the proximal ($\sim 1\,Kb$) $5'$ promoter regions of glycolytic genes specifying muscle isoforms of enzymes such as PK and enolase. Transcripts of these genes are induced about fourfold by hypoxia in cardiac and skeletal muscle (Discher et al., 1998; Webster, personal communication), but their promoters are regulated by hypoxia independently of HIF 1. Deletion and mutation analyses have identified conserved sequences in muscle type PK and in β-Eno promoters that are required for activation by hypoxia. These studies identified GC-rich elements or sequences in the muscle PK and β-Eno proximal promoters as hypoxia response elements, or HREs (figure 3.13). Protein-binding studies further revealed that transcription factors Sp1 and Sp3 bound in approximately equal amounts to the HREs in aerobic myocytes, but under hypoxic conditions only Sp1 was found to bind. Sp3 binding decreased rapidly within the first hour after exposure to hypoxia and was no longer evident after 4–8 hours in most experiments.

Since the loss of Sp3 binding correlates with increased promoter activity, it is proposed that the hypoxia-mediated depletion of Sp3 alleviates a repressor activity, thereby activating transcription from these promoters. This would mean that in muscle, hypoxia-associated increase in expression of genes for glycolytic isoforms occurs because of removal of a repressor, Sp3.

HYPOXIA-SENSITIVE FUNCTIONS OF HIF 1 AND SP3 ARE REGULATED POST-TRANSCRIPTIONALLY

In principle, the functions of HIF 1 and Sp3 could be regulated either at the transcriptional or post-transcriptional levels, so it is particularly instructive that the accumulation of HIF 1α protein and binding activity in cells exposed to hypoxia are both independent of changes in HIF 1α gene transcription, or the stability of its mRNA (Kallio et al., 1999). On the contrary, all available data suggest that HIF 1α and HIF 1β (its cofactor/binding protein ARNT) are constitutively transcribed and translated, with no known regulation in all mammalian cells tested so far.

Regulation of HIF 1α function, however, does occur. Under aerobic conditions HIF 1α is rapidly polyubiquitinated and degraded by the ubiquitin–proteasome pathway. The half-life of HIF 1α protein in well-oxygenated cells is 5–10 min. Under hypoxic conditions, ubiquitination (i.e., tagging for proteosome breakdown) does not occur; the protein is stabilized and it accumulates. Accumulated HIF 1α dimerizes with ARNT (or HIF 1β), and the complex translocates to the cell nucleus where it binds to and activates genes containing the consensus DNA sequence (figure 3.14). Aerobic ubiquitination of HIF 1α is determined by a central domain of the protein consisting of about 200 amino acids (Huang et al., 1998). When intracellular $[O_2]$ reaches a critical threshold, a specific proline residue (proline 564) in HIF 1α is oxidatively modified by a prolyl hydroxylase (PH) enzyme. The hydroxylation is necessary to make in this domain a competent binding site for a key protein, termed pVHL, for von Hippel–Landau protein; discovered in cancer research and thus known as a tumor suppressor, pVHL organizes the assembly of a protein complex that activates ubiquitin E3 ligase. The latter then ubiquinates HIF 1α targeting it for degradation. Interestingly, deletion of the proline 564-containing domain results in a stable protein that is no longer regulated by hypoxia. Oxygen sensing thus may also be a key function for an iron center contained within this domain that acts as a cofactor for the oxygen-dependent proline hydroxylase reaction (Ivan et al., 2001; Jaakola et al., 2001). Prolyl hydroxylases in general depend upon both iron and oxygen. However, collagen prolyl hydroxylases are localized within the endoplasmic reticulum, while the HIF 1α sensor appears to be cytosolic. Additionally, these two hydroxylases differ in the way they interact with oxygen. Proline hydroxylation in collagen is insensitive to a wide range of oxygen concentrations, while the HIF 1α oxygen sensor must have a higher apparent K_m for oxygen (lower apparent affinity for oxygen), allowing it to respond to subtle alternations in intracellular oxygen availability (Zhu and Bunn, 2001).

The discovery that HIF 1α is regulated by redox-dependent degradation of the protein was unexpected. Interestingly, analyses of the regulation of the hypoxia-sensitive GC-Sp3 pathway indicate that it also may be regulated at the level of protein stability. Thus Discher et al. (1998) demonstrated that whereas Sp3 protein and binding activity dropped rapidly after the exposure of cells to hypoxia, there was no change in the level of Sp3 mRNA at any time. This suggests that, like HIF 1α, Sp3 is also constitutively expressed under aerobic or hypoxic conditions but, unlike HIF 1, Sp3 is stable under aerobic conditions and preferentially degraded under hypoxia.

The two pathways for hypoxia-mediated regulation of glycolytic enzyme gene expression are summarized in figures 3.13 and 3.14. Figure 3.13 shows a hypothetical promoter with HIF 1α and GC/Sp consensus binding sites. Webster et al. (2000) propose that under aerobic conditions HIF 1α is degraded and the binding site is either vacant or occupied by other transcription factors (figure 3.13, top). The site does not contribute to transcriptional activation of the HIF 1α gene under these conditions. In the oxygenated, state members of the Sp1 family compete for binding to the GC site. Sp1 and Sp3 are the principal factors in muscle; they appear to be present in approximately equal amounts, and bind correspondingly, as estimated by in-vitro gel mobility shift assay (Discher et al., 1998). Sp1 is a transcriptional activator, whereas Sp3 represses. Therefore the activity of the site is determined by the relative contributions of each factor. With high levels of Sp3, the activity will be repressed and the hypothetical promoter containing two HREs will be weak or inactive under aerobic conditions. Under hypoxic conditions HIF 1α, represented in figure 3.13, (bottom), as a basic helix–loop–helix (B HLH) structure, is stabilized, it accumulates, associates with ARNT, occupies the ACGTGC site, and becomes a strong posi-

tive transcriptional activator. In parallel, Sp3 is degraded under hypoxia and the GC-box becomes fully occupied by Sp1, repression is relieved, and this site also becomes fully active (Webster et al., 2000).

An interesting feature of these two pathways of hypoxia-mediated gene regulation is that the mechanisms are mirror images of each other. Sp3 is a transcriptional repressor that appears to be degraded specifically under hypoxic conditions; HIF 1α is a transcriptional activator that is degraded under aerobic conditions. It is not immediately clear what selective advantage such regulatory mechanisms would convey over the more usual transcriptional regulation of genes. An advantage we and others (Webster et al., 2000) consider plausible is that regulation by protein stability allows an extremely rapid response time because new protein synthesis is not required, both transcription factors being continuously produced. This may be very important for an appropriate cell response to acute hypoxia or ischemia where aerobic pathways of energy metabolism are immediately inhibited and anaerobic energy pathways must be rapidly recruited to compensate. For reasons reviewed above, the regulated and coordinate activation of glucose metabolizing pathways (as sole sources of ATP) may be essential to survive hypoxia.

In overview, the hypoxia-sensitive expression of each of these kinds of proteins (EPO, PGK, and LDH), and of other glycolytic enzymes appears to be two-step or two-cycle systems (figure 3.14): the first cycles involve the constitutive expression of key hypoxia-sensitive transcription factors such as HIF 1 and Sp3, while the second cycles of gene expression are mediated by these transcription factors and regulate the biosynthesis of EPO, PGK, LDH, other glycolytic enzymes, and other hypoxia-sensitive gene products.

Since the expression of other proteins, such as elongation factors, may be similarly regulated, it is tempting to consider that the induction and accumulation (calibrated relative to other proteins) of EF 1α in hypoxic plant tissue and the hypoxia-sensitive proteins in turtle and rat hepatocytes are under similar two-cycle gene regulation (figure 3.15), although at this time

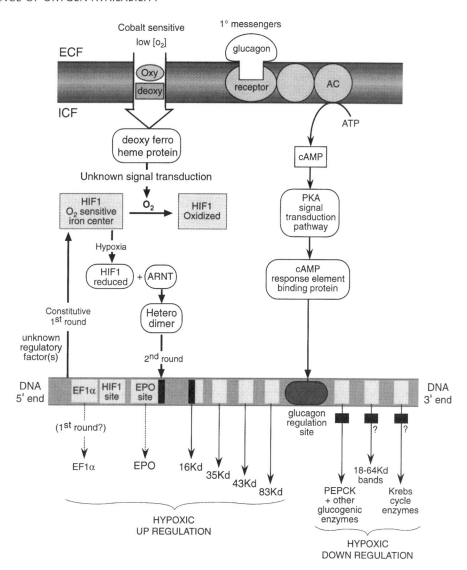

Figure 3.15. Schematic diagram of oxygen-sensing and signal transduction components thought to be involved in metabolic hypoxia defense response in turtle and rat hepatocytes. Based on the EPO model summarized in figure 3.14, it is tentatively postulated that direct sensing of molecular oxygen is mediated by a heme protein, which correlates with a first constitutive round of gene expression leading to the production of hypoxia-inducible factor 1 (HIF 1) and possibly factors involved in the rescue of mRNA translation, such as EF 1α. Under hypoxic conditions, HIF 1 is not tagged for proteosome degradation and instead is free to interact with ARNT to form the active heterodimer involved in the regulation of a second round of gene expression. These hypothetical two rounds of gene regulation are assumed to be homologous to the EPO system in EPO-producing cells. The net effects of these processes include the up-regulation of several genes (at least four proteins; elongation factors could be included in this control) with concomitant down-regulation of several others. In rat liver cells, the hypoxia-sensitive portion of this system modulates the protein kinase A (PKA) signal transduction system and down-regulates the expression of genes for PEPCK and possibly other enzymes. Summary diagram based on studies of hypoxia regulation of gene expression in turtle and rat hepatocytes. (Modified from Hochachka et al., 1996.)

such homology has not been demonstrated. Nevertheless, all the data considered together are consistent with the hypotheses (i) that iron center-based oxygen sensors and oxygen-regulated control elements are widespread and possibly universal in eukaryotes, (ii) that initial key expression products are regulatory factors, such as HIF 1 (an inducer), Sp3 (a repressor), and EF 1α (an elongation factor), and (iii) that additional hypoxia-inducible proteins in turtle liver cells are glycolytic enzymes such as PGK, pyruvate kinase (PK), and LDH, while the suppressed loci may well include genes for enzymes such as PEPCK involved in gluconeogenesis and for enzymes in the mitochondrial metabolism. The Krebs cycle is usually down-regulated under these conditions, as is the electron transfer chain (ETC). However, since the ETC components are specified in both nuclear and mitochondrial genes, their regulation is complex and requires special examination.

MITOCHONDRIAL BIOGENESIS IN HYPOXIA AND OTHER STRESSES

Adjustments in mitochondrial biogenesis and mitochondrial volume densities accompany a variety of physiological challenges, which have been reviewed by Leary and Moyes (2000). For example, increases in skeletal muscle mitochondrial content occur during chronic increases in contractile activity such as endurance exercise training, shivering thermogenesis, or chronic electrical stimulation. Additionally, hyperthyroidism, ischemia/reperfusion, cold exposure in homeotherms, and cold acclimation in ectotherms increase mitochondrial volume densities. Most of these conditions are accompanied by direct or indirect changes in metabolic rate. In the case of the mitochondrial biogenesis that accompanies myogenesis, there is no change in metabolic rate, although there is a shift in the relative importance of glycolytic and mitochondrial ATP production. As hypometabolism is a widespread hypoxia defense response (almost a hallmark of hypoxia tolerance), we might expect, and indeed it is often observed in hypoxia acclimation studies, that prolonged exposure to extremely hypoxic conditions down-regulates mitochondrial volume densities and Krebs cycle enzyme concentrations (Robin et al., 1984). In none of these examples are the primary effectors in the pathway of mitochondrial biogenesis, or the signal transduction mechanisms, established. However, an attractive hypothesis is that bioenergetic disturbances themselves alter gene expression for mitochondrial biogenesis. Possible effectors include O_2, ROSs (O_2 metabolism-linked free radicals), redox state influenced by the former and the latter, adenylates, possibly involving translocation of much of the adenylate pool from mitochondrial matrix to the cytosol, NADH or NADPH, or even ion, especially Ca^{2+}, imbalances (Leary and Moyes, 2000).

MITOCHONDRIAL BIOGENESIS REQUIRES INTEGRATION OF NUCLEAR, CYTOPLASMIC, AND MITOCHONDRIAL FUNCTIONS

While the effectors and their signaling pathways are not well known, it has been clear for some time that nuclear and mitochondrial genes are involved in generating mitochondria. Mitochondrial DNA (mtDNA) exists primarily for the expression of 13 protein subunits of the electron transfer chain (ETC) and oxidative phosphorylation system; these are but a subset of the total number of subunits required for respiratory function. The remaining coding capacity of the mtDNA genome is dedicated to the tRNAs and rRNAs required for translation by mitochondrial ribosomes. The genes encoded on both strands of mtDNA form transcripts that originate with various promoters within a relatively compact region termed the D-loop. All the rest of the proteins required for mitochondrial biogenesis are specified by nuclear genes. In addition to specifying most of the respiratory proteins, nuclear genes encode the matrix Krebs cycle enzymes, the matrix enzymes that generate key substrates and cofactors, the polymerases and auxilliary factors required for transcription and replication of mtDNA, and all the polypepetides needed for RNA processing and translation (see Scarpulla, 1996). Thus understanding the genetic control of mitochondria necessitates unraveling nuclear gene function as well as the mechanisms of communication between the two genomes.

Although the story here is still developing (figure 3.16), it is already known that central to this intergenomic integration are two key transcription factors, nuclear respiratory factors 1 and 2 (or NRF1 and NRF2, respectively). Nuclear respiratory factor gene expression is high when physiological signals call for increased mitochondrial mass (e.g., prolonged muscle work, electrical stimulation, etc.) and is low when physiological challenges are more appropriately met by down-regulation of mito-

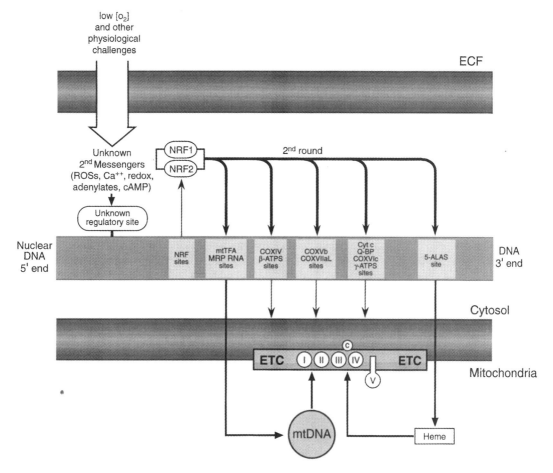

Figure 3.16. Current concepts of nuclear regulation of mitochondrial biogenesis by hypoxia and other physiological challenges such as prolonged contractile activity, exposure to hyperthyroid conditions, or exposure to hypothermia. Hypoxia or other signals are mediated via unknown second messengers and signal transduction pathway, but are known to directly influence the expression of nuclear respiratory factors (NRFs) 1 and 2 (see text). The NRFs have two categories of targets: nuclear genes for a series of proteins in the electron transfer chain (ETC) and on nuclear genes (such as mtTFA) which act as transcription factors for mtDNA genes for a smaller subset of components needed for ETC formation and function. The NRFs also regulate production of 5-aminolevulinate synthase (5-ALAS) which is a key control site in the biosynthesis of heme groups required for ETC formation. COX: cytochrome oxidase; numbers specify subunit component. Cyt: cytochrome; ATPS, ATP synthase; Q-BP, ubiquinone binding protein. (Based on summaries in Scarpulla, 1996.)

chondrial mass (e.g., hypoxia). Mitochondrial biogenesis and NRF gene expression, in other words, are directly correlated. These transcription factors have two regulatory targets: nuclear genes and mitochondrial genes. With regard to nuclear genes, functional NRF1 sites have been identified in nuclear genes encoding subunits from cytochrome c reductase and oxidase complexes and the ATP synthase (Scarpulla, 1997); complex II (succinate dehydrogenase) has also been shown to be under NRF1 and NRF2 regulation (Au and Scheffer, 1998). Nuclear respiratory factor 2 sites are involved in the regulation of genes for ETC components, such as cytochrome oxidase subunit 4 and the β subunit of ATP synthase (figure 3.16) as well as of other genes unrelated to mitochondrial function (Scarpulla, 1996).

In addition to activation of nuclear genes directly specifying ETC components, the NRFs activate genes for transcription factors for some mitochondrial genes—thus serving at least to some degree in integrating nuclear and mitochondrial genomes. One such nuclear gene product is a mitochondrial RNA processing (MRP) endonuclease, which in the mitochondria is required for mtDNA transcription. A second such nuclear gene product is the mitochondrial transcription factor A (mtTFA), which, on binding to specific mtDNA promoter sites, stimulates initiation of mtDNA transcription (figure 3.16). While these kinds of regulatory nuclear–mitochondrial interactions give us a flavor of how mitochondrial abundance is adjusted in response to hypoxia (and other physiological challenges), the finding in *Artemia* (Kwast and Hand, 1996) that hypoxia regulation of mitochondrial protein synthesis is itself initiated by intramitochondrial O_2 sensing (separate from O_2 "sensing" by cytochrome oxidase of the ETC) is instructive and clearly shows that we are dealing with more than a single and simple linear pathway from O_2 sensing at the cell boundary to the nucleus and then to mitochondrial biogenesis.

CHAPERONES AND OTHER HYPOXIA-REGULATED GENES

The above examples are not the only genes whose expression is hypoxia-dependent. Other examples of hypoxic regulation of gene expression include the cfos and cjun system (Webster et al., 1993; Mishra et al., 1998), genes for hemoxygenases (Murphy et al., 1991), genes involved in hypoxia-activated apoptosis (Graeber et al., 1996), genes for endothelial nitric oxide synthase (eNOS) (Mayer and Hemmens, 1997)), and genes for stress proteins or chaperones (Benjamine et al., 1992). The hypoxia-sensitive regulation of the cfos and cjun proto-oncogenes in rat neonatal myocytes is probably more complex than any of the examples thus far considered. (At least one rationale for using neonatal myocytes for these kinds of studies is to take advantage of a naturally evolved hypoxia or ischemia tolerance, the same rationale as was used in the above-mentioned work on turtle hepatocytes.) Both cfos and cjun are genes for transcription factors and represent two members of a family frequently referred to as classical "immediate early genes," one of the most rapidly inducible of genes in the cell; their general functional roles are to regulate growth, differentiation, and reprogramming or restructuring of cells in different physiological states. Included in this list is a key role for cfos in mitochondrial biogenesis (Xia et al., 1997). The different members of this gene family are induced to variable degree by various stimuli, and can act in synergistic or opposing manner, suggesting that both the absolute and the relative amounts of different members of the family determine their net effects (Schlingensiepen et al., 1994). The cfos and cjun protein products are separately inactive; however, as heterodimers, they form a part of the AP1 (activator protein 1) transcription factor complex and are involved in regulating the expression of a battery of other genes with AP1 binding sites in their promoter regions. This regulatory cascade is considered to orchestrate adaptive responses to various stimuli, including hypoxia, ischemia, pressure overload, stretch, and several hormones (Webster et al., 1993, 1994), all of which, if sustained, are characterized by cellular reprogramming and metabolic reorganization. Increased expression of the gene for α-actin is a good indicator of this fos/jun regulatory function in hypoxic myocytes. At least in response to hypoxia, the signal transduction pathway is protein kinase C (PKC) dependent; because jun is a sulfhydryl protein directly sensitive to hypoxia (or to redox) it is appropriate to refer to the fos/jun proteins as tertiary messengers in the overall hypoxia-initiated flow of information from the outside of the cell to the genes (figure 3.17).

The hypoxia-sensing components of this "immediate early" response system in myocytes have not been as systematically dissected as has the EPO system. Yet it is clear that if they are homologous to the EPO oxygen-sensing pathways, then the cfos/cjun regulatory system would involve three cycles of gene activation (figure 3.17). We interpret this (three-cycle) system as constituting the final step in the "rescue" phase of development of hypoxia tolerance; that is, the API-mediated regulation of genes during hypoxia is considered basic to the remolding and stabilization of the cell for sustained survival without oxygen. Interestingly, such roles—representing the epitomy of "rescue" of the cell from destructive cascades leading to hypoxic cell damage and cell death—during sustained oxygen limitation are entirely consistent with the normal normoxic roles for these proto-oncogenes in the regulation of genes for cell growth, development, and differentiation. In this frame of reference, stabilizing, restructuring, or consolidating the cell for sustained hypoxia can be viewed as a special case or a special kind of "differentiation" or de-differentiation. Although details of these processes are not yet in, there are provocative indications, arising from studies with DNA chips, of the required huge numbers of genes whose expression must be differentially regulated for reprogramming and stabilization during hypoxia exposure.

DNA MICROARRAYS: PROBING GENE RESPONSES TO O_2 LIMITATION IN HYPOXIA-TOLERANT SPECIES

For functional genomics, a number of high-throughput gene expression measurement techniques have become widely accessible to molecular physiologists (Amundson et al., 2001). Of these, DNA chips or microarrays represent one of the most powerful ways of evaluating gene expression responses during changes in physiological states. The basic idea behind the technology is quite simple: complete gene sequences or partial sequences are isolated, amplified, and then are robotically "printed" onto poly-L-lysine-coated glass slides or nitrocellulose support. Fluorescently labeled target cDNAs are prepared from whole-cell RNA from control or hypoxia-treated cells by a single round of reverse transcription in the presence of fluorescently labeled (Cyanine 3 or Cyanine 5) d-nucleotide triphosphate (either Cy3 dUTP or Cy5 dUTP). The control (Cy3, which is commonly read as a green signal by the scanning device used to quantify spot intensity) and the hypoxia-treated (Cy5, commonly recorded as red by the scanner) cDNA targets are mixed and then hybridized to the microarray. Following hybridization, the relative fluorescence of the two labels from zero-time samples are about the same (green/red ratio = 1). All changes in gene expression are expressed relative to the activity (or fluorescence) in this control state. If a gene is induced during hypoxia, and is therefore represented by more mRNA in the hypoxia-exposed cells, it will be read as a red spot by the scanner; the higher the expression, the redder the spot. Genes with equal representation in the two mixed samples will display equal fluorescence in both channels and are detected as yellow spots, while genes showing down-regulation during hypoxia will appear as green spots. In this way, the expression patterns of huge arrays of genes can be monitored quantitatively as a function of time of exposure to hypoxia or to any other environmental stressor.

The power of DNA microarray technology of course derives from its ability to interrogate

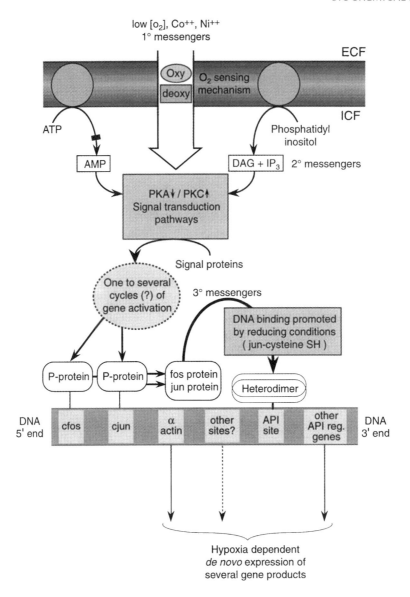

Figure 3.17. Schematic diagram of oxygen-sensing and signal transduction components thought to be involved in immediate–early gene expression responses to hypoxia in neonatal rat myocytes. It is not known whether one, two, or more cycles of gene activation are involved in the hypoxia induction of cfos and cjun. The second messenger signal transduction pathway seems to involve inositol triphosphate (IP3), diacylglycerol (DAG), and protein kinase C. The products of cfos and cjun are active as heterodimers and can be considered tertiary messengers in that their main role is to modulate the expression of additional genes further downstream in the regulatory circuit. Included in the latter regulatory targets are genes for enzymes involved in metabolic defense against hypoxia (such as enzymes in anaerobic metabolism and in metabolic suppression). (Based on Webster et al., 1994, and references quoted therein, and modified from Hochachka et al., 1996.)

huge numbers of genes at once. In so-called model organisms (those for which the complete genome has been sequenced), DNA chips are becoming available for most, or even all, of the genome of the species under study. In such species, tens of thousands of genes can be interrogated essentially at once. In so-called nonmodel organisms, that is, organisms for which genomic information is largely if not entirely lacking, the situation is not so simple for the investigator wishing to monitor changes in gene expression. Still, it is possible to use the DNA microarray approach with nonmodel organisms because many genes can be identified by sequence analysis and homology. Gracey et al. (2001) used DNA chip technology with a nonmodel organism, a goby fish (*Gillichthys mirabilis*), known to be highly tolerant to numerous environmental stresses, including hypoxia. Preparing their own DNA microarrays using 5,376 different cDNA samples, they were able to simultaneously monitor the relative expression rates of hundreds to thousands of genes in tissues of this species under normoxic conditions and during hypoxic exposures for up to 144 hours. These studies found a total of 126 distinct, hypoxia-responsive cDNAs, of which 36 were differentially expressed in hypoxia in both liver and muscle; 56 were liver specific and 34 were muscle specific. By sequence analysis, 75 of these could be identified, while the remaining "hits" are currently unidentifiable (termed novel expressed sequence tags, or ESTs). The latter were notably common in skeletal muscle, implying the existence in this tissue of a significant number of genes and proteins involved in so-far unknown hypoxia related functions. Interestingly, in comparing control versus hypoxia exposed fish, only four genes in brain tissue were differentially expressed. This result is consistent with the frequently reported preferential perfusion of brain and CNS generally during O_2-limitation periods (see chapter 4). Basically, it implies that at the cellular level the CNS is not as seriously stressed by the biologically survivable intensity of hypoxia imposed at the whole-organism level; for this reason, the main emphasis of the Gracey et al. (2001) study focused on muscle and liver.

For these two tissues, Gracey et al. (2001) identified an hypoxia-responsive gene expression pattern that seemingly is part of a complex, layered control mechanism for reorganizing cell function when O_2 is limiting. Thus in muscle and liver, the hypoxia-responsive genes were those whose protein products served in one of four categories of functions: (i) for reducing or minimizing energy production, (ii) for slowing down protein and RNA syntheses, (iii) for slowing down or turning off cell division and tissue growth, and (iv) for signal transduction processes involved in integrating all of the above. It is important to note that hypoxia-responsive expression changes could be positive or negative. For example, the expression profile in muscle was dominated by down-regulation of genes encoding proteins for the protein translation machinery (such as ribosomal proteins and some elongation factors). These down-regulation responses are presumed to be related to suppressed growth and protein turnover during hypoxic stress. Unexpectedly, Gracey et al. also found that in *G. mirabilis* hypoxia exposure results in repression of genes that encode contractile proteins (tropomyosin, myosin heavy chains, myosin light chains, and actins). Reduced expression of these genes in skeletal muscle may be associated with the decreased locomotory activity that characterizes this (and other) species during hypoxia stress. Because contractile proteins are so abundant in muscle, reduced expression of these genes may represent an especially crucial energy saving strategy during hypoxia. In addition, curtailment of protein synthesis in muscle may free-up amino acids to serve for gluconeogenic function in the liver. Under O_2-limiting conditions, liver-derived glucose is released and circulated to other tissues and organs (especially the central nervous system) and may well be critical to survival. This may explain why the gene for glucose-6-phosphatase and the genes for various enzymes in amino acid catabolism are so strongly induced in the fish's liver during hypoxia exposure.

It is perhaps not surprising that these studies also detected the induction of genes involved in signaling and coordination of hypoxia-responsive physiological processes. For example, elevated levels of mRNA for insulin-like growth factor-binding protein 1 (IGFBP-1) were detected in liver. Insulin-like growth-factor-binding protein 1 is thought to regulate the availability of insulin-like growth factors in the circulation. In other systems in chronic hypoxia, the same response is seen as a growth restriction mechanism. This kind of regulatory response, although localized to the liver, clearly influences other tissues and organs as well and thus plays an intertissue coordinating process. Additionally, and as expected from earlier studies (Webster et al., 2002), genes for intracellular signal transduction are also hypoxia-responsive. For example, Gracey et al. noted a strong induction of mitogen-activated protein (MAP) kinase phosphatase, or MKP-1. This protein attenuates the activities of a group of MAP kinases, which when phosphorylated activate a signaling cascade that stimulates cell growth. Hypoxia induction of the MKP-1 gene thus may contribute to slowing down energy-costly growth processes under O_2-limiting conditions, and this in turn may be associated with hypoxia-responsive increases (i) in expression of antiproliferation genes (e.g., transducer of Erb-B2), and (ii) in expression of genes for hemooxygenase and other enzymes involved in iron metabolism, all of which may put a brake on iron-stimulated cell growth and proliferation.

If these kinds of (up or down) hypoxia-responsive shifts in gene expression are general, they go along way to explaining the drastic (over 90%) reduction in ATP-dependent protein synthesis and protein breakdown pathway fluxes in anoxic turtle hepatocytes (Hochachka et al., 1996). What is more, these microarray studies (Gracey et al., 2001) indicate that the "rescue" phenomenon defined above represents a richly complex, multienzyme process of reorganization of cell-level function and structure. Correlated with these changes are notable increases in stability (or half-life) of individual proteins during oxygen limitation (Hand and Hardewig, 1996). In fact, stabilization probably makes the down-regulation of protein turnover "sensible" and possible. For protein synthesis, the reason for this is obvious, since a blockade of synthesis that occurred without protein stabilization would gradually deplete the pool of functional proteins in the cell. In the case of proteolysis, proteolytic blockade would be counterproductive without concomitant increase in protein half lives because it would quickly lead to hypoxic cells that were crippled from accumulations of degrading or degraded proteins. Stabilization of individual proteins may also indicate a key function for the concurrent hypoxia-dependent (Benjamine et al., 1992) induction of molecular chaperones, proteins that assist in the maintenance of native protein structure (see chapter 7).

HYPOXIA-REGULATED GENES INVOLVED IN DEFENSE AGAINST ROS

The cfos and cjun transcription factors discussed above are critically involved in the up-regulation of genes for enzymes (such as superoxide dismutases and glutathione S-transferases) functioning in detoxification of ROSs derived from oxidative metabolism (Bedoya et al., 1995; Bergelson et al., 1994; Hermes-Lima and Storey, 1993; Moffat et al., 1994; Rice, 2000; Rice et al., 1995). While these noxious metabolites are not overproduced during hypoxia or ischemia periods per se, they do represent serious problems during recovery and reperfusion. Although these problems are beyond the scope of the present analysis, it is clear that another reason for hypoxic up-regulation of cfos and cjun gene expression is to set the stage for the post-rescue phase of hypoxia tolerance; that is, to create conditions during the period of oxygen lack that should enhance survival when oxygen is again available. A similar "anticipatory" protective role is the explanation given for increased expression of enzymes of detoxification pathways during oxygen limitation periods in hypoxia-tolerant reptiles (Hermes-Lima and Storey, 1993). It is also an accepted explanation for activation of hemeoxygenase gene expression signaled by hypoxia (Murphy et al., 1991).

The cfos and cjun gene responses to hypoxia have not yet been evaluated in turtle liver cells, although they are likely to play roles at least as significant, if not more so, than in ischemic or hypoxic mammalian cells. Be that as it may, these exciting new studies in several independent lines of investigation go a long way towards explaining how hypoxia tolerant cells "know" when conditions become hypoxic or anoxic and "know" which response pathways to use to turn on hypoxia defense and "rescue" processes per se.

STABILIZING ADENYLATE CONCENTRATIONS DURING O_2 LIMITATION

An additional and important insight is that hypoxia-tolerant tissues (such as turtle liver cells and brain cortical neurons), under both normoxic and anoxic conditions, remain in energy balance. Because at steady state ATP demand and ATP supply pathways maintain the same fluxes despite the overall hypometabolism associated with O_2 limitation, the concentrations of the high-energy phosphate metabolites are usually sustained in the normal range in both cell types despite the lack of oxygen. Any perturbations that may occur are modest and probably temporary. The only known metabolite changes occur because of the requirement for anaerobic ATP-yielding pathways. Thus [glycogen] declines, while [lactate] and [H^+] rise; in some cases, [phosphocreatine] also declines, while [creatine] and [Pi] rise. In several hypoxia-tolerant cells, ATP levels are known to decline somewhat (Karumschnabel et al., 2000) or even drastically in some invertebrate cells (Hand and Hardewig, 1996) down to a new steady-state level. The net effect, however, is that adenylate concentrations during hypoxic or anoxic exposure remain relatively stable at steady-state levels that may vary between different hypoxia-tolerant systems (Hochachka et al., 1996; Lutz, 1992). This condition of matching ATP demand and ATP supply pathway fluxes seems typical of many different kinds of hypoxia-tolerant cells in a variety of species and is viewed by workers in this field as a kind of hallmark of hypoxia tolerance. It clearly contrasts with the situation in hypoxia-sensitive cells (Bickler and Buck, 1998; Karumschnabel et al., 2000; Sick et al., 1993),

which cannot maintain steady-state conditions and as a result must sustain drastic perturbation of the adenylates during oxygen lack, usually including drastic declines in ATP concentrations. Even if the decline in [ATP] is not considered the cause of cell death during oxygen limitation in hypoxia sensitive cells (Dong et al., 2001; Venkatachalam and Weinberg, 1993), the maintenance of energy balance and of stable steady state ATP concentrations in hypoxia tolerant cells are taken to be signatures of effective defense against hypoxia (Boutilier, 2000; Hochachka et al., 1996; Lutz, 1992).

MODEL OF HYPOXIA DEFENSE IN SYSTEMS TOLERANT TO HYPOXIA

From these studies, it is now possible to construct a generalized framework or working hypothesis for how hypoxia-tolerant cells respond to oxygen lack (figure 3.18). During the very early acute phases, a poorly understood hypoxia-sensing and signal transduction system orchestrates a series of molecular hypoxia defense processes, which include:

(i) a 90% or greater global decline in protein biosynthesis during oxygen lack, possibly due to low pH-mediated polysome-EF1α complexing (translational arrest), and

(ii) a generalized decline in membrane permeability ("channel arrest") and/or in firing frequency ("spike arrest") in the case of nervous tissue, and thus in the ATP demand for ion pumping.

These two processes together account for the bulk of the energy savings that allow the very low ATP turnover rates requisite for long-term hypoxia survival. These adjustments are only possible because of:

(iii) a coordinated regulation of ATP supply pathways so as to maintain balance between ATP demand and ATP supply pathways and thus to maintain stable adenylate concentrations.

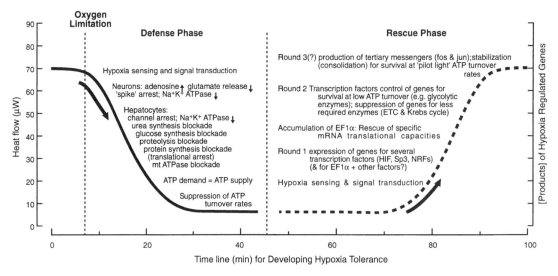

Figure 3.18. Summary model of molecular defense (left) and rescue processes (right) thought to account for the extreme tolerance to oxygen limitation expressed by cells from hypoxia tolerant species. In the left panel, probable sequences are ordered from top to bottom (indicated by direction of arrow); vertical axis is heat output of turtle hepatocytes as a kind of generalized reference. In the right panel, the temporal order of rescue processes is not as well known; although some of these processes may occur simultaneously, a possible sequence of rescue events is arranged from bottom to top (indicated by direction of arrow). Right panel vertical axis: hypoxia-induced products expressed as percent of maximum expressible response; see Hochachka et al. (1996) for magnitude in turtle hepatocytes. The time line for hypoxia tolerance is patterned after currently available information on turtle liver hepatocytes; for other systems, the time required for analogous or homologous processes may differ. Even within the same species, the time line can vary for different tissues; for example, turtle cortical neurons require longer times to mount and complete their defense phase than do turtle hepatocytes. Elongation factor accumulation to levels correlating with rescue of translational capacities in hypoxia-tolerant plant cells may require several hours. Different times may be required for hypoxia induction in hypoxia-tolerant cells such as turtle hepatocytes than in more hypoxia-sensitive mammalian cells (in part because in nature these usually occur at very different temperatures). One aspect of hypoxia tolerance that is not included in this summary or in this analysis concerns problems in recovery and reperfusion. These problems and potential solutions to them are of an entirely different nature than those involved during entry into, and survival of, oxygen lack (summarized above). See text for further details. (Modified from Hochachka et al., 1996.)

The acute or defense phase of hypoxia tolerance is considered to blend almost imperceptibly into a secondary series of processes; in the literature these are variously termed "immediate-early" gene responses (Webster et al., 1993) or acclimatory expression adjustments (Hochachka and Somero, 1984). As the combined effect of these processes is to reactivate some mRNA translational capacities and probably to consolidate and stabilize the cell at strikingly reduced ATP turnover rates, we refer to these combined processes as a rescue phase for establishing hypoxia tolerance. The rescue phase includes (figure 3.18)

(iv) constitutive one-cycle gene expression for the production of key transcription factors (such as HIF 1, Sp1, Sp3) whose functions are then regulated by hypoxia-sensitive proteolysis; one-cycle gene regulation may also allow continued production of key elongation factors and so seemingly "rescue" the cell translational capacities for specific mRNAs during continued oxygen limitation.

(v) two-cycle hypoxia-sensitive gene expression sets (probably including genes for glycolytic enzymes whose expression is up-regulated during prolonged oxygen limitation and for mitochondrial matrix enzymes such as those of the Krebs cycle, whose expression is down-regulated in hypoxia); protein products of these genes are presumably involved in stabilizing cell operations at severely suppressed ATP turnover rates during hypoxia. The gene for EF1α could be regulated by such two-cycle, rather than one-cycle, gene activation circuits.

(vi) two-cycle, hypoxia-regulated gene expression sets, including nuclear and mitochondrial genes for the ETC whose expression is down-regulated during prolonged oxygen limitation. And possibly:

(vii) more complex, two- or three-cycle hypoxia-regulated gene expression sets (such as cfos and cjun) whose products appear as tertiary messengers in the regulation of numerous other housekeeping genes involved in restructuring, consolidation, and stabilization of cell functions at the severely suppressed ATP turnover rates requisite for surviving prolonged hypoxia.

These complex regulatory phenomena, in some tissues involving expression changes in over 100 genes (Gracey et al., 2001), make it less difficult to understand features of the oxygen-limited cell such as massively suppressed proteolysis, increased protein stability, and induction of chaperone proteins, features again indicative of extensive reprogramming of the normoxic cell to generate the hypoxia-tolerant cell.

Empirically, we know that the combination of these molecular processes allows cells and tissues of hypoxia tolerant species to greatly extend the length of time they are able to survive under hypoxic or even anoxic conditions. But it is clear that summaries like those in figure 3.18 only supply key highlights and key processes of hypoxia tolerance. Further work, involving DNA chip and perhaps other analogous technologies, is required for filling in the details of such generalized maps of the nature of hypoxia tolerance—and for evaluating the molecular defense mechanisms required during recovery and reperfusion (a serious problem

area only mentioned in passing in this analysis). Equally daunting is the challenge of discovering whether or not these strategic mechanisms can be transferred from hypoxia-tolerant to hypoxia-sensitive cells—which is the Holy Grail for many hypoxia researchers in the medical field. Finally, since this summary was made possible in large part because of studies initiated with cells/tissues from species exceptionally tolerant to hypoxia, it is interesting to briefly explore the problem of how such physiological systems evolved in specific lineages.

EVOLUTIONARY PHYSIOLOGY OF HYPOXIA TOLERANCE IN TURTLES

Since the above hypoxia defense syndromes were based initially on turtle tissue studies as models of hypoxia tolerance, it is informative to inquire about how this system evolves. Unlike the evolution of the diving response in pinnipeds (chapter 4), we do not have detailed information on the evolution of hypoxia tolerance in groups such as the turtles. However, the phylogeny of these organisms is relatively well understood and there are some comparative data available on the hypoxia tolerance of other species of turtles (Ultsch, 1989). The observation that even terrestrial turtles show startling hypoxia and even anoxia tolerance early on suggested to some comparative biochemists (Bellamy and Petersen, 1968) that this entire lineage was anoxia tolerant; this would be consistent with a "once-in-a-lineage" event, all subsequent lines showing the character in question. However, examination of the phylogenetic tree in figure 3.19 is informative and does not support this speculation. Instead, it indicates (i) that the hypoxia tolerance of turtles as a group may be higher than that of sister taxa (this is indicated by data suggesting that even terrestrial species are more hypoxia tolerant than one might expect of other reptiles), but (ii) that extreme hypoxia tolerance may have evolved more than once within this lineage, possibly several times: in the aquatic Trachemys, in the aquatic Podocnemis, in Chelydra or the snapping turtles, and in Chelonia, the green sea turtles, to list four such possibilities. The

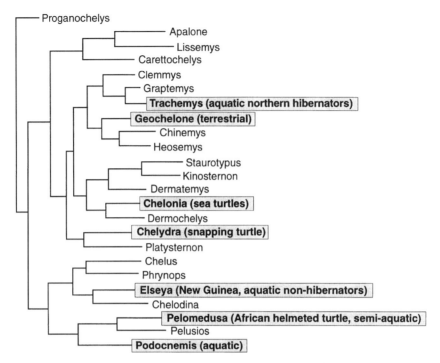

Figure 3.19. A simplified phylogenetic tree of turtles, modifed from Shaffer et al. (1997). Groups known to contain at least one or more species of hypoxia-tolerant turtles are highlighted (shaded boxes). Workers in this field consider that at least some degree of hypoxia tolerance is ancestral to turtles as a group; however, current evidence indicates striking, easily measurable differences in the expression of hypoxia defense mechanisms in different turtle groups, suggesting that many of these features are adaptable through evolutionary time. Furthermore, the spotty distribution of hypoxia tolerance within the phylogeny is consistent with multiple independent origins of hypoxia tolerance mechanisms in turtles.

latter are known to bury themselves in the mud and sands of relatively shallow water basins for "overwintering" periods of up to (if not over) two months! Additionally, in a comparison of tropical turtles, which do not hibernate, with a northern aquatic turtle that hibernates (submerges overwinter), Crocker et al. (1999) found that all four species used similar physiological defense mechanisms (which were thus deemed to represent conservative traits). However, there were important quantitative differences noted, with the northern species seemingly able to tolerate submergence-associated hypoxia most effectively (more effective or extensive expression of known hypoxia defense mechanisms). Interestingly, even subspecies of highly hypoxia-tolerant turtles vary somewhat in the effectiveness of physiological and metabolic defense mechanisms (Ultsch et al., 1999). Thus we conclude that multiple features of

molecular defense against hypoxia in turtles must be adaptable. Unlike the situation in diving mammals (chapter 4), unfortunately, at this time there is no further information on the evolution of hypoxia tolerance in this fascinating group of organisms, so the balance between physiological defense characters that are highly conservative versus those that are adaptable remains unknown. The information lacunae may soon begin to fill up, however, for at least two obvious reasons: first, because the phylogeny of this group of organisms is now rather well known (Shaffer et al., 1997), and secondly, because much of the above model in overall outline (figure 3.19) should apply not only to the Trachemys species used in the detailed molecular studies, but also to other hypoxia-tolerant turtles as well, which should speed up progress in this area.

HYPOXIA TOLERANCE IN FISHES

While there is a similar lack of detailed information on the evolution of hypoxia-tolerant physiology in many fishes, the situation here is somewhat more hopeful and interesting. This is because a larger amount of empirical (as opposed to mechanistic) information is available on hypoxia tolerance of different fish groups and of course because their phylogeny is also well understood. Figure 3.20 is a composite summary of hypothesized phylogenetic relationships of major teleost lineages (Nelson, 1994). Superimposed upon that diagram and highlighted are fish species known to be exceptionally hypoxia tolerant. Except for the Ostariophysi, within which are several groups known to be notably hypoxia tolerant, the distribution of hypoxia tolerance within the phylogeny appears sporadic. At least as a first approximation, this appears consistent with multiple independent origins of hypoxia tolerance mechanisms in teleost fishes. Additional information arises from the phylogeny of air-breathing fishes, since air breathing can be viewed as an hypoxia defense adaptation in its own right. What is more, many and possibly all, air-breathing fishes—described in a recent review as "the first diving vertebrates" (Almeida-Val and Hochachka, 1995)—display impressive hypoxia defense mechanisms similar to those described above for two cell model systems derived from aquatic turtles. Again, even a casual examination of the phylogeny of this group of fishes indicates—perhaps more clearly than in the case of the turtle example above—that air breathing as an indicator of hypoxia defense adaptation and of hypoxia tolerance has evolved numerous times within the fishes (Val and Almeida Val, 1996). While in some lineages, this may have involved common descent, in many others, it is clear that hypoxia tolerance has evolved independently. Because of the large number of fish species that are known to be hypoxia tolerant, the conclusion that hypoxia tolerance has arisen independently many times within this group of organisms is clear and compelling.

What is urgently needed (and workers in the field are waiting for this work with interest) is a detailed evolutionary analysis of hypoxia adaptations in fishes analogous to that presented for diving in pinnipeds (chapter 4). Equally important is the question of probability of parallel convergent evolution; that is, given similar environments and similar starting genotypes, how easy is it for the same or comparable complex physiologies to independently evolve over and over within a group like the fishes? The answer appears to be: strikingly easy, and the best currently known example of this is to be found in some recent penetrating studies of the origin of species in stickleback lineages.

MULTIPLE INDEPENDENT ORIGINS OF COMPLEX FUNCTIONS IN FISHES

How species originate, and indeed what constitutes a species, remain surprisingly still poorly understood questions in evolutionary biology. J.D. McPhail and E.R. Taylor and their colleagues have been probing this question for some time and their analysis of stickleback speciation bears upon our question of independent origins of similar physiological systems. The threespine stickleback is widely distributed in lowland lakes and streams throughout the Straight of Georgia in British Columbia. During the last (Fraser) glaciation, this entire area was covered with ice and later (about 13,000 years before the present, BP) was submerged by the sea. Isostatic rebound led to the present land forms about 11,000 BP. Because of this geological sequence, no lacustrine stickleback populations in this region can be older than these events, say about 12,000 years old, and many populations could well be younger. In addition, there are lacustrine populations on islands and in isolated headlands throughout the region, where the absence of primary freshwater fishes to these lakes implies that there were no dispersal routes into these areas. Islands have always been popular locations for studying issues of species origins and differentiation; these isolated lakes on isolated islands both formed during ice recession, in biological terms, are "islands" within islands. In all these cases, the presumed pattern of population establishment involved (i) an anadromous ancestral line, (ii)

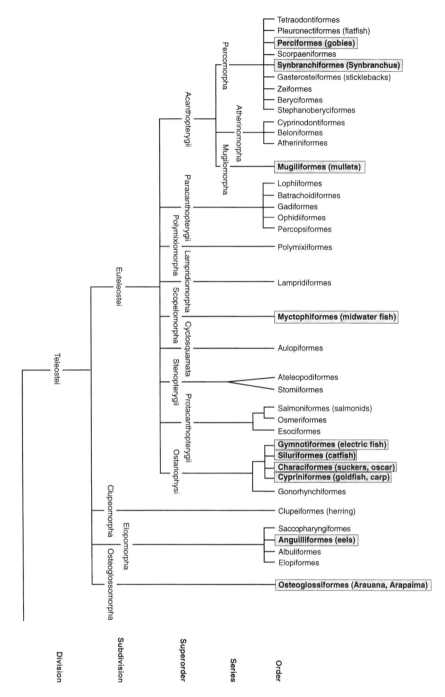

Figure 3.20. A simplified phylogenetic tree of fishes, modified from Nelson (1994). Groups known to contain at least one or more species of hypoxia-tolerant fishes are highlighted (shaded boxes). Hypoxia tolerance is very widely distributed within the phylogeny. In some cases, there is evidence that hypoxia tolerance is a highly conserved ancestral characteristic; however, the strong impression is that it has arisen independently in different lineages and in different geographical regions over and over again, raising the interesting biological question: How easy or how hard is it to evolve the same or similar suites of hypoxia defense mechanisms over and over again in different lineages independently of each other? This question is further analyzed in the text (also see figure 3.21).

stream-dwelling populations, and finally (iii) lake-dwelling populations. These sticklebacks thus should be, and, as we shall see, in fact turned out to be, ideal for the study of the evolution of species. The studies of McPhail and Taylor (see McPhail, 1991; Taylor, 1999) and those of Schluter and his students (see Rundle et al., 2000), have placed the threespine stickleback on par with Darwin's finches as unusually clear examples of speciation in action. The central observation is that ancestral morphologically conservative anadromous stickleback stock, again and again, first moved up rivers, then became isolated in newly formed lakes during deglaciation, with the same differentiation into limnetic and benthic forms appearing again and again.

One well-studied example includes such sympatric "species pairs" in six lakes on islands in the Straight of Georgia. In each case the benthic species is robust-bodied and feeds largely on (mostly invertebrate) macrobenthos in the littoral habitat; it is morphologically and behaviorally specialized for benthivory. The other species in each pair, the limnetic form, is terete-shaped; it inhabits the limnetic zone of lakes (except during breeding) and it is morphologically and behaviorally specialized for planktivory. The two species show a high degree of microhabitat partitioning during breeding in the littoral habitat, and experimental studies have demonstrated clear assortative mating between species under controlled laboratory conditions. Most recent studies show that the sexual selection mechanism is based on females preferentially choosing males that look like themselves, even if, under the experimental conditions used, the males come from a different, rather than from the same, lake (Rundle et al., 2000).

At this time functional comparisons of only anadromous versus stream dwellers are available (table 3.2). These studies confirm functionally significant changes in heart, pectoral muscle, and spleen sizes relative to body sizes in the two groups. Anadromous sticklebacks routinely perform long and sustained labriform (pectoral fin powered) swimming and all of the above adjustments would favor this kind of essentially perpetual activity. The large hearts presumably favor circulatory delivery of O_2 and fuels to the enlarged pectoral muscles used for swimming; the relatively enlarged spleen, involved in erythropoiesis, and red blood cell reservoir and storage functions, are consistent with the endurance performance lifestyle of this species. Their stream-preferring cousins, on the other hand, rely much more upon quick short bursts of swimming in their day-to-day activities and they appropriately display smaller hearts, smaller pectoral fins, smaller spleens and higher LDH A activity per gram of pectoral muscle. This species can afford to maintain smaller hearts, smaller pectoral muscles, and smaller spleens because their lifestyle relies much less upon a sustained type of swimming performance.

Unfortunately, similar functional comparisons of limnetic versus benthic sticklebacks have not been completed. However, from field observations and from general fish physiology it is safe to conclude (i) that in terms of endurance

Table 3.2. Mean (± Standard Deviation) Body Mass, Organ Sizes and Pectoral Muscle LDH Activity (U g^{-1} tissue) in Anadromous and Stream Resident Threespine Stickleback (*Gasterosteus aculeatus*)

	Anadromous	Stream resident	p value
Body mass (g)	2.23 ± 0.79	2.84 ± 0.52	NS
Pectoral muscle mass (mg)	80.0 ± 18.5	26.5 ± 10.4	< 0.0001
Heart mass (mg)	4.7 ± 0.6	2.2 ± 1.1	< 0.0001
Spleen mass (mg)	14.2 ± 6.2	5.7 ± 3.9	< 0.01
Pectoral muscle LDH activity (U g^{-1})	38.01 ± 16.85	110.12 ± 42.76	< 0.001

Unpublished data from C.A. Darveau and P.W. Hochachka. Significant differences take into account the effect of body size as a covariate (ANCOVA).

swimming the limnetics can outperform the benthics, implying fundamental adaptations of development, biochemistry, and physiology of red and white muscle, of heart, of gill, and of microvasculature; (ii) that in terms of nutrition and nutritional metabolism, the limnetics must be able to obtain all their carbon and energy needs from plankton, while the benthics enjoy the nutritional advantages (energy dense foods) of typical aquatic predators; (iii) that in terms of camouflage and mimicry, the limnetics and benthics require and indeed develop different coloration patterns; and (iv) that in terms of vision, the opsins of limnetic and benthic fishes must measurably differ from each other. Thus from first principles we can surmise that a huge amount of evolution of physiological systems underlies the ecological success of each of these species pairs (figure 3.21).

Remarkable conclusions arise from these studies: first, that similar species differentiation from anadromous ancestral forms into freshwater limnetic and benthic forms occurred multiple times in these isolated lakes on isolated islands; second, that complex embryologies, physiologies, and morphologies have arisen that underpin the multiple independent origins of these sympatric species pairs; and third, perhaps most impressive of all, this extensive evolution of physiological systems occurred within the last 12,000 or so years, since the Cordilleran ice sheet began to recede (Taylor and McPhail, 1999). How these systems arose until recently has remained controversial. However, two lines of evidence are particularly suggestive. First, the benthic and limnetic species in each lake are characterized by an unique assemblage of mtDNA haplotypes. Second, neither the limnetic nor the benthic groups form monophyletic groups among lakes. Instead, in two lakes the divergent forms are monophyletic, while in the other lakes examined divergent forms tend to cluster more closely with one another than either species does with comparable species in

other lakes (Taylor and McPhail, 1999). These observations, along with other data that are inconsistent with benthics and limnetics only diverging once in their phylogeny, taken together strongly support the conclusion that deterministic factors (especially natural or sexual selection) have driven the divergence of these species pairs and that this has occurred multiple times independently (Rundle et al., 2000).

In evolutionary biology, as already mentioned, these studies are so dramatic that threespine sticklebacks have joined the ranks of Darwin finches as particularly clear and compelling demonstrations of evolution in action. What is perhaps more surprising is that such sympatric species pairs are not unique to this phylogenetic group. For similar (i.e., history of deglaciation) reasons, similar sympatric species pairs are known to occur in the families Osmeridae, Salmonidae, and Gasterosteidae (Taylor and McPhail, 1999). Because these sympatric pairs are of recent origin (most are thought to be less than 15,000 years old) they represent unique opportunities to combine phylogenetic, ecological, and physiological approaches to the study of speciation under relatively controlled conditions. They represent unprecedented opportunities for evolutionary physiologists interested in working out pathways and mechanisms of evolution of complex physiological systems. Finally, and from our perspective, most importantly, they clearly establish the feasibility of multiple independent origins in the evolution of hypoxia tolerance in fishes and other organisms. This conclusion has far-reaching implications, since hypoxia tolerance represents a complex physiological response system whose repeated convergent evolution is analogous to the comparatively more simple independent evolutionary adaptation of unique gene products (such as the adaptation of Hbs for high-altitude function in birds discussed above).

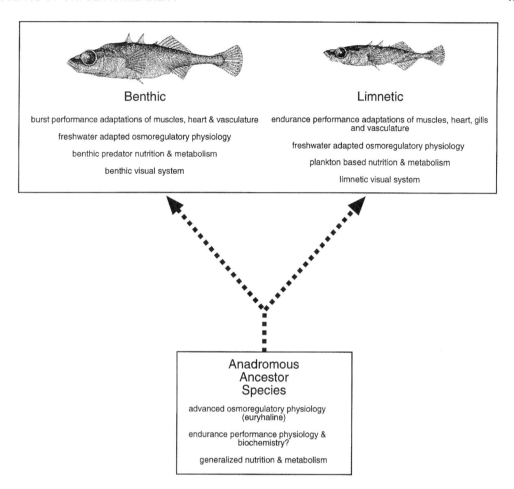

Figure 3.21. A summary of the differentiation from anadromous ancestral species of benthic and limnetic stickleback species in lakes of coastal British Columbia. Workers in this area have found that in
numerous isolated lakes, often on isolated islands, sticklebacks have consistently evolved into two incipient
species: a benthic form and a limnetic form. As far as is known, these have evolved in numerous such
lakes in North America and in North East Asia numerous times independently of each other. The amount
of time required for these speciation events can be confirmed because these lakes formed during deglaciation of these regions, about 11,000–12,000 years before the present. Since the physiologies of the benthic
and lemnitic forms clearly differ, it is difficult to avoid concluding that the independent evolution of similar
physiologies in similar environments in fishes is basically relatively straightforward. The situation is similar
to the evolution of high-O_2-affiinity Hbs for high-altitude function in widely differing groups of animals
(discussed above); however, in the Hb examples we discussed above, the exact mutations causing change in
function are frequently known, while in the complexity of integrative physiologies of hypoxia tolerance (or
benthic vs limnetic specializations), such detailed genomic information is lacking.

REFERENCES

Almeida-Val, V.M.F., and P.W. Hochachka (1995). Air-breathing fishes: Metabolic biochemistry of the first diving vertebrates. *Biochemistry and Molecular Biology of Fishes, Environmental and Ecological Biochemistry* 5: 45–55.

Amundson, S. A., M. Bittner, P. Meltzer, J. Trent, and A. J. Fornace Jr. (2001). Physiological function as regulation of large transcriptional programs: the cellular response to genotoxic stress. *Comp. Biochem. Physiol.* B, 129: 703–710.

Anderson, G.R., V.R. Polonis, J.K. Petell, R.A. Suavedra, K.F. Murty, and L.M. Matovick (1983). LDHk, a transformation dehydrogenase found in human cancer. In: *Isozymes: Current Topics in Biological and Medical Studies*. 11, pp. 155–172, ed. M.C. Rattazzi, J.G. Scandalios, and G.S. Whitt. New York: Alan R. Liss.

Au, H.C., and I.E. Scheffer (1998). Promoter analysis of the human succinate dehydrogenase iron-protein gene: both nuclear respiratory factors NRF1 and NRF2 are required. *Eur. J. Biochem* 251: 164–174.

Banfield, J.F., and C.R. Marshall (2000). Genomics and the geosciences. *Science* 287: 605–606.

Bedoya, F.J., M. Flodstrom, and D.L. Eizirik (1995). Pyrrolidine dithiocarbamate prevents IL-1-induced nitric oxide synthase mRNA, but not superoxide dismutase mRNA, in insulin producing cells. *Biochem. Biophys. Res. Comm.* 210: 816–821.

Bellamy, D., and J.A. Petersen (1968). Anaerobiosis and the toxicity of cyanide in turtles. *Comp. Biochem. Physiol.* 24: 543–548.

Benjamine, I.J., S. Horie, M.L. Greenberg, R.J. Alpern and R.S. Williams (1992). Induction of stress proteins in cultured myogenic cells: Molecular signals for the activation of heat shock transcription during ischemia. *J. Clin. Invest.* 89: 1685–1689.

Bergelson, S., R. Pinkus, and V. Daniel (1994). Intracellular glutathione levels regulate Fos/Jun induction and activation of glutathione S-transferase gene expression. *Cancer Res.* 54: 36–40.

Bickler, P.E., and L.T. Buck (1998). Adaptation of vertebrate neurons to hypoxia and anoxia: maintaining critical Ca^{++} concentrations. *J. Exp. Biol.* 201: 1141–1152.

Boutilier, R.G., and J. St. Pierre (2000). Surviving hypoxia without really dying. *Comp. Biochem. Physiol.* 126A: 481–490.

Buc-Calderon, P, V. Lefebvre, and M. van Steenbrugge (1993). *Surviving Hypoxia*, pp. 271–280, ed. P.W.Hochachka, P.L. Lutz, T. Sick, M. Rosenthal and G. van den Thillart. Boca Raton, Fla: CRC Press.

Buchner, T., D. Abele, and H.O. Pörtner (2001). Oxyconformity in the intertidal worm *Sipunculus nudus*: The mitochondrial background and energetic consequences. *Comp. Biochem. Physiol.*

Buck, L.T., and P.W. Hochachka (1993). Anoxic suppression of Na^+ K^+ ATPase and constant membrane potential in hepatocytes: support for channel arrest. *Am. J. Physiol.* 265: R1020–R1025.

Buck, L.T., P.W. Hochachka, A. Schon, and E. Gnaiger (1993). Microcalorimetric measurement of reversible metabolic suppression induced by anoxia in isolated hepatocytes. *Am. J. Physiol.* 265: R1014–R1019.

Bunn, H.F., J. Gu, L.E. Huang, J.W. Par, and H. Zhu (1998). Erythropoitin: A model system for studying oxygen-dependent gene regulation. *J. Exp. Biol.* 201: 1197–1201.

Burmester, T. (2001). Molecular evolution of the arthropod hemocyanin superfamily. *Molecular Biology & Evolution* 18: 184–195.

Burmester, T. and K. Scheller (1996). Common origin of arthropod tyrosinase, arthropod hemocyanin, insect hexamerin, and dipeteran arylphorin receptor. *J. Mol. Evol.* 42: 713–728.

Chih, C.P, M. Rosenthal, P.L. Lutz, and T.J. Sick (1989). Relationships between aerobic and anaerobic energy production in turtle brain in situ. *Am. J. Physiol.* 257: R854–R859.

Clementi, M.E., S.G.Condo, M. Castagnola, and B. Giardina (1994). Hemoglobin function under extreme life conditions. *Eur. J. Biochem.* 223: 309–317.

Crick, F. (1981). *Life Itself*, pp 1–188. Austin, Tex.: S & X Press.

Crocker, C.E., G.R. Ultsch, and D.C. Jackson (1999). The physiology of diving in a north-temperate and three tropical turtle species. *Comp. Physiol.* B 169: 249–255.

Dang, C.V. and Semenza, G.L. (1999). Oncogenic alterations of metabolism. *Trends Biochem. Sci.* 24: 68–72.

Discher, D.J., N.H. Bishopric, X. Wu, C.A. Peterson, and K.A. Webster (1998). Hypoxia regulates β-enolase and pyruvate kinase-M promoters by modulating Sp1/Sp3 binding to a conserved GC element. *J. Biol. Chem.* 273: 26087–26093.

Doll, C.J. (1993). Anoxic CNS membrane: Mechanisms of collapse and stabilization. In: *Surviving Hypoxia*, pp. 389–400, ed. P.W. Hochachka, P.L. Lutz, T. Sick, M. Rosenthal and G.van den Thillart. Boca Raton, Fla.: CRC Press.

Doll, C.J., P.W. Hochachka, and P.B. Reiner (1991). Channel arrest: implications from membrane resistance in turtle neurons. *Am. J. Physiol.* 261: R1321–R1324.

Doll, C.J., P.W. Hochachka, and P.B. Reiner (1993). Reduced ionic conductance in turtle brain. *Am. J. Physiol.* 265: R929–R933.

Doll, C.J., P.W. Hochachka, and S.C. Hand (1994). A microcalorimetric study of turtle cortical slices: Insights into brain metabolic depression. *J. Exp. Biol.* 191: 141–153.

Dudley, R. (1998). Atmospheric oxygen, giant Paleozoic insects, and the evolution of aerial locomotor performance. *J. Exp. Biol.* 201: 1043–1051.

Dong, Z. M.A. Venkatachalam, J.M. Weinberg, P. Saikumar, and Y. Patel (2001). Protection of ATP-depleted cells by impermeant strychnine derivatives—Implications for glycine cytoprotection. *Am. J. Pathol.* 158: 1021–1028.

Eckardt, K.U. (1994). Erythropoietin: Oxygen-dependent control of erythropoiesis and its failure in renal disease. *Nephron* 67: 7–23.

Fago, A., V. Carratore, G. Di Prisco, R.J. Feuerlein, L. Sottrup-Jensen, and R.E. Weber (1995). The cathodic Hb of Anguila anguila: Amino acid sequence and oxygen equilibria of a reverse Bohr effect hemoglobin with high oxygen affinity and high phosphate sensitivity. *J. Biol. Chem.* 270: 18897–18902.

Fago, A., E. Bendixen, H. Malte, and R.E. Weber (1997). The anodic hemoglobin of *Anguila anguila*: Molecular basis for allosteric effects in a Root-effect hemoglobin. *J. Biol. Chem.* 272: 15628–15635.

Firth, J.D., B.L. Ebert, C.W. Pugh, and P.J. Ratcliffe (1994). Oxygen-regulated control elements in the phosphoglycerate kinase 1 and lactate dehydrogenase A genes: Similarities with the erythropoietin 3′ enhancer. *Proc. Natl. Acad. Sci. USA* 91: 6496–6500.

Firth, J.D., B.L. Ebert and P.J. Ratcliffe (1995). Hypoxic regulation of lactate dehydrogenase A. Interaction between hypoxia inducible factor 1 and cAMP response elements. *J. Biol. Chem.* 270: 21021–21027.

Forsythe, J.S., B.H. Hang, N.V. Iyer, F. Agani, S.W. Leung , R.D. Koos, and G.L. Semenza (1996). Activation of vascular endothelial growth factor gene transcription by hypoxia-inducible factor 1. *Mol. Cell. Biol.* 16: 4604–4613.

Giere, O., J.H. Preusse, and N. Dubilier (1999a). *Tubificoides benedii* (Tubificidae, Oligochaeta)—a pioneer in hypoxic and sulfidic environments. An overview of adaptive pathways. *Hydrobiologia* 406: 235–241.

Gold, T. (1999). *The Deep Hot Biosphere*, pp. 1–235. New York: Springer-Verlag.

Golding, G.B., and A.M. Dean (1998). The structural basis of molecular adaptation. *Mol. Biol. Evol.* 15: 355–369.

Gottschalk, G. (1979). *Bacterial Metabolism*. New York: Springer-Verlag.

Gracey, A.Y., J.V. Troll and G.N. Somero (2001). Hypoxia-induced gene expression profiling in the euroxic fish *Gillichthys mirabilis*. *Proc. Natl. Acad. Sci. USA*, 98: 1993–1998.

Graeber, T.G., C. Osmanian, T. Jacks, D.E. Housman, C.J. Koch, S.W. Lowe, and A.J. Giaccia (1996). Hypoxia-mediated selection of cells with diminished apoptotic potential in solid tumours. *Nature* 379: 88–91.

Graham, J.B., R. Dudley, N. Aguilar, and C. Gans (1995). Implications of the late Paleozoic oxygen pulse for physiology and evolution. *Nature* 375: 117–120.

Grieshaber, M.K., and S. Volkel (1998). Animal adaptations for tolerance and exploitation of poisonous sulfide. *Annu. Rev. Physiol.* 60: 33–53.

Gross, S.S., and P. Lane (1999). Physiological reactions of nitric oxide and hemoglobin: A radical rethink. *Proc. Natl. Acad. Sci. USA* 96: 9967–9969.

Guppy, M., C.J. Fuery, and J.E. Flanigan (1994). Biochemical principles of metabolic suppression. *Comp. Biochem. Physiol.* 109B: 175–189.

Hand, S.C. (1991). Metabolic dormancy in aquatic invertebrates. In: *Adv. Comp. Environ. Physiol.* 8: 1–47, ed. R. Gilles. New York: Springer-Verlag.

Hand, S.C. (1993). pH and anabolic arrest during anoxia in *Artemia franciscana* embryos. In: *Surviving Hypoxia*, pp. 171–185, ed. P.W. Hochachka, P.L. Lutz, T. Sick, M. Rosenthal, and G. van den Thillart. Boca Raton, Fla.: CRC Press.

Hand, S.C., and I. Hardewig (1996). Downregulation of cellular metabolism during environmental stress—mechanisms and implications. *Annu. Rev. Physiol.* 58: 539–563.

Hardison, R. (1998). Hemoglobins from bacteria to man: evolution of different patterns of gene expression. *J. Exp. Biol.* 201: 1099–1117.

Hermes-Lima, M., and K.B. Storey (1993). Antioxidant defenses in the tolerance of freezing and anoxia by garter snakes. *Am. J. Physiol.* 265: R646–R652.

Hieter, P., and Boguski, M. (1997). Functional genomics: it's all how you read it. *Science* 278: 601–605.

Hochachka, P.W. (1986). Defense strategies against hypoxia and hypothermia. *Science* 23: 234–241.

Hochachka, P.W. (1993a). Adaptability of metabolic efficiencies under chronic hypoxia in man. In: *Surviving Hypoxia*, pp. 127–135, ed. P.W. Hochachka, P.L. Lutz, T. Sick, M. Rosenthal, and G. van den Thillart. Boca Raton, Fla.: CRC Press.

Hochachka, P.W. (1993b). Roles of the smallest metabolite—the hydrogen ion as a metabolite intermediate and a metabolic regulator. In: *Hypoxia and Molecular Medicine*, pp. 146–155, ed. J.R. Sutton, C.S. Houston and G. Coates. Burlington, Vt.: Queen City Printers.

Hochachka, P.W. (1994). *Muscles as Molecular and Metabolic Machines*, pp. 1–157. Boca Raton, Fla.: CRC Press.

Hochachka, P.W. (1998). Oxygen—a key regulatory metabolite in metabolic defense against hypoxia. *Am. Zool.* 37: 595–603.

Hochachka, P.W. (1999). The metabolic implications of intracellular circulation. *Proc. Natl. Acad. Sci. USA* 96: 12233–12239.

Hochachka, P.W., and R.A. Foreman, III (1994). Phocid and cetacean blueprints of muscle metabolism. *Can. J. Zool.* 71: 2089–2098.

Hochachka, P.W. and M. Guppy (1987). *Metabolic Arrest and the Control of Biological Time.* pp. 1–237. Cambridge, Mass.: Harvard University Press.

Hochachka, P.W., and G.N. Somero (1984). *Biochemical Adaptation*, pp. 1–521. Princeton, N.J.: Princeton University Press.

Hochachka, P.W., L.T. Buck, C.J. Doll, and S.C. Land (1996). Unifying theory of hypoxia tolerance: Molecular/metabolic defense and rescue mechanisms for surviving oxygen lack. *Proc. Natl. Acad. Sci.USA* 93: 9493–9498.

Huang, L.E., J. Gu, M. Schau, and H.F. Bunn (1998). Regulation of hypoxia-inducible factor 1alpha is mediated by an O_2-dependent degradation domain via the ubiquitin-proteasome pathway. *Proc. Natl. Acad. Sci. USA* 95: 7987–7992.

Hylland, P., S. Milton, M. Pek, G.E. Nilsson, and P.L. Lutz (1997). Brain Na^+/K^+-ATPase activity in two anoxia tolerant vertebrates: crucian carp and freshwater turtle. *Neurosci. Lett.* 235: 89–92.

Iuchi, S., and L. Weiner (1996). Cellular and molecular physiology of Escherichia coli in the adaptation to aerobic environments. *J. Biochem. (Japan)* 120: 1055–1063.

Ivan, M., K. Kondo, H. Yang, W. Kim, J. Valiando, M. Ohh, A. Salic, J.M. Asara, W.S. Lane, and W.G. Kaelin, Jr. (2001). HIFα targetted for VHL-mediated destruction by proline hydroxylation: P implications for O_2 sensing. *Science* 292: 464–468.

P. Jaakola, D.R. Mole, Y.M. Tian, M.I. Wilson, J. Gielbert, S.J. Gaskell, A. von Kriegsheim, H.F. Hebestreit, M. Mukherji, C.J. Schofield, P.H. Maxwell, C.W. Pugh, and P.J. Ratcliffe (2001). Targeting of HIFα to the von Hippel-Landau ubiquitylation complex by O_2-regulated prolyl hydroxylation. *Science* 292: 468–472.

Jackson, D.C. (1968). Metabolic depression and oxygen depletion in the diving turtle. *J. Appl. Physiol.* 24: 503–509.

Jackson, D.C. (2000). Living without oxygen: Lessons from the freshwater turtle. *Comp. Biochem. Physiol.* 125A: 299–315.

Jensen, F.B., A. Fago, and R.E. Weber (1998). Hemoglobin structure and function. In: *Fish Respiration*, pp. 1–40, ed. S.F. Perry, and B. Tufts. New York: Academic Press.

Kallio, P.J., W.J. Wilson, S. O'Brien, Y. Makino, and L. Poellinger (1999). Regulation of the hypoxia-inducible transcription factor 1alpha by the ubiquitin-proteasome pathway. *J. Biol. Chem.* 274: 6519–6525.

Keitzmann, T., H. Schmidt, I. Probst, and K. Jungermann (1992). Modulation of the glucagon-dependent activation of the PEPCK gene by oxygen in rat hepatocyte cultures. *FEBS Lett.* 311: 251–255.

Keitzmann, T., H. Schmidt, K. Unthan-Feschner, I. Probst, and K. Jungermann (1993). A ferro-heme protein senses oxygen levels which modulate the glucagon dependent activation of the PEPCK gene in rat hepatocyte cultures. *Biochem. Biophys. Res. Comm.* 195: 792–798.

Knoll, A.H., and S.B. Carroll (1999). Early animal evolution: Emerging views from comparative biology and geology. *Science* 284: 2129–2137.

Krumschnabel, G., P.J. Schwarzbaum, J. Lisch, C. Biasi, and W. Wieser (2000). Oxygen-dependent energetics of anoxia-tolerant and anoxia-intolerant hepatocytes. *J. Exp. Biol.* 203: 951–959.

Kwast, K.E., and S.C. Hand (1996). Acute depression of mitochondrial protein synthesis during anoxia: Contributions of oxygen sensing, matrix acidification, and redox state. *J. Biol. Chem.* 217: 7313–7319.

Ladoux, A., and C. Felin (1993). Hypoxia is a strong inducer of vascular endothelial growth factor mRNA expression in the heart. *Biochem. Biophys. Res. Comm.* 195: 1005–1010.

Land, S.C., and N.J. Bernier (1995). Estivation: metabolic suppression, mechanisms and models of control. In: *Biochemistry and Molecular Biology of Fishes* 5, pp. 381–405, ed. P.W. Hochachka and T.P. Mommsen. Amsterdam: Elsevier Science.

Land, S.C., and P.W. Hochachka (1994). Protein turnover during metabolic arrest in turtle hepatocytes: role and energy dependence of proteolysis. *Am. J. Physiol.* 266: C1028–C1036.

Land, S.C., and P.W. Hochachka (1995). A hemeprotein based oxygen sensing mechanism controls the expression and suppression of multiple proteins in anoxia tolerant turtle hepatocytes. *Proc. Natl. Acad. Sci. USA* 92: 7505–7509.

Land, S.C., L.T. Buck, and P.W. Hochachka (1993). Response of protein synthesis to anoxia and recovery in anoxia-tolerant hepatocytes. *Am. J. Physiol.* 265: R41–R48.

Leary S., and C.D. Moyes (2000). The effects of biogenic stress and redox balance on the expression of genes critical to mitochondrial function. In: *Environmental Stressors and Gene Responses*, pp. 209–230, ed. K.B. Storey and J. Storey. New York: Elsevier Press.

Lisa, F.D., R. Menabò, M. Canton, and V. Petronilli (1998). The role of mitochondria in the salvage and the injury of the ischemic myocardium. *Biochim. Biophys. Acta* 1366: 69–78.

Lovelock, J.E. (1979). *Gaia: A New Look at Life on Earth.* Oxford: Oxford University Press.

Lutz, P.L. (1992). Mechanisms for anoxic survival in the anoxic vertebrate brain. *Annu. Rev. Physiol.* 54: 619–637.

Lutz, P.L. and L. Manuel (1999). Maintenance of adenosine A1 receptor function during long-term anoxia in the turtle brain. *Am. J. Physiol.* 276: R633–R636.

Maxwell, P.H., C.W. Pugh, and P.J. Ratcliffe (1993). Inducible operation of the erythropoitin 3' enhancer in multiple cell lines: Evidence for a widespread oxygen-sensing mechanism. *Proc. Natl. Acad. Sci. USA* 90: 2423–2427.

McPhail, J.D. (1991). Ecology and evolution of sympatric sticklebacks (*Gasterosteus*): evidence for a species pair in Paxton Lake, Texada Island, British Columbia. *Can. J. Zool.* 70: 361–369.

Meyer, B., and B. Hemmens (1997). Biosynthesis and action of nitric oxide in mammalian cells. *Trends Biochem. Sci.* 22: 477–481.

Mishra R.R., G. Adhikary, M.S. Simonson, N.S. Cherniack, and N.R. Prabhakar (1998). Role of c-fos in hypoxia induced AP-1 element activity and tyrosine hydroxylase gene expression. *Molec. Brain Res.* 59: 74–83.

Moffat, G.J., A.W. McLaren, and C.R.Wolff (1994). Involvement of Jun and Fos proteins in regulating transcriptional activation of the human pi class glutathione S-transferase gene in multidrug-resistant MCF7 breast cancer cells. *J. Biol. Chem.* 269: 16397–16402.

Morris, S., and J. Collaghan (1998). Respiratory and metabolic responses of the Australian yabby, *Cherax destructor*, to progressive and sustained environmental hypoxia. *J. Comp. Physiol. B.* 168: 377–388.

Murphy, B.J., E.D. Robin, D.P. Tapper, R.J. Wong, and D.A. Clayton (1984). Hypoxic coordinate regulation of mitochondrial enzymes in mammalian cells. *Science* 223: 707–709.

Murphy B.J., K.R. Laderoute , S.M. Short, and R.M. Sutherland (1991). The identification of heme oxygenase as a major hypoxic stress protein in Chinese hamster ovary cells. *Br. J. Cancer* 63: 69–73.

Nelson, J.S. (1994). *Fishes of the World,* 3rd Edition, pp. 1–600. New York: John Wiley.

Nilsson, G. (1993). Neurotransmitters and anoxia resistance: Comparative physiological and evolutionary perspectives. In: *Surviving Hypoxia*, pp. 401–413, ed. J.R. Sutton, C.S. Houston and G. Coates. Burlington, Vt.: Queen City Printers.

Powers, D.A. (1972). Hemoglobin adaptations for fast and slow water habitats in sympatric catastomid fishes. *Science* 177: 360–362.

Poyart, C., H. Wajcman and J. Kister (1992). Molecular adaptation of hemoglobin functions in mammals. *Resp. Physiol.* 90: 3–17.

Reiber, C. L. (1995). Physiological adaptations of crayfish to the hypoxic environment. *Am. Zool.* 35: 1–11.

Reisser, T., W. Langutt, and H. Kersten (1994). The nutrient factor queuine protects Hela cells from hypoxic stress and improves metabolic adaptation to oxygen availability. *Eur. J. Biochem.* 221: 979–986.

Rice M.E. (2000). Ascorbate regulation and its neuroprotective role in the brain. *Trends Neurosci.* 23: 209–216.

Rice, M.E., E.J.K. Lee, and Y. Choy (1995). High levels of ascorbic acid, not glutathione, in the

CNS of anoxia-tolerant reptiles contrasted with levels in anoxia-intolerant species. *J. Neurochem.* 64: 1790–1799.

Robin, E.D., B.J. Murphy, and J. Theodore (1984). Coordinate regulation of glycolysis by hypoxia in mammalian cells. *J. Cell Physiol.* 118: 287–190.

Rouslin, W. (1991). Regulation of the mitochondrial ATPase in situ in cardiac muscle: role of the inhibitor subunit. *J. Bioenerg. Biomembr.* 23: 873–888.

Rundle, H.D., L. Nagel, J.W. Boughman, and D. Schluter (2000). Natural selection and parallel speciation in sympatric sticklebacks. *Science* 287: 306–308.

Scarpulla, R.C. (1996). Nuclear respiratory factors and the pathways of nuclear-mitochondrial interactions. *Trends. Cardiovasc. Med.* 6: 39–45.

Schlingensiepen, K.H., F. Wollnik, M. Kunst, R. Schlingensiepen, T. Herdegen, and W. Brysch (1994). The role of Jun transcription factor expression and phosphorylation in neuronal differentiation, neuronal cell death, and plastic adaptations in vivo. *Cell. Mol. Neurobiol.* 14: 487–505.

Schmidt H., and G. Kamp (1996). The Pasteur effect in facultative anaerobic metazoa. *Experientia* 52: 440–448.

Semenza, G.L., P.H. Roth, F.M. Fang, and G.L. Wang (1994). Transcriptional regulation of genes encoding glycolytic enzymes by hypoxia-inducible factor 1. *J. Biol. Chem.* 269: 23757–23763.

Semenza, G.L., B. Jiang, S.W. Leung, R. Passantino, J. Concordet, P. Maire, and A. Giallongo (1996). Hypoxia response elements in the aldolase A, enolase 1, and lactate dehydrogenase A gene promoters contain essential binding sites for hypoxia Inducible Factor-1. *J. Biol. Chem.* 271: 32529–32537.

Shaffer, H.B., P. Meylan, and M.L. McKnight (1997). Tests of turtle phylogeny: Molecular, morphological, and paleontological approaches. *System. Biol.* 46: 235–268.

Sick, T.J., M. Perez-Pinon, P.L. Lutz, and M. Rosenthal (1993). Maintaining coupled metabolism and membrane function in anoxic brain: A comparison between the turtle and rat. In: *Surviving Hypoxia*, pp 351–363, ed. J.R. Sutton, C.S. Houston and G. Coates. Burlington, Vt.: Queen City Printers.

St. Pierre, J., M.D. Brand, and R.G. Boutilier (2000). Mitochondria as ATP consumers: cellular treason in anoxia. *Proc. Natl. Acad. Sci. USA* 97: 8670–8674.

Stamler, J.S., J. Li, J.P. Eu., T.J. McMahon, I.T. Demchenko, J. Bonaventura, K. Gernert, and C.A. Piantadosi (1997). Blood flow regulation by s-nitrosohemoglobin in the physiological oxygen gradient. *Science* 276: 2034–2037.

Storey, K.B., and P.W. Hochachka (1974). Enzymes of energy metabolism from a vertebrate facultative anaerobe, *Pseudemys scripta.* Turtle heart phosphofructokinase. *J. Biol. Chem.* 249: 1423–1429.

Storey, K.B., and J.M. Storey (1990). Metabolic rate depression and biochemical adaptation in anaerobiosis, hibernation, and estivation. *Q. Rev. Biol.* 65: 145–193.

Suzuki, T., H. Kawamichi, and K. Imai (1998). A myoglobin evolved from indoleamine 2,3-dioxygenase, a tryptophan degrading enzyme. *Comp. Biochem. Physiol.* 121B: 117–128.

Taylor, A.C., J. Davenport, and J.A. Allen (1995). Anoxic survival, oxygen consumption, and hemocyanin characteristics in the protobranch bivalve, *Nucula sulcata* Brown. *Comp. Biochem. Physiol.* 112: 333–338.

Taylor, E.R. (1999). Species pairs of north temperate freshwater fishes: taxonomy, evolution, and conservation. *Rev. Fish Biol. Fisheries* 9: 281–297.

Taylor, E.R., and J.D. McPhail (1999). Evolutionary history of an adaptive radiation in species pairs of threespine sticklebacks (Gasterosteus): insights from mitochondrial DNA. *J. Linnean Soc.* 66: 271–293.

Thurman, R.G., Y. Nakagawa, T. Matsumura, J.J. Lemasters, U.K. Misra, and F.C. Kauffman (1993). Regulation of oxygen uptake in oxygen-rich periportal and oxygen-poor pericentral regions of the liver lobule by oxygen tension. In: *Surviving Hypoxia–Mechanisms of Control and Adaptation*, pp. 329–340, ed. P.W. Hochachka et al.. Boca Raton, Fla.: CRC Press.

Ultsch, G.R. (1989). Ecology and physiology of hibernation and overwintering among freshwater fishes, turtles, and snakes. *Biol. Rev.* 64, 435–516.

Ultsch, G.R., M.E. Carwile, C.E. Crocker, and D.C. Jackson (1999). The physiology of hibernation among painted turtles: The eastern painted turtle, *Chrysemys picta picta. Physiol. Zool.* 72: 493–501.

Val, A.L. (1996). Surviving low oxygen levels: Lessons from fishes of the Amazon. In: *Physiology and Biochemistry of the Fishes of the Amazon*, pp. 59–73, ed. A.L. Val, V.M. Almeida-Val, and D.J. Randall. Manaus: INPA.

Val, A.L., and V.M.F. de Almeida Val (1996). *Fishes of the Amazon and Their Environment*, pp.1–224. Berlin: Springer-Verlag.

van Holde, K. (1998). Respiratory proteins of invertebrates: Structure, function, and evolution. *Zoology (Jena)* 100: 287–297.

Vayda, M.E., C.K. Shewmaker, and J.K. Morelli (1995). Translational arrest in hypoxic potato tubers is correlated with the aberrant association of elongation factor EF-1-alpha with polysomes. *Plant Mol. Biol.* 28: 751–757.

Venkatachalam, M.A., and J.M. Weinberg (1993). Structural effects of intracellular amino acids during ATP depletion. In: *Surviving Hypoxia*, pp. 473–494, ed. J.R. Sutton, C.S. Houston and G. Coates. Burlington, Vt.: Queen City Printers.

Wang, G.L., and G.L. Semenza (1993). General involvement of hypoxia-inducible factor 1 in transcriptional response to hypoxia. *Proc. Natl. Acad. Sci. USA* 90: 4304–4308.

Wang, G.L., and G.L.Semenza (1995). Purification and characterization of hypoxia-inducible factor 1. *J. Biol. Chem.* 270: 1230–1237.

Wang, G.L., B.H. Jian, E.A. Rue, and G.L. Semenza (1995). Hypoxia inducible factor 1 is a basic-helix-loop-helix PAS heterodimer regulated by cellular oxygen tension. *Proc. Natl. Acad. Sci. USA* 92: 5510–5514.

Weber, R. (1995). Hemoglobin adaptations to hypoxia and altitude—the phylogenetic perspective. In: *Hypoxia and the Brain*, pp. 31–44, ed. J.R. Sutton, C.S. Houston, and G. Coates. Burlington,Vt: Queen City Printers.

Webster, K.A., and N.H. Bishopric (1992). Molecular regulation of cardiac myocyte adaptations to chronic hypoxia. *J. Mol. Cell. Cardiol.* 24: 741–751.

Webster, K.A., and B.J. Murphy (1988). Regulation of tissue-specific isozyme genes: coordinate response to oxygen availability in myogenic cells. *Can. J. Zool.* 66: 1046–1058.

Webster, K.A., P.W. Gunning, E. Hardeman, D.C. Wallace, and L.H. Kedes (1990). Coordinate reciprocal trends in glycolytic and mitochondrial transcript accumulations during the in vitro differentiation of human myoblasts. *J. Cell. Physiol.* 142: 566–573.

Webster, K.A., D. Discher, and N.H. Bishopric (1993). Induction and nuclear accumulation of fos and jun proto-oncogenes in hypoxia cardiac myocytes. *J. Biol. Chem.* 268: 16852–16859.

Webster, K.A., D.J. Discher, and N.H. Bishopric (1994). Regulation of fos and jun immediate-early genes by redox or metabolic stress in cardiac myocytes. *Circ. Res.* 74: 679–686.

Webster, K.A., D.J. Discher, O.M. Hernandez, K. Yamashita, and N.H. Bishopric (2000). A glycolytic pathway to apoptosis of hypoxic cardiac myocytes. In *Oxygen Sensing—Molecules to Man*, pp. 161–176, ed. S. Lahiri, N.R. Prabhakar and R.E. Forster, II. New York: Kluwer Academic/Plenum.

Wenger, R.H., and M. Gassman (1997). Oxygen(es) and the hypoxia inducible factor 1. *Biol. Chem.* 378: 609–616.

Woese, C.R., O. Kandler, and M. Wheelis (1990). Towards a natural system of organisms: proposal for the domains Archaea, Bacteria, and Eucarya. *Proc. Natl. Acad. Sci. USA* 87: 4576–4581.

Xia, Y., L.M. Buja, R.C. Scarpulla, and J.B. McMillin (1997). Electrical stimulation of neonatal cardiomyocytes results in the sequential activation of nuclear genes governing mitochondrial proliferation and differentiation. *Proc. Natl. Acad. Sci. USA* 94: 11399–11404.

Zhu, H. and H.F. Bunn (2001). How do cells sense oxygen? *Science* 292: 449–451.

4

The Diving Response and Its Evolution

EARLY LABORATORY STUDIES OF DIVING PHYSIOLOGY

Intrigued by diving mammals and birds for well over a century, biologists in the 1930s and 1940s first began to make significant progress in understanding the physiological and metabolic mechanisms now known to permit an air-breathing animal to operate successfully deep into the water column. At that time, several fundamental biological traits that seemed to correlate with diving capacity were already known; these traits included (i) an expanded blood volume and red blood cell (RBC) mass, or high hematocrit, (ii) high muscle myoglobin concentrations, and (iii) collapsible lungs in the case of deep divers such as the pinnipeds. The pioneering work of Scholander, Irving, and their colleagues (Scholander, 1940) greatly expanded this preliminary knowledge and developed the fundamental foundations of diving physiology that are now known to include three key physiological "reflexes": (i) apnea, (ii) bradycardia, and (iii) peripheral vasoconstriction and thus hypoperfusion of most peripheral tissues. Scholander referred to these physiological reflexes in combination as the "diving response," and in forced diving under laboratory conditions, he imagined the marine mammal reducing itself to a "heart, lung, brain machine." The metabolic correlates of this response included the gradual development of oxygen-limiting conditions in hypoperfused (ischemic) tissues, with attendant accumulation of end products of anaerobic metabolism (especially lactate and H^+ ions). Because peripheral tissues were hypoperfused, Scholander reasoned that most of the lactate would remain at sites of formation during the course of a simulated dive,

and that most of it would not be "washed out" of the tissues into the circulation until perfusion was restored at the end of diving. By explaining why only a small lactate accumulation is observed in blood plasma during (simulated) diving, while a post-diving peak of lactate is seen early in recovery from a (simulated) dive, Scholander used the lactate data as indirect evidence for hypoperfusion and vasoconstriction of peripheral tissues.

At first, Scholander and Irving anticipated diving would involve the Pasteur effect; that is, that energy deficits incurred by oxygen lack during diving per se would be made up by anaerobic glycolysis (with concomitant lactate accumulation). In contrast, their seminal studies of the harbor seal indicated that the post-diving oxygen debt was frequently less than the expected oxygen deficit during diving. Moreover, the amount of lactate accumulated often was substantially less than would be expected if the energy deficit were to be made up by anaerobic glycolysis. That is why as early as 1940 Scholander introduced the idea of a relative hypometabolism during diving to account for the missing lactate and the missing oxygen debt (see figure 4.1 summary of physiological and metabolic features of laboratory diving).

During the next four decades, many laboratory studies were performed which basically confirmed the earlier framework developed by Scholander and Irving (see Butler and Jones, 1982; Elsner and Gooden, 1983; Zapol et al., 1979). The key features that were observed in simulated diving studies over and over again were (i) apnea, (ii) bradycardia, (iii) peripheral vasoconstriction, (iv) low lactate accumulation during diving per se, and (v) a post-diving lactate washout peak appearing in the plasma

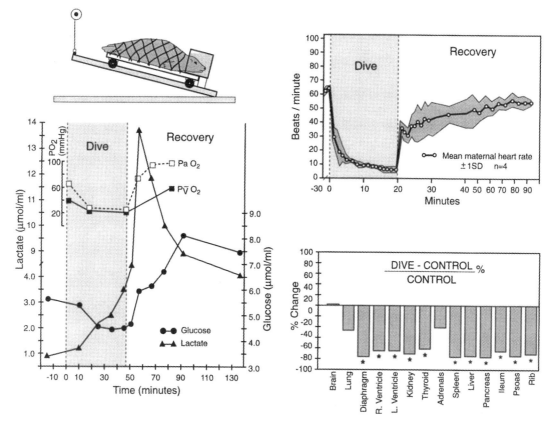

Figure 4.1. Summary of key features of the diving response in pinnipeds as assessed through simulated diving studies. Upper left shows a sketch of a typical simulated breath-hold diving experiment, which typified the field from the 1940s to the 1970s. Upper right shows representative bradycardia responses during simulated diving and recovery in adult, pregnant female Weddell seals. Lower right indicates quantitative estimates of peripheral vasoconstriction of most tissues and organs examined. The lower left panel indicates that lactate begins to build up in the plasma during the dive, but that most of the lactate formed in peripheral tissues during simulated diving is not released until recovery, when peripheral tissues are reperfused. The lactate then spilling out into the blood appears as a concentration "spike" in the plasma. Similar results were obtained over and over again in various laboratories and with various species. These summaries are taken largely from the collaborative studies by Zapol, Liggins, and Hochachka (see Hochachka, 1992 and 2000 for literature in this area).

within 1–4 min of recovery. This combination of processes became known in the literature as "the diving response." All of this quickly became pretty common knowledge (figure 4.1) and by the mid-1970s the field was slowing down, with classical laboratory analyses at a kind of point of diminishing returns. It was as if the field of diving physiology itself had entered into a breath-hold situation—awaiting new developments.

FIELD DIVING STUDIES OF THE DIVING RESPONSE

The new developments came from an unexpected direction—from field (Kooyman et al., 1980) rather than laboratory studies—and they are marked by the advent of modern field study technologies, especially of microprocessor-assisted monitoring of aquatic animals while diving voluntarily in their natural environment (Guppy et al., 1986; Hill et al., 1987). Two key differences about laboratory-simulated versus at-sea voluntary diving included the potential presence of fear in the former protocols coupled with demands of exercise in the latter. Even in early stages of voluntary diving studies, the potentially conflicting demands of diving and exercise were already emphasized (Castellini et al., 1985; Fedak, 1986; Hochachka, 1986) so when microcomputers were placed on seals to be released into the open ocean there was some uncertainty about what the data loggers would show. Carried out in the 1980s and 1990s, what these studies established can be summarized as follows (Hochachka, 2000):

(i) *Bradycardia.* Despite the possibility that demands of swimming exercise may well be anticipated to require elevated heart rates and cardiac output, seals under pretty well all conditions examined employ an easily measured, and often profound, bradycardia (figure 4.2). However, the data also exposed enormous plasticity of the response: the intensity of bradycardia could change during diving, bradycardia could be fully reversed before the end of diving, and at least in some species, underwater heart rates correlate with swim speed (with demands of exercise).

(ii) *Peripheral vasoconstriction.* Unlike laboratory studies, where direct perfusion measurements could quantify tissue/organ specific blood flow and thus quantify the intensity of peripheral vasconstriction, field studies have had to rely upon indirect evidence for this reflex during voluntary diving at sea. The most convincing studies involved injection of radiolabeled compounds after the diving response was initiated: compounds such as glucose and palmitate, which are substrates for metabolism, as well as organ-specific compounds such as inulin (clearance rate specifically determined by the kidney) required long time periods for complete equilibration in the circulation system, implying major hypoperfusion (vasoconstriction) of peripheral tissues and organs. Again, the intensity of vasoconstriction seemed to be dive specific (more intense in long-duration div-

ing) and possibly tissue/organ specific (figure 4.2).

(iii) *Hypometabolism and the aerobic diving limit (ADL).* One of the earliest and most provocative observations was that either no lactate washout or only a minimal washout peak could be observed in early post-diving interdive periods in large pinnipeds such as the Weddell seal; this was not fully consistent with earlier laboratory data where lactate washouts were almost always observed. What is more, even if a lactate washout was observed after long dives at sea, the peak was not as large as would be expected if the animal were *fully* making up the energy deficit due to O_2 limitation towards the end of prolonged diving. Two concepts arose from this work. The first was the concept of the aerobic diving limit (ADL): only if the ADL was exceeded would the diving animal be expected to display a post-diving lactate washout. The second concept was that of diving hypometabolism: in dives that were longer than the amount of time required for RMR to use up all onboard O_2 supplies (i.e., in dives longer than the ADL), the organism seemed to be relying on a suppression of energy demand (hypometabolism) as a hypoxia/ischemia defense strategy (especially as a strategy for avoiding excessive anaerobic glycolysis and excessive lactate accumulation, and hence for avoiding a long interdive period, which may otherwise be required for post-diving lactate clearance; figure 4.2).

(iv) *Physiologically controlled myoglobin (Mb) desaturation.* If the above observations were correct, they would imply that muscle Mb would not behave as a closed biochemical system (in which MbO_2 would desaturate along a hyperbolic O_2 equilibrium curve). Instead, it was predicted and observed that Mb desaturated as a linear function of time of diving (Guyton et al., 1995), implying physiological control of the process (presumably a reflection of controlled perfusion and thus controlled O_2 transfer from Hb to Mb).

(v) *Physiologically controlled spleen function.* Another early and provocative observation was that at times the spleen appeared to operate like a biological scuba tank: if the interdive period was long enough, the spleen would become expanded, filled with oxygenated RBCs. As the subsequent dive proceeded, the RBC would be gradually released into the circulation; in the Weddell seal, up to 15 min are required for the hematocrit (Hct) to reach its highest value, indicating the time at which the entire RBC mass is in the circulation (figure 4.2).

(vi) *Catecholamine regulation.* Stimulated by earlier laboratory research (Lacombe et al., 1991), a later field study with Weddell seals (figure 4.2) noted a correlation between diving and plasma concentrations of both epinephrine and norepinphrine. Catecholamines are a particularly well studied system and the background theory indicated at least several functions under sympathetic regulation during diving: vasoconstriction of peripheral arterioles, contraction of smooth muscle capsule of the spleen, titration of vagal-mediated bradycardia, inotropic effect on the heart (increased contractility), and in extreme O_2-limiting conditions, regulation of anaerobic glycogenolysis (Hochachka et al., 1995).

(vii) Field studies indicated that large seals could operate at sea for days to weeks, even up to 8 months, during which they spent as much as 90% of the time submerged. Without doubt these mammals could be called "pelagic organisms"! For species such as the northern elephant seal, up to about one-third of the dives were longer than the calculated ADL, implying a routine reliance upon peripheral tissue hypometabolism as a means for extending underwater time on a given amount of onboard oxygen. Two additional processes may play a role in assisting the energy-saving strategy of the standard dive response mechanism, especially tissue hypoperfusion: one is physiological, the second behavioral. The former involves body temperature regulation: the demonstration of regulated regional hypothermia helps to account for the field (doubly labeled water turnover) measurements of longer-than-expected submergence times as well as the low global metabolic rates measured in elephant seals at sea (Andrews et al., 1994, 1997). The behavioral feature helping to conserve energy involves swimming strategies: studies by Williams and her collaborators used onboard video cameras to monitor tail beating frequency (the motor's speedometer in diving animals). They found (Williams et al., 2000) that during deep diving up to nearly 90% of the way down is spent in a gliding (motor off) mode, not in actively swimming (motor on) mode—sinking rather than swimming is analogous to coasting downhill on a highway with one's automobile in neutral and is an obvious energy-conserving strategy. Additionally, since body composition, and hence buoyancy, of large seals varies seasonally, it is not surprising that seals shape their diving behavior to their buoyancy, and not vice versa (Webb et al., 1998).

In effect, these field studies confirmed the validity and underlined the plasticity of the overall "diving response" first elucidated in the 1930s and 1940s and greatly extended our understanding of how the diving response is used under natural diving conditions (Castellini et al., 1992; Costa, 1991, 1993; Delong and Stewart, 1991; Delong et al., 1992; Guyton et al., 1995; Hindell et al., 1992; Hochachka et al., 1995; Hurford et al., 1995; Kooyman et al., 1980; Leboeuf et al., 1989, 1992; Qvist et al., 1986; Thompson and Fedak, 1989, 1993). The most dramatic studies focused on the large seals: the Weddell in the Antarctic, the southern elephant seal in the southern oceans, and its sister species in the northern Pacific. It is not an overstatement to describe many of these studies as truly sensational. Consider the continuous time–depth monitoring of individual seals ranging over oceanic distances for months at a time (this work has been spearheaded by Costa, Leboeuf, Crocker, and their associates at the University of California in Santa Cruz [Leboeuf et al., 2000]). Consider the monitoring of heart rate, of electrocardiograms (ECGs), of body temperature (Tb), of swimming velocities, of global metabolic rates (see Andrews et al., 1994, 1997). Consider the monitoring of blood metabolites, hematocrit, tissue biochemistry, and blood endocrinological parameters during and after—spleen volume, before and after—voluntary diving at sea (Guyton et al., 1995; Hochachka et al., 1995; Hurford et al., 1995). Consider that initial studies (Guppy et al., 1986) have been made of blood metabolite fluxes

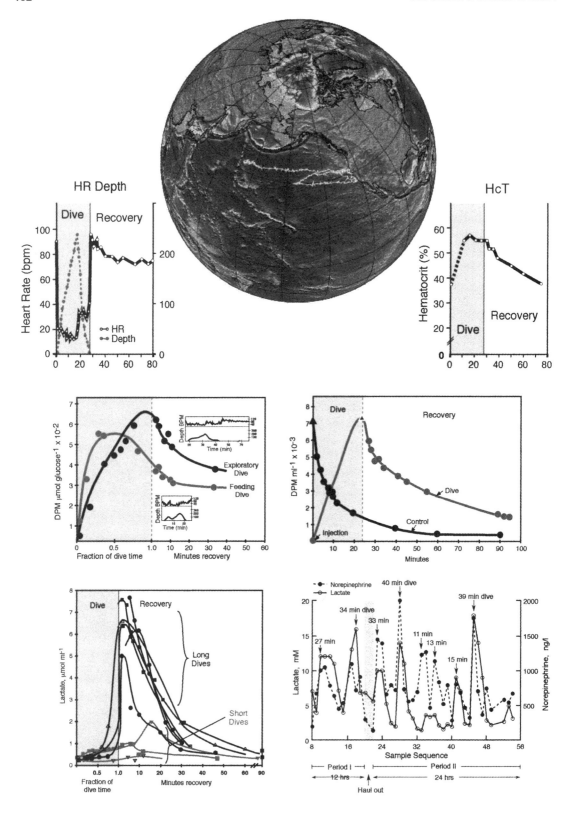

and organ-specific clearance functions (requiring at-sea injection of labeled, sometimes organ-specific metabolites and subsequent sequential blood sampling with onboard peristaltic pumps). Consider that video cameras have been installed in backpacks (Williams et al., 2000) for visual monitoring of seal activities and that current plans are on the drawing board for installing "high-tech targets" on seals in order to allow equally high-tech precision monitoring of their 3D activities at sea. For sure, "sensational" is an appropriate word for these developments. That is why biologists are filled with excitement over the success in application of early twenty-first century technologies to field studies of marine mammals.

It indeed has been an exciting period of scientific development, filled with research fermentation; but now the field of diving physiology may again be pausing and renewal is being catalyzed by two differing approaches. The first is purely experimental, tethered to the laboratory and relying on magnetic resonance imaging and spectroscopy (MRI and MRS). The second—evolutionary study of the diving response—is synthetic, linked to both field and laboratory studies. We shall consider the status of each approach separately below.

MRI/MRS—TECHNOLOGY AT THE RIGHT PLACE AND RIGHT TIME

One of the main reasons why both field and classical laboratory models of diving may be reaching points of diminishing returns is that in both cases the intellectual underpinnings are based on essentially "static" information. "Snapshot" type measurements at specific diving or post-diving states supplied the original data base for laboratory models of diving; the "forced dive" models in turn served as the framework for the field studies, which basically extended and refined them. The main conceptual contribution of all of the field studies was

Figure 4.2. Brief summary of several essential features of the diving response in pinnipeds as assessed through microcomputer-assisted monitoring of the physiology, metabolism, and behavior during voluntary diving of wild seals at sea. This summary is directly comparable to the figure 4.1 summary of simulated diving. (Upper panel, left) Representative bradycardia in the Weddell seal during a voluntary dive lasting about a half hour. (Upper panel, middle) Time–depth and geolocating data loggers allow reconstruction of migratory paths of two elephant seals from coastal California into the northwest Pacific over an 8-month migration period (courtesy of Drs. D. Costa and B. Leboeuf). (Upper panel, right) Change in hematocrit (HCT) during diving and recovery in a representative dive in the Weddell seal. (Middle panel, left) The control studies for this figure showed that radiolabeled glucose injections into Weddell seals at rest typically achieve very rapid equilibration within the blood; then replacement of "hot" or labeled glucose molecules with "cold" or unlabeled ones causes the specfic activity (disintigrations per minute or DPM per μmol glucose) to decrease down a smooth multiexponential curve (data not shown). Then, during voluntary diving at sea, a preprogrammed microcomputer is able to control the pump injection of labeled glucose after bradycardia (and peripheral vasoconstriction) have been initiated. In short or so-called feeding dives (usually less than 25 min), up to 10 or more minutes are required to get complete equilibration of label (plateaau in DPM/μmol glucose); in long or exploratory dives (usually longer than 30 min), complete equilibration did not occur until the microvasculature was fully opened (vasodilation at the end of diving). The subsequent declines in DPM per μmol glucose in both diving conditions was similar to the declines observed under resting conditions. The inset indicates dive depth profile (in meters) and heart rate in beats per min (BPM). (Middle panel right) Direct quantitative measure of kidney function (clearance of a radioactive substance) in the Weddell seal under control (nondiving) conditions compared to clearance when a preprogrammed microcomputer controlled the pump injection of labeled material after bradycardia (and peripheral vasoconstriction) had been initiated during a voluntary dive in the Weddell seal. The same results were obtained with para-aminohippuric acid or with inulin. (Lower panel, left) Representative lactate washout profiles for dives of different duration, showing that in short dives, no major lactate washout is observed. (Lower panel, right) How the catecholamines correlate with dive and recovery cycles, showing that norepinephrine concentrations in the plasma increase during every dive recorded. (All above data from Guppy et al., 1986; Qvist et al., 1986; Hochachka et al., 1995; and Hurford et al., 1995.)

to add the "plasticity" component to what was otherwise an unchanged theoretical framework.

In search of improvement and refinement of "the model" of the diving response, scientists have turned their attention to a possible technology of choice (MRI and MRS) for achieving the desired "new breakthrough." This technology has recently revolutionized conceptual frameworks in other physiological areas. Functional MRI or fMRI, for example, has hugely expanded our understanding of brain function, while MRS, through in-vivo noninvasive monitoring of metabolites and other molecules of physiological importance, has similarly enormously expanded our understanding of how cells and tissues work in vivo. Hence it was reasonable for workers interested in diving to wonder if similar successes could arise from applying this technology to diving physiology.

MRI/MRS—THE VIRTUES IN DIVING STUDIES

There are two huge advantages arising from interrogating a biological system with MRI or MRS: (i) the techniques are noninvasive and (ii) for practical purposes, they work continuously in "real time." Armed with this technology, even preliminary studies (Thornton et al., 1997a,b) uncovered an enormously rich biological tapestry that is the internal physiological and metabolic machinery of the diving seal. It can be easily understood why some biologists are enthused when comparing the vision of MRI/MRS to earlier physiological studies of the diving response in laboratory settings, so rich, so precise, and so novel are the data that can be obtained. A brief list of such information includes the following.

1. Heart function through quantitative MRI—it is possible to obtain quantitative dynamic information on cardiac output, wall thickness, and even work efficiency, beat-by-beat throughout a simulated dive-recovery sequence. These studies already indicate that flow from the heart is continuous through systole and diastole (Thornton et al., 1997a,b), unlike the situation in humans and other terrestrial mammals. What is more, at least in the short dives so far examined (with moderate bradycardia) stroke volume increases during diving, indicating some compensation for the drop in heart rate that is simultaneously occurring. When standardized to initial prediving heart rates, the more severe the bradycardia, the greater the increase in stroke volume.

2. Aortic bulb function through quantitative MRI—it is also possible to monitor in real time the dynamics of the bulbus, interrogating its role in modulating flow through systole and diastole, during diving compared to other states. Functional imaging indicates that the bulbus smooths out cardiac output over the systole diastole cycle; that is, the bulbus explains the observations described above.

3. Detailed spleen function through quantitative MRI—another important set of observations supply quantitative dynamic information on flow, spleen contraction speed and extent during diving, spleen relaxation speed and extent during recovery, and on its dynamic interactions with the rest of the circulation system. Functional imaging (Thornton et al., 2000) indicates that once the dive begins, the spleen contracts quickly (within a minute or two). Initially it empties its RBC contents into the hepatic sinus, which through fine control of the caval valve in turn meters out RBCs into the circulation. This much more complex situation (figure 4.3) explains a paradox in the current literature: a rapid catecholamine-regulated spleen emptying completed in 3–4 min (Hurford et al., 1995) but only a gradual rise in Hct, requiring 12–15 min of diving before the entire RBC mass is circulating—the original field observations of Qvist et al. (1986).

4. Perfusion adjustments of organs and tissues by quantitative MRI—it is possible, at least in principle, to obtain accurate dynamic measurements of blood flow to and from a target tissue of choice; what is more, under stable Hct conditions, a combination of flow plus oxygenation state of the venous return allows classic Fick-principle-based estimates of in-situ metabolic rate of the organ being interrogated (Li et al., 1997). Although not yet extensively explored in diving studies, it is clear that for the first time, the traditional "vasoconstrictor"

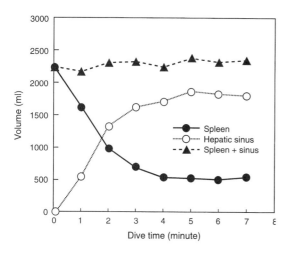

Figure 4.3. Representative set of spleen and hepatic sinus volumes, measured in vivo with MRI, during an 8 min simulated dive in a young elephant seal. The MRI images indicated that spleen emptying requires only two or so minutes. The contents are initially tranferred into the hepatic sinus and then RBCs are metered out into the blood more slowly, apparently through phrenic nerve control of the caval sphincter. Data from Thornton (2000).

component of the diving response can be monitored noninvasively and continuously throughout the diving period in more than one organ/tissue at a time. This technology obviously also allows unequivocal assessment of "continuous" versus "pulsatile" flow to specific target organs and tissues during diving (Thornton, 2000).

5. Organ- and tissue-specific biochemical responses to diving—as in more traditional models, such as humans or rats, the use of ^{31}P-MRS allows the monitoring of fundamental metabolites such as creatine (Cr), phosphocreatine (PCr), ATP, Pi, H$^+$, and H$_2$O. Additionally, and most importantly, ^{1}H-MRS can also continuously monitor the oxygenation state of muscle tissues through dive-recovery cycles by quantifying deoxymyoglobin and oxymyoglobin resonances. From this, the researcher gains insight into time-dependent dynamic metabolic modifications in specific target tissues and organs during dive recovery cycles. Using ^{31}P-MRS, such studies (Thornton, 2000) have already established that the lowest PCr concentrations occur during div-

ing hypoperfused states; the highest PCr concentrations occur during interdive hyperperfused states (figure 4.4). Such changes in [PCr], with stoichiometric (mirror image) changes in [Pi] and with stable [ATP] levels, are similar to changes occurring during work–rest–work transitions in skeletal and cardiac muscle (e.g., see Allen et al., 1997) and in both cases the change in tissue metabolic rates is a reflection of the frequently described 1:1 relationship between O$_2$ delivery by the blood ($\dot{Q}O_2$) and $\dot{V}O_2$ in muscles and other tissues as well. Careful analyses show that the drop in PCr is correlated with [H$^+$] presumably because H$^+$ drives the equilibrium to the right:

$$H^+ + PCr + ADP \rightarrow ATP + Cr$$

There are two potential sources of the H$^+$ in these diving protocols. One possibility is that the H$^+$ is lactate associated; this is considered unlikely because the dives in such studies are short and there is no significant lactate washout into the plasma. Thus the second possibility, that the H$^+$ accumulated during the diving protocol is due to CO$_2$ hydration, is considered more likely:

$$CO_2 + H_2O \rightarrow HCO_3^- + H^+$$

Extrapolating these studies to the probable situation in voluntary diving at sea indicates that CO$_2$ may have some thus far largely overlooked metabolic effects and that the time required to reestablish CO$_2$ and tissue metabolite homeostasis may well be a major determinant of surface interdive times. This role for CO$_2$ is already implied in earlier field and laboratory studies (Qvist et al., 1986), but its potential role in defining interdive surface times has been largely overlooked by later field studies of voluntary diving of pinnipeds at sea. Be that as it may, when taken together, these new experimental approaches have the potential to finally settle once and for all the extent of metabolic change between hypoperfused dive states versus hyperperfused interdive states for specific tissues and organs—reaching this goal has been a kind of Holy Grail in this field for over a half century (Scholander, 1940).

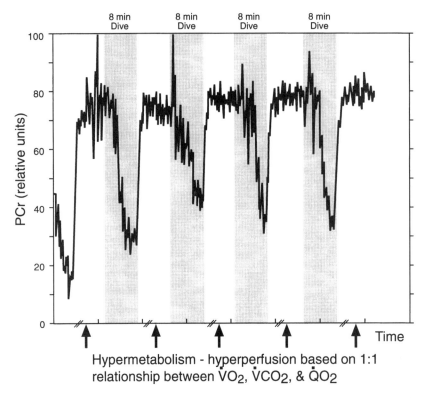

Figure 4.4. Typical in-vivo MRS measurements of [PCr] through diving and recovery cycles. PCr in relative units; dive periods are shaded and represent continuous measurements, while interdive times varied (time breaks shown on horizontal axis). Note that periods of hyperperfusion and presumably hypermetabolism (assuming a 1:1 relationship between O_2 delivery and O_2 consumption) are punctuated by periods of diving hypometabolism, when perfusion is substantially reduced. The decrease in [PCr] is thought to be caused by H^+accumulation, which shifts the creatine phosphokinase (CPK) reaction to the right $(H^+ + PCr + ADP \rightarrow ATP + Cr)$, a process linked to hydration of CO_2 formed and accumulated during diving vasoconstriction in muscle. (Data from Thornton, 2000.)

In essence, none of the above kind of information accumulated noninvasively, continuously, and in real time has ever been obtainable before by traditional physiological or biochemical research approaches. Thus such new MRI/MRS initiatives into *mechanistic* studies of the diving response in laboratory settings as a result may well have the potential to influence the research agenda into new cycles of renewal and advance in field studies as well as laboratory studies of diving physiology. A completely different approach—that exploring the evolution of the diving response—may supply a second avenue of renewal and another important research trajectory to the future. To date, the evolution of the diving response has only

been analyzed for one group of diving animals—the pinnipeds—to which we shall largely restrict our discussion.

EVOLUTION OF THE DIVING RESPONSE IN PINNIPEDS: TRADITIONAL VERSUS COMPARATIVE APPROACHES

As emphasized above, since the 1930s, physiologists working on diving have looked at the problem of evolution of the diving response in very qualitative terms and assumed that all the key components of the diving response (apnea, bradycardia, and peripheral vasoconstriction with hypometabolism of hypoperfused tissues [Butler and Jones, 1982, 1997; Hochachka and Guppy, 1987; Scholander 1940]) were biological adaptations and thus the outcome of selection-driven evolution. Other physiological characters also called adaptations to diving included greater body size, spleen size, blood volume, hematocrit, hemoglobin (Hb) concentration, and myoglobin (Mb) concentration. The reasoning behind this work was pretty intuitive. Body size influences the total onboard oxygen supply as well as mass-specific energy demands (Hochachka and Foreman, 1993; Hochachka and Guppy, 1987; Hochachka and Somero, 1984); increasing the former while decreasing the latter looked advantageous. In pinnipeds, the spleen holds and releases oxygenated red blood cells (a process under catecholamine regulation [Hochachka et al., 1995; Lacombe and Jones, 1991]), and under some circumstances can serve as a physiological "scuba tank" during diving (Hurford et al., 1995; Qvist et al., 1986); again this should be advantageous. Blood volume, RBC mass, blood hemoglobin, and muscle myoglobin concentrations are determinants of oxygen-carrying capacity (Castellini et al., 1992; Guyton et al., 1995; Hochachka, 1992); the idea that more oxygen-carrying potential should mean improved or extended diving capacity did not require an inordinate leap of faith. Thus most earlier studies implicitly or explicitly considered the above traits as "adaptations" which should improve diving performance. Scholander (1963) termed the control of bradycardia and peripheral vasoconstriction "the master switch of life" and the master switch was viewed as an elegant master adaptation. All these workers of course were using the term "adaptation" loosely and traditionally, considering any traits that aided in survival (or, in this case, any traits that were utilized during diving) as adaptations (see Johansen, 1987, for more on this approach).

The above approach, while inadequate for today's more analytical evolutionary biology (see Kirkpatrick, 1996, for example), nevertheless generated a very large data base, which was advantageous for a more quantitative analysis of the evolution of the diving response in pinnipeds. In initial examination of this issue, traditional statistical procedures were used to evaluate biological traits which correlated with diving capacity (Hochachka and Mottishaw, 1998), while to evaluate these characters in pinniped evolution more quantitatively (Mottishaw, 1997; Mottishaw et al., 1999), the method of phylogenetically independent contrast (PIC) analysis was used (Felsenstein, 1985). Nonphylogenetic data analyses run the risk of error arising from more closely related species being more phenotypically similar, which is why they should not be treated as independent data points in statistical analysis (Felsenstein, 1985). Independent contrasts use phylogenetic information to transform species data (character values of sibling species are substracted one from the other, while character values of ancestral species are assumed to be the average of the two daughter species); by this means, the physiological character data in principle become independent and identically distributed. The transformed data (standardized independent contrasts or differences) can then be used in ordinary statistical procedures (e.g., Felsenstein, 1985; Garland and Adolph 1994; Garland et al., 1992, 1993; Purvis and Rambaut, 1995). For PIC analysis it is necessary to have a phylogeny, which for pinnipeds was constructed from published relationships available in the literature. The phylogeny (figure 4.5) is consistent with both molecular and morphological evidence (Arnason et al., 1995; Berta and Demere, 1986; Berta and Wyss, 1994; Burns and Fay, 1970; De Muizon, 1976; Hochachka and Mottishaw, 1998; Lento et al., 1995; Repenning et al., 1971). Changing the tree to reflect the most highly supported alternate phylogenetic hypotheses does not qualitatively alter the results (Mottishaw et al., 1998). In short, instead of a traditional relatively qualitative evaluation of the evolution and adaptation of the diving response in pinnipeds, the issue can be addressed utilizing statistical packages that are now routine in comparative approaches to evolutionary physiology and are widely accepted as more quantitative. Let us start the analysis with bradycardia, historically considered the centerpiece of the diving response.

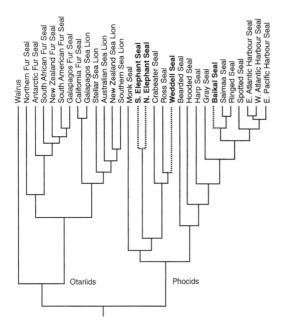

Figure 4.5. The phylogeny of the pinnipeds shown is based on morphological and molecular data. This phylogenetic tree is modified from Mottishaw et al. (1999) to highlight four outstanding species of divers. Three of these (the Weddell seal and the two species of elephant seals) are considered the "laboratory rats" in this field of research. The fourth, the Baikal seal, is substantially smaller than the former three, yet this species is capable of stunningly long (up to 1 hour) dives. Traditional statistical analyses (Hochachka and Mottishaw, 1998) as well as PIC analyses (Mottishaw et al., 1999) indicate that the data on these four species are extreme even by pinniped standards. Their exceptional diving capabilities indicate that factors other than those considered in the text (factors that are so far unknown) may be involved in extending maximum diving duration. As explained by Mottishaw et al. (1999), the above composite phylogeny is derived from many published sources (Arnason et al., 1995; Berta and Demere, 1986; Berta and Wyss, 1994; Burns and Fay, 1970; De Muizon, 1976; Lento et al., 1995; Repenning et al., 1971). Some relationships in this phylogeny are supported by both molecular and morphological evidence, whereas others, notably the relative positions of the fur seal species, are controversial (see Bininda-Edmonds et al., 1999).

CHARACTERS THAT ARE HIGHLY CONSERVATIVE IN THE PINNIPEDS

On turning attention to the relationship between diving bradycardia and diving capacity, the first thing one finds is that for species with the largest data base (such as the harbor seal, the Weddell seal, and the gray seal), the lowest heart rates (maximum bradycardia) found in the field—if not compromised by inordinate demands of swimming exercise—are similar to the lowest heart rates observed during forced laboratory diving. Harbor seals voluntarily diving at sea can depress heart rate to about 4 BPM, which is in the same range as Scholander originally found in forced diving studies. Similar maximum bradycardia values are also observed in forced versus voluntary diving in Weddell seals; in fact, to many biologists, it is axiomatic that the forced diving paradigm elicits a "maximum dive response," hence maximum bradycardia (see Hochachka and Mottishaw, 1998). These observations are important because maximum bradycardia is not always available from field studies that supply data on maximum duration diving (see Hindell et al., 1992, for example). Given this proviso (that maximum bradycardia values are similar in laboratory or field situations), the data indicate that the lowest heart rates observed during diving (maximum bradycardia) show little variation within pinnipeds (figure 4.6). As one of our colleagues put it: all pinnipeds seem to be able to suppress heart rate down to the "rock bottom"! PIC analysis of these data indicated that maximum bradycardia did not significantly correlate with dive time (figure 4.6). Similarly, there was a lack of correlation between maximum heart rates and mean or modal dive durations (see Hochachka and Mottishaw, 1998). By implication, the same considerations apply for peripheral vasoconstriction, since the two "reflexes" are mechanistically coupled.

BRADYCARDIA AND SEVERAL OTHER PHYSIOLOGICAL TRAITS ARE HIGHLY CONSERVATIVE TRAITS IN MAMMALS IN GENERAL

This surprising result contrasts with the paradigm of diving physiology defining bradycardia and peripheral vasoconstriction—the "master switch of life"—as an obvious "master adaptation" for diving. We consider that there may be two kinds of explanations for this apparent paradox. The first would interpret the result as an artifact based on too few species (figure 4.6). We do not consider this likely, since species at very different ends of the spectrum of diving duration (e.g., sea lions, which can dive for only a maximum of perhaps 7–10 min versus elephant or Weddell seals, either of which can dive for well over an hour!) show maximum bradycardia in the 4–10 BPM range. The second possibility is that the control systems for the diving response are "hard wired"; although used in—and in a sense central to—the diving response, they are also used in many other biological settings (exercise, some fear reactions, other stresses). An intriguing example comes from studies of hibernation in bears in Alaska. The bradycardia and coincident redistribution of cardiac output during hibernation are strikingly similar to what might be observed in a diving seal (Barnes et al., 1999). These data are instructive, since the phylogeny of carnivores shows that bears (Ursidae) share common ancestry with the pinnipeds (figure 4.7). Hence this physiological control system may well have been in place in common ancestors to both of these lineages. Any adaptational changes for diving per se during pinniped evolution then may have been too modest to detect with a measure as crude as heart rate against a background of much wider physiological requirements.

The concept of an ancestral trait only to these two groups is the simplest interpretation of the bradycardia data for pinnipeds, and while it may be technically sound, it is probably too narrow, because this reflex control system is used even more widely among mammals and other vertebrates. The conservative and ancestral nature of this reflex control system explains why it was recruited for purposes of controlling diving physiology several times independently in the evolution of mammals. As shown in figure 4.8, diving capabilities are expressed by Monotremes, Marsupials, and several placental mammals, and in all cases diving bradycardia with associated peripheral vasoconstrictions are the secret of diving success (Butler and Jones, 1997). Recruitment of an ancestral conservative physiological trait is the most parsimonious explanation of this repeated and independent evolution of the same processes for use during aquatic submergence. Actually, this conclusion in a sense already was appreciated by Scholander, who realized that some version of the diving response is evident almost universally among air-breathing vertebrates, including humans. In a simulated diving study with about 30 human subjects, Arnold (1985) found that most subjects displayed some diving bradycardia. One individual (a kind of "human seal?") consistently displayed profound bradycardia (down to 6 BPM!), attesting to how "hard wired" and conservative this control system is, even in our own species.

When assembled in the context of physiological control of diving, these considerations imply that bradycardia may be one of several ancestral or plesiomorphic physiological characters that—while used during, and required for, diving—have remained essentially unchanged throughout pinniped phylogenetic history. Apnea is another such conservative character that is of course a prerequisite for diving, and which is seemingly similar in all pinnipeds. This is also likely to be true for peripheral tissue hypoperfusion (because of the obligatory linkage at constant blood pressure between bradycardia and peripheral vasoconstriction) and for hypometabolism (because of the presumed link between metabolism and oxygen delivery [Hochachka and Mottishaw, 1998]). Consistent with the latter are studies on the California sea lion (Hurley, 1996), a short-duration diver, showing as much reduction in metabolic rate during trained submersion as seen in long-duration diving seals (Fedak et al., 1988).

The physiological control systems allowing regional hypothermia, used to significant advan-

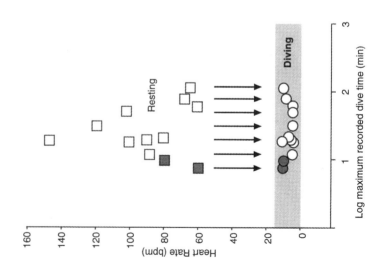

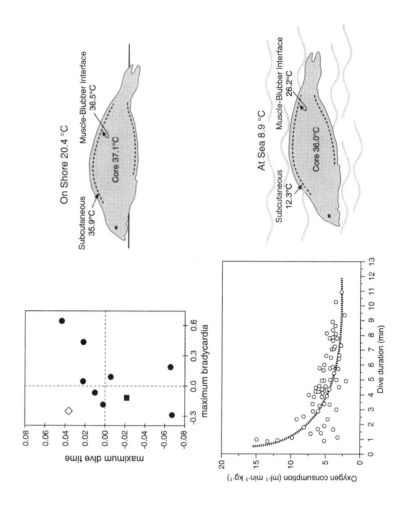

Figure 4.6 (Left panel) Relationship between maximum diving duration and degree of bradycardia expressed in several species of sea lions (dark squares and circles) and of seals (open squares and circles). It is evident that all these pinnipeds, both short-term and long-term divers, are able to activate bradycardia to about the same extent (heart rates into the range of 4–10 beats per minute). Traditional statistical analyses of these data show that there is no statistically significant correlation between degree of bradycardia achievable and the maximum length of diving possible. (The data are from the summary given in Hochachka and Mottishaw, 1998.) (Middle panel, upper) Results of a PIC analysis of the same heart rate data as in the left panel, and this also indicates that the capacity for bradycardia does not correlate with maximum diving duration. Specifically the graph shows the lack of correlation between residuals generated by regressions of log maximum dive time contrasts and maximum bradycardia contrasts on log body mass contrasts. Circles represent contrasts within the phocids (nine species), the square represents a contrast between two otariid species, and the diamond represents the root node, or contrast between phocids and otariids. The correlation was not statistically significant ($P = 0.15$). Electrocardiograms (ECGs) were in all cases used to collect heart rate data. (Modified from Hochachka and Mottishaw, 1998, and Mottishaw et al., 1999.) (Middle panel, lower) Oxygen consumption rates of gray seals as a function of dive duration, illustrating the effects of diving hypometabolism. In these protocols, metabolic rates are measured only while the animal is at the surface (where gas exchange measurements are made) and thus the data average oxygen consumption rates over dive + interdive periods of time. As indicated in the text, tissue hyperperfusion and hypermetabolism are characteristic of interdive periods. Thus the decline in metabolism as a function of dive duration is plausibly interpreted as caused by the hypometabolism of each diving period per se. (Data modified from Fedak et al., 1988.) (Right panel) Diagrammatic summary of temperature profiles in body of elephant seals at rest in normoxia, normothermia (on shore), contrasted with regional heterothermy observed during diving at sea assuming average water temperatures of 8.9°C (Data modified from Andrews, 1999; Andrews et al., 1994.)

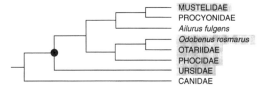

Figure 4.7. Abbreviated phylogenetic tree of a group of carnivores including the Ursidae (bears) and the pinnipeds (Otariids, Phocids, and walrus); the dark symbol indicates the last time at which the two lineages shared a common ancestor. Thermal regulatory and cardiovascular regulatory systems in the Ursidae include heterothermy (expressed during hibernation) as well as bradycardia and redistribution of cardiac output (also expressed during hibernation). Pinnipeds express both of these functional features during diving. The evolutionary implications are further reviewed in the text. (Phylogenetic information modified from Bininda-Emonda et al., 1999.)

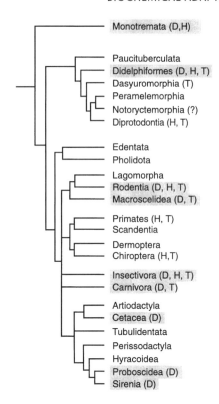

Figure 4.8. Simplified phylogeny of the mammals with groups that include species displaying significant diving capabilities (D), significant hibernation (H), and significant torpor (T) capabilities. These clusters are highlighted in the phylogenetic tree. In all three cases, the thermoregulatory systems display significant tolerance of regional or global heterothermy. In cetaceans, which are fully aquatic very capable divers, regional heterothermy is suspected but has not been studied in detail. It is interesting to note that northern artiodactyl species (reindeer, for example) display major tolerance for regional heterothermy. This is further reviewed in the text. (Phylogeny is modified from Fritz, 1998.)

tage to suppress metabolism during diving and thus to extend diving duration (Andrews et al., 1994; Butler and Jones, 1997; de Leeuw et al., 1998), may also represent ancestral characters. Fritz's (1998) analysis of the evolution of torpor and hibernation in mammals (figure 4.8) shows that mammalian groups, such as the Carnivora, capable of these extreme expressions of mammalian thermoregulatory control also include other lineages expressing significant diving capabilities. Although the cetacea are not known with certainty to fit this pattern, they share common ancestry with artiodactyls, which in northern climates are known to utilize extensive regional heterothermy as a defense against cold (Irving, 1966, 1969). Thus it is possible that the ancestral characters allowing regional heterothermy may well have been recruited for extending diving abilities by the cetaceans, just as in the case of the pinnipeds. Obviously more work is needed to explore these relationships in greater detail.

ADJUSTABLE TRAITS CORRELATING WITH DIVING NEEDS

When the PIC analyses of the diving response were extended, Mottishaw et al. (1999) found that some characters correlate well with dive time in pinnipeds. Thus if a pinniped is larger than its closest relative, it will be able to dive longer (16 phocid and 14 otariid species), as predicted from previous studies (Butler and Jones, 1982). Analysis of spleen size, using residuals (figure 4.9), shows that a pinniped with a larger spleen than its closest relative tends to display a greater diving capacity than its closest relative. The use of residuals in these statistical calculations removes the effects of body size; that is, these correlations between spleen size and diving abilities are independent of body mass changes. Similarly, pinnipeds with a larger blood volume tend to display longer maximum duration diving capacities than their closest relatives, and the same is true for [Hb] (in g per 100 ml) and whole body Hb content (calculated from Hb in g per 100 ml and total blood volume in liters) (figure 4.9). This means that for pinnipeds, independent of body size, an increase in whole-body blood volume occurs with an increase in the maximum diving capacity; similarly, an increase in Hb content corresponds with greater maximum diving duration. Interestingly, multiple regression is not individually significant for residuals of spleen weight, blood volume or [Hb], but together the model is significant. This indicates that each of the variables can explain a similar amount of the variation in dive time. However, since body size, spleen mass, blood volume, and hemoglobin content are correlated in pinnipeds, multicolinearity confounds estimation of individual coefficients of determination in a multiple regression and makes it difficult to quantify which of the characters has been most important in the evolution of longer dive duration. If each of these traits separately contributed to increasing dive time, then evolution in very different regulatory characters (organogenesis, angiogenesis, erythropoesis) would be required. Studies of other mammalian species suggest that these are independent; for example, in mammalian hypobaric hypoxia responses, hemoglobin concentration and red blood cell mass are adjusted along trajectories that are independent of blood volume, and neither is necessarily associated with spleen size (Winslow and Monge, 1987). How these characters could co-evolve in pinnipeds remains an unsolved and indeed an unexplored problem.

While these results appear to be interesting, the proviso should be emphasized that the techniques used in obtaining data on spleen mass, blood volume, and [Hb] were not always the same in all studies and that in consequence significant variation in signal/noise ratios might well be anticipated. This situation would tend to decrease rather than increase the statistical confidence levels. The fact that, despite these limitations, increased spleen size, blood volume,

and Hb content are statistically correlated in pinnipeds with long-duration diving and prolonged foraging at sea is all the more convincing. Additionally, since these correlations are based on phylogenetically independent contrasts, they demonstrate that these traits do not simply occur in certain branches of the pinniped phylogeny. Rather, across the pinniped phylogenetic tree, species that have evolved larger spleens have also evolved longer dive times and the same is true for blood volume and Hb content. Phocids tend to be longer duration divers than otariids (Hochachka and Mottishaw, 1998), but within the phocids, the longest duration divers are spread throughout the phylogeny.

Another caveat to mention parenthetically is that correlated evolution of these characters does not prove that they have been selected specifically because they promote increased dive time. Even though comparisons among species have been used to show the relationship between an organism's features and its environment (Doughty, 1996; Garland and Adolph, 1994), comparative studies are limited in untangling and sorting out events that happened in the past (Leroi et al., 1994). The correlation of these traits with maximum recorded dive time in pinnipeds, independent of phylogeny, does not address issues of origin or possibilities of correlation with other traits or other functions that are in fact selected for (Leroi et al., 1994). In contrast, careful physiological studies sometimes do allow sorting out spurious or secondary correlations and this can be well illustrated by MRI studies of seal spleen function.

THE SPLEEN STORY REVISITED

When a strong correlation between maximum dive duration and spleen size first was observed in pinnipeds, many workers in the field concluded that the spleen's main function was to act as an internal scuba tank used for extending diving time. If so, the correlation between dive duration and spleen size would be causal. Thornton et al. (2000) reexamined this problem using MRI to monitor spleen behavior during simulated diving in the elephant seal and the results were quite illuminating. Using close-to-real-time MRI imaging, the first thing that was noted was an extremely rapid contraction of the spleen (2/3 empty within 1 min) with simultaneous filling of the hepatic sinus. The hepatic sinus then displayed a decrease in signal intensity along a time course that paralleled the metering out of red blood cells into the general circulation. This transfer of blood is thought to be controlled by phrenic nerve modulation of

the caval sphincter. From the kinetics of spleen refilling, requiring at least 15–20 min after spleen contraction, it became evident that the spleen cannot be used cyclically between dive and short (2–4 min) interdive periods routinely used at sea.

Thus the question arises: Why is there such a seemingly good correlation, independent of phylogeny, between spleen size and dive duration? Thornton et al. (2000) hypothesize that

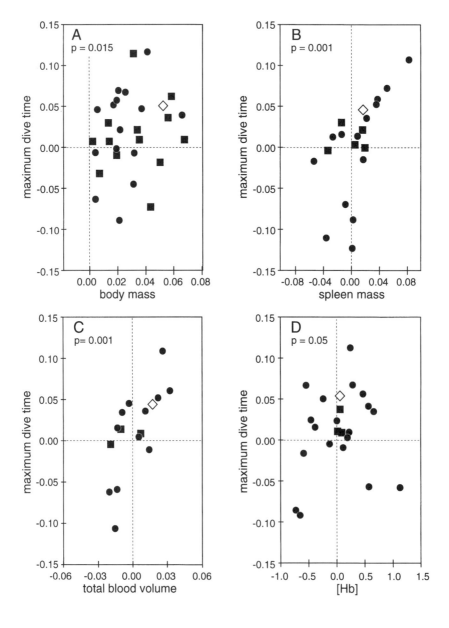

when seals are at sea, the system simply allows for the maintenance of a high circulating RBC mass during diving periods (with posssible hypoxia and ischemia developing in various parts of the animal's body) and during brief interdive periods (when O_2 stores are being replenished and circulating the entire RBC mass would seem to be advantageous, and possibly essential).

However, the blood physiological conditions for elephant seals on land differ drastically. In fact, here the opposite might be the case: with no oxygenation problems anywhere in the animal's body, circulating the complete RBC mass (hematocrits into the 70% range!) necessarily requires more energy than circulating lower viscosity blood and it may contribute to other viscosity-related problems (Teyssier et al., 1998; Thron et al., 1998). Thus the most probable real function of the enlarged spleen in long-duration divers when hauled out (on land for the elephant seals; on ice for the Weddell seals) is to avoid the viscosity-related hazards of hematocrits that approach 70% by storing a large frac-tion of the RBC mass in their huge spleens. That is, only when hauled out does splenic sto-rage of RBCs come into play, reducing the hematocrit and avoiding deleterious effects of increased viscosity when O_2 is not limiting. These new MRI data thus redefine the function of the pinniped spleen as a means of reducing blood viscosity when on land (or on ice) rather than as a means for increasing dive duration at sea. Thornton et al. (2000) argue that the corre-lation between spleen volume and dive duration is therefore spurious and purely secondary to the correlations between RBC mass/blood volume and dive duration. In contrast, no such secondary components to the correlations between dive duration and RBC mass, between dive duration and Hb content or between dive duration and blood volume are observed. In fact, the latter traits when combined represent the O_2 carrying capacity of the blood and it is understandable that, for any given set of condi-tions, the larger the O_2 carrying capacity the longer the dive duration that should be achiev-able.

Figure 4.9. Phylogenetically independent contrast analysis shows four biological characteristics, (A) body mass, (B) spleen size, (C) total blood volume, and (D) hemoglobin concentration (or indeed, hematocrit or total blood Hb content (data not shown), that correlate specifically with maximum diving capability within the pinnipeds. The meaning of these data is that, right across the pinnipeds as a species cluster, the greater the expression of any one of these characters the greater the maximum diving duration that is observed. (A) Regression of log body mass contrasts on log maximum dive time contrasts. The relationship is highly significant ($P = 0.015$). Circles represent contrasts within the phocids (17 species), the square represents a contrast between 15 otariid species, and the diamond represents the root node, or contrast between phocids and otariids. (B) Significant positive correlation between residuals generated by regressions of log maxi-mum dive time contrasts and log spleen mass contrasts on body mass contrasts ($P < 0.001$). Circles repre-sent contrasts between 14 phocid species and squares between six otariid species, with the diamond representing the root node, or contrast between phocids and otariids. (C) Significant positive correlation between residuals generated by regressions of log maximum dive time contrasts and log total blood volume contrasts on log body mass contrasts ($P < 0.001$). Circles represent contrasts between 13 phocids and squares between three otariids, with the diamond representing the root node, or contrast between phocids and otariids. (D) Significant positive correlation between residuals generated by regressions of log maxi-mum dive time contrasts and [Hb] contrasts on log body mass contrasts ($P = 0.05$). Circles represent con-trasts between 13 phocids and squares between three otariids, with the diamond representing the root node, or contrast between phocids and otariids. [Hb] is expressed as g Hb per 100 ml whole blood. Again, procedural variations in different studies are unavoidable sources of random variation in these kinds of data and would tend to reduce—not enhance—the probability of the significant correlation that was obtained. A similar positive correlation was observed for the data on whole body Hb, obtained by multi-plying measured blood volume in liters times the Hb content per liter volume of blood (see text). In all cases, species names and techniques used with each species are given in Hochachka and Mottishaw (1998). (Figure modified from Mottishaw et al., 1999.)

WHAT WE HAVE LEARNED

Given our knowledge of the mechanisms of the diving response, the present picture of their evolution leads to two general principles in the evolution of the diving response.

(1) Some physiological and biochemical characters, required and used in diving animals, are highly conserved in all vertebrates; these presumably ancestral or plesiomorphic traits are necessarily similar in all pinnipeds and include diving apnea, bradycardia, tissue-specific hypoperfusion, and hypometabolism of hypoperfused tissues.

(2) Another group of functionally linked characters are more malleable and include (i) body size, (ii) spleen volume, (iii) blood volume, and (iv) red blood cell mass and thus hemoglobin pool size. Increases in any or all of these improve diving capacity (defined as maximum recorded diving duration).

The questions arising are whether or not these principles can be accommodated by current models of molecular evolution.

CAN MOLECULAR EVOLUTION MODELS EXPLAIN ADAPTABLE PINNIPED TRAITS?

At the outset, let us be clear on one thing: current thinking in evolutionary circles assumes that selection can be an overwhelming force. Population genetics theory tells us that the response to selection depends on:

(1) the amount of phenotypic variation on which selection can act,
(2) the fraction of that variation that is heritable, and
(3) the intensity of selection.

For numerous physiological and morphological systems that have been studied quantitatively, the coefficient of variation is often about 10%

or more. Heritabilities vary widely, but a range of between about 0.3 and 0.7 is frequently reported for metabolic and physiological characters. Selection coefficients also can vary greatly; at the upper extreme are values of about 0.43. A 43% selective advantage means a selection intensity so high that individuals one phenotypic standard deviation above the mean are more than twice as fit as individuals one deviation below the mean (see Kirkpatrick, 1996).

With these sorts of values, evolutionary biologists estimate that natural selection can produce evolutionary rates in excess of 1% change in the mean value for a trait per generation. If sustained, these evolutionary conditions would take an animal the size of a mouse to that of an elephant in less than 1200 generations (Kirkpatrick, 1996). Or, in the context of diving duration, if the above conditions prevailed for a mouse- or mole-sized ancestral mammal capable of only 0.2 min diving, they could evolve this tiny mammal into a huge beast capable of at least a 200 min dive in the same 1200 generations of evolution. As pinniped phylogeny appears to extend back in time for about 20 million years, it is not hard to conclude that the observed patterns of diving capabilities within the extant pinnipeds can be easily explained by current evolutionary theory. The caveat of course is that these kinds of calculations are almost always focused onto a single trait; for situations where the evolution of two or more systems must be coordinated (as in organogenesis, angiogenesis, and erythropoiesis above) the probability and mechanisms of such coevolution remain unclear to us. Nevertheless, the answer to the question "Can molecular evolution models explain so-called adaptable biochemical and physiological traits in the time span available for pinniped phylogeny?," at least in a general sense, is: yes. Interestingly, when considering the question "Can conserved traits such as bradycardia coupled with peripheral vasconstriction be explained by modern molecular evolution theory?," the answer is not so obvious.

CAN MOLECULAR EVOLUTION
MODELS EXPLAIN CONSERVED TRAITS?

The Complexity of Conserved Systems

To put the question into perspective, we first must remind the reader of the enormous complexity of the regulatory systems involved. A hint of this is presented in figure 4.10(A), which indicates a number of major sensing, signal transduction, and effector pathways: these tell the pinniped when to activate apnea, bradycardia, and peripheral vasoconstriction. Other pathways, such as that initiated by O_2 or H^+ in the carotid body, are mainly modulatory: they tell the organism the intensity of diving response required (actually, in this case the pathway senses O_2 and H^+ and regulates the intensity of the bradycardia response relative to these parameters). At the molecular level of course each arm of this enormously complex regulatory system is made up of from several to many gene products, each interacting in a highly precise manner in order to achieve the coordinated (and evolutionarily conserved) diving response. To estimate how much negative or stabilizing selection is required to keep this system from randomly changing through phylogenetic time we need to have an estimate of the selective cost of substitutions in each of the gene products in these regulatory circuits. Of course direct information of this type basically is unavailable for the components in figure 4.10(A). However, these kinds of values are known for other comparable macromolecular systems. One such (presumably representative) example (figure 4.10(B)) is given for 16/18S rRNA by Golding (1994).

Selective Pressures Required to
Stabilize a Representative
Macromolecular Structure

Ribosomal RNAs have been used to explore the deepest branches of the phylogeny of living organisms on earth because these molecules are ubiquitous and because their primary sequences change slowly due to powerful stabilizing selection. Wishing to know how powerful, Golding (1994) examined the primary sequences for 16/18 rRNAs from 51 species, including representatives from all major branches of life. The secondary structures of rRNAs are stabilized by numerous hydrogen-bonded pairs of nucleotides, with stability of bonding being dependent upon the actual nucleotide pairs utilized and on their neighbors. In the total absence of selection, one would expect to see any base pair at any one site in the secondary structure among the 51 species, but this is not observed. Instead, most species are restricted to pairs that form strong hydrogen bonds and some sites are more conserved (are selected more strongly) than others.

When we assemble all these data together we can sketch a map of selection strength (figure 4.10(B)) where the selection coefficient for each hydrogen-bonded pair in the secondary structure of the rRNA molecule is estimated as a vertical line whose length is proportional to the strength of selection for that site. What is actually estimated is a composite parameter, $4Ns$, where N is the effective population size and s is the selective advantage of hydrogen bonding at a site. Golding (1994) found that $4Ns = 6.3$ was sufficiently large to account for complete conservation of hydrogen bonding at a site; that is, for all 51 taxa to have a hydrogen-bonded base pair at a site. If a reasonable value for N is assumed (say 16,000), then a value of $s = 0.0001$ is large enough to maintain a specific site in a sequence over long phylogenetic time periods. This means that on average a 0.01% advantage is adequate to assure the conservation of a given site in rRNA; a 1% advantage would be consistent with the conservation of about 100 such sites, which in fact is close to what is observed, with the most conservative sites tending to be located in the central part of the molecule (figure 4.10(B)).

These are highly instructive insights because similar structural constraints (requiring the conservation of weak bonding interactions at specific sites) are so commonly observed they are considered a "rule of thumb" for macromolecules such as enzymes, ion specific channels, ion exchangers, ion pumps, metabolite transporters, and ligand (signal) specific receptors. In fact, the "rule of thumb" applies pretty well across the board for all gene products, since

A

Minimum Number of Components: Carotid body O_2 Sensing -> Vagal Bradycardia

Glomus cell, carotid body:
  O_2 sensors
  O_2 signal transducers
  K^+ channels
  Na^+ channels
  Ca^{++} channels

Pathways to and within CNS:
  GABA & glycine receptors
    transducing components (for inhibitory synapses)
  Cl^- channels
  Glutamate receptors
    transducing components (for excitatory synapses)
  voltage gated Ca^{++}, Na^+, & K^+ channels

Vagus Pathway to the heart:
  ACh (muscarinic) receptors, AChE
  G_k membrane delimited proteins
  G_k activated K^+ channel
  Ca^{++}, Na^+, K^+ Channels

Minimal number of gene products: ~20
Pathway is highly conserved

Assuming 20 proteins each with 10 sites which must be conserved. Selective advantage req'd (calculated for rRNA): 10^{-4} x 20 x10 = 0.02

Conclusion: ~2% selective advantage is adequate to conserve one pathway required in the network controlling the cardiovascular system in pinnipeds

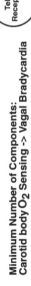

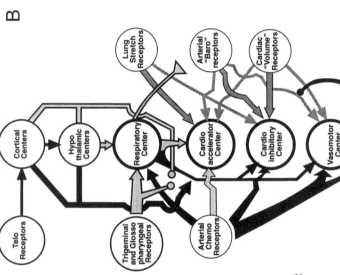

B

Cost of Site Conservation

For 51 taxa, the composite parameter $4Ns = 6.3$ where N is pop. ~ 16,000; s = selective advantage of a given H bond = ~ 10^{-4} is sufficiently large to account for conservation of hydrogen bonding at a site

Conclusion:
A selective advantage of only 0.01% is adequate to fix a given site in all 51 taxa (does this correlate with very high fidelity DNA repair targeted to rRNA genes?)

A 1% advantage could 'fix' or absolutely conserve 100 such sites

Many macromolecular structures have from a few to many sites absolutely conserved

Initial Responses
  Excitation
  Inhibition
  Occlusion
  Peripheral Preclusion

Chemoreceptor Reinforcement
  Excitation
  Inhibition
  Occlusion

Modifying Factors
  Excitation
  Inhibition

Telo Receptors
Cortical Centers
Hypo thalamic Centers
Respiratory Center
Cardio accelerator Center
Cardio inhibitory Center
Vasomotor Center
Lung Stretch Receptors
Arterial "Baro" receptors
Cardiac "Volume" Receptors
Trigeminal and Glosso pharyngeal Receptors
Arterial Chemo Receptors

Figure 4.10. (A) The diagram summarizes the integration of reflexes in initiation, development, and reinforcement of the diving response in mammals and birds. Responses are initiated by stimulation of teloreceptors and/or trigeminal and glossopharyngeal receptors. In prolonged dives, arterial chemoreceptors are activated and initiate secondary reinforcement of initial responses. The overall cardiovascular system is modified by peripheral vasoconstriction so that blood oxygen stores are delivered mainly to heart, brain, adrenals, and pregnant uterus, with the peripheral tissues gradually having to sustain oxygen-limiting conditions (Zapol et al., 1979). Arterial baroreceptors and cardiac volume receptors are instrumental in orchestrating a balanced reduction in cardiac output in concert with the redistribution of blood taking place at largely maintained blood pressure. Diagram modified from Blix (1988). Itemized on the left are the minimal number of gene products thought to be involved (Hille, 1992) in the organization of but one pathway in this complex regulatory system, that leading from the carotid body chemoreceptors to the CNS and thence the heart and serving to modulate the vagally mediated bradycardia. Assuming the same cost of conserving sequences as in rRNA (B) conserving pathways such as this (assuming for ease of estimation 10 conserved sites in each of 20 gene products forming the pathway) would require at least a 2% selective advantage. See text for further details. (B) A composite map of the strength of selection on rRNA from 51 species representing all major lines of life, with vertical lines indicating the strength of selection maintaining hydrogen-bonded base pairs in the secondary structure of 16S/18S rRNA. What is actually estimated is a composite parameter, $4Ns$, where N is the effective population size and s is the selective advantage of hydrogen bonding at a site. Golding (1994) found that $4Ns = 6.3$ was sufficiently large to account for complete conservation of hydrogen bonding at a site; that is, for all 51 taxa to have a hydrogen-bonded base pair at a site (Golding, 1994). If a reasonable value for N is assumed (say 16,000), then as shown on the left a value of $s = 0.0001$ (equivalent to a 0.01% selective advantage) is large enough to maintain a specific site in a sequence over long phylogenetic time periods and a 1% advantage could conserve 100 such sites or essentially the entire structure of the macromolecule.

their functions almost ubiquitously depend upon weak bonding interactions. Such natural-selection-based conservation of structure (i.e., of specific sites in specific sequences) of course is the basis of maintained functional specificity of macromolecules through evolutionary time and in principle should be applicable to the conservation of the regulatory pathways underlying the diving response. To indicate the flavor of the problems involved, here we will focus on only one pathway in the complex regulatory system controlling the diving response—that beginning at the carotid chemoreceptors and serving in pinnipeds to maintain diving bradycardia initiated by other (e.g., glossopharyngeal) pathways.

A Representative Conserved Control System: The Glomus Cell → Vagal Control of the Heart

The reason for focusing on this particular pathway is because it is relatively well described and we can with some confidence estimate a minimal number of gene products involved in orchestrating its role. Thus during prolonged diving, declining O_2 tensions are detected by O_2 sensors in the glomus cells of the carotid bodies; the transduction of these signals into action potentials directed towards the central nervous system (CNS) minimally requires Na^+, K^+, and Ca^{2+} channels. Numbers of synapses required in reaching key CNS control centers are unknown, but would in all cases require several to a dozen or more gene products: gamma-aminobutyric acid ($GABA_A$) and glycine receptors, transduction pathway components, and Cl^- channels mediate inhibitory synapses; glutamate or aspartate receptors, transduction pathway components, and cation channels mediate excitatory synapses. Modulation of CNS synapses would additionally require nicotinic acetylcholine (ACh), norepinephrine, adenosine, $GABA_A$, and opioid receptors. Finally, for bradycardia, this information must be transmitted from the CNS to the heart by the vagus; there muscarinic receptors for ACh, G_k-membrane-delimited signal transfer proteins, and G_k-activated K^+ channels mediate transduction processes leading to

cardiac muscle relaxation (see Hille, 1992). The net effect is the modulation or reinforcement of bradycardia already initiated by other pathways (figure 4.10(A)).

For illustrative calculations, then, an estimate of minimally 20 for the number of gene products involved in forming this particular pathway in the fine-tuning of diving bradycardia would be a safe assumption (the actual number is probably two to five times higher, especially when it is recalled that most channels and receptors are formed from more than one gene product and isoforms are frequently present; at least six genes, for example, specify alpha subunit isoforms of $GABA_A$ [Hille, 1992]). Assuming that similar selection pressures operate on each gene in this pathway as in the rRNA study of Golding (1994), then we arrive at the conclusion that about a 2% selective advantage is enough to assure that 10 sites in each of 20 proteins in the pathway will be conserved (the actual number of conserved sites may have to be substantially higher, in which event the overall selective advantage would have to be proportionately higher than 2%).

On first analysis, this looks hopeful; it suggests that modern molecular evolutionary concepts should be able to easily explain the conservation of complex (multigene dependent) control systems like those for diving apnea, bradycardia, and peripheral vasoconstriction. However, to experimental biologists, the implications are less than hopeful for two reasons. In the first place, there is the simple practical problem of this being experimentally intractable and difficult to study—signal-to-noise ratios in physiological studies almost always are in the 5–10% range. A 1–2% advantage in most studies would be undetectable. Secondly, a serious theoretical problem seems to arise because the above illustrative estimates apply to only one pathway. In contrast, the diving response is regulated by a control system involving many such pathways (figure 4.10(A)). It is unclear how far one can push these kinds of analyses, but it seems obvious that as the numbers of gene products required for given physiological systems increase towards hundreds or even thousands, the strength of selection required to conserve them unchanged through evolutionary time may rise without limit. For physiologists, this is not a very satisfying sort of relationship to contemplate but it does suggest that the problem of conserving basic regulatory systems of the diving response through pinniped phylogeny may be more difficult to explain than the appearance of so-called "adaptable" physiological traits, which in the context of this chapter probably would normally be considered central for extending diving duration capacities.

The implication is that remaining the same through long evolutionary time periods may be harder than changing; that is, conservation seems to be the general rule, while adaptive changes seem to have to be "squeezed in" within the constraints of genome sequence stability. The paradox is that known selection coefficients do not seem high enough to keep complex systems the same through phylogenetic time, yet there is observed conservation of sequences and hence of functions. Further work is clearly required in this fascinating area of modern evolutionary research.

DIVING RESPONSE PHYSIOLOGY HAS EVOLVED SEVERAL TIMES

To reiterate, from the above discussion it appears that a number of physiological and biochemical characters required and used in diving animals are highly conserved in all vertebrates; these presumably ancestral or plesiomorphic traits are necessarily similar in all pinnipeds and include diving apnea, bradycardia, tissue specific hypoperfusion, and hypometabolism of hypoperfused tissues. In contrast to such traits, another group of functionally linked characters are more malleable and include (i) body size, (ii) spleen mass, (iii) blood volume, and (iv) red blood cell mass and thus hemoglobin pool size. Increases in any or all of these improve diving capacity (defined as maximum recorded diving duration). As in our discussion in the evolution of other physiological systems (chapter 3 for example), it is interesting to inquire about how frequently these kinds of physiologies have evolved. In evolutionary terms, is it easy or difficult to evolve physiolo-

gical mechanisms for use in diving? If it were easy, one would expect diving capabilities to be widespread; if in evolutionary terms it is difficult to evolve these physiologies, diving capabilities would be found within only one or two mammalian lineages. Interestingly, even a casual examination of a mammalian phylogenetic tree (figure 4.8) shows that diving animals are distributed widely throughout the lineage— from monotremes in Australia and marsupial species in South America, to geographically more widely spread pinnnipeds, cetaceans, mustelids, and sirenians, within the placental mammals. Although from figure 4.8 it is evident that the diving response is expressed in lineages that are not closely related to each other, as far as we know today, the basic mechanisms of the diving response are similar in all of these groups. This may be understandable, given that conserved diving response components (bradycardia, peripheral vasoconstriction, and the physiological processes that necessarily follow) as well as adaptable elements (spleen, blood oxygen carrying capacity) are expressed widely, if variably, within the vertebrates. Presumably, lineage-specific differences in the evolution of the diving response arise from different assemblies of these two (adaptable vs conservative) categories of characters determining diving capabilities and from different biological imperatives (different anatomical constraints in cetaceans versus pinnipeds, for example). Because of the number of phylogenetically unrelated species that are known to express significant diving capabilities, the conclusion that diving response physiology can, and has, arisen independently many times within this group of vertebrates is clear and compelling. Although not analyzed in detail here, the same conclusions undoubtedly apply to the evolution of the diving response in birds (Butler and Jones, 1997), where the diving response mechanisms are also similar to those discussed above and where diving capabilities are expressed widely throughout the avian lineage.

Finally, it is worth pointing out that our sketch of the development of the field of diving physiology again illustrates that science progress is not a simple linear and dogged march through time; instead, things move ahead rapidly at times, more slowly at other times. New breakthroughs sometimes come unexpectedly but in many situations in science the field seems to sense when breakthroughs are "needed" and when they are more likely to occur. Some workers believe that the field of diving physiology and metabolism has now reached such a stage: its first growth phase reached an asymptote by the early 1970s; its second growth phase, catalyzed by the introduction of quantitative field monitoring strategies, exploded in the 1980s and after some 15 years of growth and fermentation, it is again at risk of reaching another point of diminishing research returns. Two new approaches with the potential for avoiding such stasis appear to be gaining momentum. On the mechanistic side, by taking advantage of being noninvasive but allowing interrogation continuously in real time, MRI and MRS analysis of the diving response appears to supply potential for new breakthroughs with improvement and refinement of our understanding of the basic machinery of diving. On the other hand is the initiative in evolutionary biochemistry and physiology, which raises our understanding of which diving traits are conservative and which are more adaptable through specific phylogenies. The potentials for interplay and interactions between these two kinds of studies (Mangum and Hochachka, 1998) raise exciting promise for the future.

REFERENCES

Allen, P.S., G.O. Matheson, G. Zhu, D. Gheorgiu, R.S. Dunlop, T. Falconer, C. Stanley, and P. W. Hochachka (1997). Simultaneous 31P magnetic resource spectroscopy of the soleus and gastrocnemius in Sherpas during graded calf muscle exercise and recovery. *Am. J. Physiol.* 273: R999–R1007.

Andrews, R.D. (1999). *The cardiorespiratory, metabolic, and thermoregulatory physiology of juvenile Northern Elephant seals (Mirounga angustirostris).* Ph.D. Thesis, University of British Columbia, Vancouver, Canada, pp. 1–123.

Andrews, R.D., D.R. Jones, J.D. Williams, D.E. Crocker, D.P. Costa, and B.J. LeBeouf (1994).

Thermoregulation and metabolism in freely diving northern elephant seals. *FASEB J.* 8: A2.

Andrews, R.D., D.R. Jones, J.D. Williams, P.H. Thorson, G.W. Oliver, D.P. Costa, and B.J. Le Boeuf (1997). Heart rates of northern elephant seals diving at sea and resting on the beach. *J. Exp. Biol.* 200: 2083–2095.

Arnason, U., K. Bodin, A. Gullberg, C. Ledje, and S. Mouchaty (1995). A molecular view of pinniped relationships with particular emphasis on the true seals. *J. Mol. Evol.* 40: 78–85.

Arnold, R.W. (1985). Extremes in human breath hold, facial immersion bradycardia. *Undersea Biomed. Res.* 12: 183–190.

Barnes, B.M., O.Toien, J. Blake, D. Grahn, H.C. Heller, and D.M. Edgar (1999). Hibernation in black bears: temperature cycles and sleep. *FASEB J.* 13: A740.

Berta, A., and T. A. Demere (1986). *Callorhinus gilmorei* n. sp. (Carnivora: Otariidae) from the San Diego formation (Blancan) and its implications for Otariid phylogeny. *Trans. San Diego Soc. Nat. Hist.* 21: 111–126.

Berta, A., and A.R. Wyss (1994). Pinniped phylogeny. *Proc. San Diego Soc. Nat. Hist.* 29: 33–56.

Bininda-Edmonds, O.R.P., J.L. Gittleman, and A. Purvis (1999). Building large trees by combining phylogenetic information: a complete phylogeny of the extant Carnivora (Mammalia). *Biol. Rev.* 74: 143–175.

Blix, A. S. (1988). Cardiovascular responses to diving. *Acta Physiol. Scand.* 571: S61–68.

Burns, J.J., and F.H. Fay (1970). Comparative methodology of the skull of the Ribbon seal, *Histriophoca fasciata*, with remarks on the systematics of Phocidae. *J. Zool. (Lond.)* 161: 363–394.

Butler, P.J., and D.R. Jones (1982). The comparative physiology of diving in vertebrates. *Adv. Comp. Physiol. Biochem.* 8: 179–368.

Butler, P.J., and D.R. Jones (1997). Physiology of diving of birds and mammals. *Physiol. Rev.* 77: 837–899.

Castellini, M.A., B.J. Murphy, M. Fedak, K. Ronald, N. Gofton, and P.W. Hochachka (1985). Potentially conflicting demands of diving and exercise in gray seals. *J. Appl. Physiol.* 58: 392–399.

Castellini, M.A., G.L. Kooyman, and P.J. Ponganis (1992). Metabolic rates of freely diving Weddell seals. *J. Exp. Biol.* 165: 181–194.

Costa, D. P. (1991). Reproductive and foraging energetics of pinnipeds: Implications for life history patterns. In: *The Behaviour of Pinnipeds*, pp. 300–344, ed. D. Renouf, London: Chapman and Hall.

Costa, D.P. (1993). The relationship between reproductive and foraging energetics and the evolution of the Pinnipedia. In: *Marine Mammals: Advances in Behavioural and Population Biology, Symposia of the Zoological Society of London*, No. 66, pp. 293–314, ed. I.L. Boyd, Oxford: Oxford University Press.

de Leeuw, J.J., P.J. Butler, A.J. Woakes, and F. Zegwaard (1998). Body cooling and its energetic implications for feeding and diving of tufted ducks. *Physiol. Zool.* 71: 720–730.

De Muizon, C. (1976). Pinniped phylogeny and dispersal. *Ann. S. Afr. Mus.* 89: 175–213.

Delong, R.L., and B.S. Stewart (1991). Diving patterns of northern elephant seal bulls. *Mar. Mammal Sci.* 7: 3619–384.

Delong, R.L., B.S. Stewart, and R.D. Hill (1992). Documenting migrations of northern elephant seals using day length. *Mar. Mammal Sci.* 8: 155–159.

Doughty, P. (1996). Statistical analysis of natural experiments in evolutionary biology: comments on recent criticisms of the use of comparative methods to study adaptation. *Am. Nat.* 148: 943–956.

Elsner, R., and B. Gooden (1983). *Diving and Asphyxia—a Comparative Study of Animals and Man*. Cambridge: Cambridge University Press.

Fedak, M. (1986). Diving and exercise in seals—a benthic perspective. In: *Diving in Animals and Man*, pp. 11–32, ed. A. Brubakk, J. W. Kanwisher, and G. Sundnes, Trondheim: Tapir.

Fedak, M.A., M.R. Pullen, and J. Kanwisher (1988). Circulatory responses of seals to periodic breathing: heart rate and breathing during exercise and diving in the laboratory and open sea. *Can. J. Zool.* 66: 53–60.

Felsenstein, J. (1985). Phylogenies and the comparative method. *Am. Nat.* 125: 1–15.

Fritz, G. (1998). Evolution of daily torpor and hibernation in birds and mammals: Importance of body size. *Clin. Exp. Pharmacol. Physiol.* 25: 736–740.

Garland, T. Jr., and S.C. Adolph (1994). Why not to do two species comparative studies: limitations on inferring adaptation. *Physiol. Zool.* 67: 797–828.

Garland, T. Jr., P.H. Harvey, and A.R. Ives (1992). Procedures for the analysis of comparative data using phylogenetically independent contrasts. *System. Biol.* 41: 18–32.

Garland, T. Jr., A.W. Dickerman, C.M. Janis, and J.A. Jones (1993). Phylogenetic analysis of covariance by computer simulation. *System. Biol.* 42: 265–292.

Golding, G.B. (1994). Using maximum likelihood to infer selection from phylogenies. In: *Non-Neutral Evolution. Theories and Molecular Data*, pp. 126–138, ed. B. Golding, London: Chapman and Hall.

Guppy, M., R.D. Hill, R.C. Schneider, J. Qvist, G.C. Liggins, W.M. Zapol, and P.W. Hochachka (1986). Microcomputer assisted metabolic studies of voluntary diving of Weddell seals. *Am. J. Physiol.* 250: R175–R187.

Guyton, G.P., K.S. Stanek, R.C. Schneider, P.W. Hochachka, W.E. Hurford, D.G. Zapol, and W.M. Zapol (1995). Myoglobin saturation in free diving Weddell seals. *J. Appl. Physiol.* 79: 1148–1155.

Hill, R.D., R.C. Schneider, G.C. Liggins, A.H. Schuette, R.L. Elliott, M. Guppy, P.W. Hochachka, J. Qvist, K. J. Falke, and W.M. Zapol (1987). Heart rate and body temperature during free diving of Weddell seals. *Am. J. Physiol.* 253: R344–R351.

Hille, B. (1992). *Ionic Channels of Excitable Membranes*. Sunderland, Mass.: Sinauer Associates.

Hindell, M.A., D.J. Slip, H.R. Burton, and M.M. Bryden (1992). Physiological implications of continuous and deep dives of the southern elephant seal (*Mirounga leonina*). *Can. J. Zool.* 70: 370–379.

Hochachka, P.W. (1986). Balancing the conflicting demands of diving and exercise. *Fed. Proc.* 45: 2949–2954.

Hochachka, P.W. (1992). Metabolic biochemistry and the making of a mesopelagic mammal. *Experientia* 48: 570–575.

Hochachka, P.W. (2000). Pinniped diving response mechanism and evolution: A window on the paradigm of comparative biochemistry and physiology. *Comp. Physiol. Biochem.* 126A: 435–458.

Hochachka, P.W. and R.A. Foreman III (1993). Phocid and cetacean blueprints of muscle metabolism. *Can. J. Zool.* 71: 2089–2098.

Hochachka, P.W., and M. Guppy (1987). *Metabolic Arrest and the Control of Biological Time*. Cambridge: Harvard University Press.

Hochachka, P.W., and P.D. Mottishaw (1998). Evolution and adaptation of the diving response: Phocids and Otariids. In: *Cold Ocean Symposia*, pp. 391–431, ed. H.O. Pörtner and R.C, Playle, Cambridge: Cambridge University Press.

Hochachka, P.W., and G.N. Somero (1984). *Biochemical Adaptation*. Princeton: Princeton University Press.

Hochachka, P. W., G.C. Liggins, G.P. Guyton, R.C. Schneider, K.S. Stanek, W.E. Hurford, R.K. Creasy, D.G. Zapol, and W.M. Zapol (1995). Hormonal regulatory adjustments during voluntary diving in Weddell seals. *Comp. Biochem. Physiol.* 112B: 361–375.

Hurford, W.E., P.W. Hochachka, R.C. Schneider, G.P. Guyton, K.S. Stanek, D.G. Zapol, G.C. Liggins, and W.M. Zapol (1995). Splenic contraction, catecholamine release and blood volume redistribution during voluntary diving in the Weddell seal. *J. Appl. Physiol.* 80: 298–306.

Hurley, J.A. (1996). *Metabolic rate and heart rate during trained dives in adult California sea lions.* Ph.D. Thesis, University of California, Santa Cruz.

Irving, L. (1966). Adaptations to cold. *Sci. Am.* 21: 94–101.

Irving, L. (1969). Temperature regulation in marine mammals. In: *The Biology of Marine Mammals* pp. 147–174, ed. H.T. Andersen, New York: Academic Press.

Johansen, K. (1987). The August Krogh Lecture: The world as a laboratory—Physiological insights from nature's experiments. In: *Advances in Physiological Research*, pp. 377–396, ed. H. McLennan, J.R. Ledsome, C.H.S. McIntosh, and D.R. Jones, New York: Plenum Press.

Kirkpatrick, M. (1996). Genes and adaptation: A pocket guide to the theory. In: *Adaptation*, pp. 125–146, ed. M.R. Rose and G.V. Lauder. San Diego: Academic Press.

Kooyman, G.L., E.H. Wahrenbrock, M.A. Castellini, R.W. Davis, and E.E. Sinnett (1980). Aerobic and anaerobic metabolism during voluntary diving in Weddell seals: Evidence of preferred pathways from blood chemistry and behaviour. *J. Comp. Physiol.* 138: 335–346.

Lacombe, A.M., and D.R. Jones (1991). Role of adrenal catecholamines during forced submergence in ducks. *Am. J. Physiol.* 261: R1364–R1372.

Leboeuf, B.J., Y. Naito, A.C. Huntley, and T. Asaga (1989). Prolonged, continuous, deep diving by northern elephant seals. *Can. J. Zool.* 67: 2514–2519.

Leboeuf, B.J., Y. Naito, T. Asaga, D. Crocker, and D.Costa (1992). Swim velocity and dive patterns in a northern elephant seal, *Mirounga angustirostris. Can. J. Zool.* 70: 786–795.

Leboeuf, B.J., D.E. Crocker, D.P. Costa, S.B. Blackwell, P.M. Webb, and D.S. Houser (2000). Foraging ecology of northern elephant seals. *Ecol. Monogr.* 70: 353–382.

Lento, G. M., R.E. Hickson, G.K. Chambers, and D. Penny (1995). Use of spectral analysis to test hypotheses on the origin of pinnipeds. *Mol. Biol. Evol.* 12: 28–52.

Leroi, A.M., M.R. Rose, and G.V. Lauder (1994). What does the comparative method reveal about adaptation? *Am. Nat.* 143: 381–402.

Li, K. C., R.L. Dalman, I.Y. Chen, L.R. Pelc, C.K. Song, W.K. Moon, M.I. Kang, and G.A. Wright (1997). Chronic mesenteric ischemia: use of in vivo MR imaging measurements of blood oxygen saturation in the superior mesenteric vein for diagnosis. *Radiology* 204: 71–77.

Mangum, C.P., and P.W. Hochachka (1998). New directions in comparative physiology and biochemistry: Mechanisms, adaptations, and evolution. *Physiol. Zool.* 71: 471–484.

Mottishaw, P.D. (1997). The diving physiology of pinnipeds: an evolutionery inquiry MSc. Thesis, University of British Columbia, Vancouver.

Mottishaw, P.D., S. Thornton, and P.W. Hochachka (1999). The diving response and its surprising evolutionary path in seals and sea lions. *Am. Zool.* 39: 434–450

Purvis, A., and A. Rambaut (1995). Comparative analysis by independent contrasts (CAIC): an Apple Macintosh application for analyzing comparative data. *CABIOS* 11: 247–251.

Qvist, J., R.D. Hill, R.C. Schneider, K.J. Falke, G.C. Liggins, M. Guppy, R.L. Elliott, and P.W. Hochachka (1986). Hemoglobin concentrations and blood gas tensions of free diving Weddell seals. *J. Appl. Physiol.* 61: 1560–1569.

Repenning, C.A., R.S. Peterson and C.L. Hubbs (1971). Contributions to the systematics of the southern fur seals, with particular reference to the Juan Fernandez and Guadalupe species. *Antarctic Res.* 18: 1–34.

Scholander, P. F. (1940). Experimental investigations in diving animals and birds. *Hvalradets Skrifter* 22: 1–131.

Scholander, P.F. (1963). The master switch of life. *Sci. Am.* 209: 92–106.

Teyssier G., J-C. Fouron, S.E. Sonesson, P. Bonnin, and A. Skoll (1998). Circulatory changes induced by isovolumic increase in red cell mass in fetal lambs. *Arch. Dis. Childhood* 79: F180–F184.

Thompson, D., and M.A. Fedak (1989). Comparison of dive behaviour and cardiac responses of free ranging harbor and grey seals. *Tenth Biennial Conf. Biol. Marine Mammals* A106.

Thompson, D., and M.A. Fedak (1993). Cardiac responses of grey seals during diving at sea. *J. Exp. Biol.* 174: 139–164.

Thornton, S.J. (2000). *Investigations into the diving response of northern elephant seals (Mirounga angustirostris) using Magnetic Resonance Imaging and Spectroscopy*. PhD Thesis, University of British Columbia, Vancouver, B.C.

Thornton, S. J., D.M. Spielman, W.F. Block, P.W. Hochachka, D.E. Crocker, B.J. Leboeuf, D.P. Costa, D. Houser, S. Kohin, L.R. Pelc, and N. J. Pelc (1997a). MR Imaging in a Diving Seal. *Proc. Intl. Soc. Magn. Res. Med.* 2: 822.

Thornton, S. J., N. J. Pelc, D.M. Spielman, J.R. Liao, D.P. Costa, D.E. Crocker, D. Houser, S. Kohin, B.J. Leboeuf, L.R. Pelc, and P.W. Hochachka (1997b). Vascular flow dynamics in a diving elephant seal (*Mirounga angustrirostris*). *Intl. Soc. Magn. Res. Med.* 2: 823.

Thornton, S.J., N.J. Pelc, D.M. Spielman, W.F. Block, D.P. Costa, D.E. Crocker, B.J. Leboeuf, and P.W. Hochachka (2000). Magnetic Resonance Imaging of northern elephant seals provides insights into the function of the phocid spleen during diving. *Proc. Natl. Acad. Sci. USA*, in review stages.

Thron, C.D., J. Chen, J. C. Leiter and L.C. Ou (1998). Renovascular adaptive changes in chronic hypoxic polycythemia. *Kidney Intern*. 54: 2014–2020.

Webb, P.M., D.E. Crocker, S.B. Blackwell, D.P. Costa, and B.J. Leboeuf (1998). Effects of buoyancy on the diving behavior of northern elephant seals. *J. Exp. Biol.* 201: 2349–2358.

Williams, T.M., R.W. Davis, L.A. Fuiman, J. Francis, B.L. Le boeuf, M. Horning, J. Calambokidis, and D.A. Croll (2000). Sink or swim: Strategies for cost-efficient diving by marine mammals. *Science* 288: 133–136.

Winslow, R. M., and C. C. Monge (1987). *Hypoxia, Polycythemia and Chronic Mountain Sickness*. Baltimore: Johns Hopkins University Press.

Zapol, W.M., G.C. Liggins, R.C. Schneider, J. Qvist, M.T. Snider, R.K. Creasy, and P.W. Hochachka (1979). Regional blood flow during simulated diving in the conscious Weddell seal. *J. Appl. Physiol.* 47: 968–973.

Zierenberg, R.A., M.W.W. Adams, and A.J. Arp (2001). Life in extreme environments: Hydrothermal vents. *Proc. Natl. Acad. Sci. USA* 97: 12961–12962.

5

Human Hypoxia Tolerance

BACKGROUND AND INTRODUCTION

The starting points for our thinking on this problem were recent studies on origins and evolution of hominids implying that the human species arose under geological conditions that were getting colder, drier and higher; that is, conditions under which endurance performance capacities and hypoxia tolerance would have been favored (Vrba et al., 1994). This aroused our interest, since biomedical researchers have long known that there are numerous mechanistic similarities in human physiology between adaptations for endurance performance and for hypoxia tolerance (Brooks et al., 1996; Green et al., 2000; Levine and Stray-Gunderson, 1996; Terrados, 1992). How physiological systems for hypoxia tolerance or endurance performance might have evolved within our phylogeny was not investigated earlier because there were few if any guidelines for tracing the evolutionary pathways of complex physiological systems in humans or other animals. In our case, initial guidelines arose from recent quantitative analyses of the variability of the diving response in pinnipeds. These studies, reviewed in chapter 4, led to two principles of evolution of the diving response that are useful as a framework for probing the evolution of complex physiological systems: (i) some physiological/biochemical characters considered necessary in diving animals are highly conserved; these traits (including diving apnea, bradycardia, tissue hypoperfusion, and hypometabolism of hypoperfused tissues) probably arose in response to factors other than—or in addition to—diving requirements and presumably

were and are maintained largely by negative or stabilizing selection (any mutations affecting them not surviving). At this stage in our understanding of diving physiology and biochemistry, we are unable to detect any correlation between these characters and diving capacity, even though they are clearly used during diving and are so important that diving bradycardia is often referred to in this literature as the "master switch of life." (ii) A few other biological "characters" or traits are correlated with long-duration diving and prolonged foraging at sea. These characters include body weight, spleen weight, blood volume, and red blood cell (RBC) mass. The larger these are, the greater the diving capacity (defined as diving duration). Since the relationships between diving capacity and any of the latter three traits are evident even when corrected for body weight, it is reasonable to conclude that these three traits—large spleens, large blood volume, and large RBC mass—are true biological adaptations that extend diving duration, probably through effects on O_2 storage and O_2 management during diving (see chapter 4 for the special case of the spleen). That is, in contrast to conserved traits such as bradycardia, these kinds of characters have evolved presumably by positive selection to enable prolonged dive times. In effect, the evolutionary physiology of the diving response thus can be described in terms of the degree of development of adaptable versus conservative categories of diving characters; that is, in terms of how these patterns change through time and how the patterns are lineage specific. Our goal in this chapter is to see if this basic framework can be applied usefully to understanding the evolution of hypoxia response physiology in our own species.

TIME AND HYPOXIA ADAPTATION OPTIONS

Anyone who has journeyed into mountains that are 2,000 or more meters high will have a sense of how debilitating hypobaric hypoxia can actually be; and, of course, the higher we go, the more severe the hypoxia, the more debilitating the effects on our physiology and performance. Many of us will also know that after some period of time at altitude, these effects are to some degree alleviated. Even more impressive on such excursions into high-altitudes are our observations of the performance of native highlanders, seemingly being far less debilitated than we might expect based on our own feelings of malaise. This is common if anecdotal knowledge for most and perhaps all of us and it represents the field of play for the disciplines of high-altitude biology, physiology, and medicine. In these disciplines, it is axiomatic that how a species deals with hypoxia, or any other selectively significant parameter, depends upon the time available for orchestrating the response. Traditionally, the time line for response is divided into three categories: acute, acclimatory, and genetic or phylogenetic. The formal relationship between these three time lines of responses (see chapter 1) begins first with sensing mechanisms, which tell the organism when the problem arises and initiate the whole hypoxia response cascade. Second, this information is transduced at various levels of organization into appropriate acute responses. Third, either the same or different sets of sensing and signal transduction pathways may be utilized to orchestrate more complex acclimatory responses. Finally fourth, any of the above—the sensing step, the signal transduction pathways, the acute response, and the acclimatory responses—during generational time:

(i) may change randomly due to genetic drift (characters arising by this means in extant lineages are not adaptations),

(ii) may change due to positive natural selection at rates proportional to selection pressures (characters arising by this process are termed adaptations), or

(iii) may be conserved or stabilized essentially unchanged by negative or stabilizing selection pressures (these kinds of characters are expressed in extant lineages as a result of common descent and are designed for function in many settings; they may be used along with (ii) above in physiologically adaptive responses to hypoxia but technically they are not hypoxia adaptations per se).

In human studies, it is of course impossible to experimentally manipulate generational time in any controllable manner. Thus the strategy of all analyses in this area is to compare human lineages (e.g., Quechuas and Sherpas) adapted to different high-altitude regions for differing periods of time to gain insight into the evolution of human hypoxia response physiology (figure 5.1). Examination of the literature shows that the acute and acclimatory responses to hypobaric hypoxia in humans are fairly well known. However, much less insight is available on how these response systems change in populations of our species through evolutionary time—the fourth process above. We shall review these different time courses of response below.

ACUTE AND ACCLIMATION RESPONSES IN LOWLAND LINEAGES

Acute responses to hypobaric hypoxia arbitrarily are defined as those occurring essentially immediately following transition from normoxia to hypoxia and continuing throughout the period required for longer term back-up responses. The latter almost by definition require restructuring and reorganization of cell and tissue function—processes that usually take from hours to days or even longer. That is why, operationally, acute hypoxia responses can be considered to be those that are based on functions of biochemical and physiological systems that are in place at the time of normoxia to hypoxia transition.

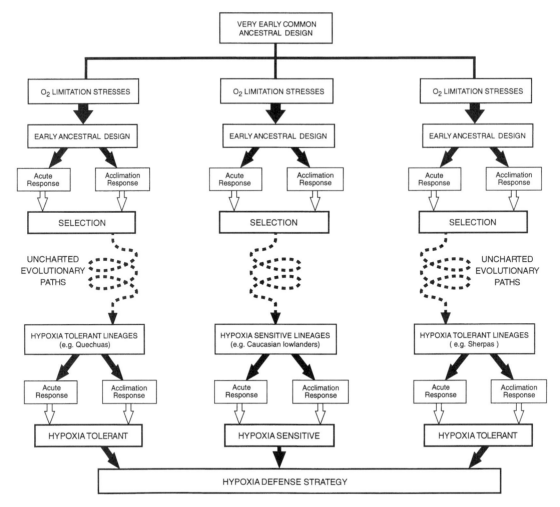

Figure 5.1. The interplay between time and adaptational options occurs in human as well as in animal evolution of physiological systems. The acute and acclimation effects on human hypoxia response physiology can be readily evaluated. However, adaptations requiring generations of time of course cannot be studied by direct manipulations in humans. All workers in this area therefore rely upon comparing human lineages adapted to hypobaric hypoxia in different regions of the world and for different time periods. Two such groups that have extensively studied in this manner are Quechuas and Aymaras from the Andes, and Sherpas and Tibetans from the Himalayas. See chapter 1 for further discussion of time and adaptation options.

Acute high-altitude studies of both human and animal models indicate that hypoxia defenses are initiated by several oxygen sensing, signal transduction pathways. For convenience, these have been summarized as five general hypoxia response systems (figure 5.2(A)–(E):

(i) Carotid body O_2 sensors initiate the hypoxic ventilatory response (HVR), which may raise the risk of alkalosis (basically by "blowing off" CO_2 reserves) but also serves to compensate for the acute oxygen shortage.

(ii) Pulmonary vasculature O_2 sensors initiate activation of the hypoxic pulmonary vasoconstrictor response (HPVR) which is thought to orchestrate adjustments in lung perfusion and in ventilation–perfusion matching.

(iii) O_2 sensors in the vasculature of other tissues activate expression of vascular endothelial growth factor 1 (VEGF1) with its receptor and thus initiate the process of angiogenesis especially in the heart and possibly the brain.

(iv) O_2 sensors in specialized kidney and liver cells activate expression of erythropoietin (EPO) and so begin the process of up-regulating red blood cell (RBC) mass.

(v) Metabolic responses to acute hypoxia, probably initially sensed by percent hemoglobin saturation of arterial blood, include attenuation of aerobic and anaerobic ATP supply pathways by regulation processes that are controversial and may or may not involve O_2 sensing by systems other than mitochondrial metabolism. However, generalized tissue-specific O_2-sensing and signal transduction pathways are involved in initial stages of tissue-specific metabolic reorganization by altering expression rates of hypoxia sensitive genes for metabolic enzymes and metabolite transporters (see chapter 3).

Even though no sharp line separates acute and acclimatory phases of hypoxia exposure, it is clear that most hypoxia response systems do not have time to go to completion during acute hypoxia. Thus, despite the above adjustments, the debilitating effects of acute hypoxia exposure are easily measurable and can be illustrated by considering an exercise protocol. On exposure to acute hypoxia (equivalent to about 4200 m altitude), there is a relatively large (20–35%) decline in $\dot{V}O_2$max in lowlanders. Furthermore, metabolic attempts to accommodate the new hypoxic conditions (which can be viewed as attempts to make up the energy deficit due to O_2 lack) are expressed as large increases in lactate accumulation in the blood during exercise (Hochachka et al., 1991; Matheson et al., 1991).

With continued exposure of lowland lineages to hypoxia (figure 5.2(A)–(E), acclimation processes:

(i) increase the hypoxia sensitivity of the HVR (at the biochemical level, this may require increasing the O_2 affinity of the O_2 sensor) and for a given hypoxic stimulus, the ventilatory response is exaggerated (Hochachka, 1994; Lahiri, 1996; Lahiri et al., 1969),

(ii) extend the HPVR (Weir and Archer, 1995) in a continued attempt to most efficiently match perfusion and ventilation, a process that sometimes comes with the cost of causing hypertension (Heath and Williams, 1981),

(iii) maintain angiogenesis coincident with blood volume expansion,

(iv) maintain erythropoiesis, thus also leading to expansion of the RBC mass, which together with (iii) above increases the O_2 delivery capacities (Harik et al., 1996; Ladoux and Felin, 1993; Ogita et al., 1994), and

(v) allow continuation of hypoxia sensitive gene function leading to significant metabolic reorganization, one expression of which is an increased carbohydrate preference during exercise (Brooks et al., 1991; Kayser et al., 1991, 1996; Levine and Stray-Gunderson, 1996).

These hypoxia acclimation processes take days to weeks to settle down at new steady states. However, when complete, hypoxia acclimations are able to compensate for the O_2 deficit of hypoxia better than acute adjustments. For example, after acclimation in lowlanders, the $\dot{V}O_2$max is still affected by hypoxia, but to a lesser degree than previously. There is less energy deficit due to O_2 lack and less postexercise blood lactate accumulation.

Parenthetically, we should mention that the whole field of lactate metabolism in high-altitude conditions has been perplexing to physiologists for two reasons. First, it was noted that the higher the altitude for acclimation, the lower the peak, postexercise blood lactate concentrations during a given exercise protocol. This observation, first noted in the early 1930s, is noncontroversial but because less lactate is found under more and more O_2-limiting conditions, the phenomenon became known as the lactate paradox (West, 1986; Hochachka, 1988). To physiologists, there was a second reason for being perplexed; namely, the observation, frequently reported, of attenuation of lactate accumulation during the hypoxia acclimation despite maintained hypoxia. The origin of the hypoxia acclimation induced *lowering* of

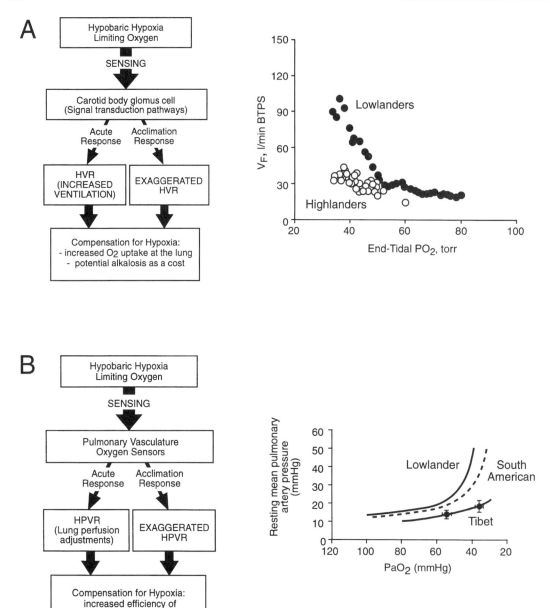

Figure 5.2

peak blood lactate concentrations relative to levels in acute hypoxia, or whether it always occurs, are both controversial (in the literature this is included in the so-called lactate paradox).

In part this controversy may result from the interplay between (i) lactate removal from the blood and (ii) its simultaneous production (by muscles) followed by release into the blood: the balance between these processes is a major determinant of plasma lactate concentrations, but the two processes can change independently of each other and may differ in different individuals (Brooks et al., 1991). Thus this source of variability could lead to differing results and confound researchers in this field. Also some interstudy differences may arise from processes occurring within exercising muscle per se. Within muscle the production of lactate always

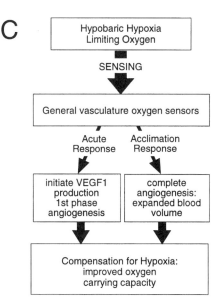

Angiogenesis and Blood Volume

Altitude	ml/kg Total Blood Volume
0	85
3700	108
4500	110
4500 (CMS)	181

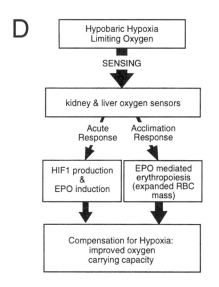

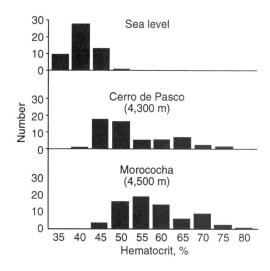

Figure 5.2. Continued

proceeds with associated release of H^+ ions and the latter in turn shift the creatine phosphokinase (CPK) equilibrium to the right:

$$H^+ + PCr + ADP \rightarrow ATP + Cr$$

As a result, decreasing [PCr] occurs with simultaneously increasing [lactate]. During the first 1–2 min of recovery after exercise, when peak blood lactate concentrations are observed, the reverse of these intracellular processes occurs, with muscle [lactate] decreasing and [PCr] increasing as its pool size is renewed. This means there is an inverse relationship between lactate clearance and PCr recovery. The process is fast in individuals with muscles rich in mitochondria, slower in mitochondria-poor muscles; and, the available data suggest that it is faster

E

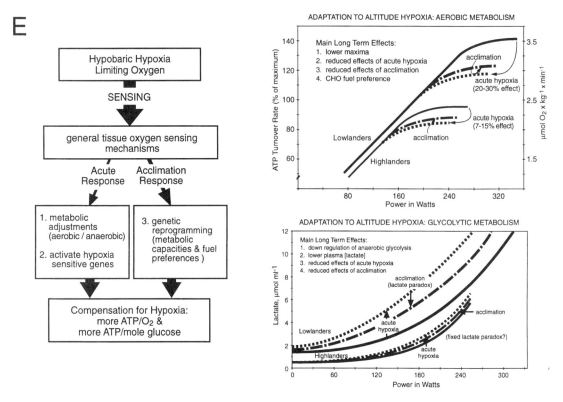

Figure 5.2. Continued

after hypoxia acclimation (consistent with lower plasma [lactate]) than during acute hypoxia exposure. Because plots of [lactate] versus [PCr] for subjects pre- and postacclimation to hypoxia should fall on the same line, the post-exercise blood lactate differences between these individuals do not represent a paradox to metabolic biochemists. They simply represent varying metabolic conditions. However, it is evident that between-study artifacts in peak lactate concentrations could easily arise because of differences in (e.g., the training or fitness states of) volunteer subjects in high-altitude research. Even though these factors clearly would influence the above [lactate]–[PCr] relationships, they are almost never taken into account in high-altitude studies, especially in the older literature. Presumably it is for these kinds of reasons that differences in results between different researchers sometimes occur and of course these may be difficult to interpret in retrospect.

In the context of this analysis, however, the key insight is that essentially all acute hypoxia

response systems in lowlanders can be further adjusted during acclimation.

ACUTE AND ACCLIMATION RESPONSES IN HIGHLAND LINEAGES

Using the above framework, the above acute and acclimatory patterns of lowlanders have been compared to those found in indigenous highlanders to evaluate change in these physiological traits through generational time. The data base arises from studies of several low- and high-altitude lineages (the Quechuas and Aymaras from the high Andes of South America; the Sherpas from Himalayan regions of Nepal; the Tibetans from the Tibetan plateau; East Africans from Kenya and other regions of the east African plateau). The studies have focused on four systems: integrated whole body physiology and metabolism, muscle metabolism at rest and during work, heart metabolism in normoxia versus hypoxia, and brain

Figure 5.2. Interplay between time and adaptive responses of five physiological systems in humans. (A) HVR (Left panel) Diagrammatic summary of the formally defined relationships between time and physiological responses (in this case, the hypoxic ventilatory response, or HVR) to environmental factors such as hypoxia. Acute responses are those which occur essentially instantaneously with environmental change; adjustments requiring some fraction of the organism's lifetime (requiring from minutes, to hours, to days to reach a new steady state) are termed acclimatory responses or acclimations. In the North American literature, the response is termed "an acclimatization" if it occurs naturally (where parameters other than the one of interest cannot be fully controlled). Only acute and acclimatory responses are possible within a given generation. However, all components of the cascade (from sensing and signal transduction to acclimatory response) can change through evolutionary time, a process defined in the literature as phylogenetic adaptation (Hochachka and Somero, 1984). See text for further details. (Right panel) HVR shown for lowlanders and highlanders, indicating severe HVR blunting in the latter (data from Winslow and Monge, 1987). V_E: ventilation volume in liters per min. (B) HPVR (Left panel) Diagrammatic summary of the formal relationships between time and the hypoxic pulmonary vasoconstrictor response (HPVR) to hypoxia. All components of the cascade (from sensing and signal transduction to acclimatory response) can change through evolutionary time, a process defined in the literature as phylogenetic adaptation and illustrated in the right panel. See text for further details. (Right panel) The HPVR for lowlanders versus indigenous highlanders, expressed as change in pulmonary artery pressure as a function of arterial oxygen tension. (See Hochachka et al., 1999, for literature in this area.) (C) Angiogenesis. (Left panel) Diagrammatic summary of the formal relationships between time and hypoxia exposure in the HIF 1-mediated production of vascular endothelial factor 1 (VEGF 1) and the initiation of angiogenesis. All components of the cascade (from sensing and signal transduction to acclimatory response) can change through evolutionary time. (Right panel). Relationship between altitude and blood volume in Peruvian natives. (Data from Winslow and Monge, 1987.) (D) Erythropoiesis. (Left Panel) Diagrammatic summary of the formal relationships between time and hypoxia exposure in the HIF 1-mediated production of erythropoietin (EPO) and the initiation of erythropoiesis. All components of the cascade (from sensing and signal transduction to acclimatory response) can change through evolutionary time. For example, the response is more robust in lowlanders and Quechuas than it is in Sherpas. See text for further details. (Right panel) Representative data indicating the relationship between altitude and red blood cell (RBC) mass. (Modified from Winslow and Monge, 1987.) (E) Metabolic responses. (Left panel) Diagrammatic summary of the formal relationships between time and hypoxia exposure in orchestrating exercise and metabolic responses to hypoxia. All components of the cascade (from sensing and signal transduction to acclimatory response) can change through evolutionary time; effects on aerobic and glycolytic contributions to whole body exercise are illustrated in right panels. (Upper right panel) Effect of acute and acclimatory exposure to hypoxia on aerobic metabolism during exericise in two human lineages (lowlanders compared to Andean and Himalayan natives). Diagrammatic summary based on lowlander and Quechua data from Hochachka et al. (1991) and Matheson et al. (1991). Main long-term effects shown in inset refer to metabolic responses in Quechuas. Adenosine triphosphate (ATP) turnover rates during exercise standardized to Quechua data. (Lower right panel) Effect of acute and acclimatory exposure to hypoxia on plasma lactate response during exercise in two human lineages (lowlanders compared to Andean and Himalayan natives). Diagrammatic summary based on lowlander and Quechua data from Hochachka et al. (1991) and Matheson et al. (1991). Main long-term effects shown in inset refer to metabolic responses in Quechuas.

metabolic organization. In addition, interpretation of these data, and the field analysis as a whole which follows below, relies on metabolic and physiological data already in the literature. Guided by the diving model (discussed in chapter 4), these studies reveal evidence that the physiology of hypoxia tolerance in humans displays both conservative and adaptable characters. Brain metabolism can serve as an example of the former and heart metabolism as an example of the latter.

BRAIN METABOLIC ORGANIZATION: A CONSERVATIVE CHARACTER IN HUMAN PHYLOGENY

To evaluate the nature of brain metabolism through generational time, these studies compared mass-specific glucose metabolic rates (using positron emission tomography, PET) in over 20 anatomically distinguishable regions of the brain in lowlanders and compared these patterns to those found in indigenous highlanders (Hochachka et al., 1995, 1996b). In all three lineages, (i) glucose is the preferred fuel of the brain, (ii) brain metabolic rates are quantitatively similar, and (iii) region-by-region comparisons indicate qualitatively similar metabolic organization (defined as "regional imaging" in figure 5.3). As these are measurements of the brain in physiological steady state, the results indicate that pathways of adenosine triphosphate (ATP) demand and ATP supply (and presumably associated regulatory mechanisms in brain ATP turnover) are all conserved in our phylogeny—an assumption running throughout these studies. In fact, studies from other laboratories indicate the above features apply for the brain in other (e.g., Japanese) lineages as well (Matsubayashi et al., 1986). Since these different human groups have been evolving separately for a significant part of our species' history, the above similarities imply that the genes specifying structure and function of the central nervous system (CNS) involved in regulated ATP demand and ATP supply pathways have been stabilized by negative selection through our phylogeny (any mutations causing change presumably being deleted). Not surpris-

ingly, human brain metabolic organization thus well illustrates a physiological character that is strikingly conserved in our evolution and whose functions appear both in normoxia and in hypobaric hypoxia.

A HIGH PROPORTION OF PHYSIOLOGICAL CHARACTERS ARE CONSERVATIVE

A key insight is that the conservative nature of human brain metabolism is by no means exceptional. Because we here are assessing traits within a single species, conservative characters are too numerous to outline in detail; suffice to emphasize that these are probably the rule. Three additional, well-worked-out examples are hemoglobin (Hb) O_2 affinity and regulation, muscle organization into different fiber types, and the cardiovascular control system used in regulation of heart and perfusion in many physiological settings (including diving, as mentioned in chapter 4). Categories of physiological traits such as these—in sum they make up most of our physiology—and the way they are used on hypoxia exposure appear common in humans no matter what the lineage or the O_2 content of the inspired air in the normal environment (Winslow and Monge, 1987).

HEART METABOLISM: EXAMPLE OF AN ADAPTABLE PHYSIOLOGICAL CHARACTER

Heart Metabolism in Lowlanders and Highlanders

Unlike the brain, the heart displays an impressively adaptable metabolic organization. In lowlanders, heart metabolism is opportunistic and it utilizes free fatty acids (FFAs), glucose, or lactate on an availability basis. To evaluate the nature of heart metabolism through generational time, studies used ^{31}P magnetic resonance spectroscopy (MRS) and compared the spectra in lowlanders to those found in indigenous highlanders in normoxia versus hypoxia. In heart, the technology is able to quantify phosphocrea-

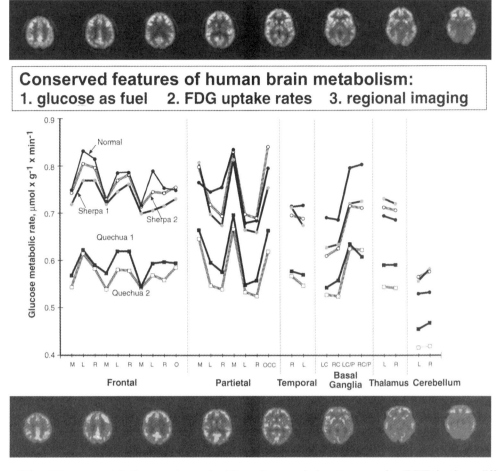

Figure 5.3. Glucose metabolic rates imaged with positron emission tomography (PET) in three different subject groups. Representative PET images (horizontal slices; frontal cortex at the top) are shown for a Caucasian lowlander (upper panel) and for a Quechua from the Andes (lower panel). Images are scaled to the same range (white, through gray, to black indicating metabolic rates ranging from about 0.8 to 0.5 μmol glucose taken up per gram per minute. Middle panel presents quantitative site-specific metabolic rates for over 20 brain regions. (Data for this figure, and brain sites identified, in Hochachka et al., 1995, 1996a,b.)

tine (PCr), ATP, and 2,3-diphosphoglycerate (2,3DPG). The DPG signals are known to derive from RBCs, while the PCr and ATP signals derive from heart tissue per se. These experiments (Hochachka et al., 1996a) showed that in indigenous highlanders, the concentration ratios of PCr/ATP were maintained at steady-state normoxic values (0.9–1) that were unusually low, about half those found in normoxic lowlanders (1.8) monitored the same way at the same time (figure 5.4). Because the creatine phosphokinase reaction functions close to equi-

librium, these steady-state PCr/ATP ratios presumably coincide with about threefold higher free adenosine diphosphate (ADP) concentrations. Higher ADP concentrations (i.e., lower [PCr]/[ATP] ratios) correlate with the K_m values for ADP-requiring kinases of glycolysis (figure 5.4) and reflect elevated carbohydrate contributions to heart energy needs. This metabolic organization was presumably selected in highlanders because the ATP yield/O_2 is 25–60% higher with glucose than with free fatty acids, the fuels usually utilized in the human heart in postfast-

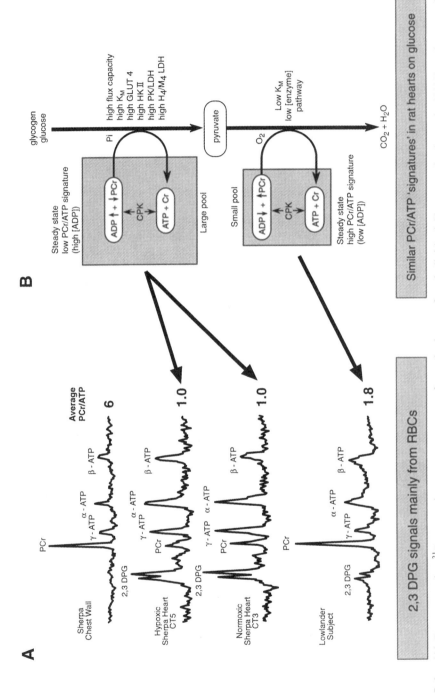

Figure 5.4. (A) Representative ^{31}P magnetic resonance spectra from the heart of an individual Sherpa under hypoxia (11%) and normoxia (room air) compared to a representative Caucasian lowlander (bottom) and the skeletal muscle of the chest wall (top). The average ratios of PCr/ATP for hearts in lowlanders (1.8) differ by nearly twofold from the values for highlanders (about 1.0). (B) Diagrammatic summary emphasizing the contribution of aerobic glycolysis to stabilizing [ADP] at steady-state concentrations high enough to satisfy the high K_M values (low ADP affinities of) phosphoglycerate kinase and pyruvate kinase. Under these steady-state conditions, the ratios of PCr/ATP are necessarily depressed below those expected when fatty acids are the preferred fuel, the situation normally found for heart metabolic organization in lowlanders. When fatty acids are the preferred or main fuel selected, the adenylate and PCr picture is dominated by mitochondrial metabolism, which displays a much higher affinity (lower K_M value) for ADP than does glycolysis. Under these steady-state conditions, the PCr/ATP ratio is necessarily elevated. (Other conditions are given in Hochachka et al., 1996a; figure modified from Hochachka et al., 1999.)

ing conditions (see Hochachka et al., 1996, for literature in this area).

Hypoxia Acclimation Effects on Heart Metabolism

Interestingly, the effects of hypoxia acclimation on heart PCr/ATP signatures also differ in the two groups. In highlanders, the PCr/ATP signature of glucose fuel preference remains stable even after four weeks of deacclimation at low altitudes, while a similar period of acclimation in lowlanders leads to a modest shift toward the highlander pattern (P.W. Hochachka and R.V. Menon, unpublished data). Studies of rats also found that hypobaric hypoxia acclimation for 3–4 weeks leads to a decrease in fatty acid oxidation capacity, with a relative increase in glucose preference as fuel for the heart (Rumsey et al., 1999). Taken together, these data indicate that heart adaptations seem to rely upon stoichiometric efficiency adjustments, improving the yield of ATP per mole of O_2 consumed, as in muscle, by increased preference for carbohydrate as a carbon and energy source (Holden et al., 1995). Together with increased blood volume and RBC mass (i.e. increased whole body O_2 carrying capacity), these adaptations lead to obvious functional advantages: dampened heart work requirements at any given altitude for a similar submaximal whole body O_2 consumption rate and level of whole body exercise. The fundamental point is that in contrast to the brain, in the heart, some component or components of the ATP supply pathways appear to be under positive selective pressure in high-altitude natives, leading to two adaptations: elevated preference for glucose as fuel for the heart and a modified hypoxia acclimation response.

ADAPTABLE TRAITS AND A HIGH-ALTITUDE PHYSIOLOGICAL PHENOTYPE

Oxygen-Sensor-Mediated Hypoxia Response Systems

Despite an overwhelmingly conservative nature to human metabolism and physiology, these studies also provide evidence for other functional responses to hypobaric hypoxia that, like heart metabolism, appear to be true adaptations in Quechuas and Sherpas. Such characters seemingly occur at all levels of organization examined and can be summarized as the same five adjustable hypoxia response systems (HRSs) discussed in lowlanders above (figure 5.5), which seem to form a common basis for the complex physiology of hypoxia tolerance (figure 5.2(A)–(E):

(i) blunted hypoxic ventilatory response (HVR) mediated by the carotid body O_2 sensor (Lahiri, 1996), serving to counteract acid–base problems arising from hyperventilation (Samaja et al., 1997);

(ii) blunted hypoxic pulmonary vasoconstrictor response (HPVR) mediated by pulmonary vasculature O_2 sensors (Weir and Archer, 1995), serving to minimize risks of pulmonary hypertension;

(iii) up-regulated expression of vascular endothelial growth factor 1 (mediated by vascular O_2 sensors [Forsythe et al., 1996]), angiogenesis and hence increased blood volume (Winslow and Monge, 1987);

(iv) maintained erythropoietin regulation of erythropoiesis (mediated by kidney O_2 sensors), and hence increased RBC mass and O_2 carrying capacity (Bunn and Poyton, 1996; Maxwell et al., 1993; Wang et al., 1995; Wenger and Gassman, 1997), and

(v) regulatory adjustments of metabolic pathways to alter fuel preferences, the ratio of aerobic/glycolytic metabolic pathways, and, in striated muscle, to attenuate concentrations of enzymes in energy metabolism (Hochachka, 1992).

Downstream Adjustable Hypoxia Response Systems

The above HRSs in turn set the stage for additional well-documented downstream effects. For example, we find that in Andean and

Himalayan natives, maximum aerobic and anaerobic exercise capacities are down-regulated. The acute effects of hypoxia (making up the energy deficit due to O_2 lack) expected from lowlanders are blunted and metabolic acclimation effects are also frequently attenuated (see, however, discussion above). The in-vivo biochemical properties of skeletal muscles, in Quechuas formed predominantly of slow-twitch fibers, are consistent with regulatory adjustments of glycolytic versus oxidative contributions to energy supply to improve the yield of ATP per mole of carbon fuel utilized. These fiber type distributions in indigenous highlanders are unchanged by acclimation and correlate with better coupling between ATP demand and ATP supply pathways (lesser perturbation of phosphate metabolite pools during rest–exercise transitions), lower lactate accumulation and improved endurance. Indeed, low lactate accumulation during exercise is one of the most characteristic metabolic features of indigenous highlanders (figure 5.2(E)), an observation first noted in the 1930s. Kenyans native to medium-altitude environments, even if not as much studied, show similar, if higher capacity, biochemical and physiological properties (adjustments at least in part based on preponderance of slow-twitch fibers in skeletal muscles); this is not evident in African Americans originating from lowland regions of West Africa, showing a much higher preponderance of fast-twitch fibers in their muscles (see Ama et al., 1986; Matheson et al., 1991; Rosser and Hochachka, 1994; Saltin et al., 1995a,b). Finally, a blunted catecholamine response to hypoxia in indigenous highlanders indicates reduced hypoxic sensitivity of sympathadrenergic control, below the normally expected desensitization on exposure of human cells to hypoxia (Antenzana et al., 1992, 1995; Mazzeo et al., 1991; Resink et al., 1996).

Compared to acute or acclimatory adjustments, these longer term (phylogenetic) adaptations appear to compensate quite well for O_2 deficits caused by hypoxia, but the advantage appears to be gained at the cost of some attenuation of maximum aerobic and anaerobic metabolic capacities. On balance the picture emerging so far is that of a high altitude physiological phenotype based on numerous similar physiological traits in different high-altitude peoples (data mainly from Andean and Himalayan natives).

Not All Hypoxia Response Systems in Indigenous High-Altitude People Are Exactly the Same

An important insight that should be added is that while overall hypoxia responses appear to involve fine tuning each of the above sensing and signal transduction pathway cascades (figure 5.5), the hypoxia defense adjustments of different high-altitude lineages are not always exactly the same. There may be two obvious explanations for this: the first is variance in physiological traits within high-altitude lineages per se and the second is simply lineage-specific change accumulated in high-altitude populations through evolutionary time. An illustration of variance within high-altitude groups comes from exercise studies of Quechuas: in one group of such subjects peak lactate concentrations were observed to be substantially lower than expected from studies in lowlanders (Hochachka et al., 1991). In a subsequent study of young Quechua farmers, completely comparable tests showed plasma lactate concentrations in a range (9–11 mM) similar to that found for many lowlanders (C. Stanley and P.W. Hochachka, unpublished data). These differences may represent physiological variance within this group either genetically based or environmentally induced. (For example, the Quechua farmers above were notably more powerfully built, and were physically stronger, than were the veterinary research assistants used in the initial studies reported by Hochachka et al. [1991] and the differences between the two groups are similar to differences noted between untrained subjects and trained athletes.) An interesting example of variance arising from between-group differences comes from studies of the HVR, which is more robust in Tibetans than in Quechuas (Strohl and Beal, 1997) or Sherpas (Lahiri et al., 1969). Also, altitude-associated birth weight perturbations are less in Tibetan than in Quechau newborns (Zamudio et al., 1993),

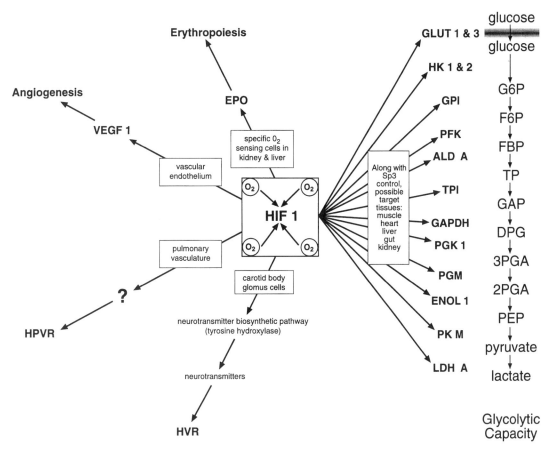

Figure 5.5. At the base of the acute hypoxia response systems (HRSs) are tissue-specific O_2-sensing systems, which in turn regulate the synthesis of hypoxia inducible factor 1 (HIF 1). HIF 1 is an O_2-sensitive transcription factor (concentration rapidly increases when O_2 is limiting); in tissue-specific manner, HIF 1 targets several different genes and so initiates the above cascades. That is why HIF 1 (controlled by tissue-specific O_2-sensing and signal transduction pathways) can be viewed as the center of these controls, with each of the five response systems showing variable degrees of tissue specificity. Studies of acute and acclimation responses of Quechuas and Sherpas in comparison with lowlanders show that all of the above hypoxia-sensitive control pathways are differentially modulated. Physiologists might think of differential modulation in highlanders vs lowlanders as control systems operating at different set points or thresholds. Abbreviations used for metabolites: G6P, F6P, FBP, TP, GAP, DPG, 3PGA, 2PGA, and PEP for glucose 6 phosphate, fructose 6 phosphate, fructose 1,6 bisphosphate, triose phosphate, glyceraldehyde 3 phosphate, diphosphoglycerate, 3 phosphoglycerate, 2 phosphoglycerate, and phosphoenolpyruvate. GLUT 1 and 3, glucose transporter isoforms 1 and 3. HK 1 and 2, hexokinase isoforms 1 and 2. GPI, glucose phosphate isomerase. PFK, phosphofructokinase. ALD A, aldolase A isoform. TPI, triose phosphate isomerase. GAPDH, glyceraldehyde 3 phosphate dehydrogenase. PGK 1, phosphoglycerate kinase isoform 1. PGM, phosphoglucomutase. ENOL 1, enolase isoform 1. PK M, pyruvate kinase, muscle isoform. LDH A, lactate dehydrogenase muscle isoform. EPO, erythropoietin. VEGF 1, vascular endothelial factor 1, a growth factor in angiogenesis. HPVR, hypoxic pulmonary vasoconstrictor response. HVR, hypoxic ventilatory response. The circled O_2 refers to O_2 sensors and signal transduction pathways leading to an inverse relationship between HIF 1 (alpha subunit) production and O_2 tension. Diagram based on various studies in the literature and modified from Hochachka et al. (1999). See chapter 3 for further discussion of O_2-sensitive genes.

and hypoxia-mediated increases in RBC mass in Andean natives are more robust than in Himalayans (Hochachka et al., 1996a). Given the length of time various high-altitude groups have been evolving separately, we would be surprised if some such differences were not found.

Hb O$_2$ Affinities Are Not Increased in Humans Indigenous to High Altitude

Most other vertebrates that tolerate extremes of high altitude display Hb homologs with increased O$_2$ affinities; as a result full saturation can be achieved at quite high altitudes (see discussion of mechanisms in chapter 3). In humans, as has been well known since the 1950s, Hb seems to be designed for "low-altitude" function because in all lineages it displays a monotonic decline in saturation with altitude (Winslow and Monge, 1987). Why this should be so has been perplexing to workers in this field, since intuitively it seemed reasonable that high-altitude humans would be selected for higher affinity Hb to facilitate O$_2$ saturation at altitude. A solution to this paradox may be proposed that arises from studies showing that the benefit of a left-shifted saturation curve is achieved only at unusually high altitudes at high work rates (Henderson et al., 2000). Since humans typically do not live above about 4500 m, there may have been little selective pressure for high-affinity Hb. At sea level or low altitudes, a left-shifted O$_2$ saturation curve is detrimental to O$_2$ unloading and leads to a decline in maximum whole body O$_2$ consumption rates. At intermediate altitudes, left shifting the O$_2$ saturation curve does not seem to have much effect on maximum aerobic metabolism. These results, along with the finding that high-altitude humans display low maximum O$_2$ consumption rates (Hochachka et al., 1991), help to explain why they have managed hypobaric hypoxia with essentially normal or lowlander types of Hb binding properties. However, as with HVR and developmental adaptations, there may be modest differences yet to be discovered in Hb O$_2$ affinity regulation between Sherpas, Quechuas, and other high-altitude natives. Given the length of time these

lineages have been evolving separately (see below), some differences in a few physiological characters are not unexpected and do not alter our impression of a high-altitude physiological phenotype based on numerous similar traits in Andean and Himalayan natives.

PHENOTYPES FOR HYPOXIA TOLERANCE AND FOR ENDURANCE PERFORMANCE

Low- and High-Capacity Forms of the Same Phenotype

Because of well-known and comparable effects of exercise and altitude, it is perhaps not surprising that most of the above *adjustable hypoxia response systems* (for convenience we will term them performance HRSs) are also found in humans adapted for endurance performance. One such similarity, already pointed out above, is the elevated preference for glucose by heart metabolism. Other common traits often include a blunted HVR and HPVR, expanded blood volume, altered expression of metabolic enzymes and metabolite transporters, fuel preference adjustments, enhanced ratio of aerobic/anaerobic contributions to exercise, and high ratios of slow-twitch/fast-twitch fibers in skeletal muscle (see Brooks, 1998; Brooks et al., 1996; Hochachka, 1999). Perhaps most telling of all is the similarly enhanced endurance found both in native highlanders (Matheson et al., 1991) and in endurance performers (Weston et al., 1999). An unusually high heart preference for glucose in fit lowlanders (J.E. Holden and P.W. Hochachka, unpublished data) means taking advantage of more ATP per O$_2$, as in Quechuas and Sherpas. This stoichiometric efficiency advantage is presumed to be the explanation for why the percent carbohydrate contribution to exercise energy demands gets higher and higher the closer to maximum the performance intensity comes, in both lowlanders (Brooks, 1998) and highlanders (Hochachka et al., 1991). In endurance athletes, who display much higher maximum aerobic capacities than do high-altitude natives, many of these series of traits appear as high-performance versions of those found in high-altitude natives, with up-regulation of heart-driven O_2 delivery and up-regulation of muscle mitochondrial volume density (of O_2 flux capacities at the working tissues) being perhaps the only serious (and largely inducible) modification to the physiological phenotype described above (Kayser et al., 1996; Saltin et al., 1995a,b).

The above comparative physiology is instructive. It indicates that the comparisons of lowlanders and highlanders under normoxia are qualitatively good descriptions of the difference between individuals who are well adapted for endurance versus those who are not (figure 5.2(E)). For example, low plasma [lactate] in exercise eliciting maximum aerobic metabolism is as characteristic of endurance performers as it is of highlanders. Or, to put it another way, the biochemical and physiological organization of both indigenous highlanders and individuals adapted for endurance performance are similar to each other, but both differ strikingly from the homologous organization in the "burst performance" phenotype. Similar contrasts emerge when East Africans (medium-altitude origins [Saltin et al., 1995a]) are compared to West Africans (lowland origins), where fast-twitch fibers form a much larger percentage of skeletal muscle (Ama et al., 1986). In the latter, exercise-induced lactate concentrations can reach very high levels, and cardiovascular adjustments play as important a role in recovery from performance as they do during performance per se (Brooks et al., 1996; Hochachka, 1994). Thus, the composite picture emerging (figure 5.6) is that of a single dominant physiological phenotype, termed for convenience the hypoxia tolerance/endurance performance phenotype, because it is at once advantageous in hypobaric hypoxia and during endurance exercise.

METABOLIC REGULATION IN ELITE ENDURANCE ATHLETES AND IN HIGH-ALTITUDE NATIVES

One of the best ways to summarize the functional properties of this phenotype is to examine the regulatory properties of energy metabolism during stresses such as exercise or hypoxia. As reviewed in our discussion on allometry (chapter 2), to evaluate the varied contributions to control of net flux, experimenters determine the fractional change in overall O_2 flux caused by a fractional change in flux through any given step or process; such fractions for different steps in the overall flux are termed control coefficients. Qualitatively, if the O_2 flux capacity of the lung, for example, is increased by 50% but only a 25% change in overall net O_2 flux is observed, the control coefficient for the lung is 0.5, equal to the fractional change in overall O_2 flux/fractional change in lung flux capacity. All the control coefficients in the pathway by definition add up to 1. In a system with a classical single rate-limiting step, say O_2 delivery, the control coefficient for that step would be essentially 1; that is, all control vested in this process.

For elite mammalian and human athletes under normoxic conditions, the control coefficients for various steps in the path of O_2 from lungs to mitochondria are in the following ranges: ventilation of alevoli (about 0.3); pulmonary diffusion (about 0.3), heart and circulation (about 0.25), and O_2 diffusion from capillaries to mitochondria (about 0.15) (see Jones, 1998; Sheel and McKenzie, 2000; Wagner, 2000). The problem with these kinds of respiratory studies is that they omit evaluation of various tissue ATPases, which in working muscle account for the bulk of ATP demand. Several recent studies (Korzeniewski, 2000; Korzeniewski and Mazat, 1996) recognize this defficiency and have identified that the control coefficient for actomyosin ATPase can be quite high. If the above control coefficients were expressed relative to ATP (or energy) turnover, rather than relative to global O_2 fluxes, and a 0.5 control coefficient is assumed for actomyosin ATPase, then the values are only half those given. An interesting study by Janeson et al. (2000) modeled working muscle as three key steps: energy supply as indexed by mitochondrial ATP synthesis and energy demand pathways as indexed by actomyosin ATPase and Ca^{2+} ATPase. They proposed that the control coefficients of the latter two ATP demand pathways fall towards zero at maximum aerobic

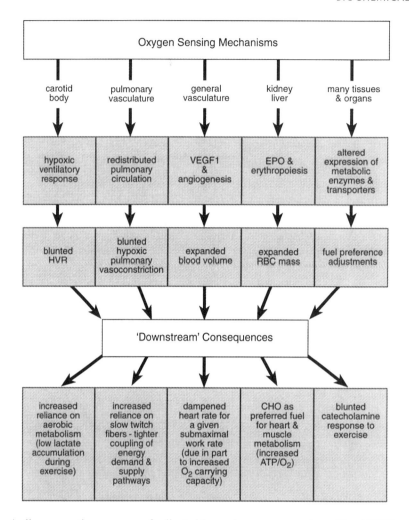

Figure 5.6. A diagrammatic summary of adjusted hypoxia response systems (the AHRS) proposed as the ancestral physiological phenotype and as a phylogenetic adaptation to hypobaric hypoxia. Summary based largely upon studies of Quechuas and Sherpas. Essentially all of the characteristics summarized here are also expressed in individuals well adapted for endurance performance. In the latter, the main modification involves an upwards regulation of mitochondrial volume densities at the working tissues (altered expression of mitochondrial metabolic enzymes and metabolite transporters above), which is why this is referred to as a "high-capacity" version of the lower capacity high-altitude phenotype. See text for further details. (Modified from Hochachka et al., 1999.)

work rates; if correct, energy supply pathways at maximum would be behaving almost like a single rate-limiting valve (with control coefficient rising towards 1). While qualitatively the trend may be correct, these workers failed to include anaerobic ATP production in their model. Why this is a problem is because the total ATP turnover rate under $\dot{V}O_2$max testing conditions is about 120% of that supported by

aerobic metabolism; the difference of course is made up by anaerobic glycogenolysis for which the control contribution of actomyosin ATPase again is very high (Thomas and Fell, 1998). What is more, if anaerobic burst work were to be imposed directly from rest, muscle actomyosin ATPases must be able to meet three- to tenfold higher total ATP turnover rates than occur under $\dot{V}O_2$max conditions (we pointed out in chapter 2 that the power input values of phosphagen and of glycogenolysis are ten-and threefold, respectively, higher than that supportable by $\dot{V}O_2max$). That means that actomyosin ATPase capacities must always exceed the mitochondrial ATP synthase capacities by huge factors. Given these conditions, and assuming for glycogenolysis an actomyosin control coefficient of about 0.5 (Thomas and Fell, 1998), more reasonable estimates of the contributions to control of the various steps in energy turnover at $\dot{V}O_2max$ in elite human athletes under normoxia can be summarized as follows: alveolar ventilation (~ 0.15), pulmonary diffusion (~ 0.15), heart and circulation (~ 0.15), aerobic cytosolic/mitochondrial metabolism (~ 0.1), anaerobic glycogenolysis (~ 0.1), actomyosin ATPase (~ 0.25), and all other energy demand pathways (~ 0.1). When acclimated to hypoxia, the control coefficients for the above O_2 delivery pathways are expected to decrease (because ventilation and circulatory O_2 delivery capacities are up-regulated, while global O_2 flux, indexed by $\dot{V}O_2max$, is down-regulated; hence fractional change of the latter/fractional change in O_2 delivery capacity must decrease). Simultaneously the control coefficients for the ATP demand pathways are expected to rise (remember that the sum of these control coefficients always is 1).

These values must be considered estimates based on studies of elite animal and human performers, but they give us a flavor of what to expect, and the question arises of how similar or different might be the control features of exercise energy turnover in native highlanders. Unfortunately, this question cannot be answered quantitatively. However, if we use normoxic lowlanders as the reference against which to compare highlanders, we can easily identify the direction in which the operational capacity of each step in energy turnover has been adjusted. Thus, in terms of such relative capacity for function, in high-altitude natives alveolar ventilation, pulmonary diffusing capacity, and circulatory O_2 delivery capacity are distinctly up-regulated. However, $\dot{V}O_2max$ in these subjects is notably down-regulated (see discussion above). Thus we can by definition, and with assurance, conclude that the control

coefficients of all of the above O_2 delivery steps will be depressed in Quechuas relative to normoxic lowlanders. On the other hand, mitochondrial ATP synthase capacities (mitochondrial volume densities), anaerobic glycolytic enzyme potentials, and muscle mass (hence total muscle actomyosin ATPase capacities) are distinctly down-regulated in Quechuas, generally in step with the decline in $\dot{V}O_2max$ and in glycolytic function (lactate production). Thus compared to the lung, heart, and circulation, their control coefficients are either similar or a bit higher than in normoxic lowlanders. According to Thomas and Fell (1998), stronger ADP control of actomyosin ATPase may underlie improved homeostasis of the adenylates and of glycolytic intermediates, including lactate; these mechanisms may also apply to improved adenylate homeostasis observed in endurance athletes and in high-altitude natives during muscle exercise (Matheson et al., 1991). So in terms of control and functional organization, the high-altitude and endurance performance phenotypes again show a general concordance.

A final key feature of these control systems should be mentioned; namely, that despite the complexity of energy supply and energy demand pathways, taken overall their function is remarkably integrated. Although, as emphasized, the exact values for control coefficients are difficult to evaluate and are dependent upon exercise conditions, it is striking how control is distributed right across all parts of the energy supply—energy demand system. (In fact the above control coefficients are given, despite uncertainty of their exact values, in order to emphasize this fundamental point.) This feature has led some workers in this area to conclude that, functionally, energy-supply–energy-demand pathways best fit models in which transition from rest to work requires simultaneous global activation of both supply and demand arms of the system, with the reverse occurring on transition from work to recovery conditions. Because of this behavior, Korzeniewski (2000) argues that the system is most accurately described as if it were a single functional unit, with all components being turned on or off at once, in differing metabolic states. Essentially the same concept was proposed by Hochachka and Matheson (1992) based on their work and other data available in the early 1990s.

The concept that the supply and demand pathways behave as a single functional unit also arises from allometric studies of the path of O_2 from air to mitochondria in a group of mammals varying in size by about three orders of magnitude. As expected, the absolute exercise and flux capacities were found to vary when comparing small to large animals; across this size spectrum, Taylor and Weibel and their coworkers found measurable adjustments and adaptations occurring at essentially every step linked in series in the functional chain from lungs to mitochondria. The concept of the entire chain being regulated as a single functional unit is thus implicit and explicit in this work (Weibel, 2000). Such convergence from different directions, from different kinds of studies, towards a remarkably similar concept is reassuring and an impressive far cry from the "single rate-limiting master valve" concept of metabolic regulation that dominated the earlier literature.

PHENOTYPIC PLASTICITY VERSUS GENETIC CONTRIBUTIONS TO VARIANCE

Always in these kinds of studies concern arises about what fractions of observed differences between different groups are due to phenotypic plasticity versus genetically based differences between the groups. The honest answer is that for complex physiologies no one knows for sure. Since the differences between acclimated and unacclimated (and trained vs untrained) individuals may be as great as the differences between genetically distinct individuals (and because acclimation responses themselves are genotype dependent), genetic versus environmental contributions to variations in these character traits are hard to quantify. In reality, most physiological studies are not properly designed to evaluate this issue, and much of the physiological literature ignores genotype, typically reporting no information at all on the genetics

of the subjects under study. Nevertheless, studies that have examined this issue (Fagard et al., 1991; Favier et al., 1996; Kirkpatrick, 1996; Moore et al., 1992; Strohl and Beal, 1996) usually find that genetic factors account for about 50% or more of the variance of these kinds of physiological systems. These values range from about 30% to 70% and the genetic contribution to variance of physiological systems includes phenotypic plasticity itself (things like trainability, hypoxia acclimation, and so forth). It is useful to remind physiologists that such estimates refer to genes affecting 50% or more of the *variance*, not the structural components, of physiological systems per se. Structural components—usually being gene products—are for practical purposes essentially 100% "genetic," which is a small but fundamental point often overlooked by physiologists (but not by pathophysiologists who well know the connection between genes and physiology). To add to our difficulties, in human evolutionary context, the percentage genetic contribution to variation in trait expression may not be the same in different lineages. The genetic contribution to variance in HVR, for example, varies in different lineages (higher in Tibetans than in Andean natives [Strohl and Beal, 1997] or Sherpas [Lahiri et al., 1969]). Given these complexities, workers in this field usually accept an arbitrary working assumption; namely, that, unless otherwise specified, the genetic contributions to the variance for physiological systems such as discussed here are similar to those already analyzed; that is, are in the 50% range. So the question arises of what genes or genotypes are actually involved in specifying the above performance HRSs.

SEARCHING FOR GENOTYPES FOR HYPOXIA-TOLERANT PHYSIOLOGICAL PHENOTYPES

With functional genomics representing a current growth industry in physiology, it is not surprising that serious interest is growing among exercise biologists in the issue of what genotypes correlate with the high altitude/

endurance performance phenotype. In consequence, several groups have recently tried to identify genetic markers of physiological phenotypes. If 50% of the variance in physiological traits is due to genetic differences, on first glance it would appear to be a simple matter to find specific alleles for the high-altitude/endurance performance phenotype. A brief review of recent analyses, however, indicates that this is not the case.

The Case for ACE

A provocative recent example is the gene for ACE (angiotensin-converting enzyme). This gene occurs in two allelic forms, termed insertion (I) or deletion (D), depending upon the presence or absence of a 287 base fragment in intron 16. ACE may affect cardiovascular coupling to exercise through formation of angiotensin II, a potent vasoconstrictor, through consequent inactivation of the vasodilator, bradykinin, and indirectly through angiotensin-mediated trophic effects on heart tissue. The D allele is associated with elevated ACE levels in serum and heart, conditions considered to predispose to hypertension, to pathological left ventricular hypertrophy, and to arteriosclerosis. The I allele in contrast correlates with lower systemic and heart ACE activity, with lower cardiac afterload, and perhaps with lesser predisposition to heart disease. A provocative publication by Montgomery et al. (1997) reported that the I allele was over-represented in a group of 33 elite British mountaineers, all of whom had been to altitudes of at least 7,000 m. In a subset of these climbers, a group who ascended to 8,000 m or higher, no individuals were homozygous for the deletion allele. The insertion (I) allele thus was reported as a "gene for human performance," and the observation seemed supported by a follow-up study a year later, when Gayagay et al. (1998) reported a similar over representation of the I allele in 64 elite rowers. These interesting findings encouraged a similar study of ACE alleles in high altitude Andean natives. These data showed (Rupert et al., 1999a) that the insertion (I) allele occurred at about twice the frequency found in

lowland Caucasians, but at about the same frequency (75–80%) as in other Amerindians. Whereas these data are consistent with anecdotal reports of reduced level of heart disease in these groups, the suggestion that ACE I is a genetic marker of (or that an II-homozygote represents a genotypic correlation with) the high-altitude physiological phenotype is made less compelling by the finding of overexpression in low-altitude Amerindians as well as in Quechuas. In none of these studies, however, were subjects selected on endurance exercise criteria; thus to this point ACE potentially remained a gene for human performance. When huge population-based studies were completed, however, no correlations between ACE alleles and any of several performance physiological characters could be found (Rankinen et al., 2000). Thus its consistent over-expression in the above mentioned studies of athletes either represents an artifact of small sample size, or in these groups the I gene may be functionally linked to some other functionally important allele that actually confers the observed physiological advantages to I-ACE allele. One possibility suggested to us by J. Rupert is that high-altitude performance may well be influenced by susceptibility to high-altitude pulmonary edema (HAPE) or high-altitude cerebral edema (HACE). The allele distributions observed by Montgomery et al. (1997) may then be founded on I-ACE correlating with HACE. Clearly more work will be required before the conflicting information in this field can be rationalized.

The Case for HIF 1 and EPO Alleles for Performance

The point of departure for another search for a genetic marker of the hypoxia physiology of high-altitude natives was the observation that native highlanders, especially the Quechuas and other natives of the Andes, gradually develop very high red blood cell (RBC) mass. Usually reported as %RBC, hematocrit values beyond the 60% range (even higher in persons sustaining Monge's disease) are not uncommon. The first step in the control system for this erythropoietic response (see figure 5.5 and discussion in chapter 3) is an O_2-sensing system located in cells in the kidney (major site) and liver (minor site). Signal transduction from this sensing step involves a transcription factor (hypoxia inducible factor 1, or HIF 1). HIF 1 is a dimer formed of α and β subunits; under hypoxic conditions (see Dang and Semenza [1999] for literature in this area), the expression of HIF 1α is increased in inverse proportion to oxygen availability. HIF 1 then has several downstream targets (genes for glycolytic enzymes, for glucose transporter, for vasculogenesis, as well as erythryopoiesis (figure 5.5).

Probably because the promoter and enhancer binding sites for HIF 1 were first worked out in studies of erythropoietin (EPO) production, the information pathway from hypoxic signal, to HIF 1 production, to HIF 1-mediated activation of EPO gene expression, and so to increased EPO production is frequently termed "the universal O_2 sensing pathway" in mammals. Since many physiological studies indicate that the hypoxia-mediated expression of this pathway is lineage specific, it was reasoned that the HIF 1 gene might be one of the genetic markers that so interested this field of research. Accordingly, a Quechua-derived cell line was used as a source of DNA and the HIF 1α and EPO genes. Although these studies have to be expanded, to this point this universal O_2-sensing system in Quechuas is seemingly 100% conserved (HIF 1α and EPO gene sequences being identical to already published Caucasian gene sequences [J. L. Rupert and P.W. Hochachka, unpublished data]). Thus it is hard to avoid the conclusion from this HIF 1 study that lineage specificity of the EPO response to hypoxia does not derive from genetic differences in the HIF 1α part of the above universal O_2-sensing pathway.

Role of β-Fibrinogen Alleles

The starting point for another study of this type again was the observation of high hematocrits in Quechuas. It is usually assumed that this response is advantageous because it increases the oxygen carrying capacity of blood.

Experimentally, this advantage in fact can be demonstrated, so the explanation is rather widely accepted. Nevertheless, the cost of this advantage is increased blood viscosity and this has always been disturbing to workers in this field. At least a partial answer to resolving this paradox is that plasma proteins, especially fibrinogens, also affect blood viscosity (through direct effects and through RBC aggregation). Elevated fibrinogen concentrations may be a risk factor in coronary and peripheral artery disease and several polymorphisms in the β-fibrinogen gene are known that affect fibrinogen concentrations. Studies by Rupert et al., 1999b found fibrinogen alleles that are associated with increased fibrinogen levels to be under-represented in Quechuas compared to two different lowland lineages (Caucasians and North American natives). These alleles could be termed "genes for the high-altitude physiological phenotype"; however, at this time there is no firm proof that they arose under directional selection for hypoxia tolerance. Hence, these data also are not as compelling as one might like.

Why Finding Alleles for Adaptive Physiological Characters Is So Difficult

Except for clear-cut cases usually of disease (such as sickle cell anemia), where a specific allele can be identified to underlie a specific phenotype, studies in this arena are often notably limited in their range. Usually for simple pragmatic reasons, the goal is not to define the genotype per se underlying the phenotype, but to find a gene marker accurately correlating with the observed phenotype. The problem is that, in contrast to a single gene marker, the physiological phenotype of interest is the product of hundreds (if not thousands) of genes and searching for the actual genes for a specific physiology (rather than a gene marker) is a much more daunting task. A variance of only a few percent in any given gene locus, when summated over hundreds of genes could add up to a large percent genetic contribution to overall variance of the integrated physiological system.

Studies of obesity along these lines are instructive. Like in the hypoxia field, researchers focusing on obesity would like to know the genetic correlates of the phenotype. As of 1997, so many genes were involved that the genotype was mapping to regions on at least 23 chromosomes; actual numbers of genes are not yet known, but clearly will be quite high (Chagnon et al., 1997). As there is no reason to expect anything much simpler in the physiology of hypoxia tolerance, it is clear that this quest in our field still has a long way to go. This should not be surprising because of the close genetic similarities of all human groups. Even in human versus chimp interspecies comparisons, to date, no one has been able to answer the question of which genes make us human (see commentary by Normille, 2001). So for now, not knowing the genotype underlying human hypoxia tolerance physiology and thus being forced to work with the physiological phenotype, should not dishearten us.

PHYLOGENETIC ORIGINS OF HUMAN HYPOXIA TOLERANCE

A Phylogeneic Tree for the Human Species

Assuming that the HRS features described above constitute the primary "solutions" of our species to "problems/requirements" of hypobaric hypoxia and/or endurance performance, the question remains of when these physiological phenotypes arose in our species' history. To explore this issue requires insight into the evolutionary pathways of our species. To this end, the above physiological analyses relied upon a simplified "phylogenetic tree" for the human species (figure 5.7) from a summary of human genetics and evolution by Cavalli-Sforza et al. (1994). The main groups whose physiological responses to hypobaric hypoxia to date have been extensively studied are shown in figure 5.7. At the outset it should be acknowledged that the age of our species is not known exactly. For the present purposes, we can assume approximately 100,000 years

(this is controversial, with some estimates based on fossil, not molecular, evidence being up to tenfold older; but if our species is older, the arguments below will be stronger). Several insights arise. First, figure 5.7 suggests that the last time Caucasians shared common ancestry with Sherpas and Quechuas was over half the age of our species. Second, the last time the Himalayan highlanders (Sherpas and Tibetans) and the Andean highlanders (Quechuas and Aymaras) shared common ancestors was equivalent to about one-third of our species history. Third, divergence times between these groups and East Africans from medium-altitude environments are even greater. Even if many details of human phylogeny remain unsettled and figure 5.7 is overly simplified, there is no doubt about our main conclusion that the lengths of separation of the Andean, the Himalayan, and the East African lineages represent large fractions of our species' history. Despite such phylogenetically deep divergences, the latter three express many similar metabolic and physiological responses to hypobaric hypoxia. Fourth, in numerous other lineages (intermediate branches in our phylogeny) the HRS features when present often are "high-performance" versions of the high-altitude phenotype. These provocative phylogenetic data are consistent with two possible interpretations.

The Convergence Hypothesis

One plausible model is that, with only modest differences, similar metabolic and physiological "solutions" arose independently by directional natural selection in the two high-altitude (Andean and Himalayan) lineages for which we have the most data and possibly in a third east African lineage for which the data are not as extensive. If so, such convergence (same characters arising independently in different lineages) would satisfy at least one of the criteria of evolutionary biology and would indicate that the above suite of physiological characters are defense adaptations against hypobaric hypoxia and arose by natural selection. Whereas this was our thinking initially (see

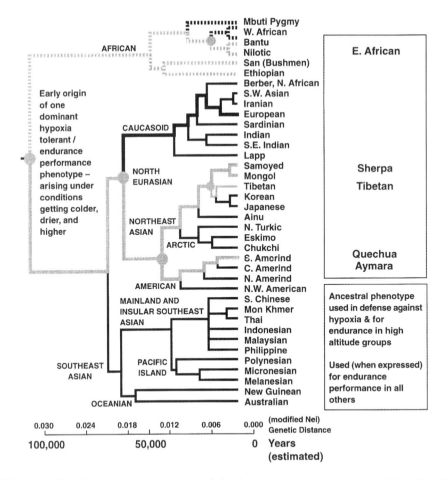

Figure 5.7. An abbreviated phylogenetic tree of the human species as summarized by Cavalli-Sforza et al. (1994) with an estimated species age of 100,000 years included as a time frame. As discussed in the text, the model proposed assumes one dominant phenotype arising early in our species history, selected simultaneously for endurance performance and hypobaric hypoxia. It is postulated that this phenotype, expressed with high frequency in high-altitude natives, is used in two settings: in defense against hypobaric hypoxia and in situations selecting for endurance. In lowland groups, when expressed, this phenotype is typical of endurance athletes and is very familiar to exercise biologists. The age estimate of our species is unsettled, but the actual age is not critical to the argument presented. The main high-altitude groups for which detailed physiological and metabolic studies are available are shown on the right. The pathways tracing each of these lineages back in time are shown in thick gray lines. Dashed lines are used for African lineages, for which many fewer data are available. Many of the reference lowlander data used in our analysis come from studies of Caucasians (thick black line traces this lineage). Solid circles identify nodes from which different lineages diverged: Sherpas versus Tibetans; Andean versus Himalayan natives; Caucasians versus Sherpas and Quechuas; West African versus East African; and African lineages versus other lineages. Such phylogenetic information shows that the last time Caucasians shared common ancestors with Sherpas and Quechuas was about half the age of our species. Similarily, Sherpas and Tibetans last shared ancestors with Quechuas and Aymara a very long time ago, about one-third the age of our species. When East Africans are considered, common ancestry with Himalayan and Andean lineages goes even a longer way back in phylogeny. The conclusion of distant divergences for these groups would be unaffected by uncertainties, which certainly exist, about details in human phylogeny. Despite such distant divergences, all five high-altitude groups (Quechua, Aymara, Sherpa, Tibetan, and East African) show numerous similarities in physiological hypoxia defense mechanisms. See text for further details. (Modified from Hochachka et al. 1999.)

discussion in Hochachka et al., 1998), the phylogenetic observations are not easily incorporated into this interpretation.

The Common Descent Hypothesis

An alternative view—hypothesis (ii)—is that the above suite of physiological and metabolic traits, the performance HRSs, while arising by directional natural selection, represents the "ancestral" condition, which would be consistent with evidence suggesting that the origin of our species occurred under conditions that were getting colder, drier, and higher. As emphasized elsewhere (Cavalli-Sforza et al., 1994; Hochachka, 1998), key environmental influences on the root of our phylogeny, on the origins of our species, go back a long way. During early phases, hominid evolution in the East African Rift was occurring under conditions of mild altitude hypoxia—ideal from a training point of view—aggravated by drier and colder climates. These conditions, where the performance HRSs would be advantageous, prevailed for the ancestors of our species, they prevailed at the origins of our species, and they prevail in parts of East Africa today. According to this model, over some 5,000 or more generations of our species history, the ancestral condition was "retained" in a down-regulated form in high-altitude groups and was "retained" in an up-regulated higher-capacity form (probably in many) groups selected for endurance performance (including Kenyan highlanders, who continue to thrive on the same plateau that served as the colder, drier, and higher place of our species' beginnings). The fact that most lineages have a significant proportion of endurance type phenotypes indicates that the ancestral condition was "retained" in many intermediate lineages in our species. In situations such as the moderate hypobaric hypoxia of East Africa, selection pressures for both hypoxia tolerance and endurance performance may well have been applied simultaneously (practical interests have provoked new detailed analysis of the interaction between endurance performance and hypobaric hypoxia [Levine and Stray-Gunderson, 1996; Weston et al., 1999]).

The Hypothesis of Common Descent with Deeper Phylogenetic Roots

A third interpretation of these data—hypothesis (iii)—considers that hypothesis (ii) is fine as far as it goes, but it may not go far enough. Hypothesis (iii) posits that many, probably most, of the physiological characters under discussion arose well before our species did. Actually, this possibility is clearly implicit in hypothesis (ii), which only refers explicitly to the hypoxia tolerance/endurance performance phenotype as having arisen by the time our species was getting started. In essence hypothesis (ii) stops where the data stop, while hypothesis (iii) extends the picture deeper into our phylogenetic past. Given that the geological conditions favoring this phenotype go back 3–4 million years into the past, it is certainly possible that much of the selection and differentiation into the hypoxia tolerance/endurance performance phenotype occurred before *Homo sapiens* arose. To this point, the two views are entirely similar. However, hypothesis (iii) additionally argues that the subsequent 5,000 or so generation of human evolution led to further directional selection in specific cases. For example, this hypothesis (Hochachka et al., 1999) considers that the high-performance versions of the ancestral phenotype (well expressed in present day, fleet-footed East Africans [Saltin et al., 1955a,b]) arose by directional selection and for this reason now differ from the low capacity highlander phenotypes (represented by Quechuas and Sherpas). We can accommodate this view, but tend to prefer hypothesis (ii) on the basis of currently available information. For example, based on present data, it appears that the main metabolic differences between native highlanders and endurance performers (even elite ones like East African runners) is in O_2 flux capacities to the working muscles. This feature could arise from adaptations at the level of the heart, for delivery of O_2 and fuels to the sites of utilization (Hochachka et al., 1996a,b) or at the level of skeletal muscles (Weston et al., 1999). Meanwhile, most of the other performance HRSs and their downstream effects appear to be more similar than different between the different groups. That is why, at least until more comparative and detailed data on hypoxia responses in endurance versus power performers in high-altitude groups, in specific African groups, and in lowlanders become available, hypothesis (ii) remains the preferred model of one phenotype arising at about the time of our species' origin. The model assumes one physiological phenotype for at least two different biological jobs: for function in hypobaric hypoxia and for endurance performance. In effect, hypothesis (ii) above predicts that the ancestral organization of our physiology was inherently very dependent upon efficient physiological O_2 delivery systems and upon "aerobic" metabolic pathways and fiber types, with relatively lesser development of, or reliance on, anaerobic metabolic systems to sustain short, intense bursts of whole body exercise.

If correct, then (in terms of the original framework for evaluating the evolution of complex physiological systems) hypothesis (ii) implies that much is determined by so called initial or ancestral conditions. Much of the evolution of metabolic and physiological systems seems to involve stabilizing or negative selection (pruning out genotypes in which the ancestral "models" are altered). Only a part of the evolution of our physiology seems to be the result of positive or directional selection for new functional capacities and fundamentally new physiological characters—the performance HRSs described above and some parallel developmental adaptations. Finally, it is satisfying to note the similarities in these interpretations of the evolution of a complex physiological system within the hominids to the picture obtained in an analysis of the diving response in pinnipeds; in one case, we are dealing mainly with, at most, a few hominid species evolving for 3–4 million years, while in the latter case, we are dealing with some 30 species whose phylogeny extends back about 20 million years (Mottishaw et al., 1999).

These studies raise the same two problems for modern molecular evolution theory that we have already encountered in the chapter 4 discussion of the evolution of the diving response—how to account for conservative and for adaptable traits in the evolution of complex physiological systems.

CAN MOLECULAR EVOLUTION MODELS EXPLAIN ADAPTABLE TRAITS IN HUMAN HYPOXIA TOLERANCE?

A Repeat Theme: The Three Factors Determining Rates of Evolutionary Change

We already know from chapter 4 that most evolutionary biologists today assume that the response to selection depends on (i) the amount of phenotypic variation upon which selection can operate, (ii) the percent variation that is heritable, and (iii) the intensity of selection. As mentioned above, most physiological studies are not designed for teasing out the values of these parameters. However, for physiological and metabolic systems in humans which have been studied quantitatively, the coefficient of variation is often well above 10%; heritabilities vary a lot, but a range of between about 0.3 and 0.7 is reported by physiological studies using family inheritance patterns or monozygotic versus dizyotic twins to quantify genetic contributions to variance in physiologcal traits; and selection coefficients as high as 0.43 are known.

Given these values, evolutionary biologists calculate that positive selection can produce evolutionary rates in excess of 1% change in the mean value for a trait per generation. As our species history goes back at least 100,000 years (early hominid phylogeny, when much of our basic physiological phenotype was being formed, goes back even further, to 3–4 million years ago), it is not hard to conclude that the observed patterns of hypoxia tolerance within the extant lineages of our human family can be easily accomodated by current evolutionary theory. Of course as in the evolution of the diving response in pinnipeds, there remains a caveat; namely, that these kinds of calculations are almost always focused onto a single trait. For situations where the evolution of two or more systems must be coordinated (as in the performance HRSs above) the probability and mechanisms of such coevolution remain obscure. Nonetheless, as before, in a general sense, the answer to the question posed appears affirmative.

CAN MOLECULAR EVOLUTION MODELS EXPLAIN CONSERVED TRAITS IN HUMAN PHYLOGENY?

The Complexity of Conserved Systems Revisited

We should not now be surprised that when considering this second issue—can conserved traits such as brain metabolic organization or such as the pathways of cardiovascular or ventilatory control be explained by modern molecular evolution theory—the answer is not so obvious. Again, for perspective, we first must remind the reader of the enormous complexity of the physiological systems involved. A hint of this arose in our earlier analysis of a number of major sensing, signal transduction, and effector pathways involved in cardiovascular control in diving animals; this control system is equally well conserved in human evolution. At the molecular level of course each arm of this enormously complex regulatory system is composed of up to 100 already identified gene products; from each protein linked in a highly precise manner with others in the pathway emerges the coordinated (and evolutionarily conserved) physiological function of cardiovascular control. In the case of the CNS, well over 200 currently known gene products are involved in pathways of ATP demand and ATP supply, in sensing, signal transduction, and regulation, and in structural integration. Conserving the emergent physiologies formed from the expression of linked function of many gene products means conserving the structure and function of gene products; that is, it means deleting most mutations which arise—this is negative or stabilizing selection. To estimate how much negative or stabilizing selection is required to keep such systems from randomly changing through phylogenetic time we again need to have an estimate of the selective cost of substitutions in each of the gene products in such integrated sequences, and since these values are unavailable for the CNS metabolic systems under discussion, we will again resort to the rRNA example.

Recalling the Magnitude of Selection Coefficients for Weak Bond Stabilization of Macromolecular Structure

Recall that the secondary structures of rRNAs are stabilized by many hydrogen-bonded pairs of nucleotides, with stability of bonding being dependent upon the actual nucleotide pairs utilized and on their neighbors (Golding, 1994). Instead of seeing any base pair at any one site in the secondary structure among the 51 species (as would be observed if there was no negative selection), in most species most sites in rRNA are restricted to pairs that form strong hydrogen bonds and some sites are more conserved (are selected more strongly) than others.

For estimating the selection coefficient for each hydrogen-bonded pair in the secondary structure of the rRNA molecule, a composite parameter, $4Ns$, was calculated, where N is the effective population size and s is the selective advantage of hydrogen bonding at a site. In the previous chapter we pointed out that $4Ns = 6.3$ was sufficiently large to account for complete conservation of hydrogen bonding at a site; that is, for all 51 taxa to have a hydrogen-bonded base pair at a site. Assuming a reasonable value for N (say 16,000), then a value of $s = 0.0001$ is large enough to maintain a specific site in a sequence over long phylogenetic time periods. This means that on average a 0.01% advantage is adequate to assure 100% conservation of a given site in rRNA; a 1% advantage would be consistent with the conservation of about 100 such sites.

In analyzing the diving response, we considered these to be instructive calculations because similar structural constraints (requiring the conservation of weak bonding interactions at specific sites) are the "rules of thumb" that apply pretty well across the board for all gene products since from mRNA onwards their functions almost ubiquitously depend upon weak bonding interactions. Such natural-selection-based conservation of structure, or of specific sites in specific sequences, is the basis of maintained functional specificity of macromolecules through evolutionary time and in principle should be applicable to the conservation of specific physiological systems in human hypoxia tolerance.

Selection Pressure Required for Stabilizing Pathways of ATP Supply and Demand in the Brain

If we assume that similar selection pressures operate on the proteins in these pathways as in conserving rRNA sequences, we can estimate s for simple multiple-component pathways (such as glucose transporter function coupled to glucose–glycogen conversion to pyruvate, a pathway involving about 15 proteins and at least that many genes). Such calculations lead to the conclusion that about a 1.5% selective advantage is adequate to assure that 10 sites in each of the 15 proteins in such a pathway in brain metabolism will be conserved (many metabolic enzymes are formed of more than one subunit and are highly conserved; hence, for this example the actual numbers of genes involved and the numbers of conserved sites per gene are substantially higher; in this event of course the overall selective advantage would have to be proportionally higher than 1.5%).

Something May Be Missing in Our Understanding of Stabilizing Selection in Evolution of Human Metabolic Physiology

At first glance, this analysis suggests that modern molecular evolutionary concepts should be able to accommodate the conservation of complex (multigene dependent) physiological systems, but unfortunately, the same problems arise as before. First, there is the practical problem of this being experimentally intractable— the accuracy of physiological measurements is usually in the 5–10% range. In most studies, a 1.5% advantage would be undetectable, which is one reason we have already seen why physiologists should turn to evolutionary studies with caution (Mangum and Hochachka, 1998). Secondly, a serious theoretical problem seems to arise because the above illustrative estimates apply to only one pathway. In contrast, human hypoxia defense mechanisms involve many such highly conserved pathways. In CNS energy supply plus energy demand pathways plus their associated controls and structures, it is easy to demonstrate over 200 genes, not the 15 or so

selected above for illustrative purposes for a simple metabolic pathway. Similarily, Iyer et al. (1999) unexpectedly found that the physiology of wound healing involves over 500 genes whose closely controlled activities rise or fall by at least two or more fold during cell activation. As in the case of genes for ATP utilization and ATP supply pathways in the CNS, the conservation of these 500+ genes for such a huge transcriptional program through long phylogenetic time in principle presents the need for equally huge stabilizing selective pressures. As before, even if we are cautious about how far we should press such analyses, it seems quite clear that as the numbers of gene products required for given physiological systems increase toward hundreds or even thousands, the strength of selection required to conserve them unchanged (to conserve the complex physiological system unchanged) through evolutionary time may rise without limit. This less than satisfying relationship suggests that the problem of conserving complex physiological systems through human phylogeny may be more difficult to achieve than the appearance of so-called "adaptable" physiological traits, which traditionally would be considered pivotal for extending tolerance of, and performance in, hypobaric hypoxia. Whereas evolutionary literature (see Ridley, 1993) has addressed this problem in general terms (with mathematical modeling) to our knowledge the selective forces required to stabilize complex physiological systems composed of hundreds or even thousands of well-defined gene products so far have never been quantified, or for that matter, even seriously addressed—a conclusion that should make young graduate students happy, since it is an obvious area still requiring a lot of research.

REFERENCES

Ama, P.M.H., J.A. Simoneau, M.R. Boulay, C.W. Serresse, G. Theriault, and C. Bouchard (1986). Skeletal muscle characteristics in sedentary Black and Caucasian males. *J. Appl. Physiol.* 61: 1758–1761.

Antenzana, A.M., J.P. Richalet, G. Antenzana, H. Spielvogel, and R. Kacini (1992). Adrenergic system in high altitude residents. *Intl. J. Sports Med.* 13: S92–S95.

Antenzana, A.M., J.P. Richalet, I. Noriega, M. Galarza, and G. Antenzana (1995). Hormonal changes in normal and polycythemic high-altitude residents. *J. Appl. Physiol.* 79: 795–800.

Brooks, G.A. (1998). Mammalian fuel preferences during exercise. *Comp. Biochem. Physiol.* 120, 89–107.

Brooks, G.A., G.E. Butterfield, R.R. Wolfe, B.M. Groves, R.S. Mazzeo, J.R. Sutton, E.E. Wolfel, and J.T. Reeves (1991). Increased dependence on blood glucose after acclimatization to 4,300m. *J. Appl. Physiol.* 70: 919–927.

Brooks, G.A., T.D. Fahey, and T.P. White (1996). *Exercise Physiology—Human Bioenergetics and Its Applications.* London: Mayfield Publishing.

Bunn, H.F., and R.O. Poyton (1996). Oxygen sensing and molecular adaptation to hypoxia. *Physiol. Rev.* 76: 839–885.

Cavalli-Sforza, L., P. Menozzi and A. Piazza (1994). *The History and Geography of Human Genes.* Princeton, N.J.: Princeton University Press.

Chagnon, Y.C., L. Perusse, and C. Bouchard (1997). The human obesity gene map: the 1997 update. *Obesity Res.* 6: 76– 92.

Dang, C.V., and G.L. Semenza (1999). Oncogenic alterations of metabolism. *Trends Biochem. Sci.* 24: 68–72.

Fagard, R., E. Bielen, and A. Amery (1991). Heritability of aerobic power and anaerobic energy generation during exercise. *J. Appl. Physiol.* 70: 357–362.

Favier, R., D. Desplanches, H. Hoppeler, E. Caceres, A. Grunefelder, H. Koubi, M. Leuenberger, B. Sempore, L. Tuscher, and H. Spielvogel (1996). Hormonal and metabolic adjustments during exercise in hypoxia and normoxia in highland natives. *J. Appl. Physiol.* 80: 632–637.

Forsythe, J. S., B.H. Hang, N.V. Iyer, F. Agani, S.W. Leung, R.D. Koos, and G.L. Semenza (1996). Activation of vascular endothelial growth factor gene transcription by hypoxia-inducible factor 1. *Mol. Cell. Biol.* 16: 4604–4613.

Gayagay, G., B.Yu, B.Hambly, T. Boston, A. Hahn, D.S. Celermajor, and R.J. Trent (1998). Elite endurance athletes and the ACE I allele—the role of genes in athletic performance. *Human Genet.* 103: 48–50.

Golding, G.B. (1994). In: *Non-neutral evolution— Theories and Molecular Data*, pp. 126–138, ed. G.B. Golding, London: Chapman and Hall.

Green, H.J., B. Roy, S. Grant, R. Hughson, M. Burnett, C. Otto, A. Pipe, D. McKenzie, and M.

Johnson (2000). Increases in submaximal cycling efficiency mediated by altitude acclimatization. *J. Appl. Physiol.* 1189–1197.

Harik, N., S.I. Harik, N.T. Kuo, K. Sakai, R.J. Przybylski, and J.C. La Manna (1996). Time-course and reversibility of the hypoxia induced alterations in cerebral vascularity and cerebral capillary glucose transporter density. *Brain Res.* 737: 335–338.

Heath, D., and D.R. Williams (1981). *Man at High Altitude.* London: Churchill Livingstone,

Henderson, K.K., W. McCanse, T. Urano, I. Kuwahira, R. Clancy, and N.C. Gonzalez (2000). Acute vs. chronic effects of elevated hemoglobin O_2 affinity on O_2 transport in maximal exercise. *J. Appl. Physiol.* 89: 265–272.

Hochachka, P.W. (1988). The lactate paradox: Analysis of underlying mechanisms. *Ann. Sports Med.* 4: 184–188.

Hochachka, P.W. (1992). Muscle enzymatic composition and metabolic regulation in high altitude adapted natives. *Int. J. Sport Med.* 13: S89–S91

Hochachka, P.W. (1994). *Muscles as Molecular and Metabolic Machines.* Boca Raton, Fla.: CRC Press.

Hochachka, P.W. (1998). Mechanism and evolution of hypoxia-tolerance in humans. *J. Exp. Biol.* 201: 1243–1254.

Hochachka, P.W. (2000). Pinniped diving response mechanism and evolution: A window on the paradigm of comparative biochemistry and physiology. *Comp. Physiol. and Biochem.* 126A: 435–458.

Hochachka P.W., and G.O. Matheson (1992). Regulating ATP turnover rates over broad dynamic work ranges in skeletal muscles. *J. Appl. Physiol.* 73: 1697–1703.

Hochachka, P.W., and G.N. Somero (1984). *Biochemical Adaptation.* Princeton, N.J.: Princeton University Press.

Hochachka, P.W., C. Stanley, G.O. Matheson, D.C. McKenzie, P.S. Allen, and W.S. Parkhouse (1991). Metabolic and work efficiencies during exercise in Andean natives. *J. Appl. Physiol.* 70: 1720–1729.

Hochachka, P.W., C. Stanley, D.C. McKenzie, A. Villena, and C. Monge (1992). Enzyme mechanisms for pyruvate-to-lactate flux attentuation: A study of Sherpas, Quechuas, and hummnigbirds. *Int. J. Sport Med.* 13: S119–S123.

Hochachka, P.W., C.M. Clark, W.D. Brown, C. Stanley, C.K. Stone, R.J. Nickels, G.G. Zhu, P.S. Allen, and J.E. Holden (1995). The brain at high altitude: Hypometabolism as a defense against chronic hypoxia? *J. Cerebral Bl. Flow Metabol.* 4: 671–679.

Hochachka, P.W., C.M. Clark, J.E. Holden, C. Stanley, K. Ugurbil, and R.S. Menon (1996a). 31P Magnetic resonance spectroscopy of the Sherpa heart: A PCr/ATP signature of metabolic defense against hypobaric hypoxia. *Proc. Natl. Acad. Sci. USA* 93: 1215–1220.

Hochachka, P.W., C.M. Clark, C. Monge, C. Stanley, W.D. Brown, C.K. Stone, R.J. Nickels, and J.E. Holden. (1996b). Sherpa brain glucose metabolism and defense adaptations against chronic hypoxia. *J. Appl. Physiol.* 81: 1355–1361.

Hochachka, P.W., H.C. Gunga, and K. Kirsch (1998). Our ancestral physiological phenotype: An adaptation for hypoxia tolerance and for endurance performance? *Proc. Natl. Acad. Sci. USA* 95: 1915–1921.

Hochachka, P.W., J.L. Rupert and C. Monge (1999). Adaptation and conservation of physiological systems in the evolution of human hypoxia tolerance. *Comp. Biochem. Physiol.* 120A: 1–17.

Holden, J. E., C. Stone, W.D. Brown, R.J. Nickels, C. Stanley, C.M. Clark, and P.W. Hochachka (1995). Enhanced cardiac metabolism of plasma glucose in high altitude natives: Adaptations against chronic hypoxia. *J. Appl. Physiol.* 79: 222–228.

Iyer, V.R., M.B. Eisen, D.T. Ross, G. Schuler, T. Moore, J.C.F. Lee, J.M. Trent, L.M.Staudt, J. Hudson Jr., M.S. Boguski, D. Lashkari, D. Shalon, D. Botstein, and P.O. Brown (1999). The transcription program in the respons of human fibroblasts to serum. *Science* 283: 83–87.

Janeson, J.A., H.V. Westerhoff, and M.J. Kushmenick (2000). A metabolic control analysis of kinetic controls in ATP free energy metabolism in contracting skeletal muscle. *Amer. J. Physiol.* 279: C813–C832.

Jones, J.H. (1998). Optimization of the mammalian respiratory system: Symmorphosis versus simple species adaptation. *Comp. Physiol. Biochem.* 120B: 125–138.

Kayser, B., H. Hoppler, H. Classen, and P. Cerretelli (1991). Muscle structure and performance in Himalayan Sherpas. *J. Appl. Physiol.* 70: 1938–1942.

Kayser, B., H. Hoppeler, D. Desplanches, C. Marconi, B. Broers, and P. Cerretelli (1996). Muscle ultrastructure and biochemistry in lowland Tibetans. *J. Appl. Physiol.* 80: 632–637.

Kirkpatrick, M. (1996). Genes and adaptation: A pocket guide to the theory. In: *Adaptation*, pp.125–146, eds. M.R. Rose and G.V. Lauder, San Diego: Academic Press.

Korzeniewski, B. (2000). Regulation of ATP supply in mammalian skeletal muscle during resting state → intensive work transition. *Biophys. Chem.* 83: 19–34.

Korzeniewski, B., and J.P. Mazat (1996). Theoretical studies on control of oxidative phosphorylation in muscle mitochondria at different energy demands and oxygen concentrations. *Acta Biotheoretica* 44: 263–269.

Ladoux, A., and C. Felin (1993). Hypoxia is a strong inducer of vascular endothelial growth factor mRNA expression in the heart. *Biochem. Biophys. Res. Commun.* 195: 1005–1010.

Lahiri, S. (1996). Peripheral chemoreceptors and their sensory neurons in chronic states of hypo- and hyperoxygenation. *Handbk Physiol.* 2: 1183–1206.

Lahiri, S., N.H. Edelman, N.S. Cherniak, and A.P. Fishman (1969). Blunted hypoxic drive to ventilation in subjects with life-long hypoxemia. *Fed. Proc.* 28: 1289–1295.

Levine, R. D., and J. Stray-Gunderson (1996). A practical approach to altitude training: Where to live and train for optimal performance enhancement. *J. Appl. Physiol.* 13: S209–S212.

Mangum, C. P., and P.W. Hochachka (1998). New directions in comparative physiology and biochemistry: Mechanisms, adaptations, and evolution. *Physiol. Zool.* 71: 471–484.

Matheson, G.O., P.S. Allen, D.C. Ellinger, C.C. Hanstock, D. Gheorghiu, D.C. McKenzie, C. Stanley, W.S. Parkhouse, and P.W. Hochachka (1991). Skeletal muscle metabolism and work capacity: a ^{31}P-NMR study of Andean natives and lowlanders. *J. Appl. Physiol.* 70: 1963–1976.

Matsubayashi, K., T. Ozawa, M. Nakashima, A. Saito, H. Fukuyama, N. Harada, and M. Kameyama (1986). Cerebral blood flow and metabolism before and after staying at high altitude. *J. Mountain Med.* 6: 51–57.

Maxwell, P. H., C.W. Pugh and P.J. Ratcliffe (1993). Inducible operation of the erythropoitin 3′ enhancer in multiple cell lines: Evidence for a widespread oxygen sensing mechanism. *Proc. Natl. Acad. Sci.USA* B90: 2423–2427.

Mazzeo, R. S., P.R. Bender, G.A. Brooks, G.E. Butterfield, B.M. Groves, J.R. Sutton, E.E. Wolfel, and J.T. Reeves (1991). Arterial catecholamine responses during exercise with acute and chronic high altitude exposure. *Am. J. Physiol.* 261: E419–E424.

Montgomery, H. M., R. Marshall, H. Hemingway, S. Myerson, P. Clarkson, C. Dollery, M. Hayward, D.E. Holliman, M. Jubb, M. World, E.L. Thomas, A.E. Brynes, N. Saeed, M. Barnard, J.D. Bell, K. Prasad, M. Rayson, P.J. Talmud, and S. Humphries (1997). Human gene for physical performance. *Nature* 393: 221–222.

Moore, L.G., L. Curran-Everett, T.S. Droma, B.M. Groves, R.E. McCullough, S.F. Sun, J.R. Sutton, S. Zamudio, and J.G. Zhuang (1992). Are Tibetans better adapted? *Intl. J. Sports Med.* 13: S86–S88.

Mottishaw, P.D., S.K. Thornton, and P.W. Hochachka (1999). The diving response and its surprisingly evolutionary path in seals and sea lions. *Am. Zool.* 39: 434–450.

Normile, D. (2001). Comparative genomics: Gene expression differs in human and chimp brains. *Science* 292: 44–45.

Ogita, H.E., T. Nakaoka, R. Matsuoka, A. Takao, and Y. Kira (1994). Rapid induction of vascular endothelial growth factor expression by transient ischemia in rat heart. *Am. J. Physiol.* 267: H1948–H1954.

Rankinen, T., L. Perusse, J. Gagnon, Y.C. Chagnon, A.S. Leon, J.S. Skinner, J.H. Wilmore, D.C. Rao, and C. Bouchard (2000). Angiotensin-converting enzyme ID polymorphism and fitness phenotype. *HERITAGE Fam. Study J. Appl. Physiol.* 88: 1029–1035.

Resink, T., L. Buravkova, E. Mirzapoyazova, E. Kohler, P. Erne and V. Tkachuk (1996). Involvement of protein kinase C in hypoxia induced desensitization of the beta-adrenergic system in human endothelial cells. *Biochem. Biophys. Res. Commun.* 222: 753–758.

Ridley, M. (Ed.) (1993). Evolution. In: *Evolution*, pp. 141–183, Cambridge, Mass.: Blackwell Scientific.

Rosser, B.W.C., and P.W. Hochachka (1994). Metabolic capacity of muscle fibers from high-altitude natives. *Eur. J. Appl. Physiol.* 67: 513–517.

Rumsey, W.L., B. Abbot, D. Bertelsen, M. Mallamaci, K. Hagan, D. Nelson, and M. Erecinska (1999). Adaptation to hypoxia alters energy metabolism in rat heart. *Am. J. Physiol.* 45: H71–H80.

Rupert, J.L, D.V. Devin, M.V. Monsolve, and P.W. Hochachka (1999a). Angiotensin-converting enzyme (ACE) alleles in the Quechua, a high altitude South American native population. *Ann. Human Biol.* 26: 375–380.

Rupert, J.L, D.V. Devin, M.V. Monsolve, and P.W. Hochachka (1999b). β-fibrinogen allele frequen-

cies in high altitude natives. *Am. J. Physical Anthropol.* 109: 181–186.

Saltin, B., H. Larsen, N. Torrados, J. Bangsbo, T. Bak, C.K. Kim, J. Svedenhag, and C.J. Rolf (1995a). Aerobic exercise capacity at sea level and at altitude in Kenyan boys, junior and senior runners compared with Scandinavian runners. *Scand. J. Med. Sci. Sports* 5: 209–221.

Saltin, B., C.K. Kim, N. Terrados, H. Larsen, J. Svedenhag, and C.J. Rolf (1995b). Morphology, enzyme activities, and buffer capacity in leg muscles of Kenyan and Scandinavian runners. *Scand. J. Med. Sci. Sports* 5: 222–230.

Samaja, M., C. Mariani, A. Prestini, and P. Cerretelli (1997). Acid-base balance and O_2 transport at high altitude. *Acta Physiol. Scand.* 159: 249–256.

Sheel, A.W., and D.C. McKenzie (2000). Hypoxemia during exercise: in health and disease. *Clin. Exercise Physiol.* 2(3): 116–127.

Strohl, K.P., and C.M. Beal (1997). Ventilatory response to experimental hypoxia in adult male and female natives of the Tibetan and Andean plateaus. In: *Women at Altitude*, pp. 154–165, ed. C. Houston, Burlington, Vt.: Queen City Printers.

Terrados, N. (1992). Altitude training and muscular metabolism. *Int. J. Sports Med.* 13: S206–S209.

Thomas, T., and D.A. Fell (1998). A control analysis exploration of the role of ATP utilization in glycolytic-flux control and glycolytic-metabolite-concentration regulation. *Eur. J. Biochem.* 259: 956–967.

Wagner, P.D. (2000). Reduced cardiac output at altitude—mechanisms and significance. *Resp. Physiol.* 120: 1–11.

Wang, G. L., B.H. Jian, E.A. Rue and G.L. Semenza (1995). Hypoxia inducible factor 1 is a basic-helix-loop-helix PAS heterodimer regulated by cellular oxygen tension. *Proc. Natl. Acad. Sci. USA* 92: 5510–5514.

Weibel, E.R. (2000). *Symmorphosis, on Form and Function Shaping Life*. Cambridge, Mass.: Harvard University Press.

Weir, E. K., and S.L. Archer (1995). The mechanism of acute hypoxic pulmonary vasoconstriction: a tale of two channels. *FASEB J.* 9: 183–189.

Wenger, R.H., and M. Gassman (1997). Oxygen(es) and the hypoxia inducible factor 1. *J. Biol. Chem.* 378: 609–616.

West, J.B. (1986). Lactate during exercise at extreme altitude. *Fed. Proc.* 49: 2953–2957.

Weston, A.R., O. Karamizrak, A. Smith, T.D. Noakes, and K.H. Myburgh (1999). African runners exhibit greater fatigue resistance, lower lactate accumulation, and higher oxidative enzyme activity. *J. Appl. Physiol.* 86: 915–923.

Winslow, R.M., and C. Monge (1987). *Hypoxia, Polycythemia, and Chronic Mountain Sickness.* Baltimore: Johns Hopkins University Press.

Zamudio, S., T. Droma, K.Y. Norkyel, G. Acharya, J.A. Zamudio, S.N. Niermeyer, and L.G. Moore (1993). Protection from intrauterine growth retardation in Tibetans at high altitude. *Am. J. Physical Anthropol.* 91: 215–224.

6

Water–Solute Adaptations

The Evolution and Regulation of the Internal Milieu

WATER AS A "FIT" MEDIUM FOR LIFE:
DIVERSE ROLES OF WATER IN
BIOLOGICAL CHEMISTRY

Life Is an Aqueous Phenomenon

The chemical reactions found in all living systems, reactions that essentially define what we mean by "life," are almost entirely aqueous phase processes that involve water-soluble reactants. Indeed, as Henderson (1913) wrote in his classic volume *The Fitness of the Environment*, the fact that water can be regarded as a (nearly) "universal solvent" makes this abundant molecule a most fit milieu for the complex metabolic systems found in organisms, systems that involve tens of thousands of different proteins and nucleic acids and vast numbers of low-molecular-mass compounds such as substrates of energy metabolism, biosynthetic intermediates, dissolved gases, and inorganic ions. The "packaging problem" faced by cells in accommodating these many different types of chemicals into a small volume of solution dictates that the solvent be extraordinarily effective. It is difficult to imagine how any solvent but water could allow the evolution of life.

Closely linked to its extraordinary solvent capacities is water's role in transporting dissolved materials throughout the organism. With the exception of air-filled channels like the tracheal systems of insects, most of the transport processes of organisms involve movement of dissolved solutes. Diffusion of solutes within water is rapid, as is the translational and rotational movement of water itself. The extensive networks of hydrogen bonds that form among water molecules and between water and solutes do not impede this dynamic move-

ment. The lifetime of a hydrogen bond between water molecules is only about one picosecond and the weak bonds that form between water and solutes have lifetimes of only about one nanosecond. Thus, water is highly mobile, as are the solutes it contains. On a larger dimensional scale, water's viscosity is permissive of flow through both large and small vessels, allowing rapid transport of dissolved materials over large distances. On a yet larger size scale, water's physical properties such as its viscosity and density allow it to be exploited by swimming organisms using a diverse suite of biomechanical inventions that support locomotion (Denny, 1993).

Water's importance in biology goes well beyond its function as a medium in which a myriad of living processes can occur. Water's physical–chemical properties have helped to shape the evolution of many of the most important features of cellular structure and function. The wide imprint of water on cellular design is a central theme of this chapter. The structures that constitute the cell—membranes of many types, assemblages of structural and enzymatic proteins, and the chromosomal apparatus—and provide the machinery for metabolic activity, transport, and gene expression, all possess properties that reflect selection based on the characteristics of water. Even the constituents of the cell that are not soluble in water have properties that reflect their evolution in an aqueous milieu. Moreover, the properties of water are manifested in the diverse suite of *micromolecules*, the low-molecular-mass organic solutes and inorganic ions that are the numerically dominant solutes of living systems. Selection of particular micromolecules for accumulation to high concentrations in the cell has not been based on criteria of "convenience," that is, on the basis of what solutes were most readily available in the environment, but rather on the grounds of how different solutes interact with water and how they affect the solubilities of certain constituents of macromolecules such as peptide backbone linkages of proteins. The evolution of micromolecular systems, like the evolution of macromolecules, reveals a high degree of natural selection based on critical aspects of water–solute interactions.

Despite its quantitative dominance among the diverse molecules present in organisms, water's profound influence on the evolution of life has arguably been a neglected aspect of studies of molecular evolution, which for the most part have emphasized macromolecules. The sections of this chapter that follow, and complementary portions of other chapters of this book, will try to remedy this shortfall in evolutionary biology. We will attempt to afford to water, the most abundant molecule of living systems (approximately 55 M in most metabolically active cells and extracellular fluids), its rightful place in the study of evolution. Through more fully appreciating the role of water in evolution, it becomes much easier to understand the importance of contemporary physiological systems for defending the status quo of the *internal milieu*—in particular, the total amount of cellular water and the types and concentrations of dissolved solutes within it—in the face of diverse types of water stress.

In this chapter, we will discuss a relatively small number of basic principles of water–solute interactions that provide a conceptual framework for understanding central aspects of macromolecular and micromolecular evolution. We will discover vital links between these two evolutionary processes through addressing the question of why the intracellular fluids have evolved to contain the types and amounts of solutes they do. The unifying view that can be developed through study of these basic principles will enable us to understand the unity that underlies the apparent diversity found in cellular fluids, in which total solute *concentration* varies by well over an order of magnitude, and solute *composition* likewise exhibits enormous variation among species. As emphasized

in chapter 1, one of the great contributions of comparative biology is to reveal the unity in principle that underlies diversity in natural systems; water–solute relationships provide an exceptionally good illustration of this philosophical point (see Somero, 2000).

Our treatment of basic principles of water–solute relationships involves a bottom-up approach that begins with a basic physical–chemical analysis of how fundamental water–solute interactions have set many of the boundary conditions for the evolution of life. We discuss how the properties of macromolecules and micromolecules alike reflect selection based on such fundamental criteria as the differential solubilities of different organic and inorganic solutes in water, and the effects that these solutes in turn have on water structure; these are two closely related issues of vast importance in cellular evolution. With these basic features of water–solute interactions established, we will then be in a position to appreciate more fully why regulation of cellular volume and the composition of the *internal milieu* demands such precision. We then can move upwards on the reductionist ladder to consider the physiological mechanisms that have evolved to enable cells to defend the appropriate solutions conditions that are "fit" for the functions of macromolecular systems. This multitiered analysis is intended to help provide answers to three primary questions about the evolution and regulation of the internal milieu:

(1) *Which* solutes are selected as constituents of the internal milieu?
(2) *Why* have these particular solutes and not others been selected for accumulation?
(3) *How* are these solutes selectively taken up, synthesized, and retained in the face of demands arising from diverse types of water stress?

A Necessary Digression: Terminology and Definitions Associated with Water–Solute Relationships

Before we further analyze water–micromolecule–macromolecule interactions, it is appropriate to introduce some of the terminology that is commonly used when biologists and chemists refer to dissolved substances in aqueous media. This terminology will provide us with a foundation on which to build much of the analysis that follows. In some cases, physiologists and physical chemists prefer to employ different terms for the same phenomenon, so the elaboration of terms given below is not just an exercise in pedantry, but rather is intended to serve primarily as a roadmap for those traversing the diverse literatures that concern water–solute relationships.

The most commonly used generic term for a dissolved substance is *solute*, and this is the term that we will employ in most contexts, for both large and small compounds, that is, for macromolecules and micromolecules. A closely related term, *cosolvent*, is often used by physical chemists when the issue in question involves a dissolved substance that either stabilizes or destabilizes the structures of macromolecules. For instance, cosolvent is often used in literature on the effects of solutes on protein stability. A more restrictive and specific term that will be employed when we discuss the osmotic relationships of organisms is *osmolyte*. Although some treatments of osmotic regulation use the term osmolyte to refer to any solute that makes a contribution to osmotic strength—and, by the nature of colligative relationships, *all* solutes are expected to do this—a more restricted definition will be used here. Thus, osmolyte will be used to refer to any inorganic or organic solute whose concentration is adaptively regulated during the process of cell volume regulation, in parallel with the osmotic stress imposed on the cell (see Somero and Yancey, 1997, p. 442). Osmolytes include certain inorganic ions. For instance, K^+ is an important osmolyte in some organisms, especially prokaryotic species. However, the predominant osmolytes in almost all types of cells are a suite of low-molecular-mass organic molecules whose properties reflect a high degree of selection based on the need to establish in the cellular water a fit milieu for macromolecular structure and function.

Units of solute concentration also require definition for, as in the case of the terminology related to dissolved substances, different units of concentration commonly are found in different literatures. Although the chemical literature customarily expresses solute concentrations in terms of the number of molecules of a single type of chemical that are present in a given volume of solution, physiologists concerned with osmotic relationships are more interested in the total number of osmotically active particles in a volume of aqueous solution. The concentrations of specific solutes typically are given in terms of their molarity (moles per liter, symbolized as M; a mole contains Avogadro's number of particles, 6.02×10^{23}). Pure water is 55.56 M; thus a liter of water contains 3.345×10^{25} molecules of water. Biological solutions seldom contain molar concentrations of chemicals other than water, so solute concentrations are more likely to be expressed as millimoles or micromoles of solute per liter of solution (mmol l^{-1} [mM] or (μmol l^{-1} [μM], respectively). An alternative expression for concentration of specific compounds is molality, moles of solute per kilogram of water. If the solutes in a solution have negligible effects on solution volume, then the molarity and molality of the solution are very similar in value (for a concise discussion of these relationships, see Potts, 1994, pp. 756–758).

Physiologists studying osmotic relationships of organisms, however, are often concerned with the total concentration of all dissolved substances, not just the concentrations of specific solutes. For expressing the total number of osmotically active particles in a solution, the concept of *osmolality* is commonly employed to refer to the osmotic pressure characteristic of a solution. One *osmole* is defined as the osmotic pressure of a 1.0 molal solution of an ideal solute. Because conditions of ideality do not pertain to the case of biological fluids, it is not possible to extrapolate precisely from chemical determinations of moles of solute per kilogram (or liter) of fluid to the osmolality of that fluid. Rather, this value must be determined empirically.

When describing how the osmotic concentrations of organisms compare to the osmolality of the surrounding solution, the following terms are employed (for reviews, see Kirschner,

1991, 1997). If the osmolality of the fluids within the organism is the same as that of the surrounding medium, then the organism is said to be *isosmotic* with its medium. If the organism has a higher osmolality than the medium, the organism is referred to as being *hyperosmotic* to its surroundings (and the medium is hypoosmotic to the organism). If the organism's total osmotic concentration is less than that of the external milieu, the organism is termed *hypoosmotic* and the medium hyperosmotic. Note that these terms and relationships refer strictly to the colligative properties of the solutions, properties that depend on the total number of particles present in a volume of solution. Whether or not the organism actually gains or loses water when hyperosmotic or hypoosmotic, respectively, is determined by the physiological characteristics of the organism, for instance, the permeability characteristics of its membranes. The tendency for water to leave or enter the cell is discussed using terms involving *tonicity*. A solution in which water tends not be to be gained or lost from cells is termed an *isotonic* solution. This solution may or may not be isosmotic. *Hypertonic* media are those that lead to loss of water from cells; *hypotonic* media are those that cause cell swelling to occur. A solution that is hyperosmotic or hypoosmotic may or may not by hypertonic or hypotonic, respectively. For example, if a cell is exposed rapidly to a solution that is hyperosmotic due to a high concentration of a nonpermeating solute, then water will be lost from the cell. That is, this solution is both hyperosmotic and hypertonic. In contrast, if the hyperosmotic solution contains a freely permeable solute (urea may approximate this condition in many cases), then the rapid entry of the solute into the cell will prevent water loss. Here, the hyperosmotic solution is not hypertonic, except for what may be a very brief period during transmembrane equilibration of the permeable solute.

We provide this somewhat lengthy treatment of terminology related to solute concentrations not to overwhelm the reader with nit-picky definitions, but to provide important conceptual tools for understanding the diverse osmotic relationships that form the focus of this chapter. It should be apparent that all of these terms

and concepts apply equally to (i) the osmotic relationships of intracellular versus extracellular fluids, as (ii) to relationships between the organism and the ambient water.

Maintaining cellular volume is a critical aspect of the environmental relationships of organisms, in both aquatic and terrestrial habitats. For aquatic species, there is a wide range of abilities to defend cellular volume as environmental salinity changes. Some species, termed *euryhaline* organisms, are widely tolerant of changes in ambient salinity, whereas other species, termed *stenohaline*, tolerate only narrow ranges of salinity. Some species, termed *osmoconformers*, allow the concentrations of the extracellular fluids to vary in parallel with ambient salinity, at least over a certain range of salinities. *Osmoregulators* closely defend the osmolality of the extracellular fluids in the face of changes in ambient salinity.

These concepts and definitions provide the vocabulary and theoretical framework for much of the analysis that follows, as we explore one of the most interesting and important aspects of life, the evolution and regulation of the internal milieu. We begin this exploration by considering a primary way in which life depends on water, namely, the role of water as a reactant in metabolic chemistry.

Water as a Reactant in Covalent Metabolic Chemistry

The generalization that water is involved in virtually all aspects of cellular chemistry applies whether we are considering reactions that involve changes in covalent bonds, which are characterized by high bond energies, or in noncovalent ("weak") chemical bonds, whose energies are of the same order of magnitude as the thermal energy of the cell. In the case of many metabolic reactions involving formation or breakage of covalent bonds, water not only plays the role of solvent, but also serves as a reactant. Thus, in both catabolic and anabolic reactions of intermediary metabolism, the addition or removal of a molecule of water is an essential event in the transformations. Removal of a molecule of water (dehydration) typically accompanies the building of larger molecules from smaller building blocks. Dehydration reactions are found in (i) the formation of peptide bonds in protein synthesis, (ii) the linking of nucleotides into nucleic acids, (iii) the combination of individual sugar molecules into oligo- and polysaccharides, (iv) the linking of fatty acids to glycerol during phospholipid synthesis, and (v) the generation of ATP from ADP and inorganic phosphate, to list but a few examples. The reactions involved in synthesizing the individual building blocks of large molecules also may involve dehydration reactions when the individual atoms of the building block are assembled, for instance, during biosynthesis of fatty acids. Conversely, the degradation of organic molecules through catabolic processes typically involves hydrolysis, the adding of a molecule of water during rupture of covalent bonds. If a catabolic process leads to complete oxidation of substrates through the electron transport system, which terminates in the cytochrome-c oxidase reaction, the final product of metabolism is water—the least toxic and least problematic end product of catabolic reactions. Thus, throughout the web of metabolic transformations found in cells, water plays key roles both as solvent and as participant in covalent chemistry.

It should be noted that, despite water's high concentration in cells, addition or removal of water through reactions involving formation or rupture of covalent bonds generally requires enzymatic catalysis. The free energy barriers to reactions involving covalent addition of water to, or its removal from, organic molecules are sufficiently large to preclude significant amounts of uncatalyzed hydrolysis and dehydration reactions at most temperatures permissive of life. At the high temperatures encountered by extremely thermophilic prokaryotes, however, hydrolysis of certain types of relatively labile covalent bonds in proteins and other biomolecules occurs at substantial rates, without the need for catalysis. These uncatalyzed and, therefore, uncontrolled hydrolytic reactions at elevated temperatures, in concert with alterations in water structure that impact noncovalent interactions between water and macromolecules, may help to set the upper thermal limits of life (Jaenicke, 2000; also chapter 7).

Water Plays Diverse Roles in Noncovalent Chemistry

It is in the context of noncovalent interactions among water, organic molecules of all types and sizes, and inorganic ions that a particularly diverse and biologically significant set of chemical interactions occurs. The diverse noncovalent interactions between water and other constituents of the cell do not, by definition, involve the formation or breakage of covalent bonds between atoms of molecules; these noncovalent reactions with water lead to no new chemical species per se. Despite this status quo in terms of the chemicals present in the cell, noncovalent water–macromolecule–micromolecule interactions play profound roles throughout biology. These interactions are of dominant importance in establishing the three-dimensional configurations and the intracellular compartmentation of the macromolecules responsible for conducting covalent chemistry. Water–macromolecule–micromolecule interactions also govern to some extent the distribution of micromolecules within the cellular water, and affect the types of structures assumed by cellular water itself. An understanding of this complex noncovalent chemistry will pave the way for the subsequent analysis of evolution of intracellular solutions, a process in which the nature of the accumulated solutes and their effects on the structure of cellular water are closely regulated to ensure the development of a solution environment that is "fit" for macromolecular structure and function.

Differential solubility: a critical aspect of water–solute interactions

When we review the many ways in which water interacts with inorganic ions and organic molecules through noncovalent bonding, we find a wide array of instances in which the *differential* solubilities of solutes are of fundamental importance. Here, differential solubility refers to that fact that inorganic ions, small organic solutes, and constituent groups of macromolecules (for instance, different amino acid side-chains) vary in their solubilities in water. Some chemicals (glycerol is a good example) are virtually infinitely miscible in water: the amount of solute in solution can be increased to nearly 100%. Other solutes, notably the acyl chains of fatty acids and the nonpolar side-chains of some amino acids, are only very weakly soluble in water. Many organic molecules are *amphipathic*: they contain both highly soluble and poorly soluble groups (phospholipids, with their polar head groups and nonpolar tails, are a good example). The occurrence of differential solubility among the chemicals found in the cellular water is not some type of evolutionary accident that was dictated by the particular types of chemicals available to early cells. Rather, natural selection has exploited the principle of differential solubility to fabricate an intracellular milieu and a set of proteins, lipids, and nucleic acids having solubility relationships that are critical for the development of cellular structures and the support of physiological processes. The pivotal importance of differential solubilities indeed is observed at all size scales of biochemistry, from the largest to the smallest constituents of the cell. Differential solubilities in water are critical for establishing the organization of large molecular assemblages such as membranes. The partitioning of *hydrophobic* ("water disliking") acyl chains of phospholipids into the interior of the membrane bilayer, while the *hydrophilic* ("water liking") headgroups partition into the aqueous phase, is one example of how differential solubilities of biomolecules are essential for establishing the three-dimensional structures of essential cellular components. Water–solute interactions also play pivotal roles in establishing the higher orders of protein structure. Differential solubilities of the side-chains of the 20 amino acids that serve as the building blocks of proteins play dominant roles in protein folding and compartmentation. Without water the tendency of unfolded polypeptide chains to assume the compact conformation of the native, functional state of the protein is low or absent. When in aqueous solution, however, the polypeptide's hydrophobic side-chains, for instance, those of the amino acids leucine, isoleucine, and valine, partition into the nonpolar interior of the folded protein,

away from water. Charged and polar amino acids, which are very hydrophilic, typically occur on or near the protein surface, in contact with solvent.

The peptide backbone linkage between amino acid residues also is hydrophilic, and approximately 50% of the peptide bonds of a globular protein lie near the surface, in contact with water. However, the relative tendency of peptide bonds to be in contact with water versus buried in the protein interior is highly dependent on the types of solutes present in solution. As discussed later in more detail, the burial of peptide backbone linkages in the nonpolar interior of a globular protein may be a favored by what are termed *osmophobic* effects. These effects involve reduced solubilities of peptide linkages in the presence of protein stabilizing solutes (see Baskakov and Bolen, 1998; Qu et al., 1998). We thus need to consider two different types of "phobias" possessed by groups on macromolecules toward the surrounding aqueous medium: osmophobic effects, deriving from the dissolved solutes, and hydrophobic effects, due to water itself. Together, these two "phobias" can be grouped under a general heading, *solvophobicity* (Qu et al., 1998).

Hydrophobic and osmophobic effects are important not only in the folding of individual polypeptide chains into compact globular proteins, but also in the assembly of multiprotein complexes. Osmophobic effects are noted, for instance, in the self-assembly of subunits of the glycolytic enzyme phosphofructokinase (PFK). Self-assembly is enhanced by the presence of stabilizing organic cosolvents such as trimethylamine-N-oxide (TMAO) (Hand and Somero, 1982). As discussed later, self-assembly driven by osmophobic effects results from the thermodynamic favorability of minimizing the surface area on the proteins that is in contact with the cosolvent.

For some multimeric proteins, hydrophobic patches on the surface of subunits serve as interaction sites that favor polymerization in aqueous solutions. To allow polymerization to occur, the organized clusters ("clathrates") of water around the hydrophobic sites must be removed. This process requires an input of thermal energy to "melt" the clathrates. Thus, the enthalpy change (ΔH) of polymerization is positive. The entropy change (ΔS) also is positive because polymerization leads to a decrease in system (water + protein) order, as the organized clathrates of water around the interacting surfaces are broken up and water enters the bulk phase of the solution. In hydrophobic interactions, the entropy change plays the dominant role in the overall free energy change (ΔG) of the process. Thus, such polymerization reactions are termed *entropy-driven processes*, in recognition of the role played by *changes in water organization* during the assembly event. It bears emphasizing again that water can play a dominant role in the energy changes that occur during a biochemical process even though water is not involved in the formation or rupture of covalent bonds. The enthalpy and entropy changes that accompany *reorganization* of water molecules may be the essential driving force of the process.

Nucleic acid structures also involve assembly events determined by differential solubilities of different molecular constituents. The stacking of purine and pyrimidine bases in the helical structures of DNA relies on hydrophobic effects, whereas the positioning of phosphate groups in contact with solvent reflects their hydrophilic nature. Secondary structures of RNA likewise are influenced by differential solubilities of polar and nonpolar constituents.

The differential solubilities exhibited by biomolecules thus should be appreciated as one of the most important aspects of the effects of water on living systems. Differential solubility is a critical principle in much of biochemical evolution, and it is a principle that is manifested in a number of contexts of adaptation to the environment. This is seen particularly clearly in the evolution of proteins in the face of different chemical and physical conditions. The amino acids selected to construct a particular protein reflect a finely tuned process that results in the generation of an appropriate three-dimensional structure and a correct balance between structural stability and flexibility—a balance termed *marginal stability*—that is essential for protein function. The marginal stability of the protein will be seen to be the consequence of complementary adaptations in the protein itself (*intrinsic* adaptations) and in the medium bathing the protein (*extrinsic* adaptations). Together, these adaptations generate a set of conditions in which the solubilities of protein side-chains and peptide backbone linkages are appropriate for the physical and chemical conditions in which the protein must function.

With these fundamental aspects of water–micromolecule–macromolecule interactions as a background, we now are prepared to analyze why evolutionary processes have led to the generation of the particular types of cellular solutions we find among the three major domains of the tree of life. This analysis will emphasize especially well the principle of "unity in diversity" that serves as a central theme of this volume.

EVOLUTION OF THE INTERNAL MILIEU: PATTERNS OF SOLUTE ACCUMULATION

Selection of Inorganic Ions

The fitness of Na^+ and K^+

The inorganic ions that are selectively accumulated in the intra- and extracellular fluids provide an appropriate starting point for analyzing the evolution and regulation of biological solutions. Inorganic ions exhibit similar patterns of accumulation across most taxa (figure 6.1, table 6.1), a similarity that pertains both to the types of inorganic ions accumulated and to their intracellular concentrations (figure 6.1). In virtually all types of cells, potassium ion, K^+, is the dominant intracellular cation, its concentration greatly exceeding that of Na^+, the major cation of extracellular fluids in multicellular organisms. The likelihood that the first cells arose in a marine environment in which the concentration of Na^+ greatly exceeded that of K^+ suggests that selective accumulation of K^+ was not simply a matter of "convenience," that is, of using the most readily available monovalent cation as the major inorganic ion of the cell. What might account for this early evolutionary decision to prefer K^+ to the more readily available monovalent cation, Na^+?

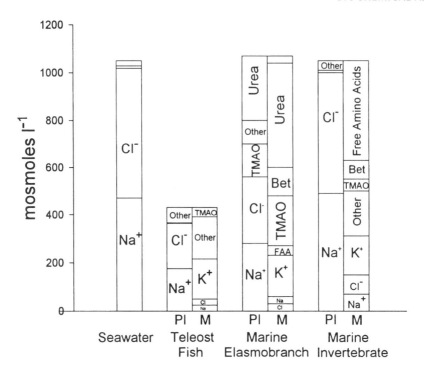

Figure 6.1. Compositions and concentrations of intracellular and extracellular fluids of selected marine animals having widely different total osmolarities. M = intracellular fluids of muscle tissue; Pl = plasma or hemolymph; TMAO = trimethylamine-N-oxide; Bet = glycine betaine; FAA = free amino acids. (Data compiled from various sources; for a comprehensive list of osmolyte compositions and concentrations in diverse species, see Kirschner, 1991; Somero and Yancey, 1997; Yancey et al., 1982.)

Differences among inorganic ions in their effects on water structure may partially explain the preference of K^+ over Na^+, as well as certain other patterns of accumulation of inorganic ions. Because potassium ion has a lower charge density than sodium ion, one positive charge for a mass of 39 daltons (Da) compared to a mass of 23 Da, respectively, K^+ is less effective at organizing water than is Na^+. In fact, potassium ion is a *water-structure-breaker* (a so-called *chaotrope*) whereas sodium ion is a water-structuring ion (a *kosmotrope*; for review, see the classic treatment by von Hippel and Schleich, 1969). Other things being equal, accumulation of K^+ will place a lower demand on water's solvent capacity than Na^+. Because solvent capacity of the cellular water is limited (see "Solvent Capacity of the Cell"), selective accumulation of K^+ rather than Na^+ may facilitate including more types of solutes, at higher concentrations, within the minute volume of water present in the cell.

Potassium ion may also have been preferentially accumulated because of its influences on proteins; K^+ has a slightly more favorable effect on protein stability than does sodium ion. In the Hofmeister Series ranking of ions in terms of their stabilizing or destabilizing effects on proteins, K^+ lies slightly to the stabilizing side of the series relative to Na^+ (von Hippel and Schleich, 1969; see figure 6.9). Potassium ion also may have more favorable effects on enzymatic activity than Na^+. Many enzymes require an inorganic ion activator, and K^+ commonly serves this role. For example, the glycolytic enzyme pyruvate kinase (PK) requires K^+ for activity; Na^+ is inhibitory of PK and many other enzymes (Bowlus and Somero, 1979).

These differences between K^+ and Na^+ in their effects on water structure, protein structure, and enzymatic activity—effects that may be intimately linked—may explain why, at the dawn of cellular evolution, one monovalent cation, K^+, was selected as the predominant

Table 6.1.   Major Classes of Osmolytes and Their Distribution among Eukaryotes, Bacteria and Archaea. Elevated Concentrations of Osmolytes Due to Freeze-Avoidance ("Freezing") or Desiccation Stress (*Artemia* Embryos) Are Included

Organism	Osmolyte

I. EUKARYOTES AND BACTERIA

A. Polyhydric alcohols (polyols) and sugars

Bacteria	trehalose, sucrose, mannitol, glucosylglycerol, mannosucrose
Algae	glycerol, mannitol, sorbitol, sucrose, glucose, volemitol, floridoside
Fungi	glycerol, erythritol, arabitol, mannitol
Vascular plants	*myo*-inositol, sorbitol, glucose, sucrose, mannitol, methyl-inositols (pinitol, etc.)
Animals	
Artemia embryos	trehalose, glycerol
Insects—freezing	glycerol, sorbitol, erythritol, sucrose
Insects—salinity	trehalose
Marine elasmobranchs	*myo*-inositol, *scyllo*-inositol
Teleosts—freezing	glycerol
Amphibia—freezing	glucose, glycerol
Mammals—kidney	sorbitol, *myo*-inositol
Mammals—brain	*myo*-inositol

B. Amino acids and amino acid derivatives

Bacteria	glutamate, glutamine, proline, ectoine, hydroxyectoine, N_α-carbamoyl-glutamate-1-amide, *N*-acetylglutaminylglutamine amide γ-amino butyrate
Algae	proline, alanine, glycine, glutamate
Vascular plants	proline
Animals	
Marine invertebrates	glycine, alanine, proline, serine, taurine, strombine, etc.
Insects (brackish water)	proline, serine
Marine cyclostomes	glycine, alanine, proline
Marine elasmobranchs	taurine, glycine, β-alanine
Amphibia	various α-amino acids
Mammals—kidney, heart, brain	taurine, glutamine

C. Methylated ammonium and sulfonium compounds

Bacteria	glycine betaine, choline-O-sulfate, proline betaine, taurine betaine, β-alanine betaine, glutamate betaine, pipecolate betaine, dimethylsulfoniopropionate (DMSP)
Algae	glycine betaine, proline betaine, choline-O-sulfate, homarine, dimethyl-taurine, taurine betaine, DMSP
Vascular plants	glycine betaine, proline betaine, β-alanine betaine, choline-O-sulfate, DMSP

continued

Table 6.1.   Continued

Organism	Osmolyte
Animals	
Marine invertebrates	glycine betaine, TMAO, proline betaine
Marine cyclostomes	TMAO
Marine elasmobranchs	TMAO, glycine betaine, sarcosine
Coelacanths	TMAO, glycine betaine
Amphibia	glycerophosphorylcholine (GPC)
Mammals—kidney, brain	glycine betaine, GPC
Birds—erythrocytes	taurine
D. Urea	
Gastropods—estivating	
Marine elasmobranchs	with methylamines
Coelacanth	with methylamines
Lungfish-estivation	
Amphibia—salinity	with methylamines
—estivation	
Mammals—kidney	with methylamines
II. ARCHAEA (see Martin et al., 1999)	
A. Inorganic ions	
Nonhalophiles	K^+, at concentrations that may exceed 0.5 M
Extreme halophiles	K^+, at concentrations that may exceed 5 M
(*Halobacteriaceae*)	

B. Polyhydric alcohols and sugars

glycerol, diglycerol phosphate, di-*myo*-inositol-1,1′-phosphate (DIP), glucosylglycerate, β-mannosylglycerate, mannosyl-DIP, 2-sulfotrehalose, α-glucosylglycerate, β-galactopyranosyl-5-hydroxylysine

C. Amino acids and amino acid derivatives

glutamate, β-glutamate, β-glutamine, N^ϵ-acetyl-β-lysine

For references to original literature, consult Somero and Yancey, 1997; Martin et al., 1999.

inorganic ion of the cell, a trait that is observed in contemporary eukaryotes, bacteria, and Archaea. The fact that cells devote a substantial fraction of their ATP turnover, through activity of the K^+-Na^+-ATPase, to maintaining a high ratio of K^+ to Na^+ in the cellular water, is a clear indication of the importance of keeping intracellular K^+ high and Na^+ low. In mammals, for example, 19–28% of ATP turnover may be in support of the activity of the K^+-

Na^+-ATPase (Rolfe and Brown, 1997; see also chapter 2).

The conjecture that K^+ is more fit than Na^+ for the role of major intracellular monovalent cation is not meant to imply that other advantages for the K^+/Na^+ gradient found across the plasma membrane are absent. The K^+/Na^+ gradient across the plasma membrane is essential for the electrical excitability of the cell. The high extracellular concentration of Na^+ is significant

in driving energetically uphill transport of dissolved organic solutes like amino acids and
sugars into cells. In fact, an initial selective
advantage of keeping concentrations of Na^+
in the cell low relative to concentrations in seawater may have related to the utility of using
the steep sodium ion gradient as a driving force
in active transport of organic molecules into
early types of cells. As is often the case in
attempts to rationalize why a particular pattern
of evolution has occurred, more than one selective advantage for a trait can be conjectured,
and the selective factor(s) of principal importance at the time of the trait's origin thus
often remain obscure (chapter 1).

Organic Osmolytes: Which Contains What?

Convergence on a few osmolyte solutions

The principle of unity in diversity that so often
applies in evolutionary biology and comparative biochemistry is well illustrated by the patterns of accumulation of organic osmolytes in
diverse taxa (figures 6.1 and 6.2; table 6.1; see
Gilles and Delpire, 1997; Kirschner, 1991, 1997;
Somero and Yancey, 1997; Yancey et al., 1982;
and chapters in Somero et al., 1992, for additional data on osmolyte distribution patterns).
Despite what might appear at first inspection to
be an enormously wide diversity of types of
organic osmolytes in different taxa, closer analysis of osmolyte accumulation patterns reveals
that only four major groups of compounds are
accumulated: (1) *Polyhydric alcohols* (polyols),
such as glycerol, and *sugars*, such as the disaccharide trehalose; (2) *Free amino acids* (such
as proline, glutamate, and alanine) and their
derivatives (for instance, taurine); (3)
Methylammonium and *methylsulfonium* solutes,
such as trimethylamine-N-oxide and dimethylsulfoniopropionate (DMSP), respectively; and
(4) *urea*. In all taxa except the halotolerant
members of the Archaea plus some extremely
halotolerant bacteria, these four classes of
organic osmolytes are the principal types of
solutes that, in conjunction with K^+, are
responsible for establishing the major portion
of intracellular osmolality. In the extremely

halophilic members of the Archaea, K^+ is accumulated to enormous concentrations, up to
approximately 5 M in extreme cases (table 6.1;
Martin et al., 1999). These organisms clearly are
outliers that represent a different way of dealing
with the type of water stress that arises from
extreme extracellular salinity. The mechanisms
and costs of this alternate strategy will be considered later, after we analyze the more common approach to osmotic adaptation, that
involving reliance on organic osmolytes to
adjust intracellular osmolality.

The occurrence of the same four basic classes
of organic osmolytes in diverse phyla (table 6.1)
suggests several things about the evolution and
biochemical effects of these osmolytes. One is
that the four commonly found classes of
organic osmolytes are more fit for accumulation
at high concentrations than are inorganic ions,
including the prevalent inorganic ion, K^+. Even
though K^+ is maintained in most cells at concentrations higher than those of most individual
organic osmolytes, an indication that the cellular machinery has evolved to work in the presence of approximately 0.1 M to 0.20 M
concentrations of K^+, the conservation of intracellular $[K^+]$ ($[K^+]_i$) during osmotic regulation
indicates that variation in $[K^+]_i$ represents a
suboptimal mechanism of osmotic adaptation,
possibly because higher or lower concentrations
of K^+ prevent K^+-dependent systems from
functioning optimally.

A second conclusion to be drawn from the
fact that only a limited suite of organic osmolytes is used by diverse taxa is that not just any
type of organic solute is fit for accumulation at
high and/or varying concentrations. The
organic compounds selected as dominant osmolytes do, in fact, have features that enable them
to be accumulated to high concentrations and,
in osmoconforming species, to be used at widely
varying concentrations, without perturbing the
structures and metabolic activities of the cell.

The chemical properties that appear to
underlie the fitness of the four classes of organic
osmolytes include the following. First, these
osmolytes are polar molecules that have *high
solubilities in water*. They can be accumulated
to high concentrations without unduly taxing
the solvent capacity of the cell. Glycerol,

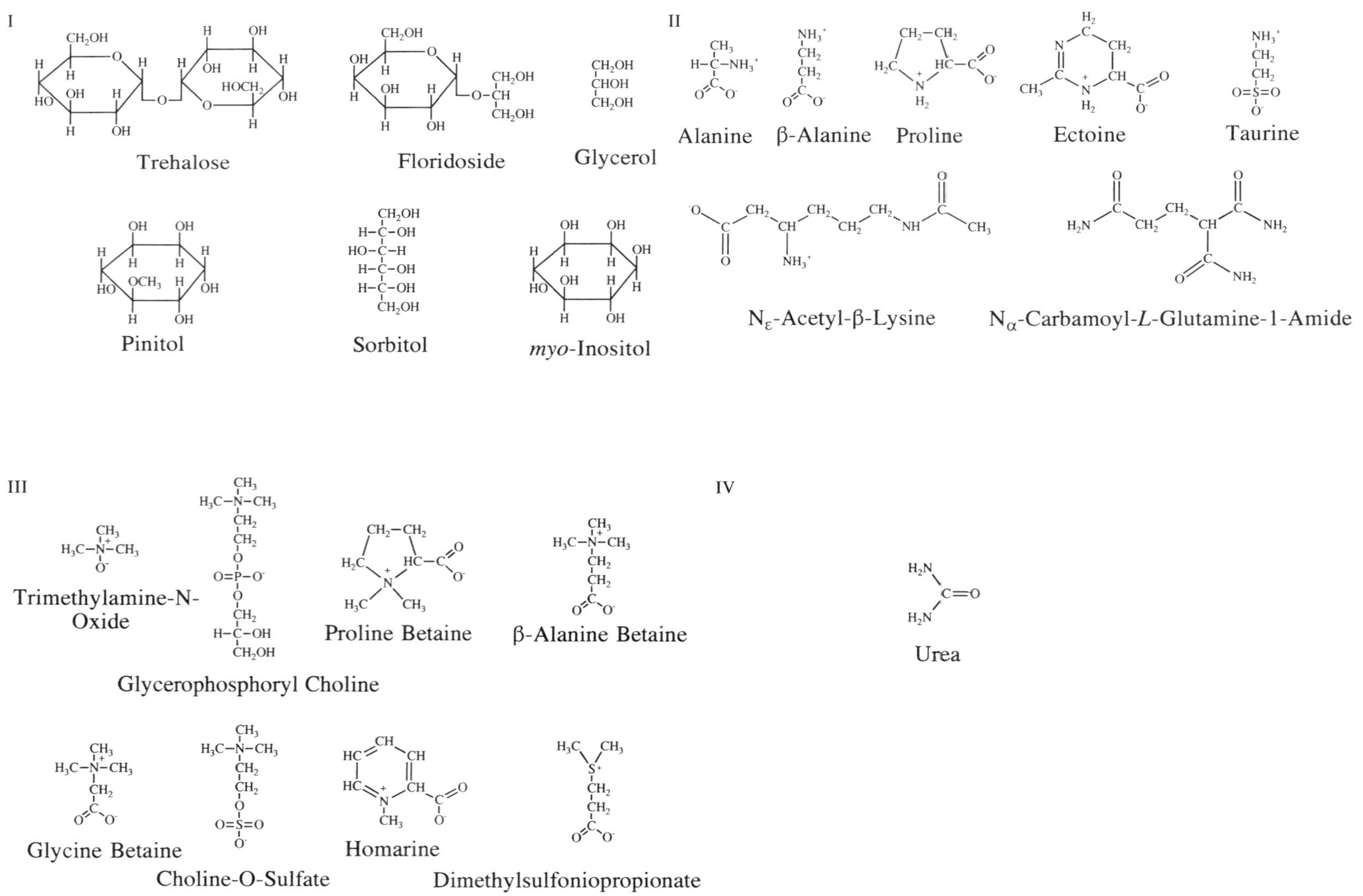

I

Trehalose

Floridoside

Glycerol

Pinitol

Sorbitol

myo-Inositol

II

Alanine

β-Alanine

Proline

Ectoine

Taurine

N_ε-Acetyl-β-Lysine

N_α-Carbamoyl-*L*-Glutamine-1-Amide

III

Trimethylamine-N-Oxide

Glycine Betaine

Glycerophosphoryl Choline

Proline Betaine

β-Alanine Betaine

Choline-O-Sulfate

Homarine

Dimethylsulfoniopropionate

IV

Urea

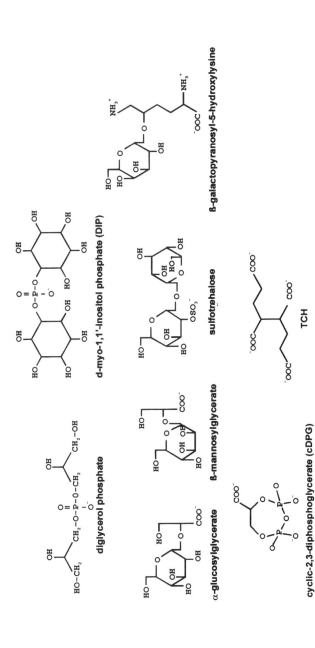

Figure 6.2. (Upper panel) The four major classes of organic osmolytes: (I) sugars and polyhydric alcohols (polyols); (II) amino acids and amino acid derivatives; (III) methylated ammonium and sulfonium compounds; and (IV) urea. (Figure modified after Somero and Yancey, 1997.) (Lower panel) Structures of charged osmolytes accumulated in extremely halophilic archaea (after Martin et al., 1999). Note that these osmolytes commonly represent a type of organic osmolyte that is found in many bacteria or eukaryotes to which a charged group has been attached. Typically, the charged group is anionic, for example, a phosphate or a carboxylate group.

which is infinitely miscible with water, is a case in point. Second, these osmolytes typically lack a *net* charge. Absence of charge is likely to reduce the tendencies of these osmolytes to interact with charged groups on macromolecules and membranes or with charged substrates and cofactors in solution. Absence of charge per se is not an absolute requirement for a solute being a good osmolyte, however. Some osmolytes, for instance, most free amino acids, are zwitterions, in which a positive charge is offset by a negative charge. Third, and following from the preceding point, if a net charge is present (glutamate, for instance), this charge is negative rather than positive. Fourth, osmolytes *lack a strongly hydrophobic region*; they have what is termed a low hydrophobic moment (see Arakawa et al., 1990; Nishiguchi and Somero, 1992). Analyses given in later sections of this chapter will account for the fitness of each of these traits of organic osmolytes in terms of physical–chemical principles of water–solute–macromolecule interactions.

A third conclusion drawn from the distribution patterns of organic osmolytes among taxa is that a substantial amount of convergent evolution has taken place in the evolutionary development of cellular osmolyte systems. The beneficial effects of most categories of organic osmolyte have been repeatedly "discovered" during evolution, as different taxa have faced a wide variety of forms of water stress. For example, the disaccharide trehalose is accumulated in plants, animals, fungi, and bacteria in response to several forms of water stress, including hyperosmotic stress resulting from increases in ambient salinity and dehydration stress arising from severe cellular desiccation during quiescent life stages. Glycerol is found in vertebrates and invertebrates, numerous vascular plants, fungi, and algae. Free amino acids are exploited by all phyla of marine invertebrates, many vascular plants, bacteria, and a few fishes and amphibians. Urea is found in elasmobranch fishes, in coelacanths (genus *Latimeria*), in certain estivating bony fishes and amphibians, and in crab-eating tropical frogs. In the mammalian kidney, urea is reabsorbed from the nephron and concentrated to high levels in the interstitial fluids of the inner medulla. This process enables the kidney to produce highly concentrated urine and, thereby, prevent excessive loss of water from the body. Unlike the other classes of organic osmolytes, urea can be highly toxic, so the strategy of using urea as an osmolyte will be seen to impose different rules from those that pertain to the other types of organic molecules that are accumulated during water stress.

Halophilic members of the Archaea: An initial look at an osmoregulatory outlier

Before we consider the rules that apply for use of organic osmolytes, it is appropriate to examine the costs and benefits of *not* using organic osmolytes for coping with water stress. Analysis of the extremely halophilic members of the Archaea will provide convincing evidence that using seemingly "cheap," readily available inorganic ions is, in fact, a very expensive strategy to follow in several respects. It is a strategy in which the choice of osmolyte entails radical modification of macromolecules and leads to a significant restriction in the range of habitats the organisms can tolerate.

We will consider the unusual osmotic characteristics of extremely halophilic archaea, members of the family *Halobacteriaceae*, at several junctures in this chapter as well as in the discussion of how organic thermoprotectant solutes contribute to adaptation to high temperatures (chapter 7). The first aspect of the osmoregulatory strategy of these species to be considered is the unusual set of osmolytes they contain: extremely high concentrations of K^+ compared to all other species, plus several organic osmolytes possessing net negative charges, which may be unique to members of the Archaea (figure 6.2). Both of these aspects of the intracellular milieu are so unusual that they suggest that the halophilic archaea have followed a unique evolutionary route in adapting to the water stress arising from the high salinity of their habitats, which include brine ponds in which saturating concentrations of NaCl occur.

As discussed above, the concentration of K^+ in cellular water is typically below 0.2 M, and $[K^+]_i$ usually is carefully regulated, even though transient increases in $[K^+]_i$ may occur during the initial phases of osmoregulation. In halophilic archaea, $[K^+]_i$ is extremely high in general and varies considerably in response to changes in ambient salinity. $[Na^+]_i$ also may be high in halophilic archaea. The approximately 5 M concentration of K^+ found in some members of the *Halobacteriaceae* would appear to tax the solvent capacity of the cell: KCl cannot be dissolved in water at this concentration. Thus, counterions other than Cl^- must be present to balance the positive charge on the potassium ion. These anionic counterions are a set of organic molecules that, in many cases, appear to be modified forms of organic osmolytes found in less salt-tolerant species (figure 6.2; Martin et al., 1999). In several cases in the extremely halophilic archaea, an uncharged osmolyte gains one or more negative charges through acquisition of a carboxylate, sulfate, or phosphate group. For instance, the commonly occurring osmolyte glycerol appears in halophilic archaea as diglycerol phosphate (DGP), which has a net charge of minus one. Trehalose, which is accumulated under diverse forms of water stress in many organisms, including some halophilic archaea, also appears as a sulfated compound, sulfotrehalose (net charge of minus three), in extremely halophilic archaea. Glucosylglycerol, a common osmolyte in cyanobacteria, has a close relative in archaea: glucosylglycerate (net charge of minus one). *Myo*-inositol, a polyol found in such diverse sites as plant cells and mammalian brain, appears as a phosphorylated disaccharide in halophilic archaea: di-*myo*-1,1'-inositol phosphate (DIP). Another phosphorylated osmolyte accumulated in archaea is cyclic-2,3-diphosphoglycerate (cDPG; net charge of minus three). This osmolyte, like DIP and certain other osmolytes found in the Archaea, may also be important as a protein-stabilizing compound, a *thermoprotectant* (see chapter 7). Another highly charged osmolyte, one identified in the thermophilic archaeon *Methanobacterium thermoautotrophicum* ΔH, is 1,3,4,6-tetracarboxyhexane (TCH), which has a net charge of minus four.

Halophilic archaea also accumulate substantial concentrations of β-amino acids, notably β-glutamate. Glutamate is a common osmolyte in all major groups of organisms, but there may be upper limits to its concentration because of its diverse roles as a metabolic intermediate. Too high a concentration of glutamate, that is, of the normally occurring form, α-glutamate, may interfere with the metabolic transformations in which this amino acid is involved. The β-form of the amino acid is less reactive, for instance, it cannot take part in transamination reactions or protein synthesis, and therefore it may be the preferred form of the amino acid for accumulation to high concentrations. β-amino acids are in fact highly stable in the cell, showing very low rates of metabolic turnover compared to the corresponding α-amino acids.

The anionic osmolytes found at high concentrations in cells of halophilic archaea provide a charge counterbalance for the high amounts of positive charge generated by potassium ion. Polyanionic osmolytes like sulfotrehalose, TCH, and cDPG allow counterbalancing of potassium's positive charge with fewer numbers of solute particles. Thus, their total concentrations typically are well below the very high $[K^+]_i$ found in extremely halophilic archaea. In a later section of this chapter we consider the effects of high $[K^+]_i$ on the proteins of these organisms and the varied roles played by polyanionic organic solutes in helping cells deal with several forms of water stress.

We now turn to a consideration of more "normal" organisms, to begin evaluating why it is generally advantageous to keep inorganic ions at low and stable concentrations and to use certain organic osmolytes as the variable solutes during osmotic stress.

OSMOLYTE COMPATIBILITY WITH MACROMOLECULAR STRUCTURE AND FUNCTION

High and Variable Concentrations of Inorganic Ions Are Perturbing of Cellular Function

To develop an understanding of the rationales underlying the selection of the particular types of organic osmolytes found in cells, it is appropriate to examine in more detail the question of why most cells do not restrict their osmoregulatory responses to adjustments in concentrations of inorganic ions like K^+. If the origin of cells took place in a marine environment in which ambient concentrations of inorganic ions were high, would it not have "made sense" to exploit these ions for volume regulation in osmoconforming cells? The concentrations of organic compounds in the environment of the first cells were no doubt very low, so extracting these compounds from seawater likely would have represented an energetically costly activity. Moreover, any useful organic molecules that could be obtained from the environment would likely have been drawn into biosynthetic or ATP-generating pathways. Many of the most prevalent organic osmolytes are important not only for their contributions to volume regulation, but also for their roles in biosynthesis and generation of ATP. For instance, free amino acids, polyols, and sugars serve as important building blocks for larger molecules (proteins, lipids, nucleotides, and storage polysaccharides) and they can be catabolized to generate ATP. Why, then, do so many organisms exploit these otherwise useful organic molecules rather than "cheap" inorganic ions as their principal osmotic agents?

An initial answer to this question is given by data found in the four panels of figure 6.3. Each data set illustrates the effects of one or more inorganic ions on the activity of a physiological process. In sum, these data provide a strong case for the lack of fitness of inorganic ions as osmolytes whose concentrations are varied under water stress.

Protein synthesis in mammalian cells

The upper-left panel of figure 6.3 shows how variations in the concentrations of KCl or K-acetate affect the incorporation of radiolabeled lysine into newly synthesized proteins in mouse L-cells (Weber et al., 1977). Both potassium salts stimulate protein synthesis up to a certain salt concentration, with the acetate salt having a higher optimal concentration and higher final degree of stimulation than KCl. Above the opti-

mal salt concentration, rates of protein synthesis fall sharply, especially in the case of KCl.

These data illustrate several important aspects of how salts can affect physiological processes. First, many processes manifest dependence on ionic strength and/or on a particular type of ion. The peak stimulation of protein synthesis by potassium acetate and KCl is found at K^+ concentrations similar to those found in most cells (figure 6.1). Second, salts differ in their effects on physiological processes. The differences observed between the chloride and acetate potassium salts show that the inorganic counterion Cl^- is substantially more inhibitory of protein synthesis than the acetate ion. Chloride ion commonly perturbs biochemical processes, and, perhaps for this reason, concentrations of Cl^- are relatively low in most types of cells compared to osmotically dominant solutes, including $[K^+]$ (figure 6.1). This fact points to a practical lesson: to perform physiological and biochemical experiments that are intended to simulate what takes place in the cell, KCl is a poor choice of salt to use in experimental media. Organic anions like acetate are much more similar to the anions found within cells than is Cl^-, and for this reason they represent a better choice for medium design.

The components of the translational machinery that are perturbed by inorganic ions include the messenger RNA (mRNA) that is being translated into protein. High salt concentrations stabilize hairpin-type secondary structure in the 5'-leader sequences of certain mRNAs, and these configurations of the message preclude access of the ribosome to the site of initiation of translation (Kozak, 1988). Not all mRNAs respond in this manner; for instance, messages for heat-shock proteins have lengthy and unstructured 5'-leader sequences that do not assume the inhibitory configurations seen for many other mRNAs in the presence of high salt (Kozak, 1988). Therefore, perturbation of the cell by high salinity may lead not only to inhibition of the overall level of protein synthesis taking place, but also to shifts in the relative amounts of different types of proteins being translated. Note that under various types of stress, the synthesis of heat-shock proteins may become dominant as an emergency

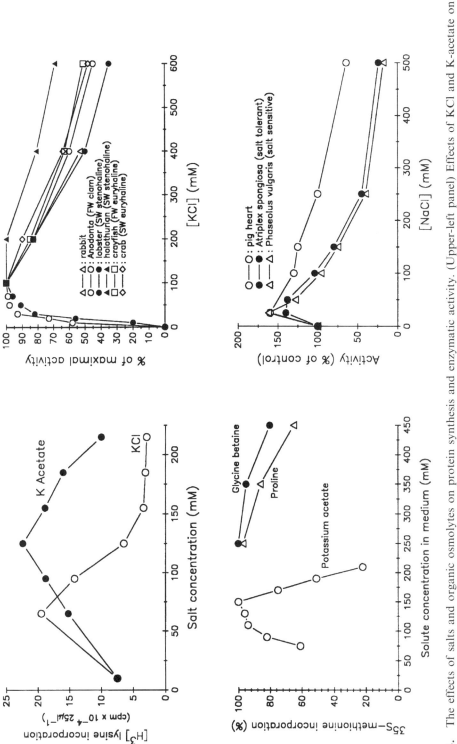

Figure 6.3. The effects of salts and organic osmolytes on protein synthesis and enzymatic activity. (Upper-left panel) Effects of KCl and K-acetate on protein synthesis by a cell-free translation system prepared from mouse L cells (after Weber et al., 1977). (Lower-left panel) Effects of K-acetate, glycine betaine, and proline on protein synthesis by a cell-free translation system prepared from wheatgerm and using wheat leaf mRNA (after Wyn-Jones, 1984). (Upper-right panel) Effects of different concentrations of KCl on the maximal velocity of pyruvate kinase reactions catalyzed by PKs isolated from animals with diverse osmotic characteristics (after Bowlus and Somero, 1979). (Lower-right panel) Effects of different concentrations of NaCl on activities of malate dehydrogenase homologs from pig heart, *Phaseolus vulgaris* (salt-sensitive plant), and *Atriplex spongiosa* (salt-tolerant plant) (after Greenway and Osmond, 1972). (Figure modified after Somero and Yancey, 1997.)

233

response to ensure that the native structures of proteins are maintained (see chapter 7).

Protein synthesis in cells of a vascular plant

The lower-left panel of figure 6.3 provides data that support the points just made about the effects of inorganic ions. It also offers an initial glimpse into the superiority of organic osmolytes for use in osmoconforming species. Here, the effects of potassium acetate and two commonly occurring organic osmolytes, glycine betaine and proline (figure 6.2), on protein synthesis in a cell-free system prepared from wheatgerm are shown (Wyn-Jones, 1984). As in the case of protein synthesis in mouse L cells, potassium acetate is stimulating of protein synthesis at concentrations in the physiological range, but inhibitory at higher concentrations. The effects of K-acetate in the wheat system are extremely similar to those found in the mammalian system, an illustration of a key point about osmolyte effects: they are generally similar for a common process (protein synthesis, in this case) across most taxa.

The effects of glycine betaine and proline differ strikingly from those of potassium acetate. Both organic osmolytes permit high rates of protein synthesis at relatively high osmolyte concentrations compared to potassium acetate. Although both organic osmolytes exhibit an optimal effect near 250 mM, even at a concentration of 450 mM protein synthesis is able to proceed at between 60 and 80% of maximal rate. Note, too, the relative effectiveness of the methylammonium osmolyte glycine betaine and the amino acid proline. As will be observed in many other contexts in the sections that follow, all organic osmolytes are not created equal.

Activity of pyruvate kinase (PK) from diverse animals

The similarity in the effects of a given solute on homologous biochemical systems from species with widely different intracellular osmolalities is shown by the data in the upper-right panel of figure 6.3. Pyruvate kinase homologs from a mammal, freshwater clam, and both stenohaline and euryhaline marine invertebrates show

extremely similar responses to KCl, despite a five- to tenfold difference in cellular osmolality among these species (Bowlus and Somero, 1979). As in the case of the protein synthetic reactions shown in this figure, potassium is activating and shows a maximal degree of activation at concentrations of 100 to 150 mM, that is, at K^+ concentrations typical of the intracellular milieu of most species.

Malate dehydrogenase activity in a mammal and plants

The lower-right panel of figure 6.3 presents data on the effects of NaCl on activity of MDH from pig heart and two vascular plants that differ in salt tolerance (Greenway and Osmond, 1972). Despite NaCl not being a physiologically appropriate salt to use to examine salt effects, these results do illustrate some important points. First, as shown by the comparison of *Atriplex spongiosa* (salt tolerant) and *Phaseolus vulgaris* (salt sensitive), the salt tolerance of the whole plant is not mirrored in differences in sensitivity to salt by homologous enzymes. The similarities of the MDHs from these differently salt-adapted plants is likely a reflection of the fact that the inorganic ion concentrations of the intracellular space in which MDH is located is highly similar in both species. Second, the effect of NaCl on the enzyme from pig heart is generally lower than in the case of the two plant MDHs. This difference could merely be a consequence of phylogeny, that is, of differences between mammalian and vascular plant homologs of a protein that have nothing whatsoever to do with adaptation to salinity.

These four experiments, performed with biochemical systems from a considerable variety of taxa, illustrate an important point: whereas inorganic ions like K^+ may be required for the activities of many physiological and biochemical processes (for instance in the case of PK, which is inactive in the absence of K^+), the curves defining the responses of these processes to variations in K^+ concentration typically show sharp optima, with activity of the process decreasing rapidly as ion concentrations surpass physiological values. The patterns of concentration-dependent activities shown in figure 6.3 document the nonsuitability of inorganic ions as osmolytes to be used at widely varying concentrations under conditions of water stress. Were euryhaline osmoconformers to rely on inorganic ions as the primary osmolyte for cell volume regulation, osmotic stress likely would lead to pervasive disruption of metabolic processes. It appears impossible to design proteins whose structures and functions are unaffected by variations in concentrations of inorganic ions. As we will learn momentarily, when euryhalinity is achieved through osmoconformity, nonperturbing organic solutes constitute the major portion of the osmolyte pool.

An Exception to the Rules: Salt-Requiring Proteins of Halophilic Archaea

There is one group of organisms that disobeys one of the most basic rules of osmotic adaptation, namely, the rule that proteins do not become differently salt-adapted in species with different internal osmolarities. As discussed above, extremely halophilic members of the Archaea are unique in accumulating enormous concentrations of inorganic ions, chiefly K^+, to attain osmotic equilibrium with their highly saline habitats. Estimated concentrations of K^+ in the cells of these extreme halophiles range up to 3–5 M, that is, up to values 20- to 50-fold higher than in "normal" cells. As the relationships illustrated in figure 6.3 suggest, proteins from "normal" species would find such high concentrations of potassium ion extremely inhibitory. In fact, concentrations of K^+ (with an appropriate organic counterion) in the range of 3–5 M might precipitate (salt out of solution) many proteins of "normal" species. At the very least, such high salt concentrations would render "normal" proteins so rigid that their functions would be severely compromised. The latter effect may explain some of the salt inhibition seen at even lower concentrations, in the range of a few tenths of a mole per liter.

The striking contrasts between the effects of salts on enzymes of extremely halophilic archaea and those of organisms in which $[K^+]_i$ lies in the more typical range of 0.1 to 0.2 M are evident from a comparison of data in figure 6.4

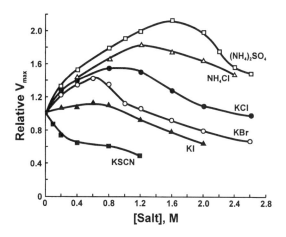

Figure 6.4. The effects of different inorganic salts on activity of malate dehydrogenase from an extremely halophilic archaeon (unpublished data of L. Borowitkza and G. Somero).

with those found in the lower-right panel of figure 6.3. Malate dehydrogenase of the extremely halophilic archaeon exhibits maximal activity at a KCl concentration near 1 M. In contrast, MDHs of pig heart and two green plants have maximal activities near 50 mM NaCl, and all three MDHs show reduced activity as salt concentration is increased up to 500 mM (figure 6.3).

The data of figure 6.4 raise additional questions. What aspects of the structures of proteins of extremely halophilic archaea account for the strong dependence of enzymatic activity on salt concentration? Why does the activation of the halophile's MDH require such a high concentration of KCl? Why does inhibition by salt occur at the highest salt concentrations measured? What accounts for the large differences in the effects of different types of salts on MDH activity of this archaeon? When we return to these questions in a later section of this chapter, we will find that their answers reflect the fact that proteins of halophilic archaea are subject to the same rules concerning water–micromolecular–macromolecular interactions that apply to "normal" organisms, despite what the marked differences in salt effects on MDHs might suggest. The unique aspect of the halophilic archaeon's solution to life at high salinity is the fact that adaptation to high internal salt has been effected by changes in protein amino acid composition. Unlike other types of organisms, the burden of adaptation has fallen on macromolecular structure, not on the composition of the internal milieu.

Compatibility of Organic Osmolytes with Biochemical Systems: Micromolecular Evolution Solves a Problem for Macromolecules

If inorganic ions at high and varying concentrations can be regarded as noncompatible with stable biochemical function, then the expression *compatible solute* is a fitting descriptor of the effects of most organic osmolytes. The expression was coined by Austen Brown (1978) to describe the types of solute effects (more appropriately, the "noneffects") that are illustrated in figure 6.5. These data illustrate why organic osmolytes, in general, are an excellent choice for use in osmotic regulation by species characterized by high and/or varying intracellular osmolalities. These data also show that organic osmolytes differ among themselves in terms of the strengths of their effects, differences that are largely independent of the biochemical system being analyzed and the phylogeny of the organism from which the study system is taken.

Michaelis–Menten constant (K_m) of phosphoenol pyruvate (PEP)

The binding of enzyme and substrate to form the enzyme–substrate (E-S) complex is the critical first step in enzymatic reactions. Binding is commonly measured by determining the apparent Michaelis–Menten constant (K_m) of ligand, the concentration of ligand (substrate or cofactor) that yields one-half the maximal velocity (V_{max}). K_m values typically are highly sensitive to physical (temperature and hydrostatic pressure) and chemical (ionic strength and pH) conditions, and because of this several types of adaptive processes function to conserve K_m values in ranges that are optimal for enzymatic activity. Although changes in amino acid sequence play key roles in setting appropriate K_m values, conserving the intrinsic binding ability of the protein often requires appropriate

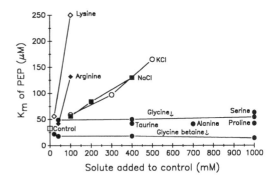

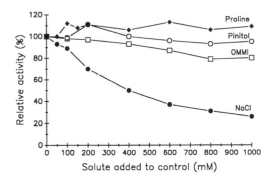

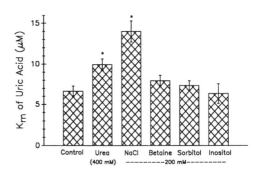

Figure 6.5. Compatibility of organic osmolytes with enzyme function. (Upper panel) Pyruvate kinase of the marine crab *Pachygrapsus crassipes*. The effects of KCl and NaCl and several organic solutes on the K_m of phosphoenol pyruvate (PEP) (modified after Bowlus and Somero, 1979). (Middle panel) Malate dehydrogenase of the mangrove (*Rhizophora mangle*). Effects of NaCl and three organic osmolytes (the amino acid proline and the polyols pinitol and OMMI) on catalytic activity (modified after Sommer et al., 1990). (Bottom panel) Effects of NaCl and four osmolytes found in mammalian kidney (urea, glycine betaine, sorbitol, and inositol) on the K_m of uric acid of uricase (modified after Yancey, 1992). (Figure modified after Somero and Yancey, 1997.)

adjustments in the milieu surrounding the enzyme. Here, we examine the roles of organic osmolytes in this important type of conservation.

In euryhaline osmoconformers, the ability to retain a stable capacity for forming the E-S complex under conditions of changing intracellular osmolarity is facilitated by use of compatible organic osmolytes (figure 6.5, upper panel). As shown for the glycolytic enzyme PK from the marine crab *Pachygrapsus crassipes*, binding of the substrate phosphoenol pyruvate to PK is strongly perturbed by inorganic salts (KCl and NaCl, which show similar effects) but is not perturbed by most of the organic solutes tested (Bowlus and Somero, 1979). Glycine, taurine, alanine, serine, and proline have similar and very minimal effects on the K_m of PEP. The methylamine glycine betaine, unlike the other organic osmolytes, slightly lowers K_m of PEP, albeit the effect is minor at the concentrations of glycine betaine likely to be found in cells (figure 6.1). These six organic compounds, then, can be viewed as compatible with PK function: they can be employed at widely varying concentrations, including concentrations up to 1 M, without having a marked effect on this kinetic parameter.

Merely by being a low-molecular-mass organic solute does not make a molecule a compatible osmolyte, however. Lysine and arginine are both strongly perturbing of binding of PEP to PK, with lysine having the stronger effect. A major distinction between lysine and arginine, on the one hand, and glycine, serine, proline, alanine, and glycine betaine, on the other, is that lysine and arginine possess a net positive charge. These two amino acids thus are able to form complexes with negatively charged solutes like PEP and other phosphorylated intermediates of metabolism, thereby reducing the effective free concentrations of these anionic substrates and cofactors in the solution bathing the enzyme. In effect, high levels of free arginine create a situation of competition between arginine residues in the ligand binding sites of proteins and free arginine in solution. Arginine residues are found in the binding sites of many enzymes

that bind phosphorylated intermediates like PEP, ADP, ATP, or NADH. High concentrations of free arginine, by competing for these anionic ligands with arginine residues found in binding sites of enzymes, make it necessary for higher total ligand concentrations to be present to keep the enzymes half-saturated with ligand. Compatible solutes, by failing to interact with negatively charged ligands, allow metabolic systems to function in the presence of lower total concentrations of anionic substrates, cofactors, and modulators than would be the case if a positively charged and, therefore, noncompatible solute like arginine were used as an osmolyte. To a certain extent, use of compatible solutes that do not form complexes in solution with charged ligands like PEP help to reduce solvent capacity problems for the cell.

Lysine also may form complexes with anionic ligands and thereby increase K_m values. In addition, lysine may have an unfavorable effect on protein structure. Because it has a considerable hydrophobic moment, it may interact with hydrophobic sites on the protein, leading to perturbation of structure. Compatible solutes lack a propensity for interacting with peptide backbone linkages or amino acid side-chains, as discussed later.

The low-molecular-mass organic molecules found in the cell may in some cases reflect selection for compatible end-products of metabolism. Certain metabolic end-products are potentially highly reactive, and these may require chemical modification to allow them to be accumulated to high levels without perturbing metabolism. An example is the glycolytic end-product octopine, which is a common terminal metabolite of anaerobic glycolysis in certain types of invertebrates (see chapter 3). Octopine is a condensation product that forms between pyruvate generated in glycolysis and arginine that is produced when arginine phosphate donates its phosphate group to ATP through the arginine phosphokinase reaction. Whereas arginine is strongly perturbing of enzymes (figure 6.5, upper panel), octopine is a compatible solute that can be accumulated to high levels without disrupting enzymatic function (Bowlus and Somero, 1979).

Activity of MDH

The responses of MDH from a vascular plant (the mangrove tree, *Rhizophora mangle*) to NaCl and three organic osmolytes (the amino acid proline and two polyols, pinitol and 1D-1-O-methyl-muco-inositol, OMMI) provide a further illustration of the compatibility of organic osmolytes with enzyme function. In this case compatibility is illustrated for the optimal velocity of the MDH reaction (figure 6.5, middle panel; Sommer et al., 1990). The three organic osmolytes, all of which are found in vascular plants, have minor effects on MDH activity, whereas NaCl is again seen to be strongly inhibitory.

K_m of uric acid for mammalian uricase

A third example of solute compatibility focuses on a mammalian enzyme, uricase, from an organ, the kidney, that experiences high and variable osmolality (figure 6.5, bottom panel; Yancey, 1992). Unlike most organs of mammals, the kidney has regions in which osmolalities may rise to very high values due to the synthesis (in liver) and excretion in the kidney of large amounts of urea during protein catabolism. Under conditions of water stress, the osmolality in the kidney's inner medulla may attain exceptionally high values for a mammal; urea concentrations alone may exceed 1–2 M (table 6.1).

The effects of five osmolytes on the K_m of uric acid for kidney uricase reflect patterns seen for solute effects on K_m of PEP for pyruvate kinase of a crustacean. Here, then, is a further illustration of the point that the effects of a solute on a protein are largely independent of the species from which the protein is derived. Sodium chloride at 200 mM is significantly perturbing, raising the K_m of uric acid by more than 100%. Urea, too, has a significantly perturbing effect on K_m, whereas the two polyols (sorbitol and inositol) and the methylamine (glycine betaine) do not. The observation that urea, unlike the other four classes of organic osmolytes, is disruptive of protein function raises several questions. First, why is this solute exploited as an osmolyte in osmotically concen-trated species like marine elasmobranchs and coelacanths? Second, in the mammalian kidney and in urea exploiting fishes, what types of adaptations are present to offset the perturbing effects of urea? Answers to these questions will substantially broaden our perspective on the evolution of the internal milieu and provide a more complete background for the subsequent physical–chemical analysis of protein–osmo-lyte–water interactions.

Counteraction Among Solutes— Algebraic Additivity of Osmolyte Effects: Urea–Methylamine Interactions

In the examples of osmolyte effects on proteins given up to this point, only a single type of osmolyte has been used in each separate treatment, for instance, in studying effects of different solutes on K_m values and enzymatic activities (figure 6.5). Because the cell contains a large number of different osmolytes, this is a simplistic in-vitro approach that may fall short of elucidating the properties of the protein as it functions in vivo. Thus, it would seem appropriate to perform in-vitro experiments with physiological mixtures of all dominant osmolytes. This more realistic approach will be seen to be especially important in cases where the effects of different osmolytes are in diametric opposition to each other.

In urea-rich fishes and in the inner medulla of the mammalian kidney, there characteristically is found a set of methylammonium solutes whose effects on proteins are opposite to those of urea (figure 6.6). Different methylamines predominate in different species. For instance, TMAO and glycine betaine are the most prevalent methylamines in elasmobranchs, and glycerophosphorylcholine (GPC) may be especially important in mammalian kidneys (figures 6.1 and 6.2). Despite interspecific differences in the types of methylamines present in cells, a common effect is noted: when urea and methylamine solutes are both included in experimental media, an *algebraic additivity* generally is observed in their influences on proteins. Thus, if urea shifts a property in one direction and a methylamine shifts it in the opposite direction, the net change in the property in a

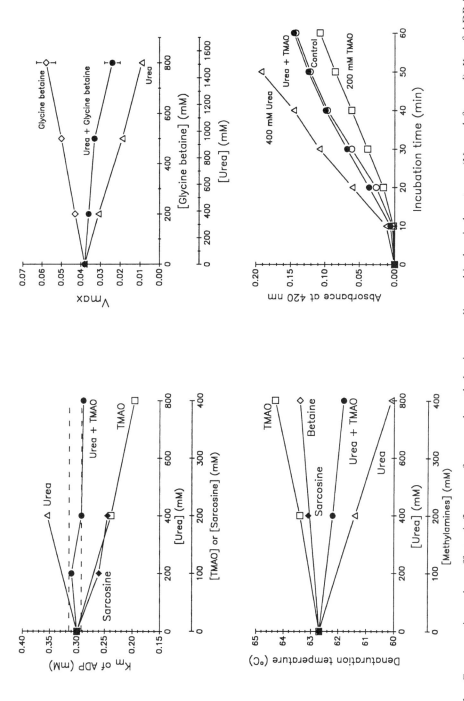

Figure 6.6. Counteracting solute effects: influences of urea and methylamines on diverse biochemical systems. (Upper-left panel) K_m of ADP for pyruvate kinase of the stingray (*Urolophis halleri*) The horizontal dashed lines bound the 95% confidence intervals for the control (no urea or methylamine) K_m value. (Figure modified after Yancey and Somero, 1980.) (Upper-right panel) Effects of urea and methylamines on the V_{max} of the reaction catalyzed by argininosuccinase from porcine kidney (unpublished data of T. Arnell, M. Blykowski, and P.H. Yancey; modified after Somero and Yancey, 1997). (Lower-left panel) Effects of urea and methylamines on thermal stability of bovine pancreatic ribonuclease (modified after Yancey and Somero, 1979). (Lower-right panel) Labeling of sulfhydryl groups of mammalian glutamate dehydrogenase by 4-chloro-7-nitobenzofurazan (Nbf-Cl), as measured by increase in absorbance at 420 nm (modified after Yancey and Somero, 1979). (Figure modified after Somero and Yancey, 1997.)

solution containing the appropriate ratio of urea and methylamines may be nil. This phenomenon has been termed *solute counteraction* (see Yancey et al., 1982).

Counteraction on enzyme function and structure

Counteracting effects of urea and methylamines have been observed for K_m values (figure 6.6, upper left) and maximal velocities (V_{max}) (figure 6.6, upper right) of enzymatic systems. For most enzymes so studied, urea increases and methylamines decrease K_m values. For V_{max}, physiological concentrations of urea often (but not always) reduce enzymatic activities, whereas methylamines often (but again not always) stimulate activity. As would be expected when algebraic additivity is present, these counteracting effects on kinetic properties are strongly dependent on the concentration ratios of the osmolytes. When the physiological ratio of the urea concentration to the total concentration of all methylamine species is employed in vitro, counteraction is typically maximal. This physiological ratio varies somewhat among species, but in most shallow-living elasmobranchs and in coelacanths, the ratio of [urea] to [Σmethylamines] is approximately 1.5:1 to 2:1.

It is noteworthy that deep-sea elasmobranchs may accumulate significantly different [urea]:[Σmethylamine] ratios than shallow-living relatives, with [TMAO] exceeding [urea] in the deepest occurring species (P.H. Yancey, personal communication). Some deep-sea teleost fishes and invertebrates (shrimp, crabs, bivalves, and anemones) also accumulate high levels of TMAO relative to shallow-living relatives (Gillett et al., 1997; Kelly and Yancey, 1999). Elevated concentrations of TMAO in deep-sea animals are viewed as a possible mechanism for offsetting the perturbing effects of elevated hydrostatic pressure on proteins (Gillett et al., 1997; Yancey and Siebenaller, 1999). Perturbation of protein structure (Yancey and Siebenaller, 1999) and function (Gillett et al., 1997) by elevated pressure can be offset by physiological concentrations of TMAO. Thus, this osmolyte may not only counteract the effects of a chemical perturbant, urea,

but also the disruption of protein function and structure by a physical variable, hydrostatic pressure.

The stabilizing effects of TMAO and the counteracting effects of urea and methylamines on protein structure have been seen in a number of studies that have employed a variety of types of proteins and different types of structure-perturbing forces. Thermal stability of proteins is reduced by urea and increased by methylamines (figure 6.6, lower left). For bovine pancreatic ribonuclease (RNase), for example, increasing concentrations of urea reduced the temperature at which heat denaturation occurred. In contrast, all methylamines studied increased the temperature of heat denaturation. The effects of the three methylamines, TMAO, glycine betaine, and sarcosine (*N*-methyl glycine), differed: the extent of stabilization was proportional to the number of methyl groups attached to the nitrogen atom, with TMAO having the strongest effect.

The opposing effects of urea and methylamines (TMAO) on protein structure are further shown by an experiment that followed the labeling of sulfhydryl (–SH) groups in a large multimeric protein, glutamate dehydrogenase (GDH) (figure 6.6, lower right). In this study, the compound 4-chloro-7-nitobenzofurazan (Nbf-Cl) was used to covalently tag –SH groups as they gained exposure to the solvent during fluctuations ("breathing") of protein structure. Proteins in solution exist in a dynamic state of structural fluctuation (see chapter 7). Numerous configurational microstates exist among the proteins in a population, and some of these configurations transiently expose to solvent side-chains that normally are buried in the protein's interior core. Conditions that tend to make proteins less rigid, for instance, elevated temperatures, extremes of pH, and structure-disrupting solutes like guanidinium hydrochloride and urea, increase the likelihood of a protein existing in a partially unfolded configuration in which buried side-chains are exposed to solvent. Conversely, physical and chemical conditions that favor a compact, rigid protein structure will lead to reduced exposure to solvent of side-chains normally found within the protein's interior. The effects of urea and TMAO on labeling of GDH illustrate these differential effects of destabilizing and stabilizing forces: 400 mM urea makes GDH more flexible and thereby allows increased access of Nbf-Cl to –SH groups, as shown by an increased rate of labeling of the protein by Nbf-Cl; TMAO at 200 mM significantly reduces the rate of labeling. When urea and TMAO are present at a 2:1 concentration ratio, the rate of labeling does not differ from the control rate (neither urea nor TMAO in solution).

TMAO and urea also have offsetting effects on the assembly of protein subunits. For instance, Tseng and Graves (1998) showed that TMAO enhanced the polymerization of microtubules and that inhibition of microtubule assembly by urea could be offset by TMAO.

These studies of protein structure, like those of urea and methylamine effects on enzyme kinetic parameters, reveal that physiological mixtures of counteracting solutes achieve essentially the same end result as use of compatible solutes: regulating cell volume through adjusting concentrations of compatible solutes or counteracting solutes (at the appropriate ratio of concentrations) conserves critical aspects of protein structure and function as well as cell volume per se.

Counteraction at the cellular level

Experimental manipulation of osmolyte concentrations in living cells has allowed a powerful extension of the types of in vitro studies discussed above. Figure 6.7 illustrates the effects of NaCl, urea, glycerol, inositol, and glycine betaine on mammalian kidney cells in culture (Yancey and Burg, 1990). The effects of these solutes on the cells were quantified by determining the colony-forming (cloning) efficiencies of the cells, defined as the number of colonies formed relative to the number of cells initially plated in culture.

Increasing the concentration of NaCl in the medium led to a steady decrease in cloning efficiency. Likewise, the two compatible solutes glycerol and inositol led to decreased cloning efficiency as their concentrations were elevated. Urea and glycine betaine showed complex indi-

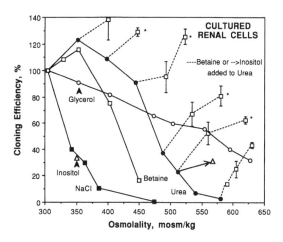

Figure 6.7. Effects of NaCl and organic osmolytes (urea, glycine betaine, inositol, and glycerol) on colony-forming (cloning) efficiency of canine kidney cells. Colony-forming efficiencies are the numbers of colonies formed per number of single cells seeded on growth plates, relative to control conditions (no test solutes added to the medium, whose osmolarity was 305 mosmolal). Open squares connected by dashed lines refer to addition of glycine betaine to cultures in which urea is also present. Asterisks indicate a 2:1 ratio of urea to glycine betaine. (Modified after Yancey and Burg, 1990.)

vidual effects as well as significant counteraction. Betaine alone at concentrations up to 50 mM increased cloning efficiency, but higher levels of betaine were inhibitory. At 50 mM and 100 mM concentrations, urea by itself increased cloning efficiency, but as in the case of betaine, increases in concentration above the optimal value were inhibitory. When betaine was added to cultures containing urea, a substantial enhancement of cloning efficiency was found in all cases. Up to conditions of 150 mM urea plus 75 mM glycine betaine, cloning efficiencies were higher than those found under control conditions (no added urea or glycine betaine and a total medium osmolality of 350 mosmolal). Counteraction of urea's effects by betaine was observed out to the highest osmolality used in the studies, 625 mosmolal, in which the concentrations of urea and glycine betaine were 275 mM and 50 mM, respectively.

These experiments with cells in culture demonstrate that the basic effects of solutes observed in simplified in-vitro systems are mirrored in many ways by the responses of intact cells to osmolytes. However, intact cells display a more complex response to solutes, for instance, a biphasic reaction to increasing concentrations of both urea and methylamines was observed.

Counteraction by organic osmolytes of effects of inorganic ions

Even though accumulation of inorganic ions such as K^+ is not a common long-term strategy during adaptation to increased salinity, transient increases in one or more inorganic ions may occur immediately after onset of hyperosmotic stress, before uptake or synthesis of organic osmolytes is completed. For example, in cells unable to maintain turgor, loss of water following exposure to hyperosmotic media will lead to increased concentrations of all solutes, including inorganic ions like K^+. During periods in which elevated levels of K^+ and other inorganic ions are transiently present in hyperosmotically stressed cells, organic osmolytes, notably certain methylamines, may confer some degree of protection of protein structure and function from perturbation by salt.

These types of protective effects are illustrated in figure 6.8, which shows how the free amino acid glycine and three methylamines, TMAO, glycine betaine, and sarcosine, affect the activity of a cyanobacterial (*Aphanothece halophytica*) ribulose-1,5-bisphosphate-carboxylase-oxygenase (RuBisCO) that has been inhibited 50% by elevated concentrations of KCl (Incharoensakdi et al., 1986). Glycine had no stimulatory effect, but instead further reduced RuBisCO activity as concentration was increased. All methylamines tested offset inhibition by KCl, and the strength of counteraction differed according to the degree of methylation of the nitrogen atom: TMAO > glycine betaine > sarcosine. Even the single methyl group of sarcosine (*N*-methyl glycine) gave this solute a protective effect that was absent with glycine itself.

Counteraction by methylamine osmolytes of salt perturbation of enzymatic activity, structures of contractile proteins, force development

by muscle fibers, and membrane-protein integrity have been reported in other studies (reviewed in Somero and Yancey, 1997). Counteraction by TMAO of the effects of high concentrations of inorganic ions also may be important in the context of freezing resistance in Antarctic fishes, which contain high concentrations of K^+, Na^+, and TMAO (Raymond and DeVries, 1998; see chapter 7). Free amino acids and their derivatives (taurine) and polyols also have been found to counteract some of the effects of inorganic ions on biochemical systems, at least in certain cases (Somero and Yancey, 1997). These instances of counteraction of the effects of inorganic ions should not be taken to imply that, in the presence of compatible organic osmolytes, the concentrations of inorganic ions such as K^+ could be allowed to vary widely during cell volume regulation. This is not the case, because in most instances the perturbing effects of inorganic ions cannot be offset by organic osmolytes. The latter solutes almost invariably play the dominant role in cell volume regulation once a new osmotic steady state is established.

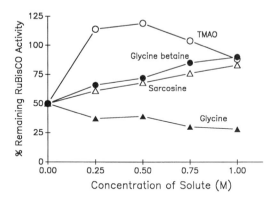

Figure 6.8. The effects of four organic osmolytes, glycerol, sarcosine, glycine betaine, and TMAO on salt-inhibited ribulose-1,5-bisphosphate-carboxylase-oxygenase (RuBisCO) activity of the cyanobacterium *Aphanothece halophytica*. The enzyme was placed in a solution containing KCl at a concentration sufficient to inhibit activity by 50%. Then, increasing concentrations of organic osmolytes were added to the assay medium, leading to restoration of activity. (Modified after Incharoensakdi et al., 1986.)

A beneficial function of urea: preventing covalent damage to DNA during hyperosmotic stress

Although most of the focus on solute effects on macromolecular systems has involved proteins, there is evidence that some of the patterns of solute accumulation reflect the dangers that high salt concentrations pose for the covalent structure of DNA. Using cultured mammalian kidney cells Kültz and Chakravarty (2001) showed that hyperosmotic stress could cause double strand breaks (dsb) in DNA. Hyperosmolality due to elevated [NaCl] in the culture medium caused the most dsb. Potassium chloride and mannitol led to less damage and, interestingly, no damage to DNA was found in cells exposed to elevated levels of urea.

The mechanisms underlying these different effects are not yet understood, but the physiological significance of urea reabsorption by kidney cells definitely is placed in a new perspective. Kültz and Chakravarty propose that the accumulation of high concentrations of urea rather than inorganic ions in kidney medullary cells under conditions in which highly concentrated urine is being produced reflects the dangers posed by inorganic ions in causing dsb. Urea, although not regarded as a compatible osmolyte in the context of protein–solute interactions, does appear to be compatible with DNA structure. The results of this study, which was the first to demonstrate the production of dsb under osmotic stress, suggest that protection of double-stranded nucleic acids, as well as proteins, may be a critical consideration in the development of osmolyte systems.

PHYSICAL CHEMISTRY OF PROTEIN–WATER–SOLUTE INTERACTIONS: PREFERENTIAL EXCLUSION AND SOLVOPHOBIA

Analysis of the physical–chemical principles underlying selection of organic osmolytes—and combinations thereof—involves a logically linked series of "why" questions. We have already addressed one "why" question above,

when we explained why organic osmolytes, rather than seemingly "cheap" inorganic ions like K^+, are the dominant solutes accumulated under water stress. The short answer to this question is that most organic osmolytes treat proteins kindly, perturbing neither structure nor function. We now are in a position to ask why most of these organic osmolytes (urea being the strong exception) are able to exert stabilizing effects on proteins and, in some cases, favorable effects on enzymatic kinetic properties like K_m values. What aspects of these osmolytes make them "fit" for accumulation at high levels within protein-rich cellular compartments? And, why are some osmolytes so much more effective than others in stabilizing proteins?

A Historical Perspective: Hofmeister and His Intellectual Heirs

The first systematic analysis of the effects of different solutes on proteins was performed by Hofmeister in the 1880s (Hofmeister, 1888). In addition to providing the first detailed evidence that salts differ in their effects on proteins, Hofmeister's data contained an important clue, but one discerned only many decades later, as to why certain types of low-molecular-mass organic molecules are especially fit for use at high concentrations during water stress. Hofmeister's pathbreaking studies showed that inorganic salts differed markedly in how they affected protein solubility in water. Some salts, for example, ammonium sulfate $((NH_4)_2SO_4)$ were strong precipitants, whereas other salts, for instance, sodium thiocyanate (NaSCN) were strong solubilizers of proteins. As more work was done to examine the effects of different salts on protein stability and solubility, a regular ranking of salts was discovered and this was termed the "Hofmeister Series" (figure 6.9). As in the case of the effects of organic osmolytes on proteins, the relative effects of different anions and cations in the Hofmeister Series were largely independent of the protein being examined. The consistency of Hofmeister Series effects on protein after protein suggested that some universal aspect of protein–water–solute inter-

⟨———Stabilizing   Destabilizing———⟩

ANIONS F^- PO_4^{3-} SO_4^{2-} CH_3COO^- Cl^- Br^- I^- SCN^-

CATIONS $(CH_3)_4N^+$ $(CH_3)_2NH_2^+$ NH_4^+ K^+ Na^+ Cs^+ Li^+ Mg^{2+} Ca^{2+} Ba^{2+}

Figure 6.9. The Hofmeister Series of ions: a ranking of organic and inorganic ions in terms of their effects on protein solubility and several features of water structure (see Collins and Washabaugh, 1985; Leberman and Soper, 1995; von Hippel and Schleich, 1969). Note that several of the stabilizing ions are incorporated into the structures of protein-stabilizing osmolytes (see text).

actions was responsible for these differential effects. Moreover, certain characteristics of the ions positioned on the stabilizing side of the Hofmeister Series allowed a new perspective to be gained on the raison d'être of compatible organic osmolytes.

This conceptual advance was made by Mary Clark (Clark, 1985), who pointed out similarities between certain of the protein-stabilizing ions of the Hofmeister Series and several chemical groups that commonly are present in organic osmolytes. For example, ammonium ion, tri- and dimethylammonium ions, and acetate ion are all constituents of organic osmolytes (figure 6.2). It would seem that the separate constituents of compatible amino acids (ammonium and acetate moieties) and methylammonium solutes could themselves have favorable effects on protein stability. Clark thus formulated a general hypothesis to account for the selection of organic osmolytes: natural selection favors accumulation of osmolytes with protein-stabilizing properties. Clark's hypothesis provided a partial answer to the question concerning why certain types of organic osmolytes are preferred in widely different species. However, it remained to be explained what physical–chemical mechanism (or mechanisms) conferred upon these osmolytes their favorable effects on proteins. Two alternatives seemed possible, a priori: stabilizers bound to proteins and thereby enhanced protein stability, or stability was conferred in the absence of binding through effects mediated by water.

Serge Timasheff made the next major contribution to this analysis (Timasheff, 1992, 1998). Through a series of elegant and extremely difficult dialysis experiments, he showed that *stabi-*

lizing osmolytes tend to be excluded from the water immediately surrounding a protein (figure 6.10). Stability thus arose from osmolyte exclusion, not binding. Using Timasheff's terminology, when a protein is bathed in a solution containing a stabilizing solute (here, the term cosolvent is commonly used in place of solute), the protein is "preferentially hydrated," that is, water, rather than a mixture of water and cosolvent, tends to coat the protein. The stabilizing cosolvent is "preferentially excluded" from the water hydrating the protein. Exclusion of the stabilizing cosolvent is not complete (figure 6.10), but there does exist a significant disparity between the concentration of the cosolvent in the water immediately adjacent to the protein and in the so-called "bulk" water of the solution. In contrast to stabilizing cosolvents, denaturing cosolvents like urea and guanidinium ion interact strongly with proteins and readily penetrate into the water surrounding the protein. Thus, binding of cosolvent is correlated with destabilization of structure.

Why should an osmolyte such as TMAO or glycine betaine that is a stabilizing cosolvent be able to enhance protein stability merely because it is excluded from the water surrounding the protein's surface? Timasheff's general answer to this question is phrased in thermodynamic terms and, for this reason, does not initially focus on the chemical mechanisms that cause preferential exclusion; these mechanisms are diverse and will be treated subsequently. The thermodynamic argument presented by Timasheff involves the change in entropy that accompanies the addition of a stabilizing cosolvent to an aqueous solution containing protein molecules. The basic argument is as follows.

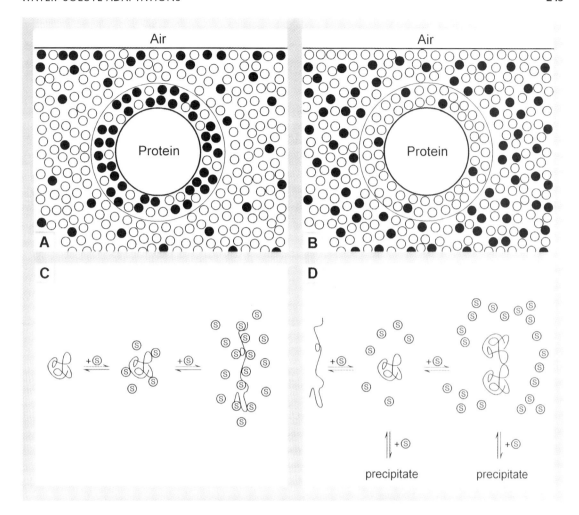

Figure 6.10. Effects of stabilizing and destabilizing solutes (cosolvents) on proteins: the "preferential hydration" model of Timasheff (1992). (A and B) An illustration of the distributions of water (open symbols) and a cosolvent (solid symbols) following equilibrium dialysis of a protein. The dialysis membrane is represented by a circle concentric with the innermost circle, which represents the surface of the protein molecule. The cosolvent in (A) is denaturing, that in (B) is stabilizing. Note in (A) that the denaturant is concentrated within the dialysis membrane, close to the protein surface, to which the denaturing cosolvent binds. Note in (B) how the stabilizing cosolvent is preferentially excluded from the area near the protein. That is, in the presence of a stabilizing cosolvent the protein is preferentially hydrated (surrounded by water, not cosolvent). Note in (B) the decidedly nonrandom distribution of stabilizing cosolvent molecules, which are forced to cluster in the volume of water outside of the hydration sphere of the protein. Stabilizing cosolvents often increase the surface tension of water and thus tend to be excluded from the air–water interface, as shown in (B). (C and D) An elaboration of the model of protein–solute effects presented in (A) and (B). In (C), a denaturing cosolvent (S) is capable of binding to the protein and favoring unfolding to the denatured state. Because the denaturant binds effectively to groups throughout the protein, for instance, to the peptide backbone linkage (the major site of binding; see Wang and Bolen, 1997) and side-chains, the more surface area exposed to solution, the more the free energy of the system is reduced. (D) shows how increasing concentrations of a stabilizing cosolvent (S), a solute that is excluded from water near the protein's surface, favor the folding of the protein into a native state and enhance polymerization of subunits into a multimeric (dimeric) state. At high cosolvent concentrations, the precipitation of the protein occurs. (Modified after Low, 1985.)

Because a stabilizing cosolvent is strongly excluded from the water near the protein's surface—for whatever underlying reason—the cosolvent must be accommodated primarily in the remaining volume of the solution. Consequently, the cosolvent is not distributed as randomly as it would be if it were to have access to the entire solution. In other words, the entropy of the solution containing the protein–cosolvent mixture is reduced because of the restricted distribution of the cosolvent. As Timasheff points out, this bad situation in terms of entropy would be made even worse if the protein were to unfold and expose additional surface area to the solvent and cosolvent. Were this to happen, an even larger fraction of the total volume of the solution would be inaccessible to cosolvent, and the entropy of the system would decrease even further. In other words, to maximize the entropy of the system (water + cosolvent + protein), the protein must attain a minimal volume (= minimal surface of contact with the medium). Stabilizing cosolvents thus favor a compact state of proteins and, as cosolvent concentration rises to very high levels, the precipitation of proteins is favored to maximally reduce the contact area between protein and the solvent plus cosolvent system.

Timasheff's dialysis experiments, as portrayed in figure 6.10, provided a precise picture of where stabilizing and destabilizing cosolvents occur in a protein-containing aqueous solution. Stabilizing cosolvents distributed away from the protein (B, D), whereas structure-destabilizing (denaturing) solutes like urea bound to the protein exergonically, favoring maximization of the protein's surface area (= maximal number of binding sites) (A, C). These experiments clearly delineated the differences between stabilizing and destabilizing cosolvents. Whatever the underlying mechanism of preferential exclusion, all stabilizing cosolvents tend to be restricted from water near the protein, whereas all destabilizing cosolvents interact favorably (exergonically) with the protein surface.

What is it about the water near the surface of a protein that tends to favor exclusion of stabilizing cosolvents? There is no single answer to this question because a number of different mechanisms may underlie the observed preferential exclusion of stabilizing cosolvents (see Timasheff, 1992, 1998). One mechanism is *surface tension*, which is the amount of energy it takes to expand a surface by unit area ($N m^{-1}$). Surface tension in water derives from the hydrogen bonding that occurs among highly polar water molecules. If the surface tension of water is enhanced by the presence of a protein, and if a particular solute tends to be excluded from water having a high surface tension, then preferential exclusion of the solute from the immediate vicinity of the protein may arise. Likewise, a cosolvent that interacts strongly with water may increase surface tension, and reduce the probability that the solute will be able to penetrate the organized water on the protein's surface. Many compatible solutes, for instance sugars and polyols, increase the surface tension of water. In fact, most compatible osmolytes, K^+ being an exception, are *kosmotropes*, water structure builders that would be expected to increase surface tension.

A second mechanism of preferential exclusion is based on the *steric properties* of the protein and cosolvent. The three-dimensional structure of the cosolvent may hinder interactions with the protein surface. High-molecular-weight cosolvents like polyethylene glycols (PEGs) and other proteins may be preferentially excluded through this steric hindrance mechanism.

A third mechanism involves *charge repulsion* between protein and cosolvent. The fact that most organic osmolytes lack a net charge suggests that this mechanism is of less general significance than the effects of surface tension and steric hindrance.

Side-Chains versus the Peptide Backbone: Which Component Is More Important in Cosolvent Effects?

The next question to be addressed carries the mechanistic analysis one step further by asking what components of proteins—the side-chains or the peptide backbone linkages—are responsible for solute effects on structure. The answer to this question, which comes from studies done by D. Wayne Bolen and his colleagues (Baskakov and Bolen, 1998; Qu et al., 1998), may seem surprising in light of the discussion given earlier about the different solubilities of the side-chains of the 20 amino acids and the importance of the hydrophobic effect in governing protein folding. Based on what has been said about the critical role played by the burial of hydrophobic groups in the interior of a protein, one might expect to find that the effects of osmolytes can be traced to the influences they have on the solubilities of nonpolar side-chains. Stabilizing cosolvents like TMAO and glycine betaine might be expected to reduce the solubilities of hydrophobic side-chains very strongly, and make their transfer into the interior of the protein even more energetically favorable. In fact, Bolen and colleagues found exactly the opposite relationship: the transfer free energies associated with move-

ment of almost all categories of amino acid side-chains from water to the interior of the protein were *less* negative in the presence of most stabilizing cosolvents (figure 6.11). In the left frame of this figure, the effects of urea, proline, sucrose, sarcosine, and TMAO on the transfer free energies (ΔG_{tr}) of side-chain from water to 1 M concentrations of the osmolytes are given. The 20 amino acids are divided into two broad classes: hydrophobic side chains (W, F, Y, L, I, P, V, M, and A: open bars) and polar/charged side-chains (T, S, Q, N, K, R, H, E, D, and G: filled bars (see Qu et al., 1998, for original data on individual amino acids). With the exception of hydrophobic side-chains in the presence of 1 M sarcosine, all of the osmolyte effects denote an increased solubility of the side-chains in the osmolyte-containing solution. In other words, insofar as amino acid side-chains are con-

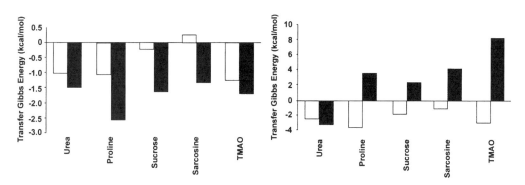

Figure 6.11. Free energy changes (transfer Gibbs free energy, ΔG_{tr}, in kcal mol^{-1}) associated with transfer of amino acid side-chains and peptide backbone linkages from water to 1 M concentrations of five osmolytes (urea, proline, sucrose, sarcosine, and TMAO). Studies were performed using a modified ribonuclease enzyme (Qu et al., 1998). (Left panel) Effects of osmolytes on side-chain transfers. Open bars represent contributions of hydrophobic side-chains (W, F, Y, L, I, P, V, M, and A); filled bars represent contributions from polar/charged side-chains (T, S, Q, N, K, R, H, E, D, and G). Note that, with the exception of hydrophobic side-chains in the presence of sarcosine, transfer into the osmolyte-containing solution is favorable (ΔG_{tr} is negative). (Right panel) Transfer Gibbs free energy changes associated with transfer of peptide backbone linkages from water to 1 M concentrations of urea and four stabilizing osmolytes. Filled bars show the total contributions of the peptide backbone; open bars show the total contribution of side-chains. The net stabilization free energy favoring folding in the presence of stabilizing osmolytes arises from the osmophobic effect with the peptide backbone of the molecule. For each of the stabilizing osmolytes, transfer of peptide backbone linkages from water to osmolyte-containing solutions is energetically unfavorable (ΔG_{tr} is positive). TMAO has by far the largest ΔG_{tr} of all solutes tested. Although not shown in this figure, the effects of urea and stabilizing osmolytes on transfers of side-chains and backbone linkages are algebraically additive (see Wang and Bolen, 1997). (Figures modified after Qu et al., 1998.)

cerned, stabilizing cosolvents, as well as urea, generally favor the unfolding of the protein (= increase in the free energy of the native protein).

This interesting discovery leaves only one potential candidate as the agent responsible for the effects of stabilizing cosolvents, the peptide bond itself. Peptide bonds, which form approximately half the surface area of a protein, exhibit significantly decreased solubility in the presence of stabilizing cosolvents (figure 6.11, right panel). In other words, the transfer of a peptide backbone linkage from water to 1 M solutions of stabilizing cosolvents entails an increase in free energy (ΔG_{tr} is positive.) Furthermore, the tendency to disfavor solubility of the peptide backbone varies among osmolytes, with TMAO having by far the greatest effect among all stabilizing cosolvents studied. Thus, it is the favorable effect on burial of peptide backbone linkages that accounts for the tendencies of stabilizing cosolvents to lead to a compact protein structure and reduced protein solubility. To use Bolen's terminology, the peptide backbone is strongly osmophobic towards stabilizing cosolvents. Urea and guanidinium, which bind to the peptide backbone and favor protein unfolding, can thus be said to represent a state of "osmophilia," the preferential binding of cosolvent to the macromolecule (figure 6.10). As would be predicted from these results, there is an algebraic additivity in the effects of stabilizing and destabilizing cosolvents on side-chain and peptide backbone solubilities (Wang and Bolen, 1997), much as seen in studies of urea–methylamine counteraction on enzymatic activity and protein stability in figure 6.6.

The thermodynamic description of protein stabilization, which involves the concept of preferential exclusion of stabilizing cosolvents, and the chemical description of osmophobicity of peptide linkages to stabilizing cosolvents represent two sides of a coin. The symmetry in these descriptions can perhaps best be appreciated by viewing osmophobicity as arising from the creation by a stabilizing cosolvent like TMAO of an aqueous phase whose structure is not favorable for hydration of the pep-

tide backbone linkage. Increases in surface tension by the cosolvent may be the physical basis for this effect. In a similar way, the water surrounding the surface of the protein tends to exclude the stabilizing cosolvent, an exclusion that again can arise from surface tension effects. In both descriptions, it is the combined effect of the protein and cosolvent on the structure of water that underlies the observed stabilization.

An Apparent Paradox Resolved: How Can Stabilizing Cosolvents Strengthen Protein Structure if They Raise the Free Energy of the Native Protein?

The effects of stabilizing cosolvents on protein structure can be summarized by considering how the addition of these solutes to a solution containing proteins affects the free energy of the system (figure 6.12). The free energy of the system is at a minimum when the native protein exists in aqueous solution (that is, in a buffer in which no stabilizing cosolvent is present): N_{aq}. When a stabilizing cosolvent is added to the system, the free energy of the native state rises to N_{os}. In part, this rise in free energy of the native protein (ΔG_4) reflects the entropic factors discussed above, that is, the nonrandom distribution of a stabilizing cosolvent in a protein-containing solution. The explanation for why the stabilizing cosolvent is able to enhance protein stability even though it raises the free energy of the native protein is shown by the energy changes that accompany protein unfolding. In aqueous solution (no stabilizing cosolvent), the positive free energy change accompanying unfolding of the protein (ΔG_1) is much smaller than the change in free energy that occurs when the protein unfolds in the presence of the stabilizing cosolvent (ΔG_3). Therefore, even though the native protein has a higher free energy when the stabilizing cosolvent is present, it is the very large increase in free energy that accompanies unfolding in the presence of the osmolyte that accounts for the enhanced stability when this cosolvent is present. This basis of stability is seen to be a reflection of a basic principle of physical chemistry: when the thermodynamic feasibility of a process

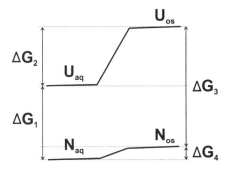

Figure 6.12. Free energy values and changes in free energy (ΔG) characterizing a system containing a protein in either an aqueous phase (aq subscripts = no added stabilizing osmolyte) or a stabilizing solute (os subscripts). Addition of a stabilizing osmolyte raises the free energy of the native protein: the $N_{aq} \rightarrow N_{os}$ transformation has a positive free energy change of ΔG_4. That is, the stabilizing cosolvent paradoxically appears to make the native protein less stable. However, the free energy changes that occur during the unfolding process differ greatly between the aqueous and osmolyte-containing systems. The transformation of the native protein in aqueous phase to the unfolded protein in aqueous phase, $N_{aq} \rightarrow U_{aq}$ involves a smaller increase in free energy (ΔG_1) than unfolding of the protein in the presence of the stabilizing osmolyte: $N_{os} \rightarrow U_{os}$ (ΔG_3). The difference in the ΔG of unfolding in aqueous and osmolyte-containing solutions, ΔG_2, accounts for the enhanced stability of the protein in the presence of the stabilizing cosolvent. (Modified from Qu et al., 1998.)

is to be evaluated, it is the *change* in free energy, ΔG, that matters, not the absolute value of the free energy of the system. To repeat this important conclusion: stabilizing cosolvents like TMAO make the free energy change of unfolding (denaturation) such a large positive number that the native state is strongly favored, despite the fact that the free energy of the native state in the presence of TMAO is higher than in a solution lacking this stabilizing osmolyte.

Common Properties of Solute and Temperature Effects: Shifting the Ensemble of Protein Microstates

In the analysis of the effects of temperature on protein structure given in the following chapter,

the importance of a protein's retaining a physiologically appropriate balance between stability and conformational flexibility is emphasized. To understand this important balancing act, that is, the conservation of *marginal stability*, it is necessary to view a protein not as a static structure, but as a dynamic entity that rapidly fluctuates among a large number of different configurations, so-called *microstates*. Protein structure is highly dynamic; the static image of a protein given by a picture of three-dimensional structure determined using X-ray diffraction fails to convey the spectrum of microstates that simultaneously exist for a protein in solution. Because an ensemble of configurational microstates of a protein is present in solution, when we speak of stability or flexibility we are referring to an average property of a population of molecules that exists in a great many different configurations at any single time.

In analyzing the effects of changes in temperature on the distribution of molecules among different microstates (see figure 7.6), it is emphasized that reduced temperature, by disfavoring unfolding of the enzyme, would be expected to reduce the number of configurational microstates in which the enzyme was sufficiently distorted to preclude high-affinity substrate binding. This effect of reduced temperature on the population of microstates favors lower K_m values, an effect of temperature seen for most enzymes. However, because the rate-limiting changes in conformation that establish k_{cat} values for many enzymes also are impeded at low temperatures due to reduced flexibility of enzyme structure, the enhancement in binding is paired with a reduction in rate of function per active site. In other words, the effect of reduced temperature on the distribution of enzymes among microstates lowers both K_m and k_{cat}.

The effects of solutes on distributions of microstates are analogous in important ways to the effects of changes in temperature (figure 6.13). A structure-stabilizing osmolyte like TMAO will favor compact, stable microstates. In the presence of a stabilizing cosolvent, the ensemble of configurational states thus includes a relatively small fraction of molecules whose

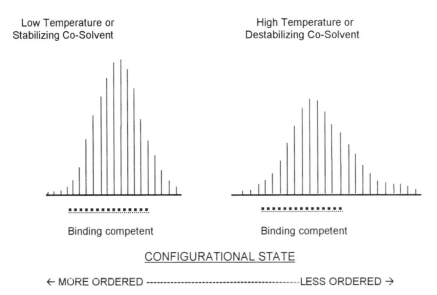

Low Temperature or   High Temperature or
Stabilizing Co-Solvent   Destabilizing Co-Solvent

Binding competent   Binding competent

CONFIGURATIONAL STATE

← MORE ORDERED --LESS ORDERED →

Figure 6.13. Effects of solutes and temperature on the distribution of configurational microstates of a protein. In the presence of a stabilizing solute like TMAO or glycine betaine (or at low temperature), the ensemble of configurational states occupied by the enzyme comprises primarily binding-competent configurations (microstates found above the dashed line). In the presence of a destabilizing cosolvent like urea (or at higher temperature), the distribution of microstates is altered: a greater spectrum of microstates is occupied by the protein, and a smaller fraction of the population of enzyme molecules exists in binding-competent configurations at any given time. More ordered states, as favored by stabilizing cosolvents and reduced temperature, are those towards the left of the two diagrams; less ordered states are to the right in each case.

three-dimensional structures are so distorted that effective binding is precluded. Through this effect on the ensemble of microstates, stabilizing cosolvents will lower K_m values. However, by enhancing enzyme stability, k_{cat} also may decrease if the rate-limiting step of the reaction involves a conformational change whose energy barriers are increased in the presence of a structure-stabilizing solute.

Because LDH-A is an enzyme for which k_{cat} depends on rates of conformational changes (Dunn et al., 1991; see also chapter 7), it is instructive to compare the effects on K_m and k_{cat} values of a strongly stabilizing solute like TMAO and a denaturing solute like urea. Baskakov et al. (1998) have shown that TMAO and urea have effects analogous to those of low and high temperatures, respectively (figure 6.14). TMAO led to a reduction in both k_{cat} and K_m of pyruvate as its concentration was increased from 0 to 0.6 M. Urea, in contrast, led to increases in both k_{cat} and K_m of pyruvate

over much of this same concentration range. Note that stimulation of catalytic activity (rise in k_{cat}) with increasing concentrations of urea was evident only up to 0.4 M urea. At higher concentrations of urea, the loosening of enzyme structure might have led to significant disruption of tertiary and quaternary structures and, therefore, to increased numbers of inactive enzyme molecules. Such denaturation would overwhelm the stimulation of activity resulting from reduced energy barriers to rate-limiting catalytic conformational changes. Note, too, that the effects of urea and TMAO are counteracting at a 2:1 (urea:TMAO) concentration ratio.

By regarding enzymes as populations of microstates rather than as existing in a single configuration, it is possible to understand more clearly how changes in physical and chemical factors influence structural stability and, thereby, kinetic properties. As is true in much of biological thought, population thinking may

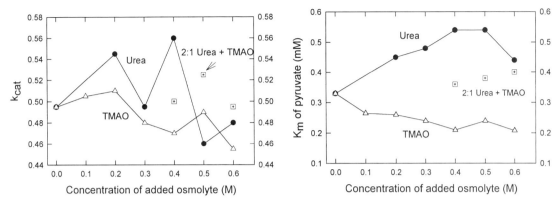

Figure 6.14. The effects of urea, TMAO, and combinations of both osmolytes on the k_{cat} (left panel) and K_m of pyruvate (right panel) for porcine LDH-A. Note that up to a concentration of approximately 0.4 M, urea increases k_{cat}, whereas TMAO is inhibitory. (Figure modified after Baskakov et al., 1998.)

clarify the nature of a study system and permit insights that essentialist thinking does not allow (see Mayr, 1982).

Unique Amino Acid Composition of Proteins of Extremely Halophilic Archaea: When Folding Requires Help from Osmolytes

The balance between stability and flexibility of protein structure that is attained in vivo is seen to arise from the complementary effects of (i) the intrinsic stability of the protein, which is determined by its amino acid sequence, and (ii) the influences of extrinsic factors, including physical variables like temperature and hydrostatic pressure, and chemical species like organic osmolytes. In most of the examples of protein–solute interactions treated up to this point, however, osmolytes have been considered largely in the context of their abilities to conserve the intrinsic properties of the protein. Thus, in a sense, compatible osmolytes "let the protein be what it is." The ability of the protein to fold into its native structure and attain its correct functional state is not dependent on the presence of osmolytes. Likewise, during osmoregulation in osmoconforming species, variations in concentration of organic osmolytes do not significantly alter protein folding.

A very different situation exists in the case of proteins of the extremely halophilic members of the Archaea. These unusual proteins can fold properly and gain activity only with the assistance of the osmolytes present in the cell. For most proteins of other organisms, the information in the primary sequence provides all of the information required to direct the folding of the protein into a compact functional enzyme or structural protein. Molecular chaperones may be required to achieve efficient folding in the crowded cytoplasm (see chapter 7), but additional extrinsic factors are not needed to allow the protein to fold into a functional state. In the extremely halophilic members of the Archaea, folding and gain of activity by proteins can only occur in the presence of high concentrations of inorganic ions, notably K^+ (figure 6.4).

The basis of this unusual salt requirement is the unique amino acid composition of proteins of these organisms. Proteins of these extreme halophiles have several distinct preferences for amino acids. Acidic amino acids (glutamate and aspartate) are present in high frequencies and basic amino acids (lysine and arginine) are reduced in frequency, giving these proteins a high negative charge. High percentages of acidic amino acids are, in fact, common in proteins of Archaea, but this unusual preference for negatively charged amino acids is most pronounced in the extremely halophilic species belonging to the family *Halobacteriaceae*. For example, the percentage contribution of aspartyl plus gluta-myl residues to ribosomal proteins is between 21 and 29% in nonhalophilic archaea, but is 54% in an extreme halophile; in contrast, ribo-somal proteins of *E. coli* have only 7% acidic amino acids (Martin et al., 1999). A second unique feature of proteins of extremely halophi-lic archaea lies in their low inherent hydropho-bicity. Strongly hydrophobic amino acids are reduced in frequency, but weakly hydrophobic amino acids are relatively abundant. How does the high net negative charge of these proteins and the relatively low propensity for hydropho-bic stabilization allow these proteins to fold into native, functional conformations? How do these unusual preferences for negatively charged and weakly hydrophobic amino acids explain the salt effects shown in figure 6.4?

To answer these questions, it is appropriate again to examine the Hofmeister Series (figure 6.9), to gain an initial sense of how the high concentrations of K^+ in the cells of extremely halophilic archaea might influence protein structure. Although potassium ion is less stabi-lizing of proteins than, for example, NH_4^+ or SO_4^{2-}, at the high concentrations of K^+ found within the cells of an extreme halophile, K^+ will exert a substantial stabilizing effect on proteins. One challenge facing extreme halophiles, then, is to prevent proteins from becoming too stable and inadequately soluble under the conditions of high solute concentration found within the cell.

The patterns of amino acid utilization found in proteins of extreme halophiles indicate how these challenges have been met. The high den-sity of negative charges on halophilic proteins due to the large numbers of $-COO^-$ groups of aspartyl and glutamyl residues tends to weaken the three-dimensional structure through charge repulsion. The fact that proteins of extreme halophiles require a substantial concentration of salt to be active is viewed as an indication that K^+ functions as a counterion to neutralize $-COO^-$ groups. Potassium ion also plays a sec-ond important role: it functions to salt-out of solution the weakly hydrophobic groups. Weakly hydrophobic side-chains have a lower tendency to partition into the interior of the protein than larger hydrophobic side-chains,

for instance, those of valine, leucine, and isoleu-cine. Thus, the inherent degree of stabilization due to the hydrophobic effect may be relatively low for proteins of extreme halophiles. How-ever, the high concentration of K^+ in the cellu-lar water leads nonetheless to an adequate ten-dency for the protein to fold into a compact, native structure. What has taken place during the evolution of the extremely halophilic archaea is the development of protein structures that have relatively low intrinsic stabilities under conditions of low ionic strength, but pos-sess the appropriate stabilities and three-dimen-sional structures for metabolic function under the conditions of high salt concentration pre-sent in the cells. The proteins of these extremo-philes thus represent an extreme case of how protein structure and function depend on the milieu in which the protein occurs. The funda-mental rules of physical chemistry dictate that the properties of any protein in solution will be shaped by its interactions with water and cosol-vents. However, it is only in the case of the proteins of the extremely halophilic archaea that the dependence of the protein on cosolvent effects is so extreme that the protein can func-tion only in the presence of physiological con-centrations of the dominant osmolyte, K^+.

REGULATION OF OSMOLYTE COMPOSITION AND CONCENTRATION

Common Solutions Are Effected Through Diverse Regulatory Mechanisms

The marked similarities among different types of organisms in the classes of low-molecular-mass organic osmolytes that are accumulated during water stress belie the variety of physio-logical mechanisms utilized to regulate intracel-lular concentrations of these solutes. A given end-result, for instance, the build-up of a com-patible solute like trehalose or glutamate, may occur by very different routes in different spe-cies. At first glance, a survey of the machinery used by different taxa to ensure that the right type of osmolyte is accumulated to the appropriate level might lead one to conclude that few unifying principles are involved in these important regulatory events. However, underlying the diversity of regulatory mechanisms are several unifying principles that are found in all species' responses to water stress. While details of mechanism may differ greatly among taxa, the principles on which these mechanisms are founded are universal and comprise the following considerations.

Economy

If a number of regulatory mechanisms are available for elevating the intracellular concentrations of organic osmolytes, the mechanism used by the cell is likely to be the one entailing the lowest energy expenditure. Thus, if uptake of an organic osmolyte from the environment is possible, and if this requires fewer ATP equivalents than de novo biosynthesis of the osmolyte, uptake pathways for transporting the externally available osmolyte may be strongly induced as the principal regulatory response. Pathways for biosynthesis of the osmolyte may be turned off, either through allosteric regulation of enzymatic activity or suppression of transcription of the genes encoding enzymes involved in osmolyte synthesis. Note that organic osmolytes that are present in the environment and are capable of being taken up by cells are termed *osmoprotectants*. This term should not be taken to imply that these solutes prevent initial shrinking of cells exposed to hyperosmotic stress, because uptake of osmoprotectants typically occurs more slowly than the rapid loss of water triggered by hyperosmotic conditions.

An especially economical solution to acquisition of organic osmolytes is to exploit metabolic end-products, metabolites that have no further use to the organism as substrates for ATP generation or as building blocks for biosynthesis. Urea would seem to be the classic example of this type of strategy, although several other organic osmolytes also are metabolic end-products or derivatives of these products, for instance, TMAO and taurine.

Metabolic accessibility

The class of organic osmolyte accumulated under water stress often reflects the metabolic capacities of the species and its access to different types of nutrients. A good example of this rule is observed in photoautotrophic species. Because of their photosynthetic potential, these organisms are capable of producing sugars and polyols through biosynthetic pathways that entail relatively low energy costs. However, photosynthetic species, especially marine algae, may be faced with limitations in availability of a critical nutrient, nitrogen. For these reasons, sugars and polyols, rather than free amino acids, typically are the primary organic osmolytes found in green plants and algae. This is a rule with many exceptions, however. For instance, salt-stressed vascular plants may accumulate high concentrations of proline (table 6.1).

Rapid responses differ from steady-state conditions

Easy-to-accumulate osmolytes that have relatively low compatibility with the biochemical machinery of the cell may appear first, as a stopgap measure, before the concentrations of more compatible osmolytes can be increased. The optimal solution to hyperosmotic stress, the accumulation of compatible organic osmolytes, is not always feasible in the short run. The initial responses of organisms may be to allow inorganic ion concentrations (chiefly K^+) to build up during the initial minutes to hours of osmotic stress, in order to preserve cell volume and, in bacteria, turgor pressure. Subsequently, as uptake and biosynthetic pathways are activated, the less-than-optimal inorganic osmolytes are replaced by compatible organic osmolytes. To understand the osmotic strategy of an organism, it is necessary to monitor the kinetics of the process, rather than to merely sample at one time point.

Tight regulatory linkages occur between pathways of accumulation and removal

To avoid what amount to futile cycles, pathways of transport and synthesis involved in accumulating organic osmolytes must be coordinated with pathways that foster removal of osmolytes from the cell. These regulatory linkages involve modulation of enzymatic activities, membrane-localized solute transporters, and gene expression. The complexity and hierarchical nature of these regulatory schemes differ substantially among organisms. This leads to wide variation among taxa in speed of response and in the extent to which integration occurs between osmoregulatory systems per se and other cellular processes that demand regulation in the face of the impact of water stress on cellular structure and function.

Regulatory Mechanisms in Bacteria

All of the principles outlined above are manifested in the responses of bacteria to changes in environmental osmolality. Because of the metabolic and ecological diversity found among bacteria, there obviously can be no single set of regulatory processes or any single family of organic osmolytes that characterizes all bacterial species. Nonetheless, despite differences in the types of osmolytes accumulated and the precise transport and synthetic pathways used, there appears to be a "bacterial" way of doing things. Below, we focus chiefly on Gram-negative bacteria like *E. coli* and *Salmonella typhimurium* that may encounter wide ranges of osmolality and highly variable access to osmoprotectants, especially when existing in soil habitats. The regulatory mechanisms that have been described in these two well-studied species provide especially good insights into the ways in which bacteria achieve rapid and effective adaptation to osmotic stress (for review, see Galinski and Trüper, 1994; Kempf and Bremer, 1998).

To appreciate the osmoregulatory problems faced by bacteria and, therefore, the particular strategies they use when faced with water stress, it is important to realize that, unlike most eukaryotic cells, bacterial cells typically must maintain a high positive turgor pressure.

Positive turgor is needed to maintain cell volume and to allow cell expansion when this is needed. The pressure required for maintaining turgor may seem surprisingly high. Thus, in Gram-negative bacteria, turgor pressure may be as high as approximately 10 atmospheres; in Gram-positive bacteria, turgor pressures of twice this magnitude have been estimated (Kempf and Bremer, 1998). These pressures may be more than 10 times the pressure in a fully inflated automobile tire. Hyperosmotic stress resulting from increased environmental salinity thus will pose threats to a bacterium's ability to maintain turgor pressure. This threat is in addition to the threats imposed to the metabolic machinery of the cell by changes in concentrations of inorganic ions resulting from efflux of water. The bacterial response to osmotic stress involves two principal phases.

Phase I: K^+ and glutamate

The initial response of bacteria to hyperosmotic stress is mounted rapidly, usually in less than one minute, and serves as a stopgap measure to defend turgor pressure and the internal milieu, thereby enabling the cell to survive until a more effective, longer term response can be completed. This initial response has two distinct components. The first event is rapid entry into the cell of K^+ from the environment, with Cl^- commonly serving as a counterion to allow electroneutrality to be maintained. Uptake of K^+ can be viewed as an emergency response that is suboptimal, but one that makes the best of a bad temporary situation. Of all monovalent cations, K^+ is apt to be least perturbing of cellular functions. Nonetheless, K^+ lacks the compatibility of organic osmolytes. Uptake of K^+ into *E. coli* cells may occur through three transporters, Kup, Trk, and Kdp (figure 6.15), whose activities are closely regulated in conjunction with changes in external osmolality. Kup is constitutively expressed and makes a minor contribution to K^+ uptake during hyperosmotic stress. The activities of Trk and Kdp are greatly increased during osmotic stress. This activation appears to involve two mechanisms: (i) direct effects on the activities of existing transporters, which is caused by changes in turgor pressure;

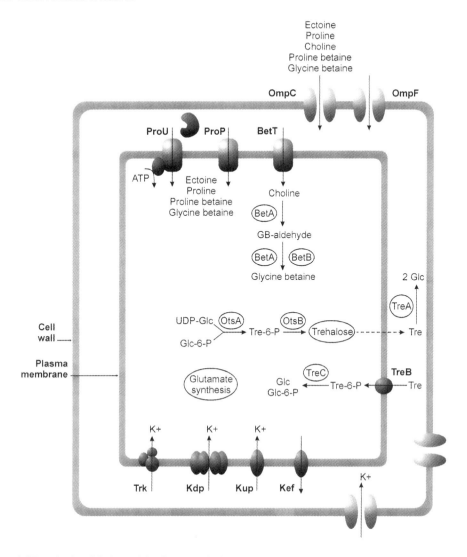

Figure 6.15. A simplified model of some of the regulatory mechanisms used by the *Escherichia coli* cell to adjust concentrations of intracellular osmolytes during osmotic stress. OmpC and OmpF are outer membrane porins that allow passage of osmoprotectants (e.g., proline and glycine betaine) into the periplasmic space. ProU and ProP are transporters responsible for selective uptake into the cytoplasm of such osmolytes as glycine betaine, proline betaine, proline, and ectoine. BetT facilitates uptake of choline, which can be transformed into glycine betaine through activities of the enzymes BetA and BetB. Trehalose (Tre) in the periplasmic space can be taken up by the cell through the TreB channel. In addition to being used as an osmolyte, trehalose can be converted into substrates for energy metabolism. In this set of conversions, trehalose is initially phosphorylated to trehalose-6-phosphate (Tre-6-P) and, then, converted to glucose (Glc) and glucose-6-phosphate (Glc-6-P) by the TreC-catalyzed reaction. Trehalose can be synthesized from uridine diphosphate glucose (UDP-Glc) and glucose-6-phosphate through the OtsA-catalyzed reaction, which yields trehalose-6-phosphate (Tre-6-P). OtsB dephosphorylates trehalose-6-phosphate to trehalose. During hypoosmotic regulation, trehalose leaks from the cell into the periplasmic space. There, the enzyme trehalase (TreA) splits trehalose into two glucose (Glc) moieties, which can be taken up by the cell for use in energy metabolism. Trk, Kdp, and Kup are potassium channels utilized to carry K^+ into the cell during early phases of osmotic adaptation (Kup is constitutive and plays a minor role; synthesis of Trk and Kdp is increased during hyperosmotic stress). Efflux of potassium ion occurs through a different channel (Kef). (Figure modified after Kempf and Bremer, 1998.)

and (ii) turgor-pressure-regulated control of expression of the operon encoding these two transporters (see Kempf and Bremer, 1998). Activation of the operon encoding the two transporters is a transient event, because accumulation of K^+ is a stopgap measure.

The second event in this initial phase of the response of *E. coli* to hyperosmotic stress is the synthesis of glutamate, which replaces Cl^- as a counterion to K^+ (figure 6.15). Increased synthesis of glutamate occurs quickly, usually within a minute of exposure to hyperosmotic stress, but it cannot occur until the initial rise in concentration of intracellular K^+ has taken place.

Phase II: Build-up of compatible osmolytes

As potassium glutamate concentrations are building up, the second phase of the osmoregulatory response is triggered: the build-up of compatible organic osmolytes. The form taken by the second phase of the process reflects the issue of "economy" mentioned above. If suitable osmoprotectant substances are in the soil water bathing the bacterium, then it will preferentially rely on these molecules for its source of organic osmolytes. If osmoprotectants are not adequately available, then synthesis within the cell of trehalose commences (figure 6.15).

Uptake of osmoprotectants. Availability of osmoprotectants in soil water varies widely and depends on several factors. Decaying organic matter is a major source of these substances, because any compatible solute released during necrosis may enter the ambient osmoprotectant pool. The transport systems for osmoprotectants expressed by bacteria may provide a clue as to the types of osmoprotectants present in soil water. Proline transporters are common. Their occurrence in many soil bacteria probably reflects the fact that vascular plants often accumulate proline during hyperosmotic stress and, later, release large amounts of this amino acid to the soil when they die and decay. Transporters for glycine betaine are present in many bacteria. Glycine betaine is a common osmolyte in plants and occurs as well in animal wastes. Organic osmolytes may be

released into the pool of osmoprotectants by bacteria themselves during hypoosmotic stress and upon death of the cells. Thus, recycling of organic osmolytes by bacteria may be important.

The nature of the osmoprotectant pool found in soil water leads to predictions about the characteristics of transport systems that would allow maximal exploitation of these solutes. First, transporters may need to have relatively *broad substrate specificities*, such that a given transporter is capable of exploiting a number of osmoprotectants. For instance, it would appear advantageous to have transporters that can recognize several different amino acids, so that the cell does not have to synthesize a separate transporter for each of the 20 amino acids. Second, because of the wide range of concentrations of any particular osmoprotectant in soil water, transporters may have to exhibit a *range of affinities* (K_m values; note: K_t is typically used to refer to the half-saturating level of substrate for a transporter; J_{max} is used instead of V_{max}). As shown for enzymes, high affinity (low K_m) is correlated with low capacity for function (low k_{cat}), and the same reciprocity is true of transporters: high affinity (low K_t) is paired with low capacity (low J_{max}). By having high-affinity–low-capacity transporters, the cell can exploit even very low ambient concentrations of an osmoprotectant. Low-affinity–high-capacity transporters allow large-scale uptake of the osmoprotectant when its ambient concentration is high. Third, because of variation in types of osmoprotectants available and in soil water osmolality, the activity and synthesis of transporters must be tightly regulated, such that the appropriate types of transporters are present at the necessary levels of activity. Regulation of transporter activity may need to be rapid in view of the rate at which soil osmolality can change, for instance, during rainfall. Like osmoprotectant influx, efflux of osmolytes from the cell must be closely regulated. For instance, removal of osmolytes from the cellular water must occur rapidly enough under hypoosmotic stress to avoid build-up of excessive turgor pressure and cell lysis.

The osmoprotectant transporters found in bacterial cell membranes have properties that are consistent with these predictions (figure 6.15). These transporters have high affinities for osmoprotectants, with K_t values in the micromolar range. Even such low concentrations of osmoprotectants are adequate to allow the cell to osmoregulate effectively at external salt concentrations of up to 1 M (Kempf and Bremer, 1998). Unlike some transporters, the osmoprotectant transporters are not inhibited in the presence of high salt concentrations. Substrate specificities of the transporters may be broad, allowing a given transporter to exploit a range of osmoprotectants. Regulation of activities of transporters is rapid and involves multiple levels: direct modulation of existing transporters and variation in numbers of transporters through close regulation of transporter-encoding genes.

Escherichia coli and *S. typhimurium* have two major transporters for osmoprotectants, the ProP and ProU systems. Both systems have broad substrate specificities. ProP can effectively transport glycine betaine, proline betaine (affinities for these two osmoprotectants are highest), proline, carnitine, ectoine, dimethylsulfoniopropionate (DMSP), homobetaine, and dimethylglycine—among others. ProP is thus well poised to exploit a variety of solutes released by plant, animal, and bacterial cells upon lysis. These and other osmoprotectants enter the periplasmic space through nonspecific porins (OmpC and OmpF; "Omp" = outer membrane protein) found in the outer membrane (figure 6.15). The genes encoding these porins are up-regulated during hyperosmotic stress and down-regulated during hypoosmotic stress. Regulation of the synthesis of these porins also involves post-transcriptional mechanisms: an antisense RNA, MicF, is a negative regulator of translation of the proteins (Pratt et al., 1996).

Regulation of ProP involves modulation of activity of existing transporters and large-scale induction of synthesis of new transporters in response to increased medium osmolality. Transcription of the gene encoding ProP (*proP*) is regulated by two promoters, both of which are activated by increased cell osmolality (see "Osmosensing and Signal Transduction").

ProU, the other major transporter in these two species of bacteria, also has broad substrate specificities, with glycine betaine and proline betaine accumulated with particular efficiency. ProU is rapidly up-regulated by more than 100-fold during salt stress, and elevated expression of *proU* persists throughout the period of osmotic stress (Kempf and Bremer, 1998).

The mechanisms that regulate the genes encoding porins, ProP, and ProU, are not fully understood. Among the mechanisms that have been proposed are direct effects of inorganic ions on DNA supercoiling, leading to altered interactions between DNA and gene regulatory proteins; and salt effects on equilibria between DNA and DNA binding-protein interactions irrespective of changes in DNA supercoiling. Despite the fact that a great many in-vitro studies have identified biochemical processes that are highly sensitive to solute concentration and composition, the biochemical components of the cell that are the primary osmosensors in vivo remain to be fully characterized. We discuss some of the known (and conjectured) mechanisms for sensing osmotic stress in a later section of this chapter ("Osmosensing and Signal Transduction").

Synthesis of Osmolytes: Trehalose Synthesis by E. coli. When adequate amounts of appropriate osmoprotectants are present in soil water, their accumulation represents an energy-efficient solution to the problems of adjusting to hyperosmotic stress. However, when soil water cannot provide osmoprotectants, then survival is likely to depend on de novo biosynthesis of one or more types of compatible osmolytes. In *E. coli* the widely occurring disaccharide trehalose is the major osmolyte synthesized. Induction of the enzymes needed for synthesis of trehalose is osmotically regulated. The *OtsBA* (osmoregulated trehalose synthesis) operon encodes two proteins of trehalose synthesis, trehalose-6-phosphate synthase, which catalyses the condensation of glucose-6-phosphate with UDP-glucose to form trehalose-6-phosphate, and trehalose-6-phosphate phosphatase, which generates free trehalose from trehalose-6-

phosphate. Osmotically induced expression of *otsBA* occurs rapidly after exposure to hyperosmotic stress and depends on activity of the transcription factor σ^S (RpoS). RpoS is a general stress response transcription factor in bacteria. It is pivotal in regulating *otsBA* expression during entry of cultures into stationary phase, when increased concentrations of trehalose are accumulated, a reflection of trehalose's importance under a wide variety of stressful conditions (Kempf and Bremer, 1998).

In osmoregulatory processes that entail increased synthesis of organic osmolytes, elevated activities of biosynthetic pathways often are effected by two mechanisms: up-regulation of the concentrations of enzymes needed for synthesis and stimulation of the activities of one or more of these enzymes by increased intracellular osmolality. Trehalose-6-phosphate synthase is strongly stimulated by potassium glutamate and certain other ions (Ström and Kaasen, 1993). Thus, accumulation of K^+ and glutamate during the first phase of osmoregulation establishes in the intracellular milieu conditions that foster a high rate of synthesis of the compatible solute trehalose, which then replaces K^+ and glutamate as the dominant contributor to the osmolyte pool. As trehalose levels build up, potassium ion is transported out of the cell (figure 6.15) and glutamate synthesis is curtailed.

In Gram-negative bacteria like *E. coli* and *S. typhimurium*, osmotic adaptation is seen as a rapid, two-phase process in which a temporary stopgap accumulation of solutes of relatively low compatibility is followed by their replacement with one or more compatible organic osmolytes that are obtained either from the environment or through biosynthesis. The reliance on external osmoprotectants is a key element in the osmoregulatory strategies of bacteria, allowing them to obtain from their environment the organic solutes needed for osmoregulation without incurring high metabolic costs of biosynthesis.

Starch–Polyol Interconversions in Marine Algae

The source of organic osmolytes that might seem most advantageous in terms of biosynthetic costs and speed of regulation would be a large osmotically inert polymer that could be stored within the cell and converted into numerous osmotically active units in the face of hyperosmotic stress. Recall that, on the basis of colligative relationships, a large polymer comprising many potential osmotically active subunits has the same effect on osmolality as one of its constituent osmolyte molecules. An osmolyte storage compound like this would enable cells to alter rapidly their concentrations of osmolytes without the need for exchange of solutes with the external milieu or for energetically costly de novo synthesis of osmolyte on each occasion.

This type of mechanism for generating and storing organic osmolytes is found in many salt-tolerant algae, in which interconversion of starch and glycerol plays a central role in osmotic adjustment. For instance, the unicellular green alga *Chlorococcum submarinum* is able to rapidly convert starch into glycerol when exposed to increased external salinity (figure 6.16, upper panel; Blackwell and Gilmour, 1991). Within several minutes after an increase in external NaCl concentration from 0.1 to 0.5 M, glycerol concentrations increase significantly and there is a concomitant decrease in cellular starch content. Note that, in this halotolerant alga, the concentration of potassium ion is strongly regulated, unlike the situation just discussed in bacteria in which transient increases in $[K^+]$ occur. The accumulation of glycerol reaches its maximal plateau value within approximately 2–3 hours after exposure to hyperosmotic stress. Decrease in starch content is essentially complete by this time. Not all of the osmotic adjustment in this species is due to glycerol, however; a minor fraction of the increase in the pool of organic osmolytes is due to proline.

When external salinity is decreased from 0.5 M to 0.1 M, there is a rapid fall in glycerol content within several minutes. Starch content appears to be restored almost immediately to the value observed prior to hyperosmotic stress (figure 6.16, lower panel). These data show that the ability to rejoin an osmolyte molecule to an osmotically inert polymer enables the cell to decrease its osmotic content very rapidly,

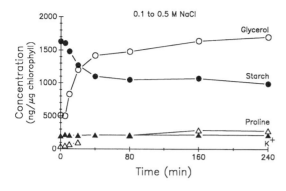

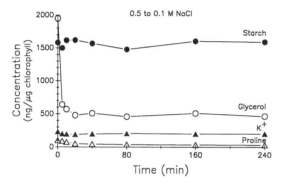

Figure 6.16. Effects of hyper- and hypoosmotic stress on osmolyte concentrations in the unicellular green alga *Chlorococcum submarinum*. (Upper panel) Exposure of cells to increased osmolality (0.1 MNaCl → 0.5 M NaCl). (Lower panel) Exposure of cells to decreased osmolality (0.5 M NaCl → 0.1 M NaCl). Figure redrawn from Blackwell and Gilmour (1991). (Figure from Somero and Yancey, 1997.)

while retaining the reduced carbon of the osmolyte within the cell.

Uptake and Synthesis of Osmolytes in the Mammalian Kidney: Coping with Salts and Urea

It is instructive to compare the mechanisms used by mammalian kidney cells to adapt to hyperosmotic stress with the osmoregulatory mechanisms used by soil bacteria exposed to high ambient osmolality. The unity in diversity so commonly found in comparative biochemistry is well illustrated by this comparison. Cells of the inner medulla of the mammalian kidney, like hyperosmotically stressed bacteria cells, (i) accumulate compatible organic osmolytes when

these are available in the external medium (blood or soil water and intestinal fluids, respectively), (ii) synthesize organic osmolytes if an external supply of these solutes is not available, and (iii) closely regulate turnover of the osmolyte pool in conjunction with the degree of water stress. Thus, common strategies of osmolyte regulation are found in mammalian and prokaryotic cells, even though the transporter molecules, the systems for sensing osmotic stress, the mechanisms of gene regulation, and the biosynthetic pathways used to accumulate organic osmolytes may differ between these taxa.

Coordinated transport, synthesis, and release of organic osmolytes in medullary cells of the mammalian kidney

The principal vehicles for accumulation and release of organic osmolytes by cells of the inner medulla of the mammalian kidney are presented in figure 6.17 (Burg et al., 1997). The classes of organic osmolytes contributing to osmoregulation in the medullary cells comprise methylammonium solutes (glycine betaine and glycerophosphorylcholine, GPC), polyols (sorbitol and inositol), and an amino acid derivative, taurine. Note that osmoregulation using free amino acids is not characteristic of kidney cells. As found in studies of bacteria such as *E. coli* and *S. typhimurium*, uptake of organic osmolytes from the medium plays a key role in adaptation to hyperosmotic stress. Glycine betaine, inositol, and taurine, if available in the extracellular water, are taken up by medullary cells. Glucose, the substrate for synthesis of sorbitol by aldose reductase, is also taken up from the blood. Choline uptake contributes to the production of GPC in a somewhat indirect fashion. Choline is first incorporated into phosphatidyl choline, which is then split by a phospholipase enzyme (PLase) to yield GPC.

The synthesis of several proteins playing key roles in osmotic regulation is increased following exposure to hyperosmotic stress (reviewed in Burg et al., 1997). Transporters for glycine betaine, taurine, and inositol all increase in abundance over a period of several hours. This up-regulation of transporter activity

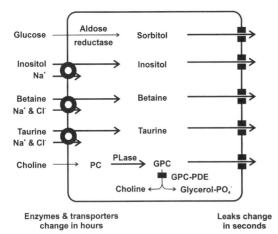

Enzymes & transporters   Leaks change
change in hours   in seconds

Figure 6.17. Regulation of organic osmolytes by cells of the inner medulla of the mammalian kidney (after Burg et al., 1997). Thick arrows denote processes that are regulated by changes in osmolality. Activities and/or concentrations of enzymes and transporters involved in uptake and synthesis of osmolytes change slowly relative to activities of leakage pathways. PLase: phospholipase, GPC-PDE: glycerol phosphorylcholine-phosphodiesterase.

depends in each case on activation of transcription of the genes encoding the transporters, as indicated by increases in synthesis of the respective mRNAs for the different transporters. The gene regulatory mechanisms that govern rate of transcription are not fully understood for any transporter. However, for the genes encoding the betaine transporter (*BGT1*) and the *myo*-inositol transporter (*SMIT*), several copies of tonicity-responsive enhancer elements (TonE) are present in the 5′-flanking region, which confer on the genes an ability to respond to hyperosmotic stress. Although the transcription factor that activates TonE has been cloned (Miyakawa et al., 1999), many details of signal transduction mechanism remain to be elucidated. It appears likely that increased intracellular concentrations of Na^+ and K^+ are pivotal in regulation expression of *BGT1*. Evidence for this hypothesis includes the observations that whereas hyperosmolal urea, a solute that readily permeates cells, fails to induce transcription of *BGT1*, high extracellular concentrations of NaCl or of a nonpermeating solute (raffinose),

which lead to cell shrinkage and, therefore, to elevated levels of inorganic ions in the cell, strongly activate transcription of this gene (Burg et al., 1997). In kidney cells, the osmosensing mechanisms that control expression of the genes encoding transporters for glycine betaine, taurine, and inositol all appear to involve effects of inorganic ions rather than membrane-localized sensors that are responsive to membrane stretch.

In medullary cells, as in bacteria, uptake of organic osmolytes from the extracellular water may be the preferred mechanism for osmoregulation when suitable solutes are available at adequate concentrations. In the acute response to hyperosmotic stress, essentially all of the increase in concentrations of glycine betaine, taurine, and inositol are the result of activation of transporters for these osmolytes. All three classes of transporters are present in the basolateral membrane of renal inner medullary cells, and all rely on transmembrane gradients in Na^+ and Cl^- for the driving force that enables the osmolytes to be transported into the cells against an unfavorable concentration gradient. Note that the glycine betaine transporter in *E. coli*, while achieving a common function, is a different type of transporter, one that is directly coupled to ATP hydrolysis to drive uptake of glycine betaine (Kempf and Bremer, 1998). Thus, evolutionary convergence in the use of glycine betaine is achieved by distinct molecular mechanisms for transport of the osmolyte into cells. In mammals, glycine betaine is obtained from the diet and synthesized in the liver and kidney cortex; it normally is present in human serum at a concentration near 38 μM (Allen et al., 1993).

The availability of osmolytes in the blood determines in part whether transcription of the gene encoding the enzyme required for synthesis of sorbitol, aldose reductase, (figure 6.17) is upregulated (Burg et al., 1997). If high concentrations of glycine betaine are available, transcription of the gene encoding aldose reductase is inhibited. When osmolyte concentrations in blood are not sufficient for osmoregulation, increased transcription of the aldose reductase gene occurs, leading to an accumulation of the mRNA and transporter. Degradation (turnover) of aldose reductase is reduced under hyperosmotic stress, which provides another mechanism for enhancing the cell's capacity for sorbitol accumulation. Like the gene for the glycine betaine transporter, the gene encoding aldose reductase is responsive to concentrations of Na^+ and Cl^- and contains the 5′-flanking region regulatory element TonE (also referred to as the osmotic response element, ORE), which is involved in sensing the osmotic status of the cell. Analysis of this regulatory element has revealed that the minimal size of the control element needed for osmotic responsiveness of the gene is 12 base pairs (Ferraris et al., 1996).

The triggers for accumulation of glycerophosphorylcholine differ somewhat from those that modulate levels of glycine betaine, sorbitol, and inositol. Unlike these other three osmolytes, GPC levels are regulated both by total osmolality and by the concentration of urea. High intracellular ionic strength is not needed to induce accumulation of GPC; rising concentrations of urea are sufficient. In contrast, urea does not affect the accumulation of glycine betaine, sorbitol, or inositol. The linkage between urea concentration and accumulation of GPC may reflect the ability of GPC to counteract the effects of urea on macromolecules. Although there have not been many studies of GPC's capacity to counteract perturbation by urea, the chemical structure of GPC, which contains three different types of protein-stabilizing components (a methylammonium unit, inorganic phosphate, and glycerol), suggests that it might function very effectively in stabilizing proteins against effects of urea. It is noteworthy that GPC is used as an osmolyte only in kidney cells, in which urea concentrations may build up to levels near one molal, depending on the amount of urea produced and the level of dehydration stress the organism is experiencing. In other organs, where urea is not present at high concentrations, dehydration does not lead to synthesis of GPC.

Glycerophosphorylcholine is produced by splitting of phosphatidyl choline (PC). Some of the phosphatidyl choline substrate is synthesized de novo from choline taken up from the blood. Phosphatidyl choline pre-existing in the cell also contributes to the substrate pool for GPC synthesis. The concentration of GPC is closely regulated, with splitting of GPC by a phosphodiesterase (PDE) playing a key role in removal of GPC from the cell. Phosphodiesterase activity increases in cells exposed to hypoosmotic stress. Efflux of GPC from medullary cells also occurs when medium osmolality is reduced.

The leakage of sorbitol, inositol, glycine betaine, and taurine from medullary cells also occurs when the osmolality of the medium is lowered. Efflux of osmolytes, part of the response known as regulatory volume decrease (RVD), is extremely rapid relative to accumulation, beginning in less than a minute following reduction in external osmolality. If efflux were not rapid, transient decreases in blood osmolality could lead to potentially lethal swelling of the cells. As discussed in more detail below (see "Osmosensing and Signal Transduction"), the speed with which RVD must be effected appears to preclude use of mechanisms that rely on changes in gene expression. Instead, post-translational modification of proteins and changes in protein compartmentation play pivotal roles in the rapid removal of osmolytes from the cell.

To summarize the important characteristics of the regulatory strategies used by kidney medullary cells, the following points bear emphasis. First, in common with the strategies found in bacteria, uptake of organic osmolytes from the water bathing the cells may be a preferred mechanism for increasing intracellular osmotic strength. This strategy may be an energy-saving approach, one that avoids expenditure of substrates and ATP for osmolyte biosynthesis, and it may permit a rapid response. Second, there is a highly coordinated, reciprocal control of osmolyte concentrations. In renal inner medullary cells, high levels of one osmolyte lead to inhibition of transcription of genes encoding transporters or biosynthetic enzymes for other osmolytes, as well as those for the specific osmolyte present at high concentrations. Third, when hyperosmotic stress is alleviated, rapid efflux of osmolytes occurs and the mRNAs encoding up-regulated transporters and osmolyte synthetic enzymes are quickly degraded. Avoiding cell swelling is likely to be critical for survival. Because the flux of water across cell membranes is rapid, removal of osmolytes during rehydration must occur quickly. Fourth, the types of solutes posing stress to the renal inner medullary cells determine in part the class of organic osmolyte that is accumulated. Whereas hypertonic stress may favor production of all of the major osmolytes found in mammalian medullary cells, rising concentrations of urea may favor the accumulation of GPC, which is likely to function as TMAO does in urea-rich elasmobranch fishes by counteracting the effects of urea on proteins. There may also be changes in relative accumulation levels under different degrees of osmotic stress; sorbitol may be more important than inositol at high osmolalities.

Heat-shock proteins may build up during hyperosmotic stress

The conjecture that a build-up of noncompatible solutes may damage proteins is supported by the finding that hyperosmotic stress of mammalian kidney cells leads to increased expression of heat-shock (stress) proteins, including hsp70 (Cohen et al., 1991). In many types of prokaryotic and eukaryotic cells, the initial effect of increased external salt concentration is a rise in intracellular levels of inorganic ions, a response that facilitates conservation of cell volume, but only at the cost of creating a solute microenvironment for proteins that may be perturbing of their structures and functions. Perturbation of protein structure by elevated concentrations of inorganic ions may, like thermal damage, require increased activities of molecular chaperones like hsp70 to restore the native states of protein. Although in both bacterial and mammalian cells the increase in concentrations of ions such as K^+ and Na^+ may be a transient stopgap measure that is used only until compatible organic osmolytes can be accumulated, damage to proteins during the period of high ionic strength might be sufficient to trigger induction of stress proteins. Thus, the rapid induction of hsps during hyperosmotic stress may be an important means for sustaining the native states of proteins during the initial phase

of osmotic adaptation. If compatible osmolytes can be accumulated rapidly at the start of the adaptation process, such that there is no need to rely initially on increased inorganic ion levels, then damage to proteins may be prevented. Support for this conjecture is given by the observation that, when organic osmolytes were supplied to the medium bathing kidney cells, the induction of hsp70 was greatly reduced (Petronini et al., 1993).

OSMOSENSING AND SIGNAL TRANSDUCTION

Common Needs and Mechanisms in Sensing and Transduction

A common problem faced by all cells that encounter water stress is detecting the need for activating the machinery required for osmoregulatory activity. To this point, little has been said about this important initial phase of the overall osmoregulatory process. We now compare the "upstream" events used by different species to initially sense the need for osmotic adaptation (*osmosensing*). Then, we examine how cells pass this information on to the gene regulatory systems and enzymatic processes that effect the osmoregulatory response (*osmosensory signal transduction mechanisms*). We will find that, whereas certain basic strategies of osmosensing and signal transduction are common to all taxa, the sophistication of the osmosensing and signal transduction mechanisms correlates strongly with the complexity of the organization of the organism.

Common to all organisms is a fundamental three-tiered sensing and signal transduction pathway (figure 6.18). This pathway comprises: (1) *primary osmosensors* that detect changes in external osmolality and transfer this information on to (2) *intracellular signaling cascades* that are activated by the osmosensors and that, in turn, regulate (3) *osmotic response elements* that modulate the activities of genes and proteins needed for the appropriate osmoregulatory response. The interspecific variation that occurs in the components of this regulatory scheme is extensive. As we move from prokar-

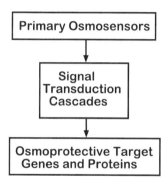

Figure 6.18. The three common elements in the osmosensory signal transduction cascade of cells: (1) osmosensors that monitor osmolality; (2) signal transduction pathways that transmit the information provided by the primary osmosensors to (3) osmotic response elements that regulate gene expression and activities of proteins (enzymes and transporters) that are essential for osmotic adaptation.

yotes to unicellular eukaryotes to complex multicellular animals, there is a parallel growth in complexity of the osmosensing and signal transduction mechanisms. And, as one might expect, there also is a parallel decrease in our level of understanding of these mechanisms as we move from relatively simple prokaryotic systems to complex eukaryotic forms. Below, we treat in some detail the available information and the current proposed models for osmosensing and signal transduction in species of varying complexity. This mode of presentation will provide a sense of how complexity in this three-tiered system has grown during the evolution of complex eukaryotes, through recruitment of different types of regulatory pathways that vary in their targets of action and their speeds of response. Furthermore, this analysis will show how, in complex eukaryotes, the integration of signaling cascades can not only activate the appropriate genes and proteins needed for osmoregulation, but can also trigger programmed cell death (apoptosis) if repair of osmotically induced damage to the cell (especially to its genome) is not adequate.

Unicellular Organisms: Bacterial and Yeast Systems of Osmosensing and Signal Transduction

We have already discussed some of the changes in gene expression and protein activity that take place when soil or enterobacteria are exposed to osmotic stress. The adaptive changes in activities of transporters for osmoprotectants and enzymes for biosynthesis of osmolytes like trehalose depend on relatively simple upstream processes that lead to conversion of information about changing external osmolality to alterations in the cellular machinery needed to adjust osmolyte levels (Csonka and Epstein, 1996). Figure 6.19(A) illustrates the basic two-component regulatory scheme found in *E. coli* and *Salmonella typhimurium*. The primary osmosensing is achieved by a transmembrane histidine kinase sensor (KdpD) that, when activated by hyperosmotic stress, phosphorylates the response regulatory protein KdpE. The phosphorylated form of KdpE binds to an *osmotic response element* in the promoter of the *kdpFABC* operon, which encodes an ion transport system. The physicochemical mechanism that enables KdpD to perceive osmotic stress is not well understood, but it might involve physical forces on the osmotically stressed membrane, as proposed for eukaryotic cells (see "Membrane-Based Osmosensors," below).

In the yeast *Saccharomyces cerevisiae*, one additional level of control is interspersed between the membrane osmosensor and the osmotic response elements of osmotically regulated genes (figure 6.19(B)). Two osmosensing membrane proteins, SLN1 and Sho1, detect shifts in osmolality and, as in *E. coli*, transmit this information to a response regulator protein (SSK1) (Ota and Varshavsky, 1993). However, unlike in *E. coli*, the phosphorylated response regulatory protein does not act as a transcription factor, but instead a mitogen-activated protein (MAP) kinase cascade is used to convey information about osmotic stress to the relevant osmotically regulated genes. This MAP kinase cascade, which comprises several different proteins, is termed the high-osmolality glycerol (HOG1) cascade because it is responsible for regulating the synthesis of glycerol under con-

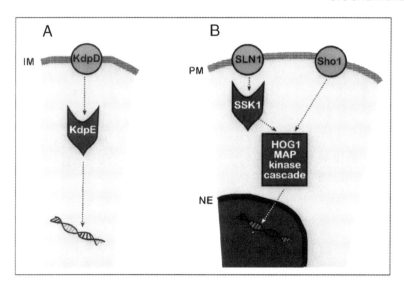

Figure 6.19. Examples of osmosensory signal transduction pathways in *Escherichia coli* (A) and the yeast *Saccharomyces cerevisiae* (B). In both species, the primary osmosensors (KdpD, SLN1, and Sho1) are transmembrane proteins. Components of the signal transduction pathways (KdpE, SSK1, and HOG1 MAP kinase cascade) are interspersed between the primary osmosensors and the chromosomes. Note that the yeast HOG1 MAP kinase cascade contains at least seven different proteins, which have been omitted from the diagram for clarity. (Figure courtesy of Dr. Dietmar Kültz.)

ditions of osmotic stress. HOG1 is the best-understood osmosensory signal transduction pathway in eukaryotes (Wurgler-Murphy and Saito, 1997). At normal osmolality, the osmosensor SLN1 is constitutively active and phosphorylates the response regulator SSK1. Phosphorylated SSK1 is active and functions to repress activities of two protein kinases. This repression shuts off the HOG1 MAP kinase pathway, thus silencing HOG1 activity. Hyperosmolality inhibits SLN1 activity, thereby leading to activation of the HOG1 pathway. When the HOG1 pathway is activated, kinases of the HOG1 system phosphorylate two transcription factors (Msn2 and Msn4). Phosphorylation favors their binding to the transcription-activating stress-response elements (STRE) of genes encoding enzymes needed for synthesis of glycerol and trehalose, glycerophosphate dehydrogenase 1, the rate-limiting enzyme for glycerol synthesis, and trehalose phosphate phosphatase, respectively (Martinez-Pastor et al., 1996). An alternative osmosensor, Sho1, also targets the HOG1 MAP kinase cascade, bypassing SSK1, and also stimulates synthesis of glycerol and trehalose.

Multicellular Organisms: Osmoregulatory Signal Transduction Pathways of Animals

A major increase in complexity of osmosensing signal transduction systems has occurred during the evolution of multicellular organisms, especially animals. Although some plants possess simple two-component osmoregulatory systems involving osmosensing histidine kinases similar to the SLN1 osmosensor of yeast (Urao et al., 1999), the systems found in animals are much more complex. Despite that fact that many aspects of these complicated regulatory cascades remain conjectural, it is worth examining some of the proposed mechanisms to illustrate the multitiered chain of information transfer that characterizes these systems, and to reveal how osmoregulatory signal transduction mechanisms exploit, and interact with, other signal transduction systems of the cell, including those of cell cycle regulation and apoptosis.

One indication of the broad differences that exist between osmoregulatory signal transduction pathways of prokaryotes and animals are the observations that no two-component systems like those of unicellular organisms (figure 6.19(A)) have been identified in animals. In fact, based on information from the genome sequences available for animals, genes for sensor histidine kinases and response regulators (e.g., KdpE) appear to be absent from animal genomes. These observations indicate that, whereas the three-phase regulatory system (figure 6.18) is present in both unicellular and multicellular organisms, many constituent elements of the systems are different between the groups.

The emerging picture of osmosensing signal transduction pathways in animal cells is as follows. Multiple sensors are employed to detect changes in osmolality and the signal transduction pathways that link the activities of these primary sensors to mechanisms for regulating gene expression and protein activity are networked in complex manners (figure 6.20). Because of the complexity of these osmosensing signal transduction networks in animals, we will first dissect each element and, then, show how it interacts with upstream and downstream constituents of the system.

1. Membrane-based osmosensors: mechanisms for "reading" the outside world

Two different types of membrane-based osmosensors have been proposed for animal cells: *extracellular solute sensors* and *membrane stretch-activated sensors*. The former sensors are conjectured to function by detecting changes in the concentration of specific ions, for instance, sodium ion, in the external fluids. There is some indirect evidence for sodium-specific sensors in animal cells, and sodium-gated cation channels have been proposed as candidates for this role. However, no direct evidence for their involvement as upstream osmoregulatory elements has yet been presented.

Membrane stretch-activated sensors, membrane-localized proteins whose activities are modulated by mechanical forces generated in the membrane due to stress, appear to be more promising candidates for the role of detecting changes in external osmolality. Whereas extracellular solute sensors will only respond to changes in concentrations of particular types of solutes, activities of stretch-activated receptors are independent of the nature of the solutes that are causing osmotic stress. Thus, stretch-activated membrane sensors detect osmolality per se, not the concentrations of particular contributors to the total osmotic pool. Although the precise nature of the forces exerted on the plasma membrane by osmotic stress remain to be elucidated in detail, it is clear that stretch-activated receptors respond to mechanical forces on the membranes, not to solute concentration per se. Thus, stretch-activated receptors are not activated by highly permeable solutes such as urea that alter cellular osmolality without changing cell volume.

Stretch-activated proteins in animal cell membranes that are candidates for osmosensing activity include mechanosensitive ion channels and the membrane-localized enzyme phospholipase A2 (PLA2). The former proteins remain to be conclusively linked to osmosensing. Activity of PLA2 is sensitive to packing of the lipid bilayer of the cell and is responsive to osmotic changes, two attributes that mark it as a prime candidate for a stretch-activated sensor (Lehtonen and Kinnunen, 1995).

Changes in the bilayer induced by osmotic stress, like changes induced by alterations in temperature (chapter 7), may alter the lateral distribution of intrinsic membrane proteins. Growth factor receptor tyrosine kinases and cytokine receptors cluster during osmotic stress, and this shift in membrane localization has been suggested to lead to activation of specific osmosensory MAP kinase pathways (Rosette and Karin, 1996). Thus, although the exact types of membrane localized proteins involved in osmosensing are not yet well understood there are several promising candidates for this role.

2. Intracellular osmosensors: detection systems that "read" the status of the intracellular milieu

Changes in external osmolality generally lead to rapid changes in cellular volume in cells that

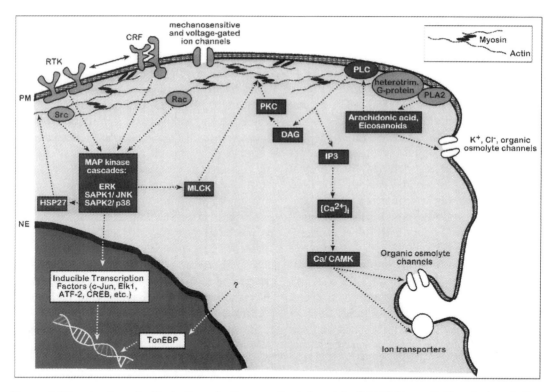

Figure 6.20. A schematic illustration of mitogen-activated protein (MAP) kinase (left) and phospholipase A2 (PLA2) dependent (right) osmosensory signal transduction pathways in vertebrate cells. Putative primary osmosensors (light gray background) and their potential relationships to MAP kinase and PLA2-dependent signal transduction pathways are shown. Important secondary elements of signal transduction cascades are also shown (dark gray background). Effectors of these pathways are transcription factors that target effector genes, ion channels, and transporters (white background). Actin and myosin, forming the peripheral cytoskeleton, could be primary sensors as well as effectors. In addition, the nonspecific clustering of growth factor receptor tyrosine kinases (RTK) and cytokine receptors (CRF) could be a primary osmosensory signal, leading to activation of MAP kinase pathways. Note that MAP kinase pathways carry information about osmotic stress from the cell surface into the nucleus to the level of gene expression, whereas PLA2-dependent pathways seem to be restricted to the cell membrane and adjacent parts of the cytosol. The TonEBP transcription factor targets a tonicity responsive enhancer element (TonE = osmotic response element, ORE) in the 5′ UTR of the *BGT1, SMIT,* and *AR* genes. These genes encode key transporters and enzymes for the accumulation of the compatible organic osmolytes glycine betaine, *myo*-inositol, and sorbitol. The signal transduction pathway that controls TonEBP activity has not yet been elucidated. (Figure courtesy of Dr. Dietmar Kültz.)

cannot generate a turgor pressure, which includes almost all types of animal cells. These rapid changes in cellular volume alter the intracellular concentrations of macromolecules and most types of micromolecules, except for those that can pass relatively freely across the plasma membrane. Cell-volume-induced changes in concentrations of both large and small molecules have been proposed as potential mechanisms for osmosensing.

The phenomenon of *macromolecular crowding*, which relates to the effects that dense packing of macromolecules, especially proteins, has on macromolecular stability and function, has been invoked as a possible mechanism for intracellular osmosensing. As discussed later in more detail ("Molecular Crowding and Excluded Volume Effects"), changing the concentrations of proteins merely through altering the amount of water in solution may significantly alter their activities (for review, see Garner and Burg, 1994). During the transient decreases in cell volume that accompany hyperosmotic stress, increased crowding could favor interactions of proteins, which, through mechanisms not yet understood, could lead to osmosensing. Some evidence for such an effect has been obtained in studies of canine red blood cells (Parker et al., 1995), but the general significance of this aspect of molecular crowding remains unclear.

Inextricably linked to macromolecular crowding during cell volume change are alterations in the concentrations of micromolecules. It thus is difficult to unambiguously attribute effects of changes in cell volume to macromolecular crowding, on the one hand, or to shifts in concentrations of small solutes such as inorganic ions, on the other. Despite this ambiguity, there is good evidence that changes in the concentrations of inorganic ions during the initial phases of cell volume regulation promote shifts in activities of proteins and genes. Some of these effects have been discussed above, for instance, in the cases of K^+ effects on regulation of the *ProU* operon in *E. coli*, and on expression of aldose reductase in mammalian kidney medulla cells (see Burg et al., 1997). We will treat solute effects on DNA structure and function in a later section (see "Osmotic Effects on DNA and Chromatin Structure").

3. Cytoskeleton-based sensors

The cellular cytoskeleton has characteristics that make it a promising candidate for a role in osmosensing. Rearrangements of cytoskeletal components such as scaffolding proteins could lead to changes in activities of signal transduction proteins, such as protein kinases and phosphatases, whose activities are governed by cytoskeletal configuration (figure 6.20). As an example, autophosphorylation of the Src tyrosine kinase depends on conformational changes in the cytoskeleton (Kültz and Burg, 1998a). Small GTPase proteins of the Rho family, for instance, Rac, are closely associated with the cytoskeleton and function as upstream elements of the SAPK1/JNK and SAPK2/p38 mitogen-activated protein kinase pathways.

Actin may play a pivotal role in cytoskeletal osmosensing and signal transduction because its state of polymerization is affected by cellular volume. Swelling leads to actin depolymerization; cell shrinkage favors polymerization (Häussinger, 1996; Hoffmann and Pedersen, 1998). Osmotic stress also influences the diameter of actin filaments (Grazi et al., 1993). Some of these effects could be the results of macromolecular crowding insofar as the concentration of actin governs its polymerization status and assembly with other types of proteins. If changes in actin structure modify the status of the peripheral regions of the cytoskeleton and lead to alterations in activities of signal transduction proteins, then actin may be viewed as an intracellular osmosensor.

To summarize, a variety of proteins involved in the cytoskeleton appear to be promising candidates for osmosensing. Identification of these proteins and elucidation of their mechanisms of action in osmosensing represent important challenges for investigation.

4. Signal transduction cascades: MAP kinases and phosphatases

Primary osmosensors, regardless of their molecular identity or localization (within the membrane, linked to the cytoskeleton, or free in the cytoplasm), regulate pathways of information transfer within the cells (figures 6.18–6.20). Most, although not all, of these transduction pathways involve protein phosphorylation and dephosphorylation reactions, that is, these pathways comprise protein kinases and protein phosphatases. This is a common design element found in a wide array of intracellular signal transduction systems. Lipids and calcium are also important elements in osmoregulatory signal transduction, much as they are in many other types of signal transduction processes.

Evolution of the complex web of signal transduction events found in osmoregulatory systems of eukaryotic cells, and animal cells in particular, appears to reflect selection for enhanced abilities for signal amplification and for signal integration (= information exchange) among different regulatory processes (figure 6.20). Of central importance are MAP kinase cascades, which are ubiquitous among eukaryotes and serve a wide range of functions associated with amplifying and integrating extracellular signals at the cellular level (Treisman, 1996). Mitogen-activated protein kinases occur as multiple paralogous isoforms throughout the eukaryotes. In vertebrates, a subgroup of MAP kinases, the stress-activated protein kinases (SAPK), appear to play key roles in osmoregulatory signal transduction. However, other categories of MAP kinases such as the extracellular signal-regulated kinases (ERKs) also are activated by osmotic stress (Kültz and Burg, 1998b). In fact, in vertebrate cells, the activities of most MAP kinases are altered during osmotic stress (Kültz and Burg, 1998b). The ubiquitous role of MAP kinases in eukaryotic osmoregulation suggests an early evolutionary origin for this mechanism of osmoregulatory signal transduction.

The multilayered pathway of MAP kinase-mediated osmoregulation in animal cells comprises MAP kinase kinase kinases (MAP3K) that phosphorylate and activate MAP kinase kinases (MAPKK). In turn, MAPKKs phosphorylate and activate MAP kinases (MAPK). Among the important substrates of MAPK are several inducible transcription factors, including Egr-1, c-Jun, ATF2, and c-Fos, and other protein kinases, including MAPKAPs, RS6K, and MLCK, that regulate gene expression, protein synthesis, and the cell cycle (Kyriakis and Avruch, 1996). Among the possible effects of these signal transduction events could be the up-regulation of synthesis in kidney inner medullary cells of the important osmolytes glycine betaine, *myo*-inositol, and sorbitol, as discussed above (Burg et al., 1997).

5. Phospholipase A2-regulated pathways

Phospholipase A2 (PLA2) is a membrane-associated enzyme that is activated by swelling in many types of cells (figure 6.20). Forces generated on the membrane by swelling may be adequate to activate PLA2, although in some cases a heterotrimeric G-protein may be needed to achieve activation. Phospholipase A2 has been conjectured to be a primary osmosensor, as discussed above, and an important element in signal transduction cascades. Phospholipase A2 cleaves fatty acids from the *sn*-2 position of phospholipids, thus providing substrates for lipoxygenase enzymes that effect synthesis of eicosanoids. The synthesis of eicosanoids, including arachidonic acid in many species, activates several types of K^+ channels and a putative Cl^- or compatible organic osmolyte channel (Hoffmann and Pedersen, 1998), leading to rapid release of osmotically active species and, thus, to restoration of normal cell volume (= regulatory volume decrease, RVD). Regulatory volume decrease normally takes place within minutes after hypoosmotic swelling commences, and the regulatory events chiefly involve regulation of enzymatic and channel protein activities; regulation of transcription is not observed in this rapid response.

In addition to modulation of activities of osmolyte-transporting channels, the number of channels in the plasma membrane may be adjusted through fusion of channel-containing intracellular vesicles with the plasma membrane. In some types of cells, for instance, rat kidney inner medullary collecting duct cells, arachidonic acid production leads to an increase in intracellular Ca^{2+} levels, presumably through activation of phospholipase C (PLC) (figure 6.20). Increased $[Ca^{2+}]_i$ is proposed to activate a Ca^{2+}/calmodulin-dependent kinase that, in turn, phosphorylates an unidentified effector protein in intracellular membrane vesicles, causing them to fuse with the plasma membrane (Kinne, 1998). The inactive osmolyte channels contained in the vesicles become active once the vesicles have fused with the plasma membrane. This mechanism for rapid enhancement of osmolyte transport is seen to depend on neither transcription nor translation, but only on the introduction into the plasma membrane of preexisting, inactive osmolyte-transporting channels. These rapid mechanisms for effecting RVD reduce the risk of cell rupture from excessive swelling. Slower-acting mechanisms, for instance, those that required alterations in gene expression, might lack the speed required to preclude cell lysis.

6. Osmotic response elements

Regulation of osmoprotective genes in animal cells is much less understood than in the case of prokaryotes. As discussed earlier, a battery of genes encoding proteins involved in osmolyte transport and synthesis is induced during hyperosmotic stress in kidney cells (figure 6.17). Pivotal in these gene regulatory events is the tonicity responsive enhancer element binding protein, TonEBP, which is up-regulated during hyperosmotic stress (Miyakawa et al., 1999). TonEBP is a transcription factor that binds to the tonicity responsive enhancer element (TonE = osmotic response element, ORE) in the $5'$ UTR of osmoprotective genes such as *BGT1* (which encodes a glycine betaine transporter), *SMIT* (which encodes a *myo*-inositol transporter), and *AR* (which encodes aldose reductase). Although TonEBP achieves a similar end-result to the hyperosmotically induced transcription factors in bacteria and yeast, it has very different properties from the analogous transcription factors in unicellular organisms. It is substantially larger, lacks any sequence similarity to the predominant unicellular osmoregulatory transcription factors, and binds to a different *cis* regulatory element on $5'$ UTR regions of the osmotically regulated genes. Thus, certain of the gene regulatory mechanisms exploited by unicellular organisms and animals to respond to hyperosmotic stress appear to represent instances of evolutionary convergence: a common physiological response, the uptake and synthesis of osmolytes needed for regulatory volume increase, is controlled at the level of the gene by transcription factors and *cis* regulatory elements that have arisen independently in these different evolutionary lineages.

OSMOTIC EFFECTS ON DNA AND CHROMATIN STRUCTURE

The observation that osmoregulatory responses frequently involve shifts in gene transcription raises an important question: Can alterations in the solute composition and concentration of the cell directly affect the structure of DNA, thereby leading to rapid changes in gene expression that are independent of complex signal transduction cascades? In considering the effects of solutes on protein synthesis (figure 6.3), it was pointed out that inorganic ions can bind to mRNA molecules, thereby altering their secondary structure and, hence, their abilities to support translation. Solute effects on DNA structure also are likely to play important roles in the responses of cells to osmotic stress. These effects will be seen to involve a much wider range of cellular processes than those involved in osmoregulation per se. Solute effects are highly varied and include shifts in DNA compaction and chromatin conformation, breaks in DNA strands, alterations in DNA repair reactions, changes in timing of the cell cycle, and activation or repression of apoptosis.

DNA Compaction Depends on Cationic Counterions

A key underlying effect of solutes on DNA structure involves changes in the compaction of DNA. The level of DNA compaction governs a wide array of DNA's functional properties, for instance, functions that depend on access by DNA binding proteins to their binding sites on DNA (for review, see Kültz, 2000). The degree of compaction of DNA depends on the concentrations of cationic counterions that neutralize the anionic phosphate groups of the DNA backbone, thereby offsetting the intramolecular charge repulsion that favors an expanded structure of DNA. In bacteria, enhanced compaction of DNA leads to what is termed *supercoiling*, a geometrical characteristic of DNA that is important in governing rates of transcription. Tightly supercoiled DNA may be transcriptionally inactive. The extent of DNA supercoiling in bacteria normally is controlled by the activities of two types of enzymes that have opposing effects on DNA compaction: Topoisomerase I loosens DNA structure, whereas DNA gyrase favors a tighter DNA configuration. The balance attained between these two influences will have major effects on the ability of gene regulatory proteins to bind to promoter regions of genes. Thus, any change in the cellular milieu that impacts the supercoiling of DNA may have pervasive effects on gene expression.

Studies of bacteria exposed to different external osmolalities have shown that DNA supercoiling is highly sensitive to osmotic stress. There is some evidence to suggest that cation-induced changes in DNA supercoiling lead to adaptive shifts in expression of osmoregulatory genes. Thus, transcription of the *proU* gene, which encodes a transporter that facilitates uptake of glycine betaine and proline (figure 6.15), may be governed in part by ion-induced changes in DNA configuration (Higgins et al., 1988). However, activation by hyperosmotic stress of transcription factors that modify supercoiling also may be critical in this regulatory event.

Solutes Affect DNA Stereoisomerization

Another key effect of solutes on DNA structure involves transitions between different stereoisomers of the molecule (for review, see Kültz, 2000). DNA molecules of randomly mixed sequence can exist in three different double-helical configurations: the A-, B-, and Z-forms. The nucleotide sequences commonly found in natural DNAs lead to a strong preference for the latter two forms, and both occur in vivo. However, the balance between B-DNA and Z-DNA is somewhat labile, and is highly sensitive to ionic strength. Both hypo- and hyperosmotic stress can lead to increased contents of Z-DNA, with potential consequences for gene expression. For instance, binding of Topoisomerase II of *Drosophila melanogaster* is substantially stronger to Z-DNA than to B-DNA. Thus, shifts from B-DNA to Z-DNA during osmotic stress could lead to alterations in Topoisomerase-mediated DNA compaction and, as a consequence of this change in DNA structure, to changes in gene expression.

The extent to which these solute-mediated shifts in DNA structure occur in vivo remains conjectural. As pointed out in numerous contexts in this book, one must beware of concluding uncritically that effects observed under in vitro conditions simulate those found in vivo. In the present context, it is important to remember that the nucleoplasm of eukaryotic cells may differ substantially in solute composition from the cytoplasm. The nuclear envelope contains a number of ion channels that control flux of ions between the cytoplasm, perinuclear space, and nucleoplasm. Thus, the nuclear envelope may be an effective protective shield for the nucleoplasm, reducing fluctuations in concentrations of DNA-perturbing solutes in the nucleoplasm that might result from osmotic stress. In light of the potential role that the nuclear envelope may play in shielding chromatin from osmotic stress, it seems likely that solute-induced changes in DNA structure in vivo are more likely to impact chromosomes of prokaryotes than those of eukaryotes.

Solutes Affect Structures of Histones and Chromatin

In eukaryotes the chromosomal organization of DNA leads to additional means by which changes in solute composition of the nucleoplasm could affect DNA structure and activity. A family of histone proteins is primarily responsible for the organization of eukaryotic DNA into the compact structure of chromatin. Binding of the positively charged (arginine and lysine-rich) histones to DNA leads to formation of nucleosome particles that, in turn, coil into strings to form the compact chromatin structure. This highly organized structure has pervasive effects on the accessibility of DNA to other molecules, notably transcription factors. The fact that about 90% of mammalian genes in differentiated cells are transcriptionally silent is due in large measure to chromatin's compact structure. Thus, osmotically induced shifts in chromatin structure raise prospects for widespread effects on gene expression and, as we will see, on the covalent integrity of DNA and the repair processes that prevent genetic damage.

The compactness of nucleosomes has been found to depend on osmolality (Bednar et al., 1995), albeit the impacts of this effect on gene expression remain to be established. Changes in chromatin structure induced by osmotic stress could be offset by alterations in histone proteins. Certain histones of mammalian cells are phosphorylated during hyperosmotic stress, and this covalent modification may affect chromatin structure (Pantazis et al., 1984). However, the most important mechanism for stabilizing the structure of chromatin during osmotic stress may be the accumulation of compatible organic osmolytes. These solutes are able to counteract the chromatin condensation seen during hyperosmotic stress, with taurine having an especially favorable effect (Buche et al., 1993).

Solutes Affect Rates of DNA Synthesis

Rates of DNA synthesis are sensitive to osmolality in both prokaryotic and eukaryotic cells. In bacteria, hyperosmolality led to a decrease in the frequency of initiation of DNA synthesis and, possibly for this reason, to an inhibition of cytokinesis (Meury, 1988). Glycine betaine was able to restore DNA synthesis, illustrating yet another benefit of relying on compatible organic osmolytes in osmoregulation. In mammalian cells, hyperosmolality has been found to both impede and increase DNA synthesis, depending on the cell types being studied and experimental conditions (Kültz, 2000).

Damage and Repair of DNA Is Important in Osmotic Stress

Osmotically induced changes in DNA compaction and chromatin structure will modify access of a wide number of proteins to DNA, including the enzymes involved in repair of damaged DNA. Although it is not known if changes in DNA configuration resulting from osmotic stress do alter access of the molecule to repair enzymes, it is known that osmotic stress caused by high [NaCl] (but not by elevated [urea]) is accompanied by accumulation of breaks in DNA strands (Kültz, 2000; Kültz and Chakravarty, 2001). The damage occurring to DNA during osmotic stress is paired with increased levels of proteins related to DNA repair, cell cycle regulation, and apoptosis. For instance, the amounts and the phosphorylation state of the tumor suppressor protein p53 increase within a few hours following onset of osmotic stress in mammalian kidney cells

(Dmitrieva et al., 2000). p53 may play a vital role in recovery from osmotic stress because it is a transcription factor that controls a number of genes that prevent damaged cells from proliferating, including genes involved in growth arrest, DNA repair, and cell cycle regulation. Rapid induction of p53 is accompanied by arrest of cells in the G2 phase of the cell cycle (Dmitrieva et al., 2000). The effect of p53 in preventing cell proliferation is of course a key reason that cancer research is so strongly focused on this transcription factor. By coupling the pathways that detect and repair damage to DNA to mechanisms involved in regulation of the cell cycle, adequate repair of damaged DNA may take place before cell division resumes. Growth arrest during osmotic stress may also free energy for use in effecting the osmoregulatory response, albeit at the expense of continued cell division.

If repair of cellular damage arising from osmotic stress is not adequate, then programmed cell death, apoptosis, may ensue (Kültz, 2000). Apoptosis leads to elimination of cells with damaged genotype. Cells with damaged DNA are genetically unstable and may undergo transformation to malignant cell types, thereby endangering the survival of the organism. In apoptosis, induction of activities of MAPK pathways may be important in mediating the program of cell death. The MAPK pathways that are activated in apoptosis also include osmotically regulated MAP kinase cascades. Thus, regulatory cascades involving MAP kinase reactions may lead to integration of signals from pathways of osmosensing and apoptosis. Increased levels of apoptosis have been observed in cells of gill epithelia of fishes exposed to osmotic stress (Wendelaar Bonga and Van der Meij, 1989).

These brief treatments of diverse osmotic effects on DNA are adequate to show that changes in the solute composition of the nucleoplasm and cytoplasm trigger a substantial number of effects on the structure and function of DNA and chromatin. These effects, which may be lethal if not reversed, are paired with regulatory responses that lead to changes in the amounts and activities of a wide range of enzymatic, transport, and gene regulatory proteins, whose activities serve to redress the osmotically induced damage to the cell's genetic system. If repair is not possible, then the regulatory systems activated during osmotic stress foster activation of programmed cell death to rid the organism of genetically damaged cells whose propagation could ultimately prove to be lethal. Adaptation to osmotic stress therefore must be appreciated as a multitiered process that involves (i) adjustments in the concentrations of osmolytes, to regulate cell volume and to provide a hospitable milieu for macromolecular function; (ii) induction of stress proteins and DNA repair mechanisms, to redress damage caused by changes in solute levels; and, if damage from stress cannot be repaired, (iii) activation of processes (apoptosis) for eliminating from the organism any cells that have been so damaged by osmotic stress as to be beyond repair and to pose a threat to the organism's survival.

SOLVENT CAPACITY OF THE CELL: SOLVING THE "PACKAGING PROBLEM" THAT ARISES FROM THE NEED TO CONTAIN SO MUCH CHEMISTRY IN SO SMALL A VOLUME

The different facets of water–micromolecule–macromolecule interactions discussed up to this point involve several of the most important ways in which water has shaped the characteristics of living systems and the ways in which the internal milieu is defended in the face of water stress. Because of water's pervasive influence on the evolution of virtually all properties of organisms, there are many other imprints of water on biological design that remain to be discussed. Below, we present in somewhat abbreviated manner several of these issues. This discussion will help us to understand more clearly how water establishes the boundary conditions for life and dictates many of the "engineering principles" that are found in the designs of cells. Of particular importance is the issue of "packaging": how to accommodate tens of thousands of chemical systems in a minute volume of water.

Although water is the most abundant molecule in the cell and may represent 80–95% of the mass of an organism, cellular water has a finite solvent capacity, and this creates a monumental "packaging problem." The problem of course arises from the vast number of metabolic reactions that must take place to support life. Each metabolic reaction is catalyzed by a specific enzymatic protein, part or all of which is hydrated. Each enzymatic reaction involves one to several substrates, cofactors, and modulators that are dissolved in the intracellular water. It seems intuitively clear that in order to package this many types of large and small molecules into a minute volume of water, the concentrations of each type of macromolecule and metabolite may have to be kept low so that excessive demands on the cell's solvent capacity do not arise. At the same time, however, the chemical activities of substrates and cofactors may need to be kept high—to ensure adequate rates of metabolism and appropriate conditions of chemical equilibrium. Another reason that cells regulate the concentrations of metabolites at low levels is because some are highly reactive and would present dangers to the cell if their concentrations were allowed to increase to high levels. Such highly reactive metabolites may need to be supplied in a chemically modified form that allows a favorable thermodynamic reactivity even when very low concentrations are present.

Below, we consider a number of different aspects of the "packaging problem," and examine characteristics of proteins and their metabolites that would seem to substantially ameliorate this problem. As a caveat for this analysis, we reemphasize an important philosophical point made at several junctures in this volume: a particular current advantage we attribute to a trait need not reflect the reason that the trait was originally selected, nor need it be the aspect of the trait that is currently of highest significance to the organism. Some of the aspects of metabolic design that facilitate "packing" complex chemistry into the water of the cell may have been selected for reasons not having to do primarily with solvent capacity. However, these solvent-capacity-related traits can at least be regarded as beneficial side effects of the original adaptation, that is, they may be exaptations in the terminology outlined by Gould and Vrba (1982) (also see chapter 1).

Kinetic Properties of Enzymes

Many functional and structural characteristics of enzymes reflect the cell's need to conduct thousands of different metabolic transformations in a limited volume of water (see Atkinson, 1969, for a lucid analysis of this issue). The ligand binding abilities of enzymes are a good example of traits that reduce the severity of the "packaging problem" arising from a finite solvent capacity. Enzymes have evolved to have high affinities for their substrates, cofactors, and modulators. Selection for high affinity probably began at the earliest stages of evolution, when proteins were faced with the need to acquire their substrates from dilute pools of metabolites. For instance, those early cells with high-affinity transporters that were best able to extract useful organic molecules from the external environment would likely have been at a selective advantage to cells with transporters having lower affinities for these molecules. Likewise, cells whose metabolic enzymes had relatively high affinities may have been capable of higher rates of metabolism, thus giving them a competitive edge over cells with lower affinity enzymes and lower rates of metabolism and growth. As metabolic systems evolved to be increasingly complex, high affinities led to an additional benefit. Because high affinity allows each individual enzymatic process to place a relatively small demand on solvent capacity of the cellular water, many thousands of different enzymes can be accommodated in the cell without overtaxing the cellular water's ability to dissolve the needed substrates. Substrate concentrations usually fall in the range of 10^{-4} M or 10^{-5} M for enzymes embedded within a pathway, but at times are somewhat higher for the first and terminal enzymatic reactions of a pathway (Srivastava and Bernhard, 1986). Of course, as discussed later, substrates, cofactors, and modulators are not evenly distributed throughout the cellular water. Adaptations that influence

where a metabolite is localized can also play important roles in conserving solvent capacity.

Although high affinities for substrates enable enzymes to function in the presence of low substrate concentrations, it is important that affinities are not so high, relative to substrate concentrations, that enzymes become saturated (function at maximal velocities). Were this to occur, increased supply of substrate could not lead to increased rates of catalysis, with the result that substrate concentrations could increase exponentially (see Atkinson, 1969). Therefore, selection has led to the development of enzymes that, while having high affinities for substrates, maintain a reserve capacity for increasing their rates of function when substrate concentrations rise. It is common for physiological concentrations of substrate to lie near or below the values of the apparent K_m for the substrate. In other words, enzymes may function near or somewhat below half-maximal velocity, thereby retaining the ability to elevate their rates of function when substrate levels rise during activation of the metabolic pathway (chapter 2). The importance of conserving K_m values in the face of physical and chemical stressors that modify enzyme–ligand binding has been emphasized at several points in this volume. The importance of conserving solvent capacity illustrates a major benefit of this prevalent pattern of conservation in enzymes' functional attributes.

Compartmentation of Enzymes

Enzymes also may reduce their demands on cellular water and enhance their efficiency of function by organizing into assemblages containing several enzymes linked to a common metabolic activity. These assemblages, termed *metabolons* (Srere, 1985), may reduce demands on the cellular water's solvent capacity for two reasons. First, this type of organization of multiple proteins may reduce the amount of water needed to hydrate the enzymes themselves, because large fractions of their surfaces are involved in protein–protein contacts rather than protein-solvent interactions. A second advantage of this type of organization of enzymes involves the issue of substrate concentration. When enzymes of coordinated metabolic function are arranged in close juxtaposition, the product of one enzyme can be passed more or less directly to the next enzyme, where it serves as a substrate. When enzymes are organized in this fashion, substrates of the pathway need not be maintained at relatively uniform concentrations throughout the cellular water, but instead can be highly localized near the enzymes of a particular pathway. The extent to which the organization of enzymes into metabolons leads to high concentrations of substrates in the vicinity of the metabolon is not fully understood. When a reaction product is released from the active site of an enzyme, some diffusion of the metabolite away from the metabolon, into the bulk water of the cytoplasm inevitably will occur. Nonetheless, it seems likely that this type of organization of linked proteins will enable an enzyme to "grab" the product of the enzyme in the previous step of the pathway before the product (= substrate) diffuses too far away from the metabolon. Moreover, there is evidence for some enzymes that products formed during catalysis may not in fact be released into the aqueous phase at all. Srivastava and Bernhard (1986) have proposed that metabolite transfer between enzyme pairs may be direct; that is, transfer may involve enzyme–enzyme interactions that entail a direct "hand-off" of product to the next enzyme of the pathway, rather than a "fumble" of the product into solution, from which the substrate must be recovered by the appropriate enzyme before it diffuses away.

Evolution of Metabolites

The "packaging problem" facing the cell has had a critical shaping influence on the evolution of metabolites as well as enzymes. In fact, the chemical forms in which some metabolites occur reflect an insurmountable barrier to enzymatic function, a barrier that has had to be surmounted through evolution of substrate structure. Although possessing capacities for catalyzing chemical reactions at high rates, enzymes are unable to shift the equilibrium of the reaction they catalyze. That is, although enzymes can lower the activation free energy

barrier ($\Delta G^{\ddagger}$) to a reaction (see chapter 7), they cannot influence the overall free energy change associated with interconversion of substrates and products. When a metabolic reaction is thermodynamically unfavorable, it would seem to be necessary to maintain a high concentration of substrate, such that the concentration gradient of substrate to product could drive the reaction in the direction of product. Such high substrate concentrations might raise problems for solvent capacity and, if the substrate is highly reactive, it could lead to side reactions and thus to chemical perturbation of the cell. The problems associated with thermodynamically unfavorable reactions have been solved in large measure through evolution of *activated substrates* whose conversions to product are thermodynamically highly favorable (see Atkinson, 1969).

A familiar example of this type of metabolite adaptation is the thiol ester derivative of acetic acid, acetyl-coenzymeA (acetylCoA). AcetylCoA has a much larger negative free energy of hydrolysis than acetate, so metabolic transformations involving the acetate ion can occur with much lower concentrations of acetylCoA than of acetate. Phosphorylated metabolic intermediates likewise allow metabolites to have high chemical potentials and occur at relatively low concentrations in the cellular water. Use of such activated intermediates enables the cell to avoid high concentrations of metabolites that can tax solvent capacity and, perhaps more important, disrupt the cell through uncontrolled chemical reactions with inappropriate molecules.

MOLECULAR CROWDING AND EXCLUDED VOLUME EFFECTS

Can In-vitro Experimentation Tell Us What Things Are Really Like within the Cell (in vivo)?

The ramifications of the "packaging problem" discussed above comprise both theoretical issues concerning cellular evolution and practical issues that involve development of strategies for conducting biologically sound experiments with cells or materials extracted from them. One of the greatest challenges facing biochemists is to design experiments that allow extrapolation from what is observed in vitro to what actually takes place in vivo. This challenge is multifaceted and involves facing a host of potential artifacts that can arise in in-vitro experimentation. Perhaps the most common artifact concerns what is almost an inevitable aspect of in-vitro experimentation: dilution of the macromolecules being studied. How can we be sure that the biochemical systems we study in dilute in-vitro solutions have the same properties they do when present within the cell? For instance, when studying the characteristics of proteins in vitro it is important to remember that, within the cell, concentrations of protein may be as high as approximately 50% in terms of wet mass. In an *E. coli* cell, the summed concentration of protein and RNA is about 300–400 mg per ml of cytoplasm (Zimmerman and Trach, 1991). If one is studying an enzyme normally found in the mitochondrial matrix, where protein concentrations are estimated to be as high as approximately 500 mg protein per gram wet mass, do the properties of the enzyme in extremely dilute experimental solutions, where only nanograms or micrograms of enzyme may be present in each milliliter of solution, resemble those of the enzyme in its natural microhabitat? For studies of certain aspects of protein structure and function, the answer to this question is likely to be "no." Although there are not a great number of data dealing with the issue of in-vitro versus in-vivo properties of proteins, the data that are available, plus theoretical considerations concerning "molecular crowding" and "excluded volume effects," provide a relatively firm basis for pessimism about using the results of in-vitro studies to predict unambiguously how the protein behaves within the cell.

Protein Stability and Activity Are Affected by Total Protein Concentration

One illustration of this type of uncertainty comes from studies of paralogs of malate dehydrogenase. The mitochondrial paralog of malate dehydrogenase (mMDH) has long been regarded as a thermally labile enzyme because of the rapid rate at which it loses activity when incubated in vitro at high temperatures in dilute buffers in which enzyme concentration is low (figure 6.21). The extreme lability of the mammalian (porcine) ortholog of mMDH at 42°C suggests that some type of extrinsic stabilization must occur in vivo if the enzyme is to have a reasonable half-life in the cell. The extrinsic factor in question may simply be other proteins. When protein concentration (bovine serum albumin, BSA) was raised towards physiologically realistic values, the stability of mMDH increased rapidly (figure 6.21) and approached that of the thermally stable paralog found in the cytoplasm, cytoplasmic MDH (cMDH) (Lin et al., 2001).

The different intrinsic stabilities in vitro of cMDH and mMDH from the same species show that evolution of protein thermal stability may involve considerations in addition to body temperature. Intrinsic stabilities of proteins may evolve to be in accord with the degree of stabilization by extrinsic factors that is characteristic of their cellular microenvironment, as well as by the needs for different classes of proteins to have different intrinsic stabilities for a number of physiological reasons (see chapter 7 for additional discussion). Highly stabilizing microenvironments such as the protein-rich mitochondrial matrix may favor selection for proteins with relatively low intrinsic stabilities, so that the proper balance between conformational flexibility and stability is attained in vivo. Within a highly stabilizing microenvironment, a protein like mMDH which has a low intrinsic stability may have the physiologically appropriate degree of flexibility to do its job well, for instance, to undergo rapid catalytic conformational changes, while retaining the right geometry for ligand binding.

Consistent with what has been observed when enzymes are bathed with high levels of stabilizing cosolvents (figure 6.6) or when orthologs of an enzyme from differently adapted species are compared (chapter 7), there is a trade-off between thermal stability and rate of function: the enhanced stability of mMDH that results from increased concentration of protein in the medium is paired with a

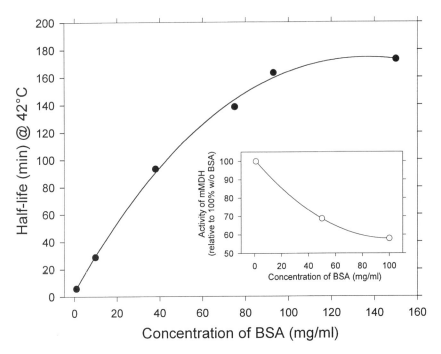

Figure 6.21. Stabilization of porcine mitochondrial MDH (mMDH) by bovine serum albumin (BSA). The half-life of mMDH at an incubation temperature of 42°C increases as the concentration of BSA in the medium is increased, but the increase in stability is correlated with a decrease in specific activity of the enzyme. (Figure modified after Lin et al., 2001.)

reduction in rate of catalysis (figure 6.21). This, then, is another illustration of the trade-off between rate of function and stability that occurs when protein stability is modified, either through intrinsic (amino acid substitutions) or extrinsic (milieu adjustments) mechanisms.

Molecular Crowding and Excluded Volume Effects Favor Protein Stability

Why does protein concentration exert such strong stabilizing influences on protein structure and, thereby, on enzymatic activity? And why can a protein such as BSA affect the stability of an unrelated enzymatic protein like MDH? To explain the effects shown in figure 6.21, another type of stabilizing influence must be introduced, one that differs from the mechanisms involving solvophobic (hydrophobic and osmophobic) effects. The primary phenomenon involved in accounting for stabilization of macromolecular structure by other macromolecules is termed the *excluded volume effect*, which is one consequence of the *molecu-*

lar crowding that characterizes the cytoplasm of all cells (for review, see Garner and Burg, 1994; Häussinger, 1996).

An excellent way to develop a sense of the crowded nature of the cytoplasm and to appreciate excluded volume effects is to study the elegant portrayals of the intracellular space that Goodsell (1993) has developed. Figure 6.22 shows the complexity of the cytoplasm of a eukaryotic cell (yeast), into which are packaged thousands of different types of proteins and a variety of organelles. This figure shows that the organization of proteins in the cytoplasm is distinctly nonrandom: many proteins are found in multiprotein complexes that serve specific functions (e.g., ribosomes, metabolons, and contractile apparatus). Scaffolding proteins may be critical for organizing proteins within the cell. One of the effects of crowding so many different proteins, nucleic acids, and membranous structures into the cell is that a significant fraction of the volume of the cell is occupied by large molecules and, consequently, is unavailable to water and the micromolecules dissolved in it. This is

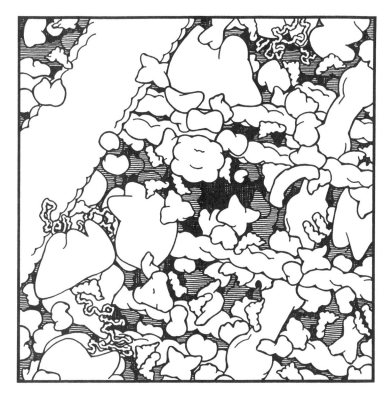

Figure 6.22. The crowded cytoplasm: a portrayal of the interior of a yeast cell. Filamentous proteins criss-cross the cell, and serve as anchorage sites for proteins. The largest filament shown is a microtubule, which runs diagonally across the upper left portion of the figure. Several actin filaments, with which a number of proteins are associated, run more or less horizontally across the cell. An intermediate filament runs diagonally across the right side of the figure. (Figure is modified after figure 5.2 in D. Goodsell (1993), *The Machinery of Life*, Springer-Verlag, Berlin, with permission. Modified figure provided by D. Goodsell.)

termed an excluded volume effect: the fraction of the cellular volume taken up by large molecular entities is excluded from penetration by water and small solutes.

One physical consequence of the excluded volume effect is that solutions crowded with macromolecules tend to be highly nonideal. In an ideal solution, a particle has access to any region of the solution. This is clearly not true for the intracellular milieu (figure 6.22). As a result of excluded volume effects, the chemical activities of both large and small solutes are considerably higher than their actual concentrations (this is another aspect of the nonideality of the intracellular milieu). The nonideal characteristics of the intracellular solution favor a minimization of excluded volume, that is, they

favor a compact, folded state for individual proteins and the aggregation of folded proteins into multiprotein complexes. The thermodynamically favorable tendency for excluded volume to be minimized should be appreciated as having parallels with the preferential hydration model developed by Timasheff (1992, 1998), in which exclusion of cosolvent from the water adjacent to the protein surface leads to minimization of protein volume. In both cases, the fraction of the total solution volume from which a particular class of molecule is excluded is minimized, leading to the most favorable state of entropy for the system, that is, to the lowest free energy state.

These effects of molecular crowding and excluded volume on protein structure can account for the stabilizing effects of increased protein concentration noted for mMDH (figure 6.21). Furthermore, because catalytic conformational changes may involve increases in protein volume, an enzyme that necessarily undergoes a volume increase during catalysis will tend to be inhibited at high protein concentrations.

The phenomenon of molecular crowding and the consequent excluded volume effects that arise from crowding raise important issues concerning protein structure and function in vivo. Other things being equal, one would predict that proteins would be more stable within their intracellular milieu than in dilute solutions—strictly because of excluded volume effects. If increased stability leads to reduced rate of function, then in vitro studies of enzymatic activity (k_{cat} values in particular) may be providing a misleading picture of what occurs in the cell.

Molecular crowding and excluded volume effects have been conjectured to play an important role in osmotic adaptation and cell volume regulation (for critical review, see Garner and Burg, 1994; Häussinger, 1996). It has been hypothesized that during exposure to hyperosmotic conditions that lead to increased concentrations of inorganic ions in the cell, molecular crowding offsets the perturbation of macromolecular function due to rising intracellular salt concentrations. Studies of hyperosmotically stressed *E. coli* cells revealed that the strong inhibition by salt (KCl) of binding of *lac* repressor and RNA polymerase to DNA noted in vitro was not evident in salt-stressed cells (Cayley et al., 1991). It was hypothesized that the cellular dehydration that accompanied hyperosmotic stress led to a sufficient increase in the chemical activities of macromolecules in the cell (excluded volume effects) to offset the effects of rising inorganic ion concentrations on the *lac* repressor–RNA polymerase–DNA interactions. However, two caveats must be raised. First, the intracellular milieu is not a chloride ion-rich solution—glutamate is preferentially accumulated as a major anion during hyperosmotic stress—so the in-vitro experiments that employed KCl may offer a misleading image of the salt inhibition that occurs in vivo. (This

caveat has been raised before, e.g., in the context of data presented in figure 6.3.) A second concern within the context of differences between in-vitro and in-vivo conditions is that, during osmotic regulation, increasing concentrations of inorganic ions like K^+ are commonly seen only during the initial phases of salt stress. As osmotic adaptation progresses, inorganic ions are extruded from the cell and compatible organic osmolytes like glycine betaine and trehalose are either taken up from the extracellular space or synthesized within the cell. It is clear, then, that in the context of osmotic adaptation and cell volume regulation, one must be cautious about attributing effects on macromolecular systems to either molecular crowding/excluded volume effects or osmolyte effects. Both types of influences may be important in governing the effects of changes in water content and solute concentration on macromolecules.

ANHYDROBIOSIS: LIFE IN THE DRY STATE

Metabolic Quiescence Is Often Paired with Desiccation

The first heading of this chapter—life is an aqueous phenomenon—notwithstanding, there are prokaryotic and eukaryotic organisms that tolerate the withdrawal of greater than 99% of the water from their cells during periods of metabolic quiescence. These organisms comprise a phylogenetically varied lot: fungi, crustaceans, nematodes, tardigrades, rotifers, and vascular plants (reviewed by Crowe et al., 1997). In each case, the organism enters a state of metabolic quiescence either as part of its normal life history, for instance, during production of seeds, cysts, or spores, or in response to environmental stress, for instance, drying or heating of the environment. Thus, whereas *metabolically active* stages of life depend absolutely on the presence of substantial amounts of water in the cell, life stages in which metabolism can be essentially halted may rely on extreme desiccation to get the organism through stressful times. The wholesale removal of cellular water can be highly advantageous when organisms enter a prolonged period of metabolic quiescence, for not only can energy stores be conserved, but the dried state of the cell may be highly resistant to a suite of environmental stresses, including extremes of temperature. *Anhydrobiosis*—life without water—thus is a form of adaptation that is found in a wide variety of taxa and used for a wide range of purposes (Crowe et al., 1997; Potts, 1994). Anhydrobiosis provides a striking example of convergent evolution, as the wide variety of taxa in which this process occurs should imply. Despite the range of different organisms in which anhydrobiosis has independently arisen during evolution, however, there may be but a single molecular "secret to success," one that has been discovered by almost all anhydrobiotes.

Before considering the mechanisms used to allow cells to survive in the dried state, it is appropriate first to examine the problems that withdrawal of water from the cell is likely to raise. Most of these potential problems should be apparent from the preceding discussions of how macromolecular structure and function are perturbed when the cellular milieu is altered. Despite its many advantages, then, anhydrobiosis poses major challenges to the structures of the macromolecules and membranes of the cell. Based on the fact that the folding and aggregation of proteins and the assembly of membranes is driven in large measure by interactions with water, that is, by the hydrophobic effect, it might appear likely that desiccation would be marked by wholesale denaturation of macromolecules and disruption of membrane integrity. This is what usually occurs in vitro when cells or isolated proteins and membranes are dried, at least when such experiments are conducted in the absence of solutes that counteract the effects of desiccation. Because only a minority of types of organisms are able to withstand extreme desiccation, the types of damage predicted from in-vitro studies and theoretical considerations are seen to be very real. Thus, we must ask what chemical properties of desiccation-resistant cells confer on them the ability to maintain native structures of macromolecules and membranes when essentially all water is withdrawn from the cells.

Water Substitutes—Trehalose and Sucrose—Protect the Cell When Water Leaves

The short answer to this question is that desiccation tolerant cells accumulate *water substitutes* that are able to maintain proteins and membranes in native states in the absence of water (Crowe et al., 1997; Potts, 1994). The water replacement hypothesis, developed most powerfully by John and Lois Crowe and their colleagues, provides a unifying explanation for anhydrobiosis in all taxa in which this phenomenon is found. The most common water substitute is trehalose, a disaccharide that we have already considered in several instances of adaptation. (Historical note: the name trehalose was given to this disaccharide in the mid-nineteenth century by M. Berthelot, who identified the unknown sugar that was present in high levels in cocoons ["trehala"] of the beetle *Larinus* [perhaps a desiccation tolerant species?] [Singer and Lindquist, 1998a].) In some plants another disaccharide, sucrose, is the predominant water substitute. The abilities of trehalose and sucrose to protect cells during desiccation might be taken to imply that any sugar or polyol osmolyte would fulfill this task. However, a number of other compatible solutes, including glycerol and monosaccharides, fail to function well as water substitutes. Thus, it is the particular disaccharide structure of trehalose and sucrose, not their constituent sugars, that gives these two molecules their abilities to protect the cell during anhydrobiosis. Note that trehalose and sucrose are not reducing sugars because they lack hemiacetal hydroxyl groups. Thus, these disaccharides do not pose the risk of entering into browning reactions with cellular proteins (see Potts, 1994). This trait of trehalose and sucrose may be a fortuitous "fringe benefit" of these molecules—an exaptation—rather than the primary selective advantage that led to their choice as water substitutes. The primary selective advantage is likely to relate to the precise steric configurations of these molecules, as discussed below.

The mechanisms that underlie the protective effects of these two water substitutes differ from the mechanisms that account for their compatibility with macromolecules under conditions of high water content. This is an important (and probably obvious) point: in the absence of water, the preferential exclusion mechanism that explains the stabilizing effects of compatible solutes in aqueous solutions cannot play any role in macromolecular stability. Instead, the mechanisms by which trehalose and sucrose stabilize proteins and membranes in the dry state involve *direct interactions* between the water substitute and the molecules being stabilized. Thus, as water content is reduced to diminishingly small values, the favorable effects of trehalose and sucrose shift from being due to their exclusion from macromolecules and membranes to their ability to engage in highly precise binding.

Membrane stabilization by trehalose: conserving the physical state and integrity of the bilayer

A clue as to the nature of trehalose's role as a membrane stabilizer comes from an observation that has been made by bakers for many centuries: to successfully rehydrate yeast to regain metabolically active ($= CO_2$-generating) cells, the dried yeast must be rehydrated in water with a temperature near 40°C. Work of John and Lois Crowe and their associates has explained this effect in terms of the influences of water content and temperature on the physical organization of the membrane bilayer. When the water surrounding a membrane is removed and no water substitute like trehalose is present, two types of damage to membranes may occur (figure 6.23). First, there may be fusion of membranes. The water layer that previously coated the phospholipid head groups of the membrane established a hydration force that led to mutual repulsion of one membrane surface from the other. The elimination of this repulsive force during dehydration allows the membranes to fuse, with damaging consequences for cellular organization.

A second important consequence of dehydration is an alteration of the physical properties of the membrane phospholipids themselves (Crowe et al., 1997). In a normally hydrated

cell, phospholipid molecules are strongly hydrated, especially at the charged headgroup region. Physical studies suggest that phospholipids in bilayers bind about 10–12 moles of water per mole of phospholipid. Through acquiring this water, the phospholipid bilayer expands and intermolecular interactions among the phospholipids are altered. For instance, swelling of the bilayer during hydration lessens chances for van der Waals interactions among the hydrocarbon (acyl) chains, and thus leads to a propensity for the phospholipids to remain in a fluid phase. Hydration of the membrane thus functions in a somewhat analogous way to an increase in membrane temperature: interactions among acyl chains are weakened, and the membrane tends to prefer a fluid rather than a gel state (see chapter 7).

As water is withdrawn from a membrane during entry into anhydrobiosis, the strengths of interactions among acyl chains increase, and a shift from the fluid to the gel state is favored. This shift is noticeable as water content is reduced below about 20% (Crowe et al., 1997). Transition temperatures (T_m), the temperatures at which the fluid (liquid crystalline) to gel conversion occurs, increase significantly during dehydration. A membrane composed of palmitoyloleoylphosphatidyl choline has a T_m of $-7°C$ when fully hydrated, but the T_m rises to approximately 60°C in the dry lipid (Crowe et al., 1997). Thus, a phospholipid membrane that would be in a fluid state at normal cell temperatures when hydrated acquires a rigid gel structure when dehydrated.

How does this shift from fluid to gel state during desiccation cause damage to the membrane, and how does the presence of trehalose or sucrose—water substitutes—prevent this damage? As the anecdote about baking technique implies, the crux of the problem occurs when dried cells are rehydrated. It is known from studies of model membranes that when phospholipid bilayers pass through the temperature range over which the gel phase is replaced by the liquid crystalline phase, transient changes in membrane permeability occur (Crowe et al., 1997). The precise mechanism responsible for this transient breakdown in the permeability barrier is not entirely clear, but it

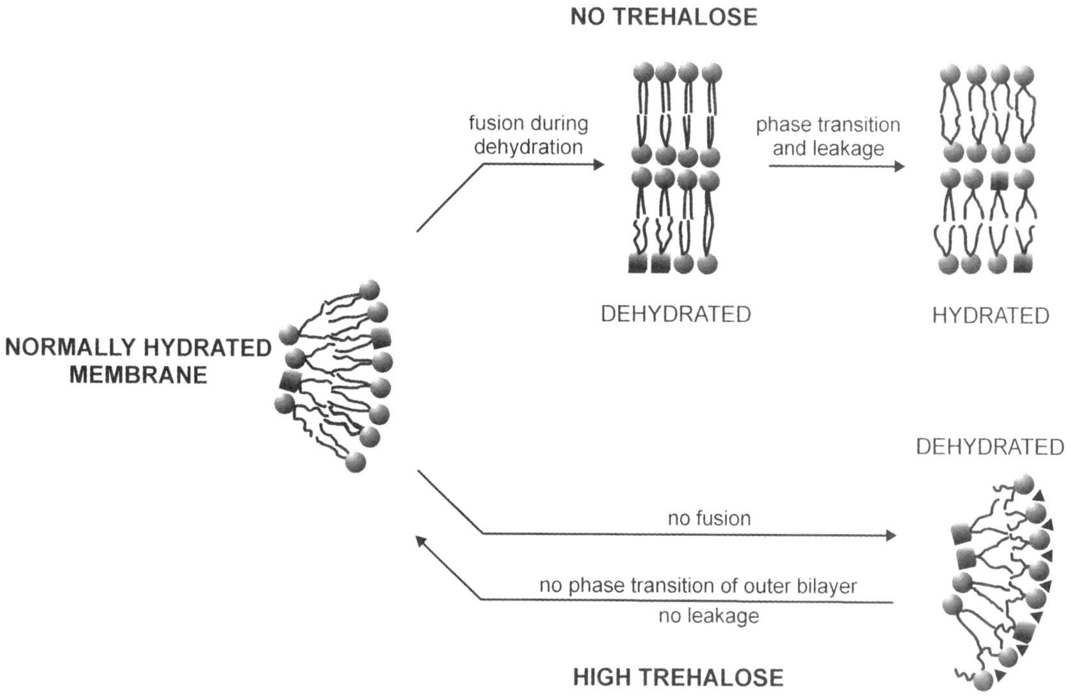

NO TREHALOSE

Figure 6.23. Protection of phospholipid bilayers by trehalose during dehydration. In the fully hydrated membrane (left), headgroups of phospholipid molecules are strongly hydrated, leading to an expanded state of the membrane and weakened interactions among acyl chains. Hydration also prevents adjacent membrane surfaces from fusing. As water is withdrawn from the system in the absence of a water substitute like trehalose (upper part), the headgroups pack more tightly and acyl chain interactions are strengthened, leading to a more rigid (gel) state of the membrane bilayer. Adjacent membranes may fuse. When a membrane dried in the absence of trehalose is rehydrated, phase transitions result and membrane integrity is lost. Leakage of materials across the membrane occurs. When the membrane is dried in the presence of trehalose (indicated by triangles, lower right), the binding of trehalose to the headgroups of phospholipids in the outer leaflet prevents membrane fusion and subsequent phase transitions during rehydration (see text for additional details). (Figure modified after Crowe et al., 1997.)

is thought to involve packing defects at the boundaries between liquid crystalline and gel phase domains. Because of the heterogeneity of phospholipid composition in membranes, there will be different local T_m values for individual domains (see figure 7.18). Thus, a domain enriched in unsaturated acyl chains will have a lower T_m value than an adjacent domain enriched in saturated acyl chains. As in the case of the effects of reduced temperature on membranes, drying of membranes can lead to changes in the lateral organization of lipid molecules, as lipids of similar T_m separate from other lipids. Lateral phase separation during chilling or drying thus predisposes the membrane to leakiness when warming or rehydration takes place. However, if (as in the case of the smart bread baker) the dried cells are warmed to a temperature above the T_m of all membrane domains, then permeability is not compromised and the cells are likely to remain viable after rehydration.

The means by which trehalose prevents loss of membrane integrity is suggested by the lower portion of figure 6.23. During withdrawal of water from a cell that contains high concentrations of trehalose, water that is lost from the phospholipid headgroups is replaced by trehalose, whose hydroxyl groups are sterically organized to allow precise interactions with the polar headgroups of phospholipids. The inter-actions between trehalose and the surface of the hemilayer of the membrane foster maintenance of the normal spacing between phospholipids that characterizes the fully hydrated membrane. By stabilizing this spacing, trehalose prevents strengthening of van der Waals interactions among acyl chains that favor formation of gel-phase domains. In short, trehalose allows the membrane to retain the balance between liquid crystalline and gel structure that it pos-sessed when fully hydrated. And, through form-ing a coating on the membrane surface, trehalose also prevents membrane fusion.

Trehalose–protein interactions: stabilization through binding, not through preferential exclusion

The mechanism by which trehalose stabilizes proteins in the dried state also involves direct interactions with the target molecule. This may seem paradoxical, because when we considered how compatible solutes achieve their protein-stabilizing effects we found that they tend to be preferentially excluded from the water sur-rounding the protein. However, when the hydration layer around the protein is removed, the rules of the game change. In the dried state, a coating of trehalose enables the native three-dimensional state of the protein to be retained.

There remains considerable uncertainly about the exact mechanism that underlies this stabilization. What is known is that hydrogen bonding is established between trehalose and the protein during drying, and this hydrogen bonding is required for stabilization (Crowe et al., 1997). Another conjecture is that trehalose enters into a vitreous (glass-like) state during dehydration, and that the protein is stabilized in its native conformation because of the restric-tions to molecular motion, that is, to unfolding of the protein, that the glass-like environment creates. However, vitrification appears to be a necessary, but not a sufficient, condition for protein and membrane stabilization (Carpenter et al., 1995). Solutes such as dextrans, that read-ily vitrify during drying, but do not appear to hydrogen bond to the surfaces of proteins, do not stabilize proteins against denaturation in

the dried state. Although the glass-like state, as opposed to a rigid crystalline state, of trehalose in a dehydrated cell is necessary, it is the hydrogen bonding between trehalose and the protein surface, and between trehalose and polar headgroups of phospholipids, that is ultimately responsible for trehalose's water sub-stitute effect. Vitrified trehalose, unlike crystal-lized trehalose, retains enough molecular motion to permit the formation of hydrogen bonds with the protein (or phospholipid) sur-face. How this interaction between trehalose and the protein leads to the latter's stabilization remains unclear. Perhaps a tightly fitting net-work of hydrogen-bonded trehalose surround-ing the protein surface inhibits structural fluctuations by the protein, much as a fish trapped in a tight-fitting net might be unable to move. This greatly increased stability would, of course, be antithetical to protein function because of the importance of confor-mational changes in protein activity. However, in the anhydrobiotic state, suppression of enzy-matic activity is desirable, and trehalose, through stabilizing proteins, may help to inhibit enzymes. Furthermore, because it is a protein stabilizer, trehalose may increase the half-lives of proteins, allowing them to persist during pro-longed periods of metabolic quiescence and be available for reactivation when the cell under-goes rehydration.

To gain a broader perspective on the roles of trehalose in adaptation to different environ-mental stresses, it is relevant to examine briefly the studies of Singer and Lindquist (1998a,b) on heat-stressed yeast (see chapter 7 for addi-tional discussion). Under heat stress, yeasts accumulate high concentrations of trehalose, much as they do under water stress. These high concentrations of trehalose in normally hydrated yeast cells are conjectured to have at least one negative consequence: they stabi-lize the conformations of partially denatured proteins, thereby preventing molecular chaper-ones (heat-shock proteins) from carrying out their repair functions. Thus, to recover from heat stress, yeast cells must lose their trehalose, in order to restore a milieu in which protein stability is of an appropriate value to allow molecular chaperones to function. Likewise, after desiccation is reversed, trehalose levels fall to low values, restoring the appropriate milieu for protein function. Trehalose, if present at high concentrations in normally hydrated cells at normal physiological temperatures, may be "too much of a good thing," and for this reason trehalose is generally accumulated to high concentrations only under conditions of environmental stress due to heat, high salinity, or desiccation.

A caveat: When is a solute "compatible"?

The concentration dependence of trehalose's effects raises a caveat about use of the expression "compatible solute." If we restrict use of this expression to cases in which the solute in question is having a negligible effect on the system, then we are adhering to the original definition of Brown (1978). However, if we are examining circumstances in which a stabilizing solute is employed at high concentrations to enhance protein stability, albeit at a cost to protein function, then "compatibility" is of a quite different sort. We examine this issue again in the context of resistance to freezing. In many terrestrial arthropods, high concentrations of glycerol or trehalose prevent ice formation within cells, yet at these elevated levels these polyols are likely to inhibit enzymatic activity because of their stabilizing effects on protein structure (chapter 7).

Kinetics of water replacement

For both membranes and proteins the kinetics of water replacement remains a mystery. For instance, at what stage during entry into anhydrobiosis does trehalose (or sucrose) change from being a preferentially excluded solute to a protein-binding solute? When does the water surrounding polar headgroups of phospholipids give way to trehalose as a water substitute? Although evidence suggests that the water substitute role is assumed only quite late in the dehydration process, much remains to be discovered about the kinetics of anhydrobiosis.

Absorbing Water Vapor: Another Function of Sugar and Polyol Osmolytes

Much as certain sugar and polyol osmolytes can protect cells when extreme desiccation occurs, accumulation of other representatives of this class of osmolyte may facilitate avoiding desiccation in the first place. Soil arthropods of the order Collembola are able to use sugars and polyols to draw water into the body from air with low relative humidity (RH) (Bayley and Holmstrup, 1999). Soil arthropods typically encounter relative humidity near 100% in the pores among soil particles that they inhabit. At this RH, the animals maintain an osmotic concentration in their hemolymph that renders them slightly hyperosmotic relative to the water vapor pressure in the surrounding air, thereby ensuring that they can absorb water as needed. However, because their exoskeletons are highly permeable to water, any decrease in RH of the air is likely to lead to loss of water from the body. In fact, RH need only fall below approximately 99.4% to trigger loss of water. Soil arthropods thus could face lethal levels of desiccation, unless some mechanism was available to prevent exit of water across the exoskeleton—or to allow the organism to enhance its ability to imbibe water from the air in the surrounding soil.

By subjecting the Collembola species *Folsomia candida* to air with an RH of 98.2% for seven days, it was possible to follow the flux of water between the insects and the surrounding air, and to track adaptive responses that occurred in the hemolymph. During the first day at low RH, the animals dehydrated quickly, losing about one-third of their initial water and shrinking in volume. Under these shrunken conditions, the insects were essentially moribund. The increase in hemolymph osmotic pressure resulting from this water loss brought the animals into osmotic balance with the air. Then, an increase in hemolymph osmolality commenced, enabling the animal to establish an osmotic gradient that favored uptake of water into the organism from the air, despite its reduced relative humidity. The solutes responsible for this increase in osmolality were glucose and *myo*-inositol. As these solutes built up in the hemolymph, the animals regained, over the six-day recovery period, essentially all of the water they lost during the first day. The combined concentrations of glucose and *myo*-inositol represented about 8% of the animals' dry weight. Upon return to air with 100% RH, the levels of glucose and *myo*-inositol fell to basal levels within 24 hours, thereby preventing undue swelling of the insects. This use of compatible osmolytes to regulate the osmolality of body fluids in order to allow extraction of water from the air illustrates yet another way in which these solutes contribute to regulation of cell (body) volume.

WATER HELPS DEFINE THERMAL RELATIONSHIPS AND THERMAL BOUNDARY CONDITIONS OF LIFE

The properties of water have such pervasive influences on living systems that some aspect of the physics and chemistry of water is almost certain to trickle into each chapter of this volume. As a prefatory note to the following chapter on temperature effects, it is useful to review the thermal properties of water, and see how these relate to the thermal relationships of organisms. This brief review of the effects of temperature on water will serve to introduce the key roles played by water in establishing the thermal sensitivities of organisms and in setting the temperature limits for life.

Water has a high *heat capacity*. Because of this, addition to an organism of heat from the environment or from metabolic reactions tends not to lead to rapid changes in body temperature. Water's heat capacity thus favors substantial thermal buffering, at least in the case of multicellular organisms of sufficient mass. Water has the highest *heat of vaporization* (H_{vap}) of any known liquid: 44.0 kJ at 25°C. Because of its high H_{vap}, evaporative cooling involving losses of small amounts of water enables large amounts of heat to be ducted from the body. Ducting of heat from the body through evaporative cooling thus leads to a relatively modest threat of desiccation compared to what a coolant with lower H_{vap} would impose.

The density of water and the manner in which its density changes with temperature are well-understood aspects of water's importance in biology. Water has its maximal density at suprafreezing temperatures (near 4°C for pure water), allowing ice to form on the top of a body of water. Ice on the surface of a body of water tends to insulate the water below and impede further loss of heat and freezing. Water's expansion on freezing leads to a pressure sensitivity of the freezing point, because elevated hydrostatic pressure inhibits any process that occurs with an increase in volume. The reduction in freezing point at elevated pressures reduces the danger of freezing for deep-living hypoosmotic marine teleosts from high latitudes. These fishes may contain lower concentrations of antifreeze proteins than shallow-living species (chapter 7).

The dissociation of water into hydrogen (hydronium, H_3O^+) and hydroxyl ions is temperature dependent. As temperature is increased, dissociation of water is enhanced, such that the pH and pOH of a solution fall with rising temperature. Because of the large number of biological processes that are affected by changes in pH, the temperature–pH relationship is an important aspect of adaptation to temperature.

Water's properties may contribute in several ways to setting the upper thermal limits for life. Some organisms, notably the hyperthermophilic members of the Archaea, withstand temperatures near 100°C, the one-atmosphere boiling point of water. And, as illustrated by hyperthermophilic archaea from deep-sea hot springs, even higher temperatures can be tolerated when elevated hydrostatic pressures keep water in a liquid state at temperatures that exceed the boiling point of water at one atmosphere. However, even though high pressures can be used to keep water in a liquid state at high temperatures, no successful culturing of cells has been possible above 113°C (Jaenicke, 1991, 2000).

One limitation to life at higher temperatures comes from the roles played by water in stabilizing the higher orders of protein structure. Hydrophobic interactions seem likely to be pivotal in this regard. Because hydrophobic stabilization of proteins involves positive changes in enthalpy—heat is needed to disrupt the cages of water surrounding hydrophobic groups so they can be buried in the protein's interior— the hydrophobic effect tends to be enhanced as temperature is increased over a certain range. However, at temperatures near the apparent upper limits of life the organization of water becomes so reduced that cages of organized water around exposed hydrophobic groups have difficulty forming (Jaenicke, 2000). Thus, the entropy change occurring during the burial of hydrophobic groups ceases to be a strong driving force for the hydrophobic effect. The loss of hydrophobic stabilization at elevated temperatures may be a major determinant of the upper temperatures for life.

The exclusion of stabilizing solutes from the water adjacent to proteins may also be reduced as temperature is increased, although this effect of temperature on water's properties is not well understood. The preferential exclusion mechanism for protein stabilization, like hydrophobically based stabilization, thus could be temperature dependent and cease to make a strong contribution to protein stability at high temperatures.

The role of water in governing the upper thermal limits for life also is based on covalent transformations in which water is a reactant. As emphasized earlier in this chapter, the removal of a molecule of water from reactants is common in diverse biosynthetic reactions, including the polymerization of amino acids into proteins and nucleotide triphosphates into nucleic acids. The breakdown of biomolecules often involves hydrolysis, and increased temperatures generally enhance these hydrolytic reactions. The thermal stabilities of many biomolecules, for instance, certain amino acids and ATP, become limiting at high temperatures. Calculations suggest that ATP hydrolysis becomes a critical limiting factor for life at temperatures between 110°C and 140°C (Leibrock et al., 1995; Jaenicke, 2000). Thus, at temperatures near 110°C, both the covalent and the noncovalent chemistries of water that are so critical for life are altered to the extent that life based on an abundance of liquid water ceases to be possible.

We see, then, that the properties of water influence a vast number of the characteristics of life, ranging from the selection of low-molecular-mass solutes that are "fit" for life, to the nature of the forces that drive folding of proteins and organization of membranes, to the thermal limits at which life is possible. It is hoped that the treatment given to water relationships in this chapter has helped to highlight the pervasive physiological significance of the most abundant molecule found in organisms and has succeeded in illustrating the central role that water plays in biological evolution.

REFERENCES

Allen, R., S. Stabler, and J. Lindenbaum (1993). Serum betaine, *N,N*-dimethylglycine and *N*-methylglycine levels in patients with cobalamin and folate deficiency and related inborn errors of metabolism. *Metabolism* 42: 1448–1460.

Arakawa, T., J.F. Carpenter, Y.A. Kita, and J.H. Crowe (1990). The basis for toxicity of certain cryoprotectants. *Cryobiology* 27: 401–415.

Atkinson, D.E. (1969). Limitation of metabolite concentrations and the conservation of solvent capacity in the living cell. In: *Current Topics in Cellular Regulation* 1: 29–43. New York: Academic Press.

Baskakov, I.A., and D.W. Bolen (1998). Forcing thermodynamically unfolded proteins to fold. *J. Biol. Chem.* 273: 4831–4834.

Baskakov, I., A. Wang, and D.W. Bolen (1998). Trimethylamine-N-oxide counteracts urea effects on rabbit muscle lactate dehydrogenase function: A test of the counteraction hypothesis. *Biophys. J.* 74: 2666–2673.

Bayley, M., and M. Holmstrup (1999). Water vapor absorption in arthropods by accumulation of myo-inositol and glucose. *Science* 285: 1909–1911.

Bednar, J., R.A. Horwitz, J. Dubochet, and C.L. Woodcock (1995). Chromatin conformation and salt-induced compaction: three-dimensional structural information from cryoelectron microscopy. *J. Cell Biol.* 131: 1365–1376.

Blackwell, J.R., and D.J. Gilmour (1991). Physiological response of the unicellular green alga *Chlorococcum submarinum* to rapid changes in salinity. *Arch. Microbiol.* 157: 86–91.

Bowlus, R.D., and G.N. Somero (1979). Solute compatibility with enzyme function and structure: Rationales for the selection of osmotic agents and end-products of anaerobic metabolism in marine invertebrates. *J. Exp. Zool.* 208: 137–152.

Brown, A.D. (1978). Compatible solutes and extreme water stress in eukaryotic micro-organisms. *Adv. Microbial Physiol.* 17: 181–242.

Buche, A., P. Colson, and C. Houssier (1993). Organic osmotic effectors and chromatin structure. *J. Biomol. Struct. Dyn.* 8: 601–618.

Burg, M.B., E.D. Kwon, and D. Kültz (1997). Regulation of gene expression by hypertonicity. *Annu. Rev. Physiol.* 59: 437–455.

Carpenter, J.F., S. Prestrelski, and T. Arakawa (1995). Separation of freezing- and drying-induced denaturation of lyophilized proteins using stress-specific stabilization. 1) Enzyme activity and calorimetric studies. *Arch. Biochem. Biophys.* 303: 456–464.

Cayley, S., B.A. Lewis, H.J. Guttman, and M.T. Record, Jr. (1991). Characterization of the cytoplasm of *Escherichia coli* K-12 as a function of external osmolarity. Implications for protein-DNA interactions *in vivo*. *J. Mol. Biol.* 222: 281–300.

Clark, M.E. (1985). The osmotic role of amino acids: discovery and function. In: *Transport Processes, Iono- and Osmoregulation*, pp. 412–423, ed. R. Gilles and M. Gilles-Baillien. Berlin: Springer-Verlag.

Cohen, D., J. Wasserman, and S. Gullans (1991). Immediate early gene and HSP70 expression in hyperosmotic stress in MDCK cells. *Am. J. Physiol. (Cell Physiol.)* 261: C594–601.

Collins, K.D., and M.W. Washabaugh (1985). The Hofmeister effect and the behavior of water at interfaces. *Q. Rev. Biophys.* 18: 323–422.

Crowe, J.H., L.M. Crowe, J.E. Carpenter, S. Prestrelski, F.A. Hoekstra, P. Araujo, and A. Panek (1997). Anhydrobiosis: cellular adaptation to extreme dehydration. In: *Handbook of Physiology, Section 13: Comparative Physiology*, Vol. II, pp. 1445–1477. ed. W. Danztler. New York: Oxford.

Csonka, L.N., and W. Epstein (1996). Osmoregulation, In: *Escherichia coli and Salmonella typhimurium: Cellular and Molecular Biology*, pp. 1210–1223, ed. F.C. Neidhardt, I.I. Curtiss, J.L. Ingraham, E.C. Lin, K.B. Low, B. Magasanik, W.S. Reznikoff, M. Riley, M. Schaechter, and H.E. Umbarger. Washington, D.C.: American Society for Microbiology.

Denny, M.W. (1993). *Air and Water: The Biology and Physics of Life's Media*. Princeton University Press.

Dmitrieva, N., D. Kültz and M.B. Burg (2000). High NaCl, but not urea increases p53 in inner medullary collecting duct (mIMCD) cells. *FASEB J.* A716.

Dunn, C.R., H.M, Wilks, D.J. Halsall, T. Atkinson, A.R. Clarke, H. Muirhead, and J.J. Holbrook (1991). Design and synthesis of new enzymes based on the lactate dehydrogenase framework. *Phil. Trans. R. Soc. Lond. B.* 332: 177–184.

Ferarris, J.D., C.K. Williams, K.-Y. Jung, J.J. Bedford, M.B. Burg, and A. Garcia-Perez (1996). ORE, a eukaryotic minimal essential osmotic response element: the aldose reductase gene in hyperosmotic stress. *J. Biol. Chem.* 271: 18318–18321.

Galinski, E.A., and H.G. Trüper (1994). Microbial behavior in salt-stressed ecosystems. *FEMS Microbiol. Rev.* 15: 95–108.

Garner, M.M., and M.B. Burg (1994). Macromolecular crowding and confinement in cells exposed to hypertonicity. *Am. J. Physiol.* 266 (*Cell Physiol.* 35): C877–C892.

Gilles, R., E. Delpire (1997). Variations in salinity, osmolarity, and water availability: vertebrates and invertebrates. In: *Handbook of Physiology, Section 13: Comparative Physiology*, Vol. II, pp. 1523–1586, ed. W. Danztler. New York: Oxford.

Gillett, M.B., J.R. Suko, F.O. Santoso, and P.H. Yancey (1997). Elevated levels of trimethylamine oxide in muscle of deep-sea gadiform teleosts: a high-pressure adaptation? *J. Exp. Zool.* 279: 386–391.

Goodsell, D. 1993. *The Machinery of Life*. New York: Springer-Verlag.

Gould, S.J., and E.S. Vrba (1982). Exaptation—a missing term in the science of form. *Paleobiology* 8: 4–15.

Grazi, E., C. Schwienbacher, and E. Magri (1993). Osmotic stress is the main determinant of the diameter of the actin filament. *Biochem. Biophys. Res. Commun.* 197: 1377–1388.

Greenway, H. and C.B. Osmond (1972). Salt responses of enzymes from species differing in salt tolerance. *Plant Physiol.* 49: 256–259.

Hand, S.C., and G.N. Somero (1982). Urea and methylamine effects on rabbit muscle phosphofructokinase. *J. Biol. Chem.* 257: 734–741.

Häussinger, D. (1996). The role of cellular hydration in the regulation of cell function. *Biochem. J.* 313: 697–710.

Henderson, L.J. (1913). *The Fitness of the Environment*. Boston: Beacon Press.

Higgins, C.F., C.J. Dorman, D.A. Stirling, L. Waddell, I.R. Booth, G. May, and E.

Bremer (1988). A physiological role for DNA supercoiling in the osmotic regulation of gene expression in *S. typhimurium* and *E. coli. Cell* 52: 569–584.

Hoffmann, E.K., and S.F. Pedersen (1998). Sensors and signal transduction in the activation of cell volume regulatory ion transport systems. *Contrib. Nephrol.* 123: 50–78.

Hofmeister, F. (1888). On the understanding of the effect of salts. Second report. On regularities in the precipitating effects of salts and their relationship to their physiological behavior. *Naunyn-Schmiedebergs Arch. Exper. Path. Pharmakol. (Leipzig)* 24: 247–260.

Incharoensakdi, A., T. Takabe, and T. Akazawa (1986). Effect of betaine on enzyme activity and subunit interaction of ribulose-1,5-bisphosphate carboxylase/oxygenase from *Aphanothece halophytica. Plant Physiol.* 81: 1044–1049.

Jaenicke, R. (1991). Protein stability and molecular adaptation to extreme conditions. *Eur. J. Biochem.* 202: 715–728.

Jaenicke, R. (2000). Stability and stabilization of globular proteins in solution. *J. Biotech.* 79: 193–203.

Kelly, R.H., and P.H. Yancey (1999). High contents of trimethylamine oxide correlating with depth in deep-sea teleost fishes, skates, and decapod crustaceans. *Biol. Bull.* 196: 18–25.

Kempf, B., and E. Bremer (1998). Uptake and synthesis of compatible solutes as microbial stress responses to high-osmolality environments. *Arch. Microbiol.* 170: 319–330.

Kinne, R.K. (1998). Mechanisms of osmolyte release. *Contrib. Nephrol.* 123: 34–39.

Kirschner, L. B. (1991). Water and ions. In: *Comparative Animal Physiology: Environmental and Metabolic Animal Physiology*, pp. 13–107, ed. C.L. Prosser. New York: Wiley-Liss.

Kirschner, L.B. (1997). Extrarenal mechanisms in hydromineral balance and acid-base regulation in aquatic vertebrates. In: *Handbook of Physiology, Section 13: Comparative Physiology.* Vol. I, pp. 577–622, ed. W. Dantzler. New York: Oxford.

Kozak, M. (1988). Leader length and secondary structure modulate mRNA function under conditions of stress. *Mol. Cell. Biol.* 8: 2737–2744.

Kültz, D. (2000). Osmotic regulation of DNA activity and the cell cycle. In: *Environmental Stressors and Gene Responses*, pp. 157–179, ed. K.B. Storey and J. Storey, New York: Elsevier.

Kültz, D., and M.B. Burg (1998a). Intracellular signaling in response to osmotic stress. In: *Cell Volume Regulation*, pp. 94–109, ed. F. Lang. Basel: Karger.

Kültz, D., and M.B. Burg (1998b). Evolution of osmotic stress signaling *via* MAP kinase cascades. *J. Exp. Biol.* 201: 3015–3021.

Kültz, D., and D. Chakravarty (2001). Hyperosmolality in the form of elevated NaCl but not urea causes DNA damage in murine kidney cells. *Proc. Natl. Acad. Sci. USA*, 98: 1999–2004.

Kyriakis, J.M., and J. Avruch (1996). Protein kinase cascades activated by stress and inflammatory cytokines. *Bioessays* 18: 567–577.

Leberman, R., and A.K. Soper (1995). Effect of high salt concentrations on water structure. *Nature* 378: 364–366.

Lehtonen, J.Y.A., and P.K.V. Kinnunen (1995). Phospholipase A_2 as a mechanosensor. *Biophys. J.* 68: 1888–1894.

Leibrock, E., P. Bayer, and H.-D. Lüdemann (1995). Non-enzymatic hydrolysis of ATP at high temperatures and high pressure. *Biophys. Chem.* 54: 175–180.

Lin, J.J., T.H. Yang, B.D. Wahlstrand, P.A. Fields, and G.N. Somero (2001). Phylogenetic relationships and biochemical properties of the duplicated cytosolic and mitochondrial isoforms of malate dehydrogenase from a teleost fish, *Sphyraena idiastes. J. Mol. Evol.*, in press.

Low, P.S. (1985). Molecular basis of the biological compatibility of nature's osmolytes. In: *Transport Processes, Iono- and Osmoregulation*, pp. 467–477, ed. R. Gilles and M. Gilles-Ballien. Berlin: Springer-Verlag.

Martin, D.D., R.A. Ciulla, and M.F. Roberts (1999). Osmoadaptation in Archaea. *Appl. Environ. Microbiol.* 65: 1815–1823.

Martinez-Pastor, M.T., G. Marchler, C. Schüller, A. Marchler-Bauer, H. Ruis, and F. Estruch (1996). The *Saccharomyces cerevisiae* zinc-finger proteins Msn2p and Msn4p are required for transcriptional induction through the stress-response element (STRE). *EMBO J.* 15: 2227–2235.

Mayr, E. (1982). *Growth of Biological Thought.* Cambridge, Mass.: Harvard University Press.

Meury, J. (1988). Glycine betaine reverses the effects of osmotic stress on DNA replication and cell division in *Escherichia coli. Arch. Microbiol.* 149: 232–239.

Miyakawa, H., S.K. Woo, S.C. Dahl, J.S. Handler, and H.M. Kwon (1999). Tonicity-responsive enhancer binding protein, a novel Rel-like protein that stimulates transcription in response to hypertonicity. *Proc. Natl. Acad. Sci. USA* 96: 2538–2542.

Nishiguchi, M.K., and G.N. Somero (1992). Temperature- and concentration-dependence of compatibility of the organic osmolyte β-dimethyl-sulfoniopropionate. *Cryobiology* 29: 118–124.

Ota, I.M., and A. Varshavsky (1993). A yeast protein similar to bacterial two-component regulators. *Science* 262: 566–569.

Pantazis, P., M.H. West, and W.M. Bonner (1984). Phosphorylation of histones in cells treated with hypertonic and acidic media. *Mol. Cell Biol.* 4: 1186–1188.

Parker, J.C., P.B. Dunham, and A.P. Minton (1995). Effects of ionic strength on the regulation of Na/H exchange and K-Cl cotransport in dog red blood cells. *J. Gen. Physiol.* 105: 677–699.

Petronini, P., W. De Angelis, A. Borghetti, and K. Wheeler (1993). Effect of betaine on HSP70 expression and cell survival during adaptation to osmotic stress. *Biochem. J.* 293: 553–558.

Potts, M. (1994). Desiccation tolerance of prokaryotes. *Microbiol. Rev.* 58: 755–805.

Pratt, L.A., W. Hsing, K.E. Gibson, and T.J. Silhavy (1996). From acids to *osmZ*: multiple factors influence synthesis of the OmpF and OmpC porins in *Esherichia coli*. *Mol. Microbiol.* 20: 911–917.

Qu, Y., C.L. Bolen, and D.W. Bolen (1998). Osmolyte-driven contraction of a random coil protein. *Proc. Natl. Acad. Sci. USA* 95: 9268–9273.

Raymond, J.A., and A.L. DeVries (1998). Elevated concentrations and synthetic pathways of trimethylamine oxide and urea in some teleost fishes of McMurdo Sound, Antarctica. *Fish. Physiol. Biochem.* 18: 387–398.

Rolfe, D.F.S., and G.C. Brown (1997). Cellular energy utilization and molecular origin of standard metabolic rate in mammals. *Physiol. Rev.* 77: 731–758.

Rosette, C., and M. Karin (1996). Ultraviolet light and osmotic stress: activation of the JNK cascade through multiple growth factor and cytokine receptors. *Science* 274: 1194–1197.

Singer, M.A., and S. Lindquist (1998a). Thermotolerance in *Saccharomyces cerevisiae*: the Yin and Yang of trehalose. *Trends Biotech.* 16: 460–468.

Singer, M.A., and S. Lindquist (1998b). Multiple effects of trehalose on protein folding *in vitro* and *in vivo*. *Mol. Cell* 1: 639–648.

Somero, G.N. (2000). Unity in diversity: A perspective on the methods, contributions, and future of comparative physiology. *Annu. Rev. Physiol.* 62: 927–937.

Somero, G.N., and P.H. Yancey (1997). Osmolytes and cell volume regulation: physiological and evolutionary principles. In: *Handbook of Physiology, Section 14: Cell Physiology*. Vol. II, pp. 1445–1477, ed. W. Danztler. New York: Oxford.

Somero, G.N., C.B. Osmond, and C.L. Bolis (1992). *Water and Life: A Comparative Analysis of Water Relationships at the Organismic, Cellular, and Molecular Levels*. Berlin: Springer-Verlag.

Sommer, C., B. Thonke, and M. Popp (1990). The compatibility of D-pinitol and ID-1-O-methyl-muco-inositol with malate dehydrogenase. *Bot. Acta* 103: 270–273.

Srere, P. A. (1985). The metabolon. *Trends. Biochem. Sci.* 10: 109–110.

Srivastava, D.K., and S.A. Bernhard (1986). Metabolite transfer via enzyme-enzyme complexes. *Science* 234: 1081–1086.

Ström, A.R., and I. Kaasen (1993). Trehalose metabolism in *Escherichia coli*: stress protection and stress regulation of gene expression. *Mol. Microbiol.* 8: 205–210.

Timasheff, S.N. (1992). A physicochemical basis for the selection of osmolytes by nature. In: *Water and Life: A Comparative Analysis of Water Relationships at the Organismic, Cellular, and Molecular Levels*, pp. 70–84, ed. G.N. Somero, C.B. Osmond, and C.L. Bolis. Berlin: Springer-Verlag.

Timasheff, S.N. (1998). Control of protein stability and reactions by weakly interacting cosolvents: the simplicity of the complicated. *Adv. Protein. Chem.* 51: 355–432.

Treisman, R. (1996). Regulation of transcription by MAP kinase cascades. *Curr. Opin. Cell Biol.* 8: 205–215.

Tseng, H.-C., and D.J. Graves (1998). Natural methylamine osmolytes, trimethylamine N-oxide and betain, increase Tau-induced polymerization of microtubules. *Biochem. Biophys. Res. Comm.* 250: 726–730.

Urao, T., B. Yakubov, R. Satoh, K. Yamaguchi-Shinozaki, M. Seki, T. Hirayama, and K. Shinozaki (1999). A transmembrane hybrid-type histidine kinase in *Arabidopsis* functions as an osmosensor. *Plant Cell* 11: 1743–1754.

von Hippel, P.H., and T. Schleich (1969). The effects of neutral salts on the structure and conformational stability of macromolecules in solution. In: *Structure and Stability of Biological Macromolecules*, pp. 417–574, ed. S.N.

Timasheff and G.D. Fasman. New York: Marcel Dekker.

Wang, A., and D.W. Bolen (1997). A naturally occurring protective system in urea-rich cells: Mechanism of osmolyte protection of proteins against urea denaturation. *Biochemistry* 36: 9101–9108.

Weber, L.A., E.D. Hickey, P.A. Maroney, and C. Baglioni (1977). Inhibition of protein synthesis by Cl⁻. *J. Biol. Chem.* 252: 4007–4010.

Wendelaar Bonga, S.E., and J.C.A. Van der Meij (1989). Degeneration and death, by apoptosis and necrosis, of the pavement and chloride cells in the gills of the teleost *Oreochromis mossambicus. Cell Tissue Res.* 255: 235–243.

Wurgler-Murphy, S.M., and H. Saito (1997). Two-component signal transducers and MAPK cascades. *Trends Biochem. Sci.* 22: 172–176.

Wyn-Jones, R.G. (1984). Phytochemical aspects of osmotic adaptation. *Rec. Adv. Phytochem.* 18: 55–78.

Yancey, P.H. (1992). Compatible and counteracting aspects of organic osmolytes in mammalian kidney cells *in vivo* and *in vitro*. In: *Water and Life: A Comparative Analysis of Water Relationships at the Organismic, Cellular, and Molecular Levels*, pp. 19–32, ed. G.N. Somero, C.B. Osmond, and C.L. Bolis. Berlin: Springer-Verlag.

Yancey, P.H., and M.B. Burg (1990). Counteracting effects of urea and betaine on colony-forming efficiency of mammalian cells in culture. *Am. J. Physiol.* 258 (*Regulatory Integrative Comp. Physiol.* 27): R198–R204.

Yancey, P.H., and J.F. Siebenaller (1999). Trimethylamine oxide stabilizes teleost and mammalian lactate dehydrogenases against inactivation by hydrostatic pressure and trypsinolysis. *J. Exp. Biol.* 202: 3597–3603.

Yancey, P.H., and G.N. Somero (1979). Counteraction of urea destabilization of protein structure by methylamine osmoregulatory compounds of elasmobranch fishes. *Biochem. J.* 182: 317–323.

Yancey, P.H., and G.N. Somero (1980). Methylamine osmoregulatory compounds in elasmobranch fishes reverse urea inhibition of enzymes. *J. Exp. Zool.* 212: 205–213.

Yancey, P.H., M.E. Clark, S.C. Hand, R.D. Bowlus, and G.N. Somero (1982). Living with water stress: the evolution of osmolyte systems. *Science* 217: 1212–1222.

Zimmerman, S.B., and S.O. Trach (1991). Estimation of macromolecular concentrations and excluded volume effects for the cytoplasm of *Escherichia coli. J. Mol. Biol.* 222: 599–620.

7

Temperature

TEMPERATURE RELATIONSHIPS: BASIC QUESTIONS, DEFINITIONS, AND MODES OF ANALYSIS

Biogeographic Patterning Indicates That Temperature Is a Major Determinant of Habitat Suitability

Anyone versed in biogeography, indeed anyone even moderately familiar with natural history, is aware that the distribution patterns of organisms commonly reflect gradients or discontinuities in temperature. This type of temperature-related—and, by implication, temperature-*caused*—patterning is seen in both aquatic and terrestrial habitats, in both spatial and temporal contexts, and among all types of organisms. Thus, in moving from lower to higher latitudes, species replacement patterns are ubiquitous and may involve the replacement of one species in a genus by another (a *congener*). Species replacement is also seen along vertical gradients in temperature at a given latitude, for instance, along gradients characteristic of transitions from subtidal to intertidal marine habitats and from low to high elevations in mountainous regions. Mobile animals commonly select a preferred temperature, using a variety of strategies including seasonal migrations by aquatic and terrestrial animals, diurnal vertical migrations in marine and freshwater habitats, and selection of the appropriate period of the day for foraging and predation in terrestrial animals.

The pervasiveness of these temperature-related patterns of organismal distribution indicates that the effects of temperature on organisms are universal among taxa and of sufficient magnitude to impose strict limits on where life

can occur, even when other environmental factors would seem permissive of life. Indeed, temperature affects essentially every aspect of an organism's physiology, from the basic structures of the macromolecules that are responsible for catalysis and information processing to the rates at which chemical reactions occur. One index of the scope and magnitude of temperature's effects on biological systems is the fact that no species can withstand, at least when in a metabolically active state, cell temperatures spanning the full range of temperatures found in the biosphere—from slightly above 100°C in geothermal hot springs to ∼ −80°C in high-latitude and high-altitude terrestrial habitats. Through evolutionary processes, each species has eked out a particular thermal niche, within which it may function well, but outside of which it may fail to survive.

Accounting in mechanistic terms for these commonly observed linkages between habitat temperature and biogeographic patterning is one of the principal goals of this chapter. To realize this goal, a twofold scheme of analysis will be used. First, we will delineate in considerable detail how temperature perturbs the structural and functional properties of organisms. Here, we ask, "What is the nature of thermal stress?" Secondly, we will describe how modifications at the physiological, biochemical, and molecular levels alter the thermal sensitivities of organisms during both multigenerational evolutionary adaptation and phenotypic acclimatization during an individual's lifetime. Here, we will be asking, "How do organisms adapt to thermal stress?" Through this twofold mode of analysis, it is hoped that a sound mechanistic basis can be provided for explaining major features of current biogeographical patterning and for predicting how future changes in temperature might impact the biosphere.

Some Important Terminology

In order to analyze properly the thermal relationships of diverse organisms, it is first necessary to define the terminology used to describe how changes in ambient temperature influence body (or cell) temperature. An especially important aspect of an organism's thermal relationships is the degree to which it can maintain its body temperature independent from the ambient temperature. If an organism is successful in decoupling changes in ambient temperature from alterations in body temperature, then it is less susceptible to direct thermal perturbation, and it may select its habitat with less regard for thermal considerations than in the case of a strict thermal conformer.

Organisms whose body temperatures conform to the temperature of the milieu, whether this is air or water, are termed *ectotherms* (*ecto* is the Greek prefix for "outer" or "outside"). Aquatic species generally are strict ectotherms because they lack anatomical and physiological means for maintaining a thermal gradient between the medium and the body. A primary source of the difficulty faced by aquatic ectotherms in avoiding thermal equilibration with their medium is the requirement for gas exchange at respiratory surfaces. Metabolically produced heat is lost rapidly at respiratory surfaces during uptake of O_2 and elimination of CO_2 and other waste products such as ammonia. Exceptions to strict ectothermy among aquatic organisms are rare; only birds, mammals, and several species of "warm-bodied" (regionally endothermic; see below) fishes succeed in maintaining a stable gradient of temperature between medium and body core. Terrestrial ectotherms like reptiles and insects may have temperatures considerably different from air temperature as a result of behavioral thermoregulation, anatomical and physiological factors (for instance, heat-generating sites within certain flying insects), and locomotory activity. However, with the exception of mammals, birds, and a few types of insects that are

able to achieve stable body temperatures (*homeothermy*) by a combination of heat generation (*endothermy*) and close control of heat exchange with the environment, most terrestrial species also are essentially ectothermic. Ectotherms frequently are referred to as *poikilothermic* (from *poikilo*, which is Greek for "varied") when their body temperatures change in concert with the ambient temperature. Strictly speaking, the terms ectotherm and poikilotherm are not synonymous. In principle, an ectotherm might be able to use behavioral means to select a stable body temperature, that is, it may avoid being poikilothermic. However, it is common to see these two terms used interchangeably. The term *heterotherm* generally is reserved for endotherms that elect to change their body temperatures as environmental conditions dictate. For instance, hummingbirds may allow their body temperatures to fall considerably at night, when foraging is not possible, in order to conserve energy reserves. Hibernators likewise allow body temperatures and, thus, rates of metabolism, to fall during seasons when active life is precluded by environmental conditions of temperature and food availability. *Regional heterothermy* is an expression used to describe a strategy, typically in an endothermic species, in which thermal gradients are present, for instance, between the deep core and the appendages. In effect, all endotherms are likely to be regionally heterothermic, for a number of reasons. For instance, in cold climates it may be advantageous to allow the extremities (hands, flippers, feet) to run at cooler temperatures than the body core, in order to preserve metabolically generated heat. Suffice it to say that the terminology used to describe thermal relationships more commonly reflects ideal cases than what actually transpires in the real world. Nonetheless, for most of our purposes, this terminology is a necessary and important foundation for the analyses to follow.

Thermal Tolerance Ranges Vary Greatly: Stenotherms and Eurytherms

Species differ enormously in the *range* of body temperatures they can tolerate, as well as in the *absolute* temperatures at which they can live.

Some species, for instance Antarctic fishes of the teleost suborder Notothenioidei, which normally live between approximately 2°C and −1.86°C, the freezing point of seawater, and die of heat death at temperatures above 4°C, are markedly *stenothermal* (*steno* is Greek for "narrow"). Ten to twenty million years of evolution in what was basically an ice-water bath appears to have led to the loss of ability to cope with higher temperatures; even prolonged acclimation cannot broaden the thermal tolerance range of these extraordinary stenotherms (see Eastman, 1993). Other aquatic species, including many intertidal organisms that experience long periods of emersion during low tide, commonly withstand variations in temperature of 20–30°C on a daily basis, and encounter even wider thermal ranges on a seasonal basis. These species are extremely *eurythermal* (*eury* is Greek for "wide"). Eurythermal invertebrates and fishes from temperate zone habitats may remain metabolically active at temperatures as low as those at which Antarctic fishes can survive, that is to say, temperatures only a few degrees Celsius above zero, and also withstand temperatures as high as those characteristic of avian and mammalian core body temperatures. If we broaden the definition of eurythermy to include organisms that tolerate transitions from metabolically active states to states of physiological quiescence, then the most extreme eurytherms may be desert lichens whose cell temperatures and states of hydration vary enormously on diurnal and seasonal bases (see Louw and Seely, 1982). Cell temperatures may fluctuate by close to 100°C between cold nights and hot days. If we even further broaden the concept of eurythermy to include effects created only in the laboratory, then we can list rotifers and tardigrades as the most thermally tolerant metazoans. When desiccated, they can survive temperatures close to absolute zero (0 K) and well over 100°C. Removal of cellular water and transition to a state of metabolic quiescence appear to be obligatory conditions for the most extreme patterns of eurythermy found in the biosphere, observations that emphasize the pivotal role of liquid-state water in metabolically active living systems (see chapter 6). A number of other mechanisms that underlie the wide differences among species

in thermal tolerance range will be examined throughout this chapter.

From Molecules to Politics: Studies of Thermal Relationships May Assist Predictions About Effects of Global Change

The strong and frequently dominant role that temperature plays in governing the distribution patterns of organisms provides compelling motivation for analyzing the basic effects of temperature on living systems at all levels of biological organization, from basic molecular processes to the ecosystem. Such analysis will not only provide insights into major patterns of evolutionary adaptation, but will also offer indications as to how future changes in temperature due to global warming are apt to impact the distributions and physiological status of organisms. There is, then, a practical reason of substantial economic and, thus, political significance for furthering our understanding of thermal effects on organisms.

To achieve an analysis of thermal biology that spans the full spectrum of topics from molecular evolution to broad-scale ecological and climate change issues, we will attempt to maintain a distinct view of the "forest" even as we engage in minute dissection of some of its individual "trees." Thus, woven throughout the following analysis are three questions that are of both "academic" and "practical" interest in the study of effects of temperature. One question relates to the optimal values of temperature-dependent physiological and biochemical traits. At what temperatures does a system work best—and why? A second question, one that may be experimentally difficult to address, concerns the minimal amount of change in temperature that is sufficiently perturbing of the system to make some type of adaptive response advantageous. A third question, one that follows from the two preceding issues, concerns how close to their thermal tolerance limits contemporary organisms are now living. All three questions can be seen to apply at the level of the whole organism and for traits at lower levels of biological organization such as organ function, protein synthesis, and ATP generation. These three questions will be recurring themes throughout this chapter, and in at least some instances the answers given to them will speak directly to concerns about global climate change.

The question about optimal values for traits will be approached in a strictly empirical manner, and will not entail Panglossian discussions of what might be the ideal characteristics of a trait in "the best of all possible worlds." Our approach to the question of optimal values will involve analysis of the quantitative values of temperature-sensitive traits, and will identify the values (or ranges of values) that recur in differently thermally adapted species. These patterns of conservation in the quantitative values of traits will reveal how diverse physiological and biochemical systems have evolved to attain highly similar physiological and biochemical abilities at their respective body (cell) temperatures, despite the fact that temperature has strong effects on the traits in question. In this context, "optimal" will be equated to the quantitative properties of traits that diverse species have converged on through processes of adaptation to temperature.

The second of these three recurring themes, that concerning the issue of when changes in temperature start to "hurt," is a tricky one, both logically and experimentally. However, it represents an important issue that merits close scrutiny. To provide a basis for predictions about the effects of climate change on organisms, it is important to discern what can be termed *threshold effects* of temperature: the minimal amounts of change in temperature that appear sufficiently perturbing of some aspect of biological activity to favor selection for adaptive change. How much change in temperature is needed before organisms are, in some important way, "hurt" sufficiently to jeopardize their existence in their current habitat, or at least render their performance suboptimal? It is important to examine the fundamental logic of the study of threshold effects of temperature in order to gain a sense of what is possible in this type of analysis, and what is not. It is difficult to experimentally determine the minimal amount of increase (or decrease) in temperature that is sufficiently perturbing to

favor adaptive change. In nature, it is likely to be impossible to reconstruct in fine detail the thermal histories of organisms during their evolution, to establish how much change in temperature was responsible for the thermal characteristics of contemporary traits. Laboratory "evolution" experiments exploiting species like bacteria with short generation times might be able to provide insights into this question, however (Mongold et al., 1996). Nonetheless, even in naturally occurring adaptive processes, it is possible to draw strong inferences about the amount of change in temperature that appears to have been *at least enough* to favor adaptive changes in different species. For instance, if we find compelling evidence for adaptive differences between species whose maximal body temperatures lie, say, 5°C apart, then we may decide to conclude that an increase in temperature of this magnitude has been sufficient to favor adaptive change. This conclusion does not, of course, mean that a temperature change of only 1, 2, 3, or 4°C could not also favor adaptive change. That temperature changes of only one to a few degrees Celsius can be important is demonstrated by several observations, including (i) the discovery that the circadian oscillators driving biological clocks in reptiles, insects, and fungi can be entrained by very slight differences in temperature cycles (Liu et al., 1998); (ii) that changes in water temperature of only 2–3°C can lead to large changes in the feeding rates of seastars on their mussel prey (Sanford, 1999); (iii) that minor increases in water temperature can cause extensive bleaching of coral reefs and trigger the heat-shock response (Gates and Edmunds, 1999; Sharp et al., 1997), and (iv) that multidecadal increases in seawater temperature of about 2°C are correlated with—and possibly causative of—major faunal shifts in intertidal and subtidal habitats (Barry et al., 1995; Sagarin et al., 1999; see Hughes, 2000, for review).

The logical and empirical facets of the analysis of threshold effects will be developed more fully when comparisons are made between confamilial and congeneric species that are found in habitats that differ only slightly in temperature. These comparisons of differently adapted, yet closely related, species will provide us with an especially strong empirical base for predicting how global climate change will impact organisms.

Tightly linked to the question about threshold effects of temperature change are several other questions that bear on the abilities of organisms to cope with alterations in their habitat temperatures. Do some organisms now live so close to the upper limits of their thermal tolerance ranges that rising temperatures will lead to their disappearance from current habitats and shifts in their overall distribution range? How much phenotypic plasticity is available to allow acclimatization to temperature change, thus enabling species to "stay put" despite increases in habitat temperature? How rapidly can species adapt genetically to a new temperature? These questions, too, are themes in the analysis to follow.

Exploiting the Comparative Approach to Study Adaptation to Temperature

From these initial considerations of temperature's influences on organismal distribution patterns, it follows that temperature-adaptive changes at the molecular, cellular, and physiological levels of biological organization are likely to represent a ubiquitous feature of biological evolution. The temperature-linked biogeographic patterning found in nature thus is a clear manifestation not only of temperature's pervasive effects on all organisms, but also of organisms' success in adapting to thermal variation.

We will employ the comparative approach to study these adaptations, using as examples homologous systems from differently thermally adapted organisms. The logic of the comparative analysis we will use parallels in an important way the logic that is commonly exploited by cellular and molecular biologists to deduce basic elements of cellular design. Much of the progress in biology during the past several decades has been made using laboratory-generated mutants that have allowed researchers to gain insights into how many cellular processes work. Selective modification of some component of a system through mutation is an extremely effec-

tive way of determining what the particular component's role is. For example, introducing a single amino acid substitution into a protein using the method of site-directed mutagenesis may yield novel insights into structure-function linkages in proteins. Identical logic applies in well-designed comparative studies. Here, naturally occurring variations of a given structure are examined to learn how differences at the structural level support adaptively important modifications in function. It will become clear through the comparative analyses presented in the following sections of this chapter that deducing basic structure–function linkages in molecular and cellular systems may be especially favored by using the comparative approach.

A second key point is that the success of the comparative approach usually depends on the judicious selection of study organisms. Apples must be compared to apples, if clear conclusions are to be drawn. The effects of phylogeny per se must be distinguished from the results of natural selection and adaptation. Both of these themes, which have been discussed in chapter 1, will be woven through the analysis that follows.

The Need for Complementary Reductionist and Integrative Analyses in Thermal Biology

To conclude this overview of basic aspects of thermal biology and of the appropriate methods for its study, one of the philosophical points central to this book's approach to biological adaptation merits emphasis. To achieve a broad, multilevel analysis of temperature's effects on organisms and of organisms' adaptive responses to thermal perturbation, it is necessary to conduct a dual type of analysis, one involving a reductionist's approach, and one that is integrative and synthetic. Initially, it is important to adopt a reductionist approach and dissect the cell into its individual components—its proteins, membranes, nucleic acids, low-molecular-weight organic solutes, protons, water, and so forth—in order to address two complementary questions. First, how is a particular class of cellular constituents such as proteins affected by temperature? This analysis will enable us to appreciate in fine detail how temperature perturbs the constituent in question. The next question in this reductionist context asks: What "raw material" is available for adaptive change in this particular constituent of the cell and how rapidly can this "raw material" be exploited?

It also is crucial to adopt an integrative approach, one that succeeds in linking together the effects of temperature on different constituents of the cell, so that the interplay among these constituents in achieving adaptation to temperature can be appreciated. Attaining the appropriate functional and structural states of macromolecular systems commonly involves changes in the macromolecules themselves (adaptations in *intrinsic* macromolecular properties) plus alterations in the milieu in which they occur (*extrinsic* adaptations). This statement pertains both to aqueous phase systems, in which the activities of protons, inorganic ions, and small organic molecules may play significant roles in establishing the properties of macromolecules, and to lipid-based systems like cellular membranes, in which the activities of proteins are governed by the particular types of phospholipids and sterols they interact with. Much of the message about adaptation of macromolecules lies in the medium that surrounds them. There is a further important outcome of integrative analysis that takes into account the complexity of biological systems and the complementary roles of intrinsic and extrinsic adaptations: this mode of analysis not only places evolutionary change and physiological regulation in a more realistic context, but also offers important caveats about the design of experiments in which in-vitro analysis of macromolecules attempts to discern what occurs in vivo. While the simplification of reductionist approaches is often necessary to determine how an individual component of the cell is affected by temperature, the characteristics of that component in its normal physiological milieu can only be discerned if the medium used for in-vitro studies simulates the normal intracellular microenvironment. Comparative and integrative analyses provide important guidelines for putting the "bio" back into biochemistry.

In conclusion, because temperature affects essentially everything that a cell contains and does, this environmental variable serves as a major driving force in evolution. The pervasive nature of temperature's effects dictates that we examine each of the fundamental constituents of cells, beginning with proteins, to understand the nature of thermal perturbation and the characteristics of the adaptive responses erected by organisms to cope with thermal effects.

PROTEINS AND TEMPERATURE

Temperature Adaptation of Proteins

Why are rates of enzymatic reactions so strongly dependent on temperature?

Perhaps the most familiar biological effect of temperature is its influence on the rates at which living processes occur. For ectothermic species that are poikilothermic, rates of respiration, feeding, growth, and locomotion may be strongly influenced by changes in environmental temperature on both daily and seasonal time scales. Heterothermic birds and mammals likewise experience large temperature-induced changes in metabolic rates when their body temperatures fall or rise, for instance during entry into or termination of bouts of torpor. Such effects of temperature on rates of biological activity are quantified by calculating the temperature coefficient or Q_{10} of the process, the effect that a $10°C$ ($10\,K$) change in temperature has on the rate in question:

$$Q_{10} = (k_1/k_2)^{10/(t_1 - t_2)}$$

Here, k_1 and k_2 are rate constants determined at high and low temperatures, t_1 and t_2, respectively.

For many processes such as rates of respiration and enzymatic activity, Q_{10} values near two or slightly higher are observed when thermal effects are studied within the species' normal ("physiological") range of body temperatures. Outside this normal range, Q_{10} values may deviate sharply from values near two. At high temperatures at which lethal effects may ensue, Q_{10} values may be less than one, indicating that increases in temperature are damaging the system in question and leading to what may be an irreversible loss of function. We will see several examples of sharp reductions in Q_{10} at elevated temperatures when we consider the physiological and biochemical factors that establish organisms' thermal tolerance limits. At relatively low temperatures, Q_{10} values may become much larger than two. These high Q_{10} values may be indicative of a change in the properties of the underlying biochemical systems, such that the energy barriers to the process in question are increased. Thus, discontinuities in Q_{10} values, which often are shown especially clearly when data are plotted on Arrhenius axes (log of rate versus reciprocal of absolute temperature), are frequently indicative of underlying perturbations of the structures that support the rate process in question. However, even within the normal range of body temperatures through which a stable Q_{10} is observed, the biochemical apparatus of the cells that is responsible for establishing the temperature sensitivity of reaction rates is by no means in a constant structural state. Q_{10} values often represent the net effect of temperature on a complex suite of underlying events.

The concept of activation energy

There would seem to be a simple answer to the question asking why metabolic rates depend so strongly on temperature. The temperature dependence of chemical reaction rates stems from the fact that the reactivity of molecules typically depends on their kinetic energy. Thus, because temperature is a measure of the level of kinetic energy most frequently occupied by the molecules of a system, changes in temperature will affect rates of biological reactions. Higher kinetic energy translates into higher chemical reactivity.

This answer, however, is but a partial and rather qualitative explanation for the Q_{10} values observed in biological reactions, as shown by the following calculation. A 10°C (10 K) change in temperature represents a relatively minor change in the most frequent level of kinetic

energy possessed by the molecules of the system. Recall that the absolute temperature scale must be employed in computing kinetic energies. Thus, at 25°C (298 K) a 10°C change in temperature represents only a 10/298th ($\sim 3\%$) change in the average level of kinetic energy. How can an approximately 3% change in energy be translated into a doubling of reaction rate?

The answer to this question involves an important principle of physical chemistry that was developed by the Swedish Nobel laureate Svante Arrhenius (1856–1927), after whom the Arrhenius plot is named. Arrhenius pointed out that the distribution of kinetic energies among the molecules in a population follows a Maxwell–Boltzmann function (figure 7.1), and it is important to consider not only the most frequently occurring energy level in the population (a measure of temperature), but also energies that are much higher than average, for these are the energies that are most relevant to

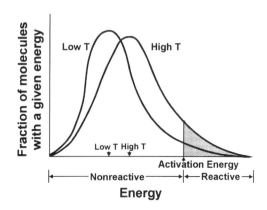

Figure 7.1. The concept of activation energy. Energy distribution curves (Maxwell–Boltzmann distribution functions) are shown for a population of molecules at two different temperatures. The most frequently occupied energy state provides an estimate of the temperature of the system. For a molecule to be chemically reactive, it must possess an energy level equal to or greater than the activation energy (E_a), which remains the same at the two temperatures. As heat is added to the system, the most frequently occupied energy state (= temperature) rises slightly, but the fraction of the population of molecules with energy level equal to or greater than E_a increases greatly.

reaction rates. Thus, only a small fraction of the molecules in a population are apt to have sufficient energy to be reactive at biological temperatures. These are the molecules possessing kinetic energy equal to or exceeding the *activation energy* (E_a), the minimal level of energy required for the reaction to occur (figure 7.1). Arrhenius demonstrated that the fraction of the population of molecules that has an energy equal to or greater than E_a rises with temperature much more quickly than the increase in the most probable level of kinetic energy, the temperature, would suggest. Thus, a 10 K increase in temperature, while representing only a 3% rise in the level of kinetic energy most frequently occupied by the population, may lead to a doubling of the number of molecules having energies equal to or greater than the activation energy. Thus, Q_{10} values near two can be explained.

What events in enzymatic catalysis are rate limiting and responsible for Q_{10} effects?

The explanation of Q_{10} effects just presented is rather typical of treatments found in most textbooks, in which a relatively simplified thermodynamic explanation, based on energy distribution patterns, is developed to account for effects of temperature on reaction rates. Such treatments of temperature effects, while correct overall, are abstract and nonmechanistic—a necessary property of thermodynamic explanations—and will be seen to be incomplete in important ways. In particular, thermodynamic treatments that eschew discussions of underlying mechanisms are unable to provide an explicit account of what steps in an enzyme-catalyzed reaction are rate limiting and, thus, responsible for Q_{10} effects.

In order to determine which events are of primary importance in establishing Q_{10} values, it is necessary to analyze a second key facet of the concept of activation energy, its role in governing the catalytic prowess of enzymes. Enzyme-catalyzed reactions occur at rates many orders of magnitude greater than uncatalyzed rates, a reflection of the abilities of enzymes to greatly lower activation energies.

Temperature determines the fraction of a population of molecules with energy equal to or greater than E_a, but enzymes determine the actual value of E_a. Enzymes "set the bar" to rates of biochemical reactions. At any given temperature, then, the lower the energy of activation is, the larger will be the proportion of molecules that are reactive. Thus, Arrhenius' concept of activation energy is central to answering two distinct and extremely important questions in physiology and biochemistry: "Why are enzymes capable of driving chemical transformations at such rapid rates at biological temperatures?" and, "Why are rates of enzymatic activity so dependent on temperature?" We will see below that these two questions are both rooted in a common phenomenon, namely, the essential roles of changes in protein three-dimensional structure (*conformation*) during enzyme function.

The canonical view concerning how enzymes achieve their extraordinarily high catalytic activities has evolved considerably in recent years. The advent of new methodologies for "dissecting" enzymatic reactions into separate events has allowed biochemists to understand more fully why enzymes are such efficient catalysts, and what individual step in an enzymatic reaction is the rate-limiting event. These analyses have involved a broad spectrum of techniques, including methods to allow measurement of the rates at which covalent chemistry occurs between ligands, and means for making precise determinations of the conformations of the *apoenzyme* (enzyme lacking bound ligands) and *holoenzyme* (enzyme with bound ligands)— and of the speed with which these conformations can be interconverted. For many enzymes, characterization of the three-dimensional structures of apo- and holoenzymes has allowed an extremely detailed picture to be developed of the conformational changes that accompany the catalytic cycle, beginning with the binding of substrates and ending with the release of products. These new methods show that the events occurring during the catalytic process are complex and are inadequately represented by the conventional description of an enzymatic reaction:

enzyme + substrate → enzyme–substrate

complex→activated complex→

enzyme–product complex →

enzyme + products

Although this conventional portrayal of enzymatic catalysis is correct in overall form, it fails to suggest the dynamic nature of the enzyme's structure during the catalytic cycle. Furthermore, this description of enzymatic catalysis implies that the rate-determining step in the overall four-step reaction shown is the second step, the one in which the bound substrate progresses to an activated state. One major conclusion from recent studies of enzyme function is that the rate-governing event in the overall catalytic cycle may not be the actual conversion of substrate to product, that is to say, changes in the covalent bonds of the reactants, but instead may be the rate at which conformational changes occur during binding and release of ligands. In effect, the activation energy barrier to forming or breaking covalent bonds may not be what sets the rate of a multistep enzymatic reaction like the one portrayed above. Evolution has led to extraordinarily efficient active sites in which covalent chemistry occurs with remarkable speed. The effectiveness with which enzymes drive covalent chemistry arises from the establishment in the holoenzyme of an appropriate microenvironment (termed the *catalytic vacuole*; see Dunn et al., 1991) for allowing reactants to undergo rapid chemical transformation to products. What commonly sets the rate of the overall, multistep enzymatic reaction is the much slower rate at which the enzyme changes conformation during either the formation of the holoenzyme complex or the release of products (figure 7.2).

In summary, we can integrate the century-old concept of activation energy with this newer view of enzyme function as follows. Whereas the remarkable abilities of enzymes to catalyze high rates of covalent chemistry at biological temperatures are due to enzymes' abilities to reduce activation energies of chemical reactions, for many and perhaps most enzymes, the required changes in enzyme conformation that are needed to create the catalytic vacuole where this covalent chemistry can take place are not able to keep pace with the rate at which conversion of substrate to product can occur. This new perspective on the rate-determining events in the catalytic process has important implications in several contexts, including the thermal relationships of central focus in this chapter. By looking in detail at certain enzymes for which we possess data on the key roles played by conformational changes in controlling rates of enzymatic function, we can illustrate contemporary views of enzyme structure–function relationships, and also understand how evolutionary processes may lead to adaptive changes in the rates at which enzymes work.

Lactate dehydrogenase: a model enzyme for studying adaptation to temperature

The glycolytic enzyme lactate dehydrogenase (LDH) has been thoroughly "dissected" to characterize the conformational changes that occur during substrate binding and product release (figure 7.2, middle panel). In addition, the covalent chemical transformations that occur within the catalytic vacuole, subsequent to formation of the ternary (LDH–substrate–cofactor) complex are well understood (Dunn et al., 1991). Lactate dehydrogenase catalyzes the interconversion of pyruvate and lactate, using the cofactors NADH and NAD$^+$, respectively. Note that it is arbitrary whether we call pyruvate or lactate the "substrate" of the LDH reaction. The predominant isoform of LDH found in vertebrate skeletal muscle, LDH-A, typically works in the pyruvate reductase direction. We will focus on this isoform of LDH, so our treatment will regard pyruvate as substrate and lactate as product. Note that LDH is a tetramer, so it is more descriptive to refer to LDH-A as A_4-LDH; the latter designation will be used in the following analysis.

The overall changes in conformation of an individual subunit of A_4-LDH are shown in the middle panel of figure 7.2. Entry of

NADH and pyruvate into the binding pocket leads to changes in the three-dimensional configuration of the enzyme, with movement of two loop regions (darkened lines within the structure) playing an important role in establishing the catalytic vacuole. The movements of these two loop regions are somewhat analogous to the closure of two doors that separate the catalytic vacuole from the surrounding medium. Once within the catalytic vacuole, the conversion of pyruvate to lactate and NADH to NAD^+ occurs rapidly, typically within one to a few milliseconds.

To understand more fully how A_4-LDH carries out its functions and, thereby, to build a framework for subsequent analyses of how these functions can be adaptively modified during evolutionary adaptation to temperature, it is necessary to dissect the catalytic vacuole in more detail. The enzyme–ligand interactions that occur within the catalytic vacuole of A_4-LDH are shown in the bottom panel of figure 7.2. Pyruvate is anchored in the active site through interactions with several residues, including arginine-171 and histidine-193. (Note: The numbering given to residues of LDH-A sequences varies somewhat among publications because of additions or deletions of residues between species, and because of errors made in early determinations of the LDH-A sequence [see Abad-Zapatero et al., 1987].) The positive charge on Arg-171 interacts with the negatively charged carboxyl group of pyruvate, helping to orient the substrate correctly within the catalytic vacuole. His-193 also forms a charge–charge interaction with pyruvate, one that is dependent on the pH of the cell. For pyruvate to bind to LDH, His-193 must be protonated. Conversely, lactate can bind only to the unprotonated form of histidine. Because the pK of the imidazole group on histidine is near the pH of the cell (pH_i), changes in pH_i induced by temperature or physiological activity can have large effects on formation of the enzyme–substrate complex. We will discuss the key role of His-193 in the temperature dependence of substrate binding in a later section (see "Temperature–pH Interactions").

The conversion of substrate to product also requires immobilized water molecules within the active site and an appropriate charge environment to facilitate the transfer of electrons and hydrogens to pyruvate. After pyruvate is bound, its reduction to lactate involves addition of two electrons, one proton, and one hydride ion (H^-). NADH provides the electrons and hydride ion; the proton comes from the imidazole ring of His-193. The rate-determining step in the *covalent* chemistry taking place in the catalytic vacuole is that of hydride transfer, which occurs at a rate of approximately $750\,s^{-1}$ at room temperature for bovine A_4-LDH (Dunn et al., 1991).

It is seen, then, that the catalytic power of A_4-LDH arises from the precise juxtaposition within the catalytic vacuole of the reactive groups on the substrate, cofactor, and enzyme. Because of the importance of these precise alignments for catalysis, the three-dimensional structure of the catalytic vacuole is very strongly conserved in evolution. In fact, the geometry defining enzyme–ligand interactions within the catalytic vacuole appears virtually identical in all orthologs of LDH (Deng et al., 1994). This is an extremely important finding in the context of potential mechanisms of enzyme evolution: adaptive changes in kinetic properties, such as adaptations related to temperature, generally cannot be achieved through altering the chemistry that takes place within the catalytic vacuole of the ternary complex. Essentially complete conservation of active site residues is required for a given type of catalysis, such as interconversion of pyruvate and lactate, to be possible, so adaptive change in sequence must occur in other regions of the enzyme.

The temperature-adaptive interspecific variations in kinetic properties discussed below are possible only because the rate at which covalent bonds in pyruvate and NADH are formed and broken turns out not to determine of the rate of LDH function. As emphasized above, the rate-determining event in the overall catalytic sequence is the change in conformation that occurs during ligand binding (or product release). Thus, although enzymes are remarkably effective in reducing the activation energy

Catalytic vacuole

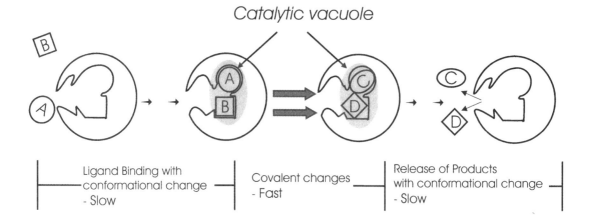

| Ligand Binding with conformational change - Slow | Covalent changes - Fast | Release of Products with conformational change - Slow |

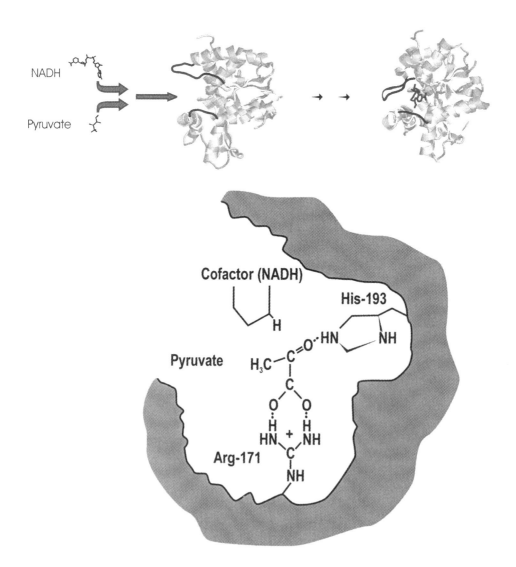

barriers to chemical reactions involving the formation and rupture of covalent bonds, activation energy barriers to conformational changes may prevent the rate of an enzymatic reaction from reaching the full potential represented by the extremely rapid rates of covalent chemistry that occur in the catalytic vacuole. Bovine LDH-A at 25°C falls short by a factor of approximately three: the velocity of the rate-limiting conformational change is only about one-third the rate at which pyruvate is converted to lactate in the catalytic vacuole.

Interspecific variation in k_{cat} values

If rates of catalytic conformational changes are the rate-determining steps in many classes of enzymatic reactions—and the prevalence of conformational changes in enzymatic activity suggests this may be a broadly important relationship—then interesting consequences follow in the context of thermal biology. First, as long as the rates of catalytic conformational changes remain rate-limiting at different temperatures, the Q_{10} values of enzymatic reactions may be due largely to effects of temperature on conformational changes rather than on the covalent chemistry involved in substrate to product conversions. Second, for enzymes of cold-adapted species, a potential evolutionary route for enhancing rates of catalytic activity to compensate for reduced temperature might involve development of enzymes with the ability to undergo catalytic conformational changes

more rapidly. That is, the energy barriers to catalytically essential conformational changes may be lowered, thereby allowing compensation for reduced thermal energy and increased solvent drag on movements of the protein. This strategy of adaptation may be the *only* route available because, as mentioned in the preceding section, the covalent chemistry that occurs within the catalytic vacuole is likely to be invariant among orthologs of an enzyme (Deng et al., 1994). As will be addressed later, however, this scenario lacks a certain degree of symmetry because it begs an important question: Why wouldn't all organisms, whatever their body temperatures, benefit from having enzymes with the lowest possible energy barriers to catalytic conformational changes?

We begin our investigation of temperature-compensatory modification of enzymatic function by considering how the catalytic performance of orthologs of A_4-LDH varies among species that have evolved at widely different temperatures. The initial criterion we employ to quantify catalytic performance is the *catalytic rate constant* (k_{cat}) of the reaction, the rate at which substrate is converted to product per active site per unit time. For the pyruvate reductase reaction catalyzed by A_4-LDH, k_{cat} is expressed as the number of molecules of pyruvate reduced per second per active site. k_{cat} is the best index for evaluating how rapidly an enzyme can work if it is provided with unlimited and non-inhibiting amounts of substrates. Even though enzymes generally do not encounter

Figure 7.2. The catalytic vacuole and the role of conformational changes in catalysis. (Upper panel) The cartoon portrays the (i) substrate binding events, (ii) covalent chemistry (conversion of substrates to products) taking place within the catalytic vacuole, and (iii) release of products by an enzyme. Binding of substrates (A and B) is accompanied by changes in conformation of the enzyme, leading to the generation of a catalytic vacuole within which the covalent chemistry takes place (conversion of A + B to products, C + D). Following formation of products, the conformation of the enzyme again changes, allowing release of products from the enzyme. The rate of conversion of A + B to C + D may be severalfold higher than the rates of the conformation changes that accompany binding and release. (Middle panel) The conformational changes accompanying binding of NADH and pyruvate by lactate dehydrogenase. The darkened regions of the enzyme represent loop structures that undergo large displacements during ligand binding. Only a single subunit of the tetrameric enzyme is illustrated. (See figure 7.5 for additional details on LDH structure.) (Bottom panel) The catalytic vacuole of LDH. Shown are the residues that interact with substrate (pyruvate) and cofactor NADH (for clarity, only a portion of NADH is shown). See text for explanation.

such high substrate concentrations within the cell, it is useful to employ k_{cat} as a measure of how fast an enzyme could, in theory, drive a specific biochemical reaction. We will later provide a more integrated perspective of enzyme function when the dual requirements for rapid rate of catalysis and effective binding are juxtaposed.

Figure 7.3 illustrates values of k_{cat} for orthologs of A_4-LDH from vertebrates adapted to temperatures between $-1.86°C$ (Antarctic notothenioid fishes) and approximately 37–42°C (mammal, birds, and a thermophilic reptile) (Fields and Somero, 1998). All k_{cat} values either were determined at 0°C or, when measurements were made at higher temperatures, k_{cat} values at 0°C were obtained by extrapolation using a Q_{10} of two. The key fact that emerges from these data is that, despite the likelihood that all orthologs of LDH-A have identical catalytic vacuoles in their ternary complexes, large temperature-related differences in k_{cat} exist. At the extreme, the k_{cat}'s of LDH-A orthologs of Antarctic notothenioid fishes are approximately four to five times higher than the k_{cat}'s of mammalian, avian, and thermophilic reptilian orthologs at 0°C. The interspecific differences in k_{cat} are not indicative of a "lower" versus "higher"

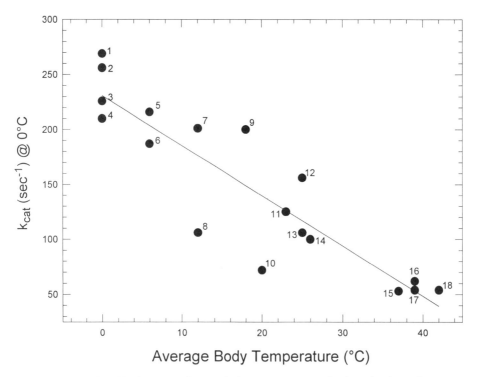

Figure 7.3. The relationship between the catalytic rate constant (k_{cat}) and adaptation temperature for A_4-LDH orthologs from differently thermally adapted vertebrates. Species studied were: four Antarctic notothenioids, *Parachaenichthys charcoti*, (1) *Lepidonotothen nudifrons*, (2) *Champsocephalus gunnari*, (3), and *Harpagifer antarcticus* (4); two South American notothenioids, *Patagonotothen tessellata*, (5) and *Eleginops maclovinus* (6); a temperate rockfish, *Sebastes mystinus* (7); a halibut, *Hippoglossus stenolepis* (8); a temperate barracuda, *Sphyraena argentea* (9); the dogfish, *Squalus acanthias* (10); a subtropical barracuda, *Sphyraena lucasana* (11); a temperate goby fish, *Gillichthys mirabilis* (12); the bluefin tuna, *Thunnus thynnus* (13); a tropical barracuda, *Sphyraena ensis* (14); the cow, *Bos taurus* (15); the chicken, *Gallus gallus* (16); the turkey, *Meleagris gallopavo* (17); and the desert iguana, *Dipsosaurus dorsalis* (18). Linear regression: $y = -4.6x + 231$; $r^2 = 0.81$. (Figure modified after Fields and Somero, 1998.)

vertebrate distinction: k_{cat} varies regularly among fishes adapted to different temperatures. These data, plus those from comparisons of other sets of enzyme orthologs from differently adapted species (see Somero, 1995, 1997, for review), show that interspecific differences in k_{cat} are a reflection of evolution in different thermal conditions, rather than a consequence of the evolutionary lineage to which a species belongs. The relationship between adaptation temperature and k_{cat} is found in all branches of the evolutionary tree. For example, highly temperature-tolerant members of the domain Archaea ("hyperthermophiles" or "ultrathermophiles") found in geothermal springs and other extremely hot environments possess enzymes with extremely low catalytic activities, at least when measurements are made at the moderate temperatures at which mesophilic species live (Jaenicke, 1991, 2000).

To understand the ultimate and proximate causes of why organisms adapted to high temperatures "fail" to have enzymes that function as rapidly as enzymes of cold-adapted species— at least when measurements are conducted at a common temperature—it is necessary to cast the analysis of adaptive variation in k_{cat} values in a broader context, one that involves other kinetic properties plus the issue of protein structural stability. Before making this analysis, however, it is relevant to consider how interspecific variation in k_{cat} values of enzymes contributes to adaptation to temperature at the level of metabolic function. How effectively do the higher k_{cat} values of orthologs from cold-adapted species help these organisms overcome the chilling effects of low temperatures on metabolic rates? Are differences in enzymatic performance manifested at higher levels of biological organization?

Adaptive variation in k_{cat} and metabolic compensation to temperature in ectotherms

There is a large and somewhat contentious literature dealing with the question of how fully the respiratory rates of ectotherms can be adjusted to offset Q_{10} effects on metabolic reactions, a process known as *temperature compensation of metabolism*. Metabolic compensation

has most commonly been studied by quantifying the effects of temperature on rates of oxygen consumption by differently adapted and differently acclimated ectotherms. In some but not all cases, the rates of respiration of the cold-adapted or cold-acclimated individuals are higher, especially at low temperatures of measurement, than the rates of warm-adapted or warm-acclimated forms. This difference in respiratory rate commonly has been referred to as metabolic cold adaptation (MCA; see Clarke, 1991). However, as discussed by Clarke (1991), Holeton (1974) and Zimmermann and Hubold (1998), attempts to quantify metabolic compensation at the level of whole organism respiration are generally plagued by serious experimental and interpretive problems. For instance, in interspecific studies, comparing highly active species with sluggish species may lead to erroneous conclusions about compensation in whole organism respiration rate (for review, see the insightful analysis of Zimmermann and Hubold, 1998). An actively swimming pelagic polar fish, when compared to a sluggish demersal tropical fish, may seem highly cold-adapted. Yet, when a relatively sluggish polar fish is compared to an active tropical or temperate species, the polar fish may exhibit no apparent metabolic compensation. The physiological states of experimental organisms, such as their feeding status and level of excitement due to experimental manipulation, also affect rates of respiration and may lead to experimental artifacts. For these reasons, comparisons of metabolic activity must be designed as carefully as possible to involve "apples to apples" comparisons in which the effects of adaptation or acclimation to temperature can be teased out from a myriad of other factors that influence rates of respiration. It would seem advisable to design experiments in which an organ whose metabolic activity is unlikely to be affected by factors such as activity, diet, or handling stress is studied in order to isolate effects of adaptation to temperature from these influences.

Brain would seem to offer the potential for satisfying this criterion of sound experimental design. Brain is likely to have to perform similarly in all fishes, regardless of level of locomotory activity or general ecological character-istics such as benthic versus pelagic habitat. Metabolic activities in brain also are strongly defended in the face of poor nutritional conditions, so the feeding state of organisms is not as likely to influence levels of enzymatic activity in brain as it might activities in liver or muscle (see, e.g., the study of dietary effects on enzymatic activity in different organs of fish by Yang and Somero, 1993). In fact, studies of oxygen consumption of brain slices in vitro revealed a high degree of temperature compensation in the metabolism of Antarctic notothenioid fishes (Somero et al., 1968). The question as to whether this compensation is due to a "better" enzyme (higher k_{cat}) or to elevated enzyme concentrations has recently been addressed (figure 7.4; Kawall et al., 2001).

As the data in figure 7.4 indicate, a substantial degree of metabolic compensation is noted: activities of LDH and citrate synthase (CS), a Krebs citric acid cycle enzyme, in brains of Antarctic notothenioid fishes are two- to three-fold higher than in tropical fishes, at a common measurement temperature. Although there are no k_{cat} data available for the CS orthologs of these species, the difference in LDH activity between the two groups compares closely with the differences in k_{cat} between A_4-LDHs of Antarctic notothenioids and warm-adapted fishes such as the tropical barracuda *Sphyraena ensis* (point #14 in figure 7.3) and bluefin tuna (point #13). Therefore, it appears that cold-adapted and warm-adapted species contain similar numbers of LDH molecules, and that differences in mass-specific enzymatic activity are due to differences in k_{cat} among orthologs. "Better," rather than "more," may describe enzymatic mechanisms of metabolic compensation to temperature. Note that this conjecture applies not only to differently adapted species, but also to populations of a single species that are adapted to different thermal conditions (Place and Powers, 1979; Powers et al., 1993; Watt and Dean, 2001). An example of this type of genetic patterning is found for the killifish *Fundulus heteroclitus* (Place and Powers, 1979; reviewed in Powers et al., 1993), in which a sharp latitudinal gradient in two allelic variants of lactate dehydrogenase-B

(LDH-B) occurs. The "northern" and "southern" allozymes have kinetic properties that reflect adaptation to the different thermal conditions of their habitats.

In the case of the comparisons of LDH and CS given in figure 7.4, when activities are extrapolated to normal body temperatures of the two groups of species using experimentally determined Q_{10} values for the two reactions, metabolic compensation is seen to be substantial, although not complete. At $0°C$, LDH and CS activities in brains of Antarctic fishes are only about one-half the activities characteristic of tropical fishes at $25°C$. Why enzymatic compensation to temperature is incomplete is not known. Life at low temperatures may reduce certain metabolic costs, allowing life to occur with lower rates of energy turnover. For instance, reduced costs for maintaining transmembrane ion gradients may exist due to lower flux rates of ions through membranes. Costs of protein turnover may be reduced at low temperatures if the lifespans of proteins are increased at low temperatures. These, however, are conjectures that remain to be tested. It is clear that the more efficient enzymes of cold-adapted species allow relatively high rates of catalysis without a concomitant increase in the total number of enzymes in the cells. This mechanism of evolutionary compensation to low temperature would lead to energy savings compared to an alternate mechanism that was based on elevated enzyme concentrations in the cold.

Mechanisms of compensation may differ between evolutionary adaptation and acclimation/acclimatization

Although brains of differently thermally adapted species appear to contain similar numbers of LDH molecules, differently acclimated or acclimatized individuals of a species have been observed to alter the amounts of enzyme in their cells (Hazel and Prosser, 1974; Sidell, 1977). These temperature-compensatory adjustments in enzymatic activity typically entail altering concentrations of a given isoform of a protein, not the induction of a new isoform with different kinetic properties. That is, k_{cat} does

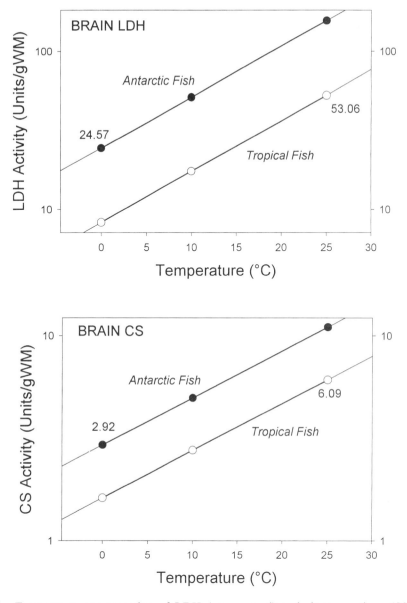

Figure 7.4. Temperature compensation of LDH (upper panel) and citrate synthase (CS) (lower panel) activity in brains of Antarctic notothenioid fishes and tropical fishes. Enzymatic activity in homogenates of brain was measured at a common temperature, 10°C, and extrapolated to the approximate habitat temperatures of the species (0°C for Antarctic fish and 25°C for tropical species) using experimentally determined Q_{10} values. Activities at habitat temperatures are indicated in the figure. Despite substantial temperature compensation, an approximately twofold difference in activity persists at habitat temperatures for both enzymes. (Data from Kawall et al., 2001).

not vary with acclimation or acclimatization states, even though the amount of enzymatic activity in the cell changes substantially (Activity = k_{cat} × [enzyme]).

The relative roles played by adjusting the rate of enzyme synthesis versus changing the rate of protein turnover are not known in a general sense, albeit both processes are likely to contribute to setting the intracellular concentration of an enzyme during acclimation or acclimatization. Work with *Fundulus heteroclitus* has demonstrated that levels of messenger RNA production (transcription) vary between northern and southern populations as a consequence of differences in the regulatory regions of the *ldh-b* gene in these populations (Schulte et al., 2000). Thus, even though adaptive differences in kinetic properties may exist for allozymes of northern and southern populations of *F. heteroclitus* (Place and Powers, 1979; Powers et al., 1993), adjustments in the level of gene expression also make an important contribution to establishing temperature-compensatory differences in enzymatic activity.

How can protein structure be modified to adjust k_{cat} values?

Having seen that adjustments in k_{cat} values contribute to offsetting the Q_{10} effects of temperature on metabolic rates of species evolutionarily adapted to different temperatures, we now return to a mechanistic mode of analysis and examine how these adjustments in k_{cat} might be achieved. From what was presented earlier, it is reasonable to hypothesize that differences in k_{cat} among orthologs must arise from differences in the rates at which catalytically essential conformational changes take place. The challenges, then, are to identify the regions of the enzyme that govern the rates of these conformational changes and determine how specific amino acid substitutions in or near these regions can alter the speed with which an enzyme can change its three-dimensional structure.

Variation in sequence among orthologs differs greatly among regions of an enzyme. Some regions show identical sequences in all orthologs, whereas other parts of the molecule are extremely variable in sequence. The conservation seen in the covalent chemistry of a particular class of enzymatic reaction is reflected in a strong conservation of the amino acid residues that interact directly with substrates and cofactors. For all classes of enzymes for which data on sequences of orthologs from different species are available, there is virtually complete conser-

vation of sequence for regions of the enzyme that contain the residues that form the catalytic vacuole. For A_4-LDH orthologs, there is especially strong conservation in the sequence of the *catalytic (specificity) loop* (figure 7.5). This region of the enzyme contains residues that interact with ligands, and, during formation of the ternary complex, the catalytic loop undergoes the largest displacement of any region of the enzyme, approximately 15 Å (Gerstein and Chothia, 1991). Other regions of the LDH-A subunit that undergo substantial changes in orientation during substrate binding and product release are the C-terminal helix, αH, and the $\alpha 1G$-$\alpha 2G$ helix (figure 7.5). In effect, the catalytic loop, αH, and the $\alpha 1G$-$\alpha 2G$ helix can be viewed as "doors" that close down during binding to lock pyruvate and NADH within the catalytic vacuole. In fact, it is these very changes in enzyme conformation that bring about a reorientation of the catalytically essential residues of the enzyme to create a catalytic vacuole in the ternary complex.

Because of the need to maintain appropriate geometry for substrate binding within the catalytic vacuole, these parts of the LDH molecule appear "off-limits" for generating temperature-adaptive change in k_{cat}. If some or all regions of the "doors" that close over the substrate and cofactor to generate the catalytically active ternary complex cannot be varied, what about the "hinges" that link these "doors" to the remainder of the enzyme? Might there be a means to alter these "hinge" regions so as to modify the energy requirements entailed in forming the ternary complex? More flexible "hinges" might allow more rapid movement of key elements of secondary structure, such as the catalytic loop, αH, and the $\alpha 1G$-$\alpha 2G$ helix, and, thereby, to higher k_{cat} values.

There is evidence that such "hinge" regions can be important sites of adaptation to temperature. The $\alpha 1G$-$\alpha 2G$ helix is linked to a beta sheet region (β-J) of the enzyme by a loop of 22 residues that may influence the freedom of movement of the $\alpha 1G$-$\alpha 2G$ helix (figure 7.5). The movement of $\alpha 1G$-$\alpha 2G$ may, in fact, be the rate-limiting step in catalysis (Dunn et al., 1991). This loop has an extremely high degree of variation in sequence among species, so it can be termed a hypervariable loop (Fields and Somero, 1998). The high degree of variation in sequence among orthologs could be due to two factors: either the region is of limited importance in enzyme function and stability—and thus is relatively free to vary neutrally among species—or the hypervariable loop plays an important role in determining rates of movement of helix α1G-α2G. The logic to use in distinguishing between these two hypotheses is straightforward: if variation in sequence of the hypervariable loop is such that the more cold-adapted enzymes have amino acid residues facilitating a higher degree of loop flexibility (and, by implication, lower energy barriers for movement of helix α1G-α2G), then the observed sequence variation is likely to be temperature-adaptive and not neutral with respect to function.

When the sequences of hypervariable loop regions are examined, it is found that the most cold-adapted A$_4$-LDH orthologs, those of Antarctic notothenioid fishes, contain high levels of glycyl residues relative to orthologs of warm-adapted fishes, birds, and mammals. Glycyl residues introduce a high level of configurational entropy into a protein because they restrict rotation around peptide bonds the least of any residue. Thus, the finding that five glycyl residues occur in the hypervariable loops of Antarctic notothenioid fishes, whereas only two or three glycyls are present in A$_4$-LDH orthologs of more warm-adapted species, is consistent with selection for a more flexible "hinge" in these cold-adapted orthologs. In addition, the residues found in the hypervariable loop of A$_4$-LDHs of Antarctic fishes tend to be relatively hydrophilic. This difference, too, could affect the conformational flexibility of the enzyme because the hypervariable loop interacts with the N-terminal region of an adjoining subunit (figure 7.5). If subunit–subunit interactions are reduced, then freedom of movement of the α1G-α2G helix might be enhanced. It has been demonstrated in studies of LDH-A orthologs of barracuda fishes (genus *Sphyraena*) that a single substitution in the N-terminal region of the molecule at a site that is involved in subunit–subunit interactions is sufficient to alter the thermal stability and kinetic

properties (both k_{cat} and Michaelis–Menten constant, K_m) of the enzyme (Holland et al., 1997).

Studies using laboratory-generated mutants of LDH support the conclusions drawn from analysis of naturally occurring variation in k_{cat} among orthologs. Site-directed mutagenesis of bacterial LDHs has created variants in which reduced rates of conformational changes led to significantly lower values of k_{cat} (Dunn et al., 1991). Site-directed mutagenesis experiments with A$_4$-LDHs of fishes have shown that substitutions that affect the freedom of movement of certain of the "doors" that close during formation of the ternary complex, for example, the C-terminal helix (αH) and the α1G-α2G helix, can alter kinetic properties. One substitution within each of these sequence regions of an Antarctic notothenioid A$_4$-LDH converted this cold-adapted enzyme to a variant having kinetic properties similar to those of a temperate fish (P.A. Fields, unpublished observations).

In summary, knowledge of the refined three-dimensional structure of A$_4$-LDH (Abad-Zapatero et al., 1987), in conjunction with information on the sequences of many orthologs of the enzyme, permits structural interpretations of interspecific differences in LDH function. One of the most important conclusions from such analyses is that amino acid substitutions responsible for adaptation of kinetic properties like k_{cat} *never* appear to occur in regions of the molecule that form the catalytic vacuole. Rather, substitutions appear to affect the local flexibility of regions of the molecule that govern the energy barriers to catalytically essential conformational changes. Substitutions that constrain movement of these regions of the enzyme may impede essential conformational changes; substitutions that make the "hinges" more flexible may allow conformational changes to occur more rapidly, leading to elevations in k_{cat}.

Why aren't k_{cat} values of all orthologs as high as possible?

As mentioned earlier, there is an apparent paradox associated with the scenario presented

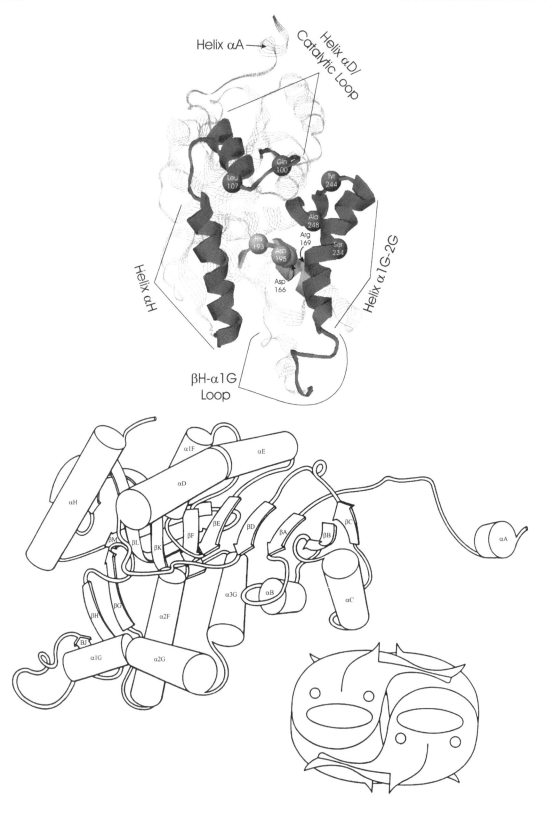

above for adaptation of k_{cat} values to temperature. If we view alterations in k_{cat} values from the perspective of adaptation to low temperatures, then it seems reasonable to view as adaptive any sequence changes that facilitate higher k_{cat} values. However, evolutionary adaptation to temperature also involves acquiring abilities to function at higher body temperatures. For instance, the so-called higher vertebrates—birds and mammals—are assumed to have evolved from lower vertebrate ancestors whose body temperatures were well below 37–39°C. During the evolution of birds and mammals, enzymes seem to have become "poorer" in that there appears to have been a decrease in k_{cat} values (figure 7.3).

There would seem to be two possible explanations for this evolutionary trend. First, to turn the discussion of temperature compensation around, it might have been advantageous for birds and mammals, as well as other high-body-temperature organisms like thermophilic reptiles, to evolve less efficient enzymes to retard metabolic rates and thereby offset the rate-enhancing effects of elevated body temperatures. Whereas too little metabolic flux may be a danger for a species with a low body temperature, too great a rate of metabolism could be problematic for an organism with a high body temperature. Thus, it could be conjectured that, in the face of abundant thermal energy, it would be disadvantageous to possess enzymes with inherently high k_{cat} values. This conjecture is suspect in light of the fact that the control of rates of enzymatic activity can be effected quite readily by changing the number of enzyme molecules in the cell. Thus, a "smart" mammal or bird might want to develop enzymes with high k_{cat} values so it could support its high metabolic rate by synthesizing relatively small numbers of enzyme molecules and, thereby, save considerable energy in protein synthesis.

What we regard as a more reasonable interpretation of the low k_{cat} values of enzymes of higher vertebrates and of warm-adapted species in general, including hyperthermophilic members of the Archaea, involves a more integrated view of the structure–function relationships of enzymes. To develop this perspective, it is necessary to return to the overall sequence of events involved in enzymatic catalysis and to look at other steps in enzymatic processes where temperature perturbs the system and where adaptive change might be required. This analysis will identify other features of enzymes that manifest adaptation to temperature, and will allow a more complete synthesis to be developed concerning how kinetic properties and structural stability are linked.

Figure 7.5. Three-dimensional structure of A_4-LDH. (Top panel) A single subunit of the A_4-LDH tetramer. The major structural elements that are important in catalytic conformational changes and subunit interactions are indicated. The amino acid residues involved in binding and catalysis are numbered. Structural elements undergoing large (up to 15 Å) displacements during binding of cofactor and substrate are darkened and include: (i) the helix αD/catalytic loop, (ii) helix α1G-2G, (iii) helix αH, and (iv) the βH-α1G loop. Helices αD, α1G-2G, and αH function somewhat like doors that close down over the bound ligands, to generate the catalytic vacuole of the ternary complex. The loop connecting beta sheet J and helical region α1-G also undergoes a large change in orientation. Regions of subunit interaction include αA (N-terminal helix) and portions of helix α1G-α2G and other nonmarked regions of the structure. The remaining regions of the enzyme are indicated using lighter lines. (Figure modified after Fields and Somero, 1998.) (Lower panel) Another view of the structure of a single subunit of LDH-A, showing the helical and beta-sheet elements, and a cartoon quaternary structure. The Kama Sutra fish aggregation portrays the arrangement of the four subunits of the active tetrameric form of the enzyme. The "tail" of each subunit includes helix αA (N-terminal helix); the lower jaw contains helix α1G-α2G. (Modified after Abad-Zapatero et al., 1987.)

Enzymes exist as ensembles of conformational states

Textbook diagrams of enzymes are apt to portray the apoenzyme as existing in a single, binding-competent conformation, "waiting" for the entry of substrate(s) into the active site, so that the catalytic cycle can commence. Formerly, it was common to view the enzyme as a "lock" waiting for the insertion of the "key," the substrate. This static picture of enzyme structure fails to do justice to the true situation that characterizes enzymes in solution. Rather than occurring in a single, binding-competent conformation, enzymes exist in an *ensemble of conformational states* (Bai et al., 1996; Hilser et al., 1998) due to the fact that proteins have a considerable degree of flexibility or, to employ more precise terminology, they possess a considerable level of *conformational (configurational) entropy* (figure 7.6). Among the many conformational states present will be those that are permissive of ligand binding—configurations that allow access of ligands to the binding pocket—and others that either do not allow binding or function relatively poorly in this capacity. Fluctuation among these conformations is rapid, so that a single enzyme molecule may "flicker" between binding-competent and binding-incompetent conformations. For enzymes like A_4-LDH that undergo large changes in three-dimensional structure during binding (figure 7.2, middle panel; figure 7.5), fluctuations in the positions of structures like the catalytic loop, helix αH, and the $\alpha 1G$-$\alpha 2G$ helix will change the binding competency of the

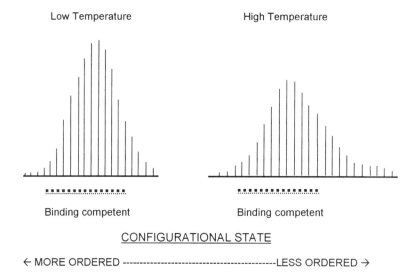

CONFIGURATIONAL STATE

← MORE ORDERED ---LESS ORDERED →

Figure 7.6. Proteins exist in an ensemble of configurational microstates. At any given instant, only a certain fraction of a population of enzyme molecules possesses the configuration required for effective binding of substrates and cofactors (dashed lines beneath distribution curves). As temperature is elevated (compare left and right distribution curves), the protein has access to increased numbers of conformations, many of which are unable to bind ligands or bind ligands weakly. Therefore, elevations in temperature may reduce an enzyme's ligand binding ability whether or not the actual bonds formed between the enzyme and ligand in the catalytic vacuole are stabilized or destabilized by changes in temperature.

The effect of a change in temperature on the ensemble of conformational states may differ between relatively rigid and relatively flexible proteins. A flexible protein from a cold-adapted species may be more perturbed by increases in temperature than a warm-adapted species' ortholog of this same protein. However, at the different species' respective physiological temperatures, it is conjectured that a similar fraction of the total population of protein molecules will occur in a binding-competent conformation. Conservation of ligand binding ability is, then, proposed to be due to the similar ensembles of conformations found at normal body (cell) temperatures for different orthologs.

enzyme because the orientations of these groups determine whether or not NADH and pyruvate have easy access to the binding site. A wide range of accessibilities to the binding site is expected because of structural fluctuations in A_4-LDH, and the overall binding affinity (association constant) of a substrate represents an average of the binding abilities of all conformational states.

When temperature is brought into the picture, the role of configurational entropy looms especially large. As shown in figure 7.6, increasing temperature broadens the array of conformations accessible to an enzyme and additional conformations that disallow binding may be formed. To a first approximation, then, increasing temperature is predicted to reduce the average binding ability of the enzymes in a population. Furthermore, the relatively flexible proteins of low-temperature-adapted species are apt to be more perturbed than orthologs of more warm-adapted species, which are more rigid and thus have higher energy barriers to conformational changes.

Trade-offs exist between binding (K_m) and k_{cat}

The facts that (i) proteins exist in solution in an ensemble of conformational states and (ii) the inherent flexibility of an enzyme may influence its catalytic and binding properties provide a helpful frame of reference for interpreting differences in both k_{cat} values and apparent Michaelis–Menten constants (K_m) among orthologs. Because the equation defining K_m for any enzyme–ligand pair may contain rate constants in addition to those defining the true dissociation constant of the enzyme–ligand complex, apparent K_m values often do not provide quantitative estimates of binding ability (for LDH, see Powers, 1987). However, for purposes of relating k_{cat} and K_m to structural flexibility, it is satisfactory to use apparent K_m as an approximate index of the affinity between enzyme and substrate or cofactor. A *low* value for K_m indicates *high* affinity for the ligand in question; a high value denotes weak binding.

Comparisons of K_m values for orthologs of enzymes from differently thermally adapted species generally reveal a common pattern: increases in measurement temperature cause increases in K_m for all orthologs, but at the normal body (cell) temperatures of differently adapted species, K_m values are highly conserved. This relationship is illustrated for the K_m of pyruvate (K_m^{PYR}) for A_4-LDH in figure 7.7. For each ortholog, increasing temperature of measurement increases K_m^{PYR} (figure 7.7, upper panel). However, at any given temperature of measurement the value of K_m is lowest for the ortholog of the most warm-adapted species and highest for the most cold-adapted species (figure 7.7, lower panel: K_m^{PYR} at 10°C). Because of this displacement of the K_m^{PYR} versus temperature relationships for the A_4-LDH orthologs of differently thermally adapted species, substantial conservation of K_m^{PYR} occurs at physiological temperatures (figure 7.7, lower panel: K_m^{PYR} at upper limit of body temperature). Enzymes of highly eurythermal species like the tidepool goby *Gillichthys seta*, which may encounter temperatures from less than 10°C to over 40°C in its shallow habitat in the Gulf of California, have especially flat K_m^{PYR} versus temperature relationships (Fields and Somero, 1997). Its less eurythermal congener, *Gillichthys mirabilis*, which is unlikely to have a body temperature above 32–35°C, has an A_4-LDH with a sharper temperature dependence of K_m^{PYR} at higher temperatures of measurement.

How can these differences in the relationship between temperature and K_m^{PYR} for orthologs of LDH-A be explained mechanistically? From the discussions of catalytic vacuole geometry and amino acid sequences given earlier, we can eliminate one potential mechanism: interspecific differences in K_m values cannot be explained in terms of the chemical bonds that form between ligands and amino acid side-chains in the catalytic vacuole of the ternary complex. The catalytic vacuole is conserved among species, so adaptive change in K_m and k_{cat} must be achieved by modifying aspects of enzyme structure other than the sequence and three-dimensional structure of the catalytic vacuole itself.

By combining elements of the conformational ensemble model for protein structures in solution (figure 7.6) with the observations that flexibility-related differences in k_{cat} occur

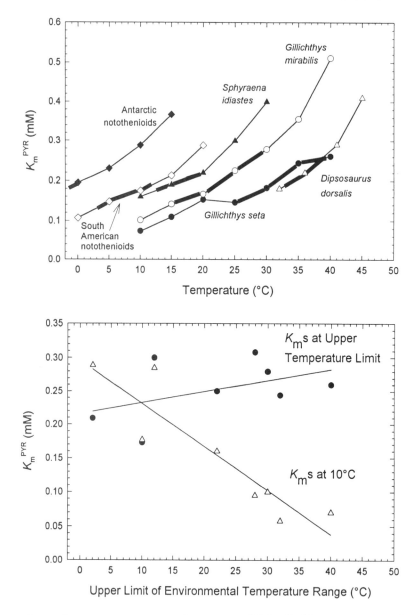

Figure 7.7. Effects of assay temperature on the apparent Michaelis–Menten constant of pyruvate (K_m^{PYR}) for A$_4$-LDH orthologs of differently thermally adapted vertebrates. (Upper panel) K_m^{PYR} versus measurement temperature for orthologs of Antarctic and South American notothenioid fishes, a barracuda fish (*Sphyraena idiastes*), two goby fishes (*Gillichthys mirabilis* and *Gillichthys seta*) and the desert iguana (*Dipsosaurus dorsalis*). Thick line segments indicate the approximate ranges of body temperatures of the species. (Lower panel) K_m^{PYR} measured at 10°C (open triangles) and K_m^{PYR} at the species' upper limits of body temperature (filled circles) for eight teleost fishes. Species shown, from left to right across the abscissa, are an Antarctic notothenioid, a South American notothenioid, a cold-adapted scorpaenid (*Sebastolobus alascanus*), *Sphyraena idiastes*, a subtropical barracuda (*Sphyraena lucasana*), *Gillichthys mirabilis*, a warm-adapted goby (*Coryphopterus personatus*), and *Gillichthys seta*. Note how the decrease in K_m^{PYR} at 10°C with increasing adaptation temperature leads to a conservation of K_m^{PYR} at physiological temperatures. (Data from Graves and Somero (1982), Holland et al., 1997, and Fields and Somero, 1997, 1998.)

among orthologs of LDH-A, a model can be developed that at once accounts for three phenomena: (i) variation in K_m with temperature for any single ortholog, (ii) differences in the absolute values of K_m among orthologs, and (iii) covariation between k_{cat} and K_m when different orthologs are compared. At any single temperature of measurement, the ensemble of conformational states that characterizes an enzyme will be defined by the inherent structural flexibility of the protein. If, within this ensemble of conformational states, there exist states that are both permissive of and nonpermissive of ligand binding, it would be expected that, at a common temperature of measurement, an enzyme from a cold-adapted species would exhibit lower affinity for a ligand than an ortholog from a warm-adapted species (figure 7.6). The more flexible structure of the ortholog of the cold-adapted species would allow fluctuations of the protein to occur more readily, and a lower fraction of the total population of enzyme molecules would exist in a binding competent state. As measurement temperature is increased and the distribution of conformational states broadens, a reduced proportion of the population of enzymes is expected to be in binding-competent conformations, and all orthologs would show reductions in affinity for substrates (figures 7.6 and 7.7). At normal body temperatures, it is hypothesized that a relatively stable proportion of the population of enzyme molecules exists in binding competent conformations for all species, as suggested by the conservation in K_m at these temperatures.

This analysis leads to a view of enzyme evolution that can be said to involve a "trade-off," and that may resolve the apparent paradox of loss of catalytic power (reductions in k_{cat}) during evolution in high-body-temperature species. In effect, this view of enzyme evolution is a reflection of the principle that few, if any, traits exist in isolation, such that properties of one trait can be modified independently of effects on other traits of the system. (The embedding of several rate constants within the expression for apparent K_m is one illustration of this principle.) For enzymes, it is important to remember that three interrelated traits are critical and

must be retained, regardless of the temperatures at which the enzyme functions. First, enzymes must possess sufficient *structural stability* to allow persistence of a functional conformation at physiological temperatures, yet their structures must be flexible enough to allow catalytically essential conformational changes. Second, they must *catalyze metabolic transformations at high rates*. Third, they must be able to *recognize and bind the appropriate ligands* under physiological conditions of ligand concentration. What the above discussion of enzyme structure in solution has shown is that these are three properties that evolve in concert. At any given temperature, the enzyme's structure must permit adequate binding and catalytic function. The highly flexible proteins of cold-adapted species, at these species' low body temperatures, possess adequate flexibility to support high k_{cat} values, and a sufficient proportion of the population of enzymes exists in binding-competent conformations to allow effective binding of ligands at the low ligand concentrations characteristic of most substrates and cofactors. As temperature increases, cold-adapted enzymes tend to lose their binding abilities relatively rapidly, as evidenced by sharp upswings in K_m values with rising temperature. Furthermore, as discussed below under the heading of "The Heat-Shock Response," thermally induced unfolding may lead to denaturation of an enzyme. The more rigid enzymes of high-body-temperature species, at these organisms' higher cell temperatures, are able to retain effective binding ability because their less flexible structures ensure that a high proportion of the enzymes in the population occur in a binding-competent state, even at high temperatures. This, then, is the "trade-off": the retention of binding ability is achieved only at the cost of some reduction in k_{cat}. Not only is binding ability conserved by these changes in structural flexibility, but the potential for heat-induced denaturation of the protein also is reduced.

In summary, during protein evolution at different temperatures, selection favors the accumulation of amino acid substitutions whose effects are manifested by adaptive changes in stability and kinetic properties. Of overarching importance is the maintenance of the geometry of the catalytic vacuole, with retention of appropriate levels of mobility in those regions of the enzyme that change orientation during formation of the vacuole. The enzyme must have requisite stability to exist in conformations that allow ligands to have access to the binding site on the enzyme. Stability must not be too great, however, if rate-determining changes in enzyme conformation are to occur with sufficient speed to support an adequate level of metabolic flux. And, linked to both of these aspects of function is the requirement that proteins be adequately stable to avoid rapid denaturation under cellular conditions of temperature and chemical composition.

Protein flexibility and activation energy parameters

To extend the discussion of linkages between conformational flexibility and kinetic properties, we will next examine activation energy parameters, which have frequently been used to characterize responses of proteins to temperature in the contexts of evolutionary adaptation and acute thermal effects (Low et al., 1973). According to absolute reaction rate theory developed by Henry Eyring and others, the rate-governing energy barrier to a chemical reaction is the *activation free energy*, symbolized as $\Delta G^{\ddagger}$. Following conventional thermodynamic treatment, $\Delta G^{\ddagger}$ comprises an enthalpy term ($\Delta H^{\ddagger}$) and an entropy term ($\Delta S^{\ddagger}$):

$$\Delta G^{\ddagger} = \Delta H^{\ddagger} - T\Delta S^{\ddagger}$$

The activation enthalpy is derived from the slope of an Arrhenius plot of log V_{max} versus the reciprocal of absolute temperature, and is related to the Arrhenius activation energy

$(E_a)_+$ as follows: $\Delta H^{\ddagger} = E_a - RT$. Thus, $\Delta H^{\ddagger}$ is proportional to the Q_{10} of the reaction and provides a measure of the amount of energy required to form the activated ternary complex.

If the hypothesized linkage between changes in localized structural flexibility, rates of catalytic conformational changes, and k_{cat} is correct, we would expect to find that the A_4-LDH orthologs of cold-adapted species would have low $\Delta H^{\ddagger}$ values because less energy is required to drive the rate-limiting conformational changes. Strictly on the basis of the size of $\Delta H^{\ddagger}$, then, enzymes of cold-adapted species would be expected to have lower values of $\Delta G^{\ddagger}$ than orthologs of warm-adapted species. However, in view of the less ordered ensemble of conformations that cold-adapted proteins adopt at any given temperature, relative to warm-adapted orthologs, the activation entropy term, $\Delta S^{\ddagger}$, for a cold-adapted enzyme is predicted to *higher* because of the required increase in system order during the catalytic conformational changes involved in formation of the ternary complex. This relatively large negative activation entropy for a cold-adapted ortholog counterbalances the effect of a low $\Delta H^{\ddagger}$ on $\Delta G^{\ddagger}$. Thus, because $\Delta G^{\ddagger} = \Delta H^{\ddagger} - T\Delta S^{\ddagger}$, the differences between orthologs in $\Delta H^{\ddagger}$ and $\Delta S^{\ddagger}$ are strongly offsetting ("compensating") in their effects on $\Delta G^{\ddagger}$.

As the data in Table 7.1 reveal, an A_4-LDH ortholog from a highly cold-adapted Antarctic fish (*Pagothenia borchgrevinki*) is characterized by lower values of $\Delta H^{\ddagger}$ and larger negative values of $\Delta S^{\ddagger}$ relative to the ortholog of a mammal. These observations are fully consistent with the hypothesis that cold-adapted proteins are more flexible than warm-adapted orthologs and exist in a higher state of config-

Table 7.1. Activation Energy Parameters: a Comparison of a Cold-Adapted Fish and a Mammal[1]

	$\Delta G^{\ddagger}$ (cal mol^{-1})	$\Delta H^{\ddagger}$ (cal mol^{-1})	$\Delta S^{\ddagger}$ cal mol^{-1}°C^{-1}	k_{cat} (relative)
Pagothenia (-2°C)	14,000	10,470	-12.7	1.00
Rabbit	14,340	12,550	-6.4	0.54

[1]Calculations for 5°C; see Somero and Siebenaller, 1979. $\Delta G^{\ddagger} = \Delta H^{\ddagger} - T\Delta S^{\ddagger}$.

uration entropy. Differences in $\Delta G^{\ddagger}$ among orthologs are relatively small, of the order of a few hundred calories per mole, relative to the differences that would be predicted by the differences in either $\Delta H^{\ddagger}$ or $\Delta S^{\ddagger}$ alone. Although seemingly small, these interspecific differences in $\Delta G^{\ddagger}$ are adequate to yield temperature-compensatory adaptations in k_{cat} because of the exponential relationship between k_{cat} and $\Delta G^{\ddagger}$.

Thresholds for adaptation: How much change in temperature is needed to favor adaptive change?

This question addresses an important issue in the context of physiological determinants of biogeographic patterning, for it concerns the relationship between thermal optima for proteins and the abilities of organisms to exploit habitats with different ranges of temperature. It is also a relevant question in the context of global climate change. Thus, will the increases in global temperature of a few degrees Celsius that are predicted to occur over the next several decades be adequate to significantly perturb proteins (and other biochemical and physiological systems) and thus have significant effects on organisms and their distribution patterns? There is already evidence that temperature-linked shifts in organismal distribution patterns have accompanied climate change (see Hughes, 2000). However, there remains uncertainty about the mechanistic causes of these trends, for instance, the role of thermal perturbation of proteins.

To address questions about thresholds of thermal perturbation and adaptation, a critical first step is to select appropriate species (or populations of conspecifics) for comparison. One obvious requirement is that the species to be compared are ones that have evolved in thermal conditions (e.g., habitat thermal maxima) that differ only slightly, perhaps by one to a few degrees Celsius. If mechanistic analysis of adaptations is to be attempted, good experimental design dictates optimizing signal-to-noise ratios: one must design experiments in which amino acid substitutions playing a temperature-adaptive role can be discerned from sequence variation not related to temperature. This requirement logically demands that one examine proteins from species that are at once adapted to different temperatures, yet not so evolutionarily diverged that the background noise in protein sequence is too high to permit determination of the temperature-adaptive differences in sequence. Confamilial and congeneric species may provide especially suitable study systems for examining these sorts of fine-scale temperature adaptations. Congeners in particular often occur in habitats that differ relatively slightly in temperature as a consequence of latitude, depth in the water, or elevation on land. And, because of relatively short divergence times, only minimal amounts of difference in amino acid sequence may exist among orthologous proteins of congeners.

Studies of A_4-LDH orthologs of confamilial and congeneric fishes have shown that differences in maximal habitat temperature of only a few degrees Celsius are sufficient to favor adaptive change. Moreover, temperature-adaptive change in function or stability may require only a single amino acid substitution. The A_4-LDH orthologs of barracuda fishes (genus *Sphyraena*) exhibit the type of variation in kinetic properties that has been noted in comparisons of widely different vertebrates (figure 7.8). Values of k_{cat} and K_m^{PYR} differ among barracuda congeners according to the patterns observed in comparisons of polar, temperate, and desert species (figure 7.7). In view of the fact that the barracuda congeners differ in midrange and maximal habitat temperatures by approximately 3–8°C, it is reasonable to conclude that these differences in temperature are enough to favor selectively important changes in A_4-LDHs. Whether even smaller differences in maximal habitat temperature could lead to adaptive variation in A_4-LDHs remains to be determined. Also, because different proteins may have different sensitivities to thermal perturbation, threshold effects may differ from protein to protein.

The amounts of change in sequence that underlie the different kinetic properties of A_4-LDH orthologs of barracuda congeners are small (Holland et al., 1997). Only a single difference in sequence (at position 8) distinguishes

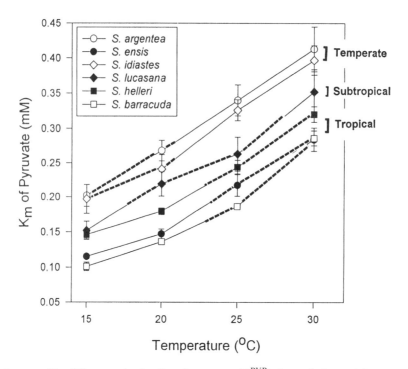

Figure 7.8. Interspecific differences in the K_m of pyruvate (K_m^{PYR}) for orthologs of A_4-LDH of congeneric barracuda fishes (genus *Sphyraena*) adapted to temperate (*S. argentea* and *S. idiastes*), subtropical (*S. luca-sana*) and tropical (*S. ensis, S. barracuda,* and *S. helleri*) waters. Habitat (body) temperature ranges of each species are indicated by dashed line segments. (Figure modified after Holland et al., 1997.)

the orthologs of the south temperate species *Sphyraena idiastes* and the subtropical species *Sphyraena lucasana.* The other ortholog sequenced, that of the north temperate species *S. argentea,* differed from the orthologs of *S. idiastes* and *S. lucasana* by four substitutions. The mechanism by which the substitution at position 8 exerts its effects on kinetic properties is suggested by the previous discussion of catalytic conformational changes and by the role played by the N-terminal region of the subunit. The N-terminal region (the "tail" shown in the lower panel of figure 7.5) interacts with an adjoining subunit's α1G-α2G region (part of the "lower jaw" shown in figure 7.5). As discussed earlier, the α1G-α2G helix undergoes a substantial shift in position during formation of the ternary complex, and this conformational change may be rate-limiting for catalysis. If the interaction of the N-terminal region of one subunit with the α1G-α2G region of the adjoining subunit is weakened, then the rate of cata-

lysis may increase. In the case of the orthologs of *S. idiastes* and *S. lucasana,* the occurrence at position 8 of an aspartyl residue in the former species in place of the asparagine found in *S. lucasana* could favor a weakening of this interaction because position 8 is brought into close contact with an aspartyl-containing region on the adjoining subunit. The charge repulsion that results from the aspartyl–aspartyl interaction would be expected to weaken the interaction between the N-terminal region of one subunit and the α1G-α2G helix of the adjoining subunit. This weakened interaction could make the movement of the α1G-α2G helix less energetically costly, leading to a low k_{cat} value.

Fishes of the teleost suborder Notothenioidei provide another example of how relatively small differences in temperature may favor evolutionary changes in kinetic properties. A_4-LDH orthologs of Antarctic members of this suborder also illustrate how different amino acid sequences can produce similar kinetic properties

(Fields and Somero, 1998). Notothenioid fishes are the dominant members of the fish fauna of the Antarctic Ocean (see Eastman, 1993, for a masterful account of the biology of these fascinating organisms). The suborder comprises several families that have radiated to fill a wide spectrum of niches. Studies of A_4-LDH orthologs of these species have, as discussed above, revealed aspects of the structural changes that underlie adaptation of proteins to low temperatures. These studies also have shown that A_4-LDH orthologs of South American confamilials of the family Nototheniidae, whose body temperatures differ from those of Antarctic notothenioids by only a few degrees, have kinetic properties that are distinctly more warm-adapted (figures 7.3 and 7.7). As in the case of the A_4-LDH orthologs of barracuda, only a small number of amino acid substitutions underlie these functional differences (Fields and Somero, 1998). Moreover, identical kinetic properties can arise from different sequences. There is "more than one way to skin the cat" when it comes to selection of sequence changes that adapt a protein to a new temperature. Lastly, the notothenioid A_4-LDHs have taught another lesson: although all A_4-LDHs of Antarctic notothenioids are very similar in K_m and k_{cat} values, they differ substantially in global stability, as indexed by temperatures of heat denaturation (Fields and Somero, 1998). Thus, as discussed in the next section of this chapter, the linkage between protein stability and function is complex, and the differences in structural stability that lead to adaptation of kinetic properties may not necessarily be linked to differences in overall—that is, global—stability of the protein. Likewise, differences in the amino acid sequence that favor shifts in global stability need not always change kinetic properties (Fields and Somero, 1997).

Conspecifics have also proven useful in discerning the difference in temperature needed to foster adaptive change and the amounts of sequence change needed to generate this adaptation. Powers et al. (1993) have shown that in the killifish *Fundulus heteroclitus* only one or two amino acid substitutions are sufficient to explain the differences in kinetics and thermal stability of LDH-B variants in northern and southern populations of the species. In one comparison of LDH-B variants, the only difference in structure was a hydroxyl (–OH) moiety due to the substitution of a serine residue for an alanine. The absence of the –OH group eliminated a polar interaction between subunits, resulting in decreased thermal stability.

To summarize, studies of differently thermally adapted confamilial, congeneric, and conspecific organisms have shown that temperature differences of a few degrees Celsius have sufficient effects on proteins to favor adaptive change. Although studies to date have focused on only a few classes of proteins, the ubiquitous effects of temperature on protein conformation are such that many, and perhaps most, proteins are likely to exhibit a similar "threshold" for perturbation and adaptive change.

Protein stability: proteins are only marginally stable at physiological temperatures

The intimate linkage between conformational flexibility and protein function carries an important implication for the evolution of protein stability: to function quickly and with accuracy, proteins cannot become too rigid, at least in those regions of the molecule that are involved in recognizing ligands and that undergo changes in conformation during the catalytic cycle. Selection thus prevents proteins from acquiring the highest degree of structural stability that would be possible in principle (e.g., for T_4 lysozyme, see Shoichet et al., 1995). A demonstration of the brakes that evolution applies to acquisition of stronger protein structures is given by numerous studies in which site-directed mutagenesis has been used successfully to "toughen-up" a protein's structure. In nature, such "engineering" is disfavored because of the likely negative impacts on function that would result from undue stiffening of the enzyme's structure.

Because of the requirements for conformational changes during function, proteins are only *marginally stable* (Jaenicke, 1991, 2000). This conclusion would seem to follow logically from the discussion of structure–function relationships given earlier. However, when one does a bonding energy budget analysis of proteins, it is nonetheless quite remarkable how fine a balance exists between stabilizing and destabilizing forces. If the effects of destabilizing forces such as configurational entropy (see below) are subtracted from the stabilizing forces due to hundreds of noncovalent bonds, a *net* stabilization free energy results that is equivalent to only a few stabilizing weak bonds. The folding of proteins is a delicate balancing act in which stabilizing and destabilizing forces are almost, yet not quite, equivalent.

Several forces contribute to the balance between stabilization and destabilization. Stabilizing forces include *the hydrophobic effect*, the tendency for nonpolar side-chains such as those of valine, leucine, isoleucine, and tryptophan to be buried within the protein, largely out of contact with water. *Ionic interactions, hydrogen bonds*, and *van der Waals interactions* also help to stabilize the native structures of proteins. Destabilizing forces arise from several factors. Primary among these factors is the decrease in *configurational entropy* that accompanies the folding of the disorganized polypeptide chain into a compact, highly ordered and functional protein. The Second Law of Thermodynamics, which states that all closed systems tend towards maximal entropy, presents an obvious challenge to protein folding. This challenge is met, that is to say, the Second Law is upheld despite the formation of an ordered and compact folded protein structure, by the large increase in entropy (ΔS) that accompanies the burial of hydrophobic groups within the interior of a protein. Why should this event, which is key to the generation of the highly ordered protein structure, occur with an increase rather than a decrease in entropy? The answer requires the introduction of a second critical component of the protein folding process, water.

When hydrophobic side-chains of amino acids are in contact with water, they can only be accommodated in the aqueous phase if water structure is altered. Water near nonpolar groups forms what are sometimes referred to as "cages" or "clathrates" around these groups. Water molecules in these "cages" possess a relatively high amount of structure compared to the bulk water of the solution. It should be clear, then, why an increase in the entropy of the *sys-*

tem—the protein plus the surrounding aqueous phase—occurs during burial of hydrophobic groups. As the nonpolar groups are transferred to the interior of the protein, they shed their organized cages of water, and the resulting increase in entropy of the aqueous phase more than counterbalances the reduction in configurational entropy that occurs during formation of the native folding state of the protein itself. The enthalpy change (ΔH) that accompanies burial of nonpolar residues or sidechains is unfavorable because thermal energy is needed to "melt" the cages of water around hydrophobic groups. This positive enthalpy change has an important consequence: the hydrophobic effect contributes more to protein stabilization at high than at low temperatures. In contrast, ionic interactions and hydrogen bonds exhibit increased stability as temperature is reduced. Thus, the effects of changes in temperature on protein structure are complex because of the opposite responses of different classes of stabilizing forces to changes in temperature. One consequence of the different thermal responses of hydrophobic interactions and other classes of bonds is that proteins typically exhibit a temperature of maximal stability (defined as the temperature at which the negative free energy change, ΔG, of folding is maximal) that is above $0°C$. It follows, then, that proteins exhibit cold denaturation as well as heat denaturation.

Global protein stability (usually) correlates with evolutionary adaptation temperature

Because of the strong and differential effects of temperature on all classes of noncovalent bonds, and because the net free energies of stabilization of globular proteins are so low, it is expected that protein structural stability will be subject to stringent modulation during evolutionary adaptation. We will see that this prediction is upheld for global stability, as it has been for the balance between flexibility and stability that exists for the regions of the protein that undergo large changes in conformation during function. However, these two aspects of protein stability need not be inextricably linked.

We first consider global stability, as commonly measured by temperatures of heat denaturation. Strong correlations between protein stability and adaptation temperature have been observed for several sets of orthologs (e.g., collagen: Bailey, 1968; malate dehydrogenase: Dahlhoff and Somero, 1993a; pyruvate kinase: Low and Somero, 1976; for review, see Somero, 1997). This relationship is illustrated for eye lens crystallins of a wide range of vertebrates (figure 7.9). In this study, the physical method of circular dichroism (CD) spectroscopy was used to follow loss of secondary structure (McFall-Ngai and Horwitz, 1990). Circular dichroism spectroscopy monitors unfolding of helical and beta sheet structures, and thus provides a highly accurate image of structural unfolding. Eye crystallins comprise a variety of types of proteins, including several enzymatic proteins (LDH is a crystallin in some species), which are recruited in the visual system

for a very different type of function from the metabolic roles they normally serve. The strong correlation between resistance to unfolding of secondary structure and evolutionary adaptation temperature shows how tightly protein stability is modulated during evolution. Note that differences in temperatures of unfolding should not be taken to imply that different total amounts of secondary structure are present in different orthologs. In fact, orthologs from differently adapted species may have the same amounts of secondary structure even though they differ in global stability. It is the interactions within the tertiary and quaternary structures that may govern global stability.

A caveat relating to methodology needs to be introduced at this point. A method commonly used for examining thermal stability of enzymatic proteins entails monitoring the loss of catalytic activity as a function of time of incubation at a denaturing temperature. Although in most cases a positive correlation between resistance to denaturation and adaptation temperature has been observed, in some instances this relationship has not been found. There are some cases in which heat denaturation occurred more rapidly for orthologs from warm-adapted species (Fields and Somero, 1998; Holland et al., 1997) and warm-adapted populations of a single species (Place and Powers, 1984) than for cold-adapted orthologs. However, the apparent "failures" of these proteins to adapt their stabilities to temperature may be artifactual. Slight and reversible unfolding of enzymes may lead to aggregation and precipitation of enzymes that otherwise would be able to refold into active conformations. Because of this aggregation artifact, losses of catalytic activity during incubation at high temperatures may not provide an accurate estimate of net free energies of stabilization. For this reason, physical methods like CD spectroscopy and calorimetry are to be preferred when the global structural stabilities of sets of orthologs are assessed.

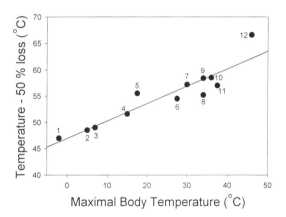

Figure 7.9. Thermal stabilities of eye lens crystallins of differently thermally adapted vertebrates. The temperature (°C) at which 50% loss of secondary structure occurred, as measured using CD spectroscopy, is given as a function of the maximal body temperature of each species. Species: (1) *Pagothenia borchgrevinki* (Antarctic fish), (2) *Coryphaenoides armatus* (deep-sea fish), (3) *Coryphaen-oides rupestris* (deep-sea fish), (4) *Oncorhynchus mykiss* (rainbow trout), (5) *Cebidichthys violaceus* (tidepool fish), (6) *Rana muscosa* (frog), (7) *Alticus kirkii* (Red Sea fish), (8) *Rana erythraea* (frog), (9) *Gekko gecko* (lizard), (10) *Rattus norvegicus* (rat), (11) *Tropidurus hispidus* (reptile), and (12) *Dipsosaurus dorsalis* (desert iguana). (Figure modified after McFall-Ngai and Horwitz, 1990.)

Kinetic adaptations need not be reflected by differences in global stability

During the past several years, there has been intense interest in studying the determinants of protein thermal stability. One of the outcomes of this work has been the development of a more refined view of the linkages between kinetic properties and protein stability. In particular, it has become apparent that adjustments in the conformational mobility of regions of enzymes that are key to catalytic activity, for instance the catalytic loops of enzymes like LDH, can be achieved by amino acid substitutions that do not alter global protein stability (Hernández et al., 2000; Jaenicke, 2000). Furthermore, site-directed mutagenesis methods have been used successfully to alter global protein stability without changing catalytic activity, although the success rates of these studies have often not been high (Giver et al., 1998; Jaenicke, 2000; Shoichet et al., 1995).

What these studies suggest in the context of adaptation of proteins to temperature is that global stability and kinetic properties governed by localized flexibility of the "working parts" of an enzyme may evolve independently. Whereas selection may favor higher global stability and reduced flexibility of the "working parts" of a protein during evolution at elevated temperatures, the two processes may or may not be linked to a common set of amino acid substitutions. For example, increased global stability may be established by stronger subunit–subunit interactions, whereas decreases in configurational entropy of the key "working parts" of an enzyme may be due to substitutions that affect mobility of catalytic loops and other elements in the protein whose configurations are essential for binding ligands and initiating the catalytic cycle.

Because of this decoupling of global stability, on the one hand, and localized balance between flexibility and stability of the "working parts" of a protein, on the other, the evolution of global stability may exhibit substantially more variation among similarly adapted orthologs than is seen in kinetic properties (K_m and k_{cat}). For kinetic properties the strong conservation that is seen among orthologs adapted to a common range of temperatures is hypothesized to be due to a common level of conformational mobility in the regions of the enzyme that are responsible for establishing the energy changes of binding and catalysis. That orthologs with similar

kinetic properties can have widely different global stabilities suggests that some threshold level for global stability is important, but increases in stability above this threshold may not matter— they may have no selective importance—as long as they do not influence the flexibilities of the regions of the protein that govern K_m and k_{cat}.

An illustration of a lack of correlation between habitat temperature and protein stability is given by LDHs of porcelain crabs (genus *Petrolisthes*) (Stillman and Somero, 2001). Among the 22 congeners studied, there was no significant overall correlation between habitat temperature and thermal stability (indexed by loss of catalytic activity or denaturation of secondary structure, as monitored with CD spectroscopy). However, for most of the LDH orthologs studied, their global stability was extremely high. The temperatures required for a 50% loss of enzymatic activity during a 10 min incubation period ranged between 65° and 76°C, denaturation temperatures much higher than those seen for any vertebrate LDHs. One interpretation of these findings is that the ancestral LDH of these crabs may have acquired a very high global stability, and that as the porcelain crabs diverged and colonized different habitats, there was no negative consequence of this high stability on LDH function. Thus, in contemporary porcelain crabs found in widely different habitats in which maximal temperatures range from approximately 15°C to 42°C, LDH global stability is similar and adequate to allow avoidance of denaturation in even the most heat-adapted congeners.

Structural bases of adaptive change in thermal stability of proteins

Above, we showed how a finely modulated balancing act between stabilizing and destabilizing forces yields marginally stable protein structures. We now examine in more detail how the same types of noncovalent interactions are used in differently thermally adapted proteins to achieve appropriate levels of structural stability. The adaptive changes discussed below are relevant to both global protein stability and to the establishment of the appropriate balance between stability and flexibility required for the "working parts" of the protein structure, the elements that undergo large changes in conformation during activity.

As is frequently the case in analyses of mechanisms of adaptation, looking at an extreme case of adaptation can be particularly helpful in discerning general rules. Recent studies of enzymes of thermophilic organisms, especially hyperthermophilic members of the domain Archaea, have provided especially clear illustrations of how shifts in amino acid composition finely tune protein stability. Proteins of these extremophiles exhibit the highest thermal stabilities known—they may retain their native conformations and activities at temperatures of 100°C and slightly higher—and it was no doubt hoped by the biochemists who set out to study these unusual molecules that some new "trick" had been discovered during evolution of these extremeophiles to achieve such extraordinary stabilities. Studies since the 1980s have shown, however, that there is no special mechanism that underlies the unusual thermal stabilities of proteins of hyperthermophilic organisms. Rather, studies of their sequences and three-dimensional structures have shown that the folding rules already well understood for "normal" proteins can explain the increased stabilities of these molecules.

The following conclusions have been reached about the mechanisms that underlie the enhanced resistance to heat denaturation of thermophilic enzymes. One key finding is that there is no evidence that disulfide bridges (cysteine–cysteine linkages; S−S bonds) are exploited by these proteins to increase thermal stability. This finding may appear surprising at first glance. A priori, it might seem that disulfide bridges, by introducing a covalent bond into the folded protein structure, would be an ideal mechanism for enhancing thermal stability. However, disulfide bridges occur only infrequently in proteins found in intracellular compartments, whether or not the organism is adapted to high or low temperatures. It may be that the rigidity introduced by disulfide bridges reduces a protein's ability to undergo the changes in conformation required for rapid enzymatic function. Genetically engineered proteins into which a disulfide bond has been introduced may undergo distortions in conformation in order to accommodate the S−S bond, and these changes in an enzyme's geometry may impede catalytic activity. Disulfide bonds are found in some extracellular proteins. These typically are small, monomeric enzymes that function in extracellular microenvironments that are less conducive to structural stability than the intracellular fluids. In these microenvironments, these small proteins may require the unusual stabilities conferred by S−S linkages.

Enhancement of structural stability in proteins of thermophiles, then, is achieved primarily by altering the types and numbers of noncovalent interactions that stabilize the molecules and by modifying the changes in configurational entropy that accompany folding and unfolding. Surveys of a number of orthologous proteins in thermophiles and mesophiles have led to some general conclusions about the types of amino acid substitutions that are most prevalent in enhancing thermal stability (Haney et al., 1999). The particular route taken to enhance stability varies from protein to protein, however. The following types of substitutions seem most important.

1. *Increases in charged residues.* The addition of one or more ionic interactions, for instance, between residues of arginine and glutamate, is a common mechanism for enhancing protein thermal stability. Ionic interactions form with a significant negative ΔG; they are the strongest type of noncovalent bond between amino acid side-chains that can occur in a protein. (Interactions between charged amino acids and inorganic ions such as Ca^{2+} can also strongly enhance stability.) A comparison of the protein-coding regions of the genomes of thermophilic and mesophilic archaea of the genus *Methanococcus* (Haney et al., 1999) revealed an 8% increase in fully charged residues (arginine, lysine, glutamate and aspartate; note: as discussed later in the context of temperature–pH relationships, histidine is a partially charged amino acid). The primary type of change leading to increase in charge involved substitution of a charged residue for a polar but uncharged residue. Substituting charged amino

acids with relatively large side-chains could not only facilitate ionic interactions and hydrogen bonding, but could also lead to strengthened hydrophobic interactions, for instance, in the case of lysine. Arginine residues, too, are increased in thermophilic proteins; in fact, shifts from lysine to arginine were observed in the comparison of congeners of *Methanococcus*. Arginine can form multiple ionic interactions due to its resonance structures, thereby facilitating interconnected salt bridges in the thermophilic protein.

2. *Losses of uncharged-polar amino acids*. One of the strongest trends noted in the comparisons of thermophilic and mesophilic archaea was a reduction in the contributions of uncharged-polar amino acids (serine, threonine, asparagine, and glutamine). Although some of the uncharged-polar amino acids were replaced by charged amino acids, in most cases, uncharged-polar amino acids were replaced by hydrophobic amino acids. Thus, the net contribution of hydrogen bonding to protein stability was reduced, and the role of hydrophobic interactions was increased. These shifts in relative importance of different classes of stabilizing forces follow from the thermodynamic analysis presented earlier. Thus, whereas hydrogen bonding is weakened at elevated temperatures, hydrophobic interactions are stabilized, at least up to temperatures at which significant water structure remains.

3. *Increases in bulky hydrophobic side-chains*. Not only is there a trend towards a higher percentage of hydrophobic amino acids in proteins of thermophiles, in addition there is a shift to larger, bulkier hydrophobic side-chains. For instance, Haney et al. (1999) observed shifts from glycine to alanine, leucine to isoleucine, and methionine to leucine. Increased percentages of bulky hydrophobic side-chains and the replacement of uncharged-polar side-chains both have been found to lead to an increase in the percentage of the protein's volume occupied by amino acid residues. The comparisons of proteins of congeners of *Methanococcus* showed that, in a typical thermophilic protein, the equivalent of 20 additional methylene ($-CH_2-$) groups was present. Tighter packing of residues within the protein's interior would facilitate van

der Waals interactions and, thus, thermal stability.

4. *Adjustments in configurational entropy*. Bulkier side-chains also affect configurational entropy by reducing the degrees of freedom of movement of side-chains in the unfolded state. Adjustment of the configurational entropy of the unfolded state of a protein is an important component of adaptation to temperature. Consider the effects of a common stabilizing substitution, replacement of a glycine residue by an alanine residue. This substitution only involves the replacement of a hydrogen atom ($-H$) by a $-CH_3$ group, leading to an increase in mass of merely 14 daltons. However, even in a protein with a mass of many thousand daltons, a single substitution of this type can lead to a large change in thermal stability (Matthews et al., 1987). There in fact may be two explanations for this enhancement of stability. One mechanism involves entropy changes during folding or unfolding. Substitution of a $-CH_3$ for a $-H$ reduces the number of configurations accessible to the unfolded protein. Glycine residues permit relatively free rotation around a peptide bond. Thus, they present much lower steric hindrance to conformational changes and allow a protein to attain a larger number of conformational states than any other amino acid residue. The potential increase in entropy during unfolding is thus greatest when a glycine residue is present at a site. It follows from this fact that replacing a glycine with another residue that reduces the number of configurations possible in the unfolded state will lower the entropy change during unfolding and favor stabilization of the folded state. In addition, replacement of a glycine by an alanine residue will increase the hydrophobic effect due to the addition of the nonpolar $-CH_3$ group.

5. *Reduced potential for damage to covalent bonds*. The discussion to this point has largely emphasized the roles played by noncovalent interactions in stabilizing proteins. For extreme thermophiles like the hyperthermophilic members of the Archaea, damage to covalent bonds is also a threat. Deamidation and peptide backbone cleavage at sites where asparagine and glutamine residues are present can occur at the

high temperatures encountered by hyperthermophiles. These deamidation reactions can be catalyzed by threonine and serine. Thus, the reductions in asparagine, glutamine, threonine and serine (i.e., in uncharged-polar residues) found in hyperthermophiles can be regarded as a mechanism for avoiding thermal damage to covalent bonds.

What has emerged from the analysis of proteins of thermophilic organisms is the realization that no new rules have been needed to allow protein-based processes to occur at temperatures up to 113°C, the highest temperature that hyperthermophilic archaea are known to withstand. Likewise, studies of proteins of cold-adapted, psychrophilic species, both prokaryotic and eukaryotic, have demonstrated that shifts among a common set of stabilizing forces can provide cold-adapted proteins with the structural characteristics they require for function at low thermal energy (Feller and Gerday, 1997). The increased structural flexibility that is conjectured to be important for cold-adapted proteins appears to be generated by evolutionary changes that, in many ways, are the mirror-image of those outlined above for thermophiles. Reduced hydrophobicity, increased surface polarity and clustering of glycine residues near functional domains are apparent in many cold-adapted proteins. In addition, reductions in proline content, especially in loops and turns linked to mobile elements of secondary structure, are common (Feller and Gerday, 1997; Fields and Somero, 1998). Another change noted in some proteins of cold-adapted species is the addition or lengthening of disorganized surface loop regions that enhance protein–solvent interactions and reduce the compactness of the protein's structure.

In summary, a common set of thermodynamic rules governing protein folding applies across the full spectrum of temperatures permissive of life, and it is the fine-tuning of protein sequences using these rules that allows cells as different as those of Antarctic ectotherms and hot-spring archaea to conduct many of the same types of enzymatic processes at temperatures that differ by up to 115°C.

Protein stability in vitro may misrepresent stability in vivo

Data on thermal stability of proteins derive almost exclusively from work done in vitro with highly dilute proteins bathed in an aqueous milieu that differed in major ways from the normal intracellular medium of the protein under study. As emphasized later in this chapter and in discussions of protein–water–solute interactions in chapter 6, numerous aspects of the solution in which a protein is dissolved may strongly influence its stability. Substrates and cofactors, which typically enhance protein stability when present in the medium, are usually not present in media used to study protein thermal stability. Salt composition and concentration and pH values typically are non-physiological. Phenomena such as molecular crowding and stabilization by nonbinding organic osmolytes contribute importantly to protein stability in the cell (chapter 6), and these effects, too, are usually ignored in studies of heat denaturation. Thus, one must use caution in evaluating data on protein stability obtained in vitro under nonphysiological conditions. Although such data are likely to be valid for providing an index of the *relative* stabilities of orthologs of a protein from differently adapted species, these data may not reflect the protein's *absolute* stability under in vivo conditions. Putting this another way, simplified in vitro studies may allow determination of the relative *intrinsic stabilities* of orthologs of a protein, while failing to account for the influences on stability of *extrinsic stabilizers* that may be important in vivo.

Extrinsic stabilization from low-molecular-mass "thermoprotectants." The intrinsic stability of a protein reflects selection for an amino acid sequence that confers on the protein the appropriate balance between rigidity and flexibility that is required for physiological function under the thermal conditions facing the organism. This being said, the stability of the protein in vivo may be modulated by extrinsic factors, including pH, which varies with temperature, and low-molecular-mass organic osmolytes, whose concentrations may be temperature-dependent. Certain "thermoprotec-tant" osmolytes appear to be especially impor-tant for hyperthermophilic members of the Archaea, cells that can be cultured at tempera-tures as high as 113°C. Less heat-tolerant spe-cies, including some eukaryotes, may also accumulate one or more organic osmolytes for thermoprotectant function (see below). However, it is the hyperthermophilic members of the Archaea that provide some of the most interesting examples of use of thermoprotec-tants to enhance protein stability (Martin et al., 1999).

One illustration of the use of thermoprotec-tants is given by a study of a thermophilic archaeon, *Methanothermus fervidus*, that toler-ates temperatures as high as 85°C, but whose proteins do not exhibit a high level of intrinsic thermal stability (Hensel and Konig, 1988). Stabilization of proteins within the cell appears to be mediated by the accumulation of high concentrations of an organic solute, cyclic-2,3-diphosphoglycerate (cDPG), which is the major anion of the cell. Cyclic-2,3-diphosphoglycerate greatly increased the resistance of the archae-on's proteins (glyceraldehyde-3-phosphate dehydrogenase and malate dehydrogenase) to heat denaturation in vitro, conferring upon the two enzymes a level of stability that seemed sufficient to protect the proteins under in-situ conditions of high temperature. Curiously, cDPG did not exert similar stabilizing effects on a homolog of glyceraldehyde-3-phosphate dehydrogenase from a mammal. This finding suggests that the proteins of the archaeon may be specially adapted to benefit from the effects of cDPG. This discrepancy in solute effects between isoforms of a protein is an unusual observation because the effects of stabilizing and destabilizing solutes on proteins are usually independent of the isoform of protein being examined (chapter 6).

Other organic solutes found in thermophilic archaea likely play roles as thermoprotectants, although there have been few in vitro studies in which the effects of these solutes on protein stability have been tested. Among the putative thermoprotectants in hyperthermo-philic archaea is di-*myo*-inositol-1,1′-phosphate (DIP) (see figure 6.2 for the structure of this compound). This is synthesized only at high culture temperatures, presumably temperatures at which intrinsic protein stability becomes marginal and extrinsic stabilizers (thermo-protectants) become necessary for survival of the cells. Thus, in the hyperthermophile *Methanococcus igneus*, DIP does not begin to accumulate until growth temperature exceeds 80°C (Ciulla et al., 1994). Regulation of synth-esis of DIP at high temperatures may be a direct consequence of Q_{10} effects on a key enzyme in the synthetic pathway. Although the first two reactions in the pathway of DIP synthesis have rather typical activation energies, approxi-mately 15 and 12 kcal mol^{-1}, the final enzyme in the pathway, DIP synthase, has an extremely high activation energy, approximately 30 kcal mol^{-1}. As growth temperature is increased, DIP synthase activity rises very rapidly, and any inositol-1-phosphate (I-1-P) produced by the first enzyme in the pathway, inositol-1-phos-phate synthase, would be drawn towards DIP synthesis and away from alternate routes, for instance, hydrolysis of I-1-P to *myo*-inositol for incorporation into lipids.

Low-molecular-mass extrinsic stabilizers appear capable of broadening the thermal range over which cells can operate, at least in the case of the hyperthermophilic members of the Archaea. Eurythermality by these organ-isms thus may be based in large measure on mechanisms that allow the concentrations of thermoprotectants to be modulated in accord with the requirements of proteins for extrinsic stabilization. The fact that thermoprotectants may only be synthesized under conditions of extreme heat stress may be an indication that, at lower temperatures at which the intrinsic sta-bilities of proteins are adequate, the additional stability conferred by high concentrations of extrinsic stabilizers is maladaptive for protein function. In addition, the energy costs of synthesizing thermoprotectants may warrant their synthesis only under severest conditions when they are needed to preserve protein integ-rity.

Total protein concentration may affect protein stability.   Although low-molecular-mass solutes may play important roles in enhancing stabilities of proteins in certain organisms, protein concentration per se may be the most general enhancer of stability under in-vivo conditions, as a consequence of "molecular crowding" effects (chapter 6). Comparisons of thermal stabilities determined in vitro using low concentrations of protein may provide a misleading picture of stability in vivo, especially when the protein in question normally occurs in a cellular compartment with an especially high concentration of protein, for instance, the matrix of the mitochondrion. Proteins compartmentalized in protein-rich microenvironments like the mitochondrial matrix may require *low* intrinsic stabilities in order to avoid becoming too rigid for effective function when present in their normal intracellular milieu. The mitochondrial paralog of malate dehydrogenase (mMDH) is an extremely labile protein when studied in vitro in solutions with low protein concentration. However, when the concentration of protein (bovine serum albumin) was elevated toward the levels expected in the mitochondrial matrix, the stability of mMDH rose to a value similar to that characteristic of the cytosolic paralog, cMDH, which has a higher intrinsic stability (Lin et al., 2001). In keeping with the relationship between enzyme stability and rate of function that has been documented in this volume, the maximal velocity of the reaction catalyzed by mMDH decreased as enzyme stability rose.

The joint evolution of proteins and the solution in which they occur is an issue within evolution that we treat at numerous junctures in this volume. The types of effects noted for enzymes of *M. fervidus* and paralogs of MDH show that joint evolution of proteins and solutes may be of broad importance in adaptation to temperature. Data such as these also have a practical lesson for us: they show that the complexity of the intracellular milieu must be carefully evaluated when designing and interpreting experiments done in vitro. All partners in the evolutionary process must be considered if the nature of physiological adaptation is to be appreciated. This point brings us to one of the most striking differences exhibited by proteins under in-vitro versus in-vivo conditions: the extent to which the primary structure of the protein is able to direct its folding into the three-dimensional conformation needed for function.

Molecular Chaperones and the Heat-Shock Response

Help is needed to direct protein folding and compartmentation

The description of protein folding developed earlier in this chapter is a thermodynamic analysis in which only two components of the cell were considered: the protein that is undergoing folding and the water that bathes it as it folds. Two critical assumptions are implicit in this description of folding. First, all information needed to direct the folding of a protein is contained in the protein's amino acid sequence, its primary structure. Second, the energy changes that favor acquisition of the folded state involve only the interactions taking place (i) between residues within the protein and (ii) between the protein and water. In other words, thermodynamic forces are viewed as *necessary and sufficient* to translate the information given in the primary structure into a properly folded, functional protein.

Christian Anfinsen (1916–1995) performed landmark (and Nobel Prize-winning) studies that provided unequivocal support for this model of folding. Anfinsen denatured proteins by incubating them in high concentrations of denaturing solutes like urea. After restoring solution conditions that favored the native structure, he monitored the enzyme's progress in regaining catalytic activity (Anfinsen, 1973). His studies showed that an unfolded protein could find a productive refolding pathway that led to regeneration of an active enzyme, at least if given enough time to "try" a number of folding pathways. It is conjectured that the number of potential configurations that a protein can occupy during folding exceeds the number of stars in the Universe, so finding the right pathway is a nontrivial challenge to an unfolded (or a newly synthesized and not yet folded) protein. These important studies led to the paradigm that protein folding in the cell occurs spontaneously, without any need for assistance. Furthermore, these early in-vitro studies suggested that protein–protein and protein–water interactions were all that were required for driving the folding process.

It should be noted that Anfinsen cautioned readers that the simplified model that his in-vitro studies generated might not represent what actually occurs within the cell—a warning that proved to be correct. It now is clear that this simplified perspective on protein folding and maturation is incomplete in important ways. The thermodynamic arguments are correct, but the complexity of the cellular milieu creates a folding environment so different from that used in folding studies performed in vitro that assistance is required for proteins to fold properly and find their ways to the sites within the cell where they belong.

Molecular chaperones: assistants to protein maturation in the cell

One of the major discoveries in biochemistry and cell biology during the latter part of the past century is that a diverse suite of proteins known as *molecular chaperones* play essential roles in the folding and compartmentation of proteins in all types of cells (Ellis, 1996a,b; Ellis and van der Vies, 1991; Parsell and Lindquist, 1993). In essence, molecular chaperones allow the thermodynamic rules of protein folding that were discovered under in-vitro conditions to be followed in the complex, crowded environment of the cellular fluids. Molecular chaperones are encoded by a number of gene families, and they vary considerably in mass. The naming of chaperones of eukaryotic cells is commonly based on their mass as expressed in kilodaltons (kDa). Some bacterial chaperones have names derived from their functional roles, which were discovered prior to the identification of homology between the eukaryotic and bacterial orthologs. Furthermore, because the initial chaperones to be discovered were induced by high temperature and for this reason were called heat-shock proteins (hsp's), the acronym "hsp" is used somewhat generically to refer to both heat-inducible and constitutively synthesized chaperones. For instance, chaperones with masses near 70 kDa are referred to as members of the hsp70 class of chaperones. These chaperones are orthologous to bacterial chaperones of the DnaK class. Different types of chaperones occur in different species and within different cellular compartments. However, in spite of their diversity in size and site, chaperones perform a common and critical set of roles: they help to guide protein folding and compartmentation throughout the life of a cell, and, when the cell is subjected to stresses that denature proteins, chaperones play vital rescue missions that restore unfolded proteins to their native, functional states.

Synthesis of molecular chaperones may be constitutive or stress-induced. Several size classes of molecular chaperones are synthesized constitutively to facilitate the housekeeping functions associated with protein synthesis and maturation. All organisms contain constitutively expressed chaperones, and the ubiquitous occurrence of these proteins is strong reason to believe that they appeared very early in evolution. Orthologs of some classes of molecular chaperones are found in prokaryotes and all eukaryotes.

The synthesis of some constitutively expressed chaperones may be elevated during stress, and other isoforms of molecular chaperones are expressed only in response to stress. Elevated expression of chaperones in response to heat stress is called the *heat-shock response* (Feige et al., 1996; Lindquist, 1986; Parsell and Lindquist, 1993). However, because these heat-induced chaperones are used in the face of a variety of types of physical and chemical stress, for instance, exposure to alcohols, heavy metals, hypoxia, hyperoxia, and ultraviolet light, they sometimes are referred to as *stress proteins*, and their induction by diverse stresses can be termed the *stress response*. The common element in all of these types of stress is damage to protein structure. Like their close relatives the constitutively expressed chaperones, stress proteins facilitate recovery of native structure by helping to prevent aggregation of denatured proteins and by facilitating refolding along productive folding pathways (figure 7.10).

The history of study of molecular chaperones is rather fascinating and merits at least a brief review. The initial discovery that heat shock was able to modify gene expression was made

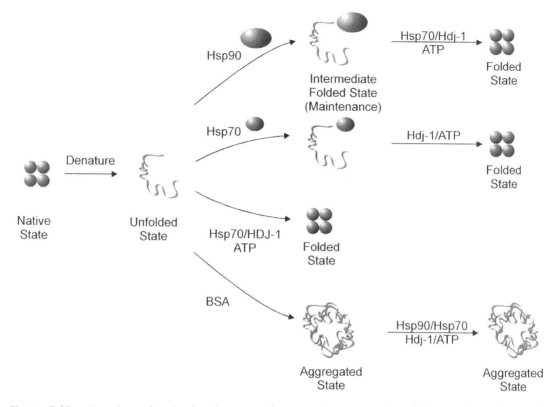

Figure 7.10. Functions of molecular chaperones in preventing aggregation of denatured proteins and in assisting refolding to the native state. A native protein is denatured into an unfolded state, whose subsequent fate is governed by the availability of molecular chaperones, co-chaperones (Hdj-1), and ATP. In the absence of adequate chaperoning activity, the unfolded protein may aggregate with other proteins (bovine serum albumin, BSA, is shown as playing this role in vitro) and form an insoluble mass that is refractory to chaperone-assisted renaturation (lowest pathway). If hsp70 + ATP + the co-chaperone Hdj-1 are all present, the unfolded protein may refold to the native folded state (next to bottom pathway). If either Hsp90 or Hsp70 alone is present, a complex between the unfolded protein and a chaperone may form and prevent further unfolding and aggregation (maintenance steps). For the hsp70-protein complex, provision of ATP + Hdj-1 allows refolding. For the hsp90-protein complex, refolding may depend on supply of hsp70 + ATP + Hdj-1. (Modified after Morimoto and Santoro, 1998.)

by Ritossa in 1962, in a study of the puffing of giant salivary chromosomes in *Drosophila*. It was another 12 years before Tissières et al. (1974) demonstrated that a specific group of proteins, which they termed heat-shock proteins, was encoded by the genes activated by heat shock. In the topsy-turvy world of explosive growth in molecular biology during this time, the sequences of the heat-shock genes and their promoters were completed before the nature of the proteins' functions were discovered (Ellis, 1996b; Lindquist, 1986). It was only in the mid-1980s that the phenomenon of chaperoning was elucidated. Since that time, more than 15,000 papers on molecular chaperones and the heat-shock response have appeared. However, despite the importance of the heat-shock response in coping with environmental stress, only a small fraction of these publications concern the function of the heat-shock response in adaptation (for review see Feder, 1999; Feder and Hofmann, 1999).

Before considering in detail the roles of heat-shock (stress) proteins in helping organisms cope with extremes of environmental temperature, it is important to examine more closely the basic activities of molecular chaperones in assisting the folding and compartmentation of proteins under normal cellular conditions (Hartl, 1996). This analysis will bring into clearer focus the nature of thermal stress on cells and the defensive functions that are required of stress-induced chaperones. The importance of molecular chaperones is shown by their occurrence in every type of protein-synthesizing cell, in every species. Whenever protein synthesis occurs, even under conditions in which no environmental stress is present, there exists a danger of improper folding and maturation. During protein synthesis, the nascent polypeptide chain extends from the polysome complex, into the surrounding aqueous medium. Until the nascent polypeptide is able to fold in upon itself, the possibility exists that it may interact with another nascent polypeptide or with an unfolded protein in its environment. The thermodynamic rules governing protein folding apply just as strictly to interprotein interactions as to intraprotein interactions, and to nonproductive interactions leading to nonfunctional proteins as to productive interactions leading to the native, functional state. Interprotein interactions between nascent polypeptides, which lead to clusters of aggregated, nonfunctional polypeptides, would be damaging and perhaps lethal for the cell. One role of protein chaperones, then, is to prevent inappropriate interactions between mutually attractive, geometrically complementary surfaces—hence the name "chaperone" is well chosen (Ellis and van der Vies, 1991).

Molecular chaperones prevent these interactions in at least two different ways. Some chaperones, for instance those belonging to the 70 kDa family (hsp70 and its relatives) bind to unfolded proteins at hydrophobic sites, thereby shielding these sites from interactions with other unfolded proteins and preventing inappropriate aggregation from occurring. Splitting of ATP bound to hsp70-type chaperones releases the bound polypeptide, at least transiently, which affords it an opportunity to fold. Binding and release may go on for many cycles, during each of which an ATP is split as the nascent polypeptide "tries" a new configuration of folding. The requirement for ATP

is an indication that, within the complex, protein-rich milieu of the cell, the thermodynamic rules governing protein folding under dilute in-vitro conditions can no longer support "cost-free" maturation of proteins, which is driven strictly by the favorable changes in free energy that accompany folding. Energy must be supplied by hydrolysis of ATP to ensure that folding occurs along what are termed *productive folding pathways*—those folding events that lead to the native state—and that inappropriate misfolding and aggregation are avoided. Protein maturation in vivo thus requires substantially more energy than folding under simplified in-vitro conditions. Operating the chaperone machinery significantly increases the cost of producing proteins. And, as we will see later, increased costs of chaperoning under conditions of heat stress may play an important role in thermal relationships of organisms.

Folding of nascent polypeptides in the cell may involve cooperativity among different classes of chaperones, for instance those of the hsp70 and hsp90 size classes, and one or more types of *co-chaperones* such as Hdj-1, a member of the hsp40 family (figure 7.10; see Ellis, 1996a; Morimoto and Santoro, 1998). Co-chaperones influence molecular chaperones' affinities for unfolded proteins and alter the ATPase activities of chaperones that require hydrolysis of ATP for their function. Under cellular conditions, hsp70, hsp90, and Hdj-1 may all be important for folding of a nascent polypeptide or renaturation of a heat-damaged protein. Binding of either hsp90 or hsp70 alone may hold the partially unfolded protein in an intermediate folded state, preventing aggregation or further unfolding. When Hdj-1 is included in the complex, ATP-dependent renaturation of the unfolded protein can occur. Note that, in this model of renaturation, once the protein forms an aggregated state (lowest pathway in figure 7.10), the "rescue team" of hsp70 + hsp90 + Hdj-1 + ATP is unable to restore the native conformation. Thus, it is essential that chaperones act rapidly to prevent the formation of aggregates.

Another mechanism of chaperone function involves entry of the unfolded protein into a "box" where folding can occur in relative isolation, away from other unfolded proteins. This type of chaperone activity is effected by chaperones such as hsp60 and grp. These are multimeric chaperones, involving up to 16 individual subunits in the complete chaperone complex. In essence, the unfolded protein enters into the box, the lid is closed, and the protein gets to "try out" different conformations until it "finds" the thermodynamically stable conformation of the native state. The absence of other proteins in its microenvironment eliminates the danger of inappropriate aggregation. In a very real sense, chaperones like hsp60 provide a folding environment similar to that created during in-vitro folding experiments of the sort devised by Anfinsen. As in the case of hsp70-type chaperones, however, splitting of ATP is required for the chaperoning activity of hsp 60 and grp.

Protein chaperones are also important in helping to guide proteins into the cellular compartment in which they belong, a process known as *compartmentation*. Binding of a chaperone to a newly synthesized protein may serve to keep the protein in a largely unfolded state. By remaining in a relatively linear as opposed to a globular configuration, the protein can be transported through a membrane, into the compartment (e.g., the mitochondrion) where the protein normally occurs. Once within its proper compartment, the protein is directed along a productive folding pathway through assistance by additional chaperones, which may be isoforms that are specific for the intracellular compartment in question (Pilon and Schekman, 1999).

In summary, the normal processes of molecular chaperoning during protein synthesis and compartmentation are key elements in ensuring that the fundamental thermodynamic relationships governing protein folding can be followed under the conditions that occur in vivo. Inappropriate interprotein interactions are avoided and the correct intraprotein interactions take place. Even though refolding of a denatured protein under dilute in-vitro conditions may not require ATP, protein folding within the cell exacts a high payment for ensuring that only productive folding occurs. Protein synthesis is one of the most ATP-costly processes occurring in cells, and the synthesis and use of molecular chaperones may represent a substantial—albeit as yet unquantified—fraction of this cost. During environmental thermal stress, the costs of ensuring that proteins acquire and retain their native states increase even further, as the heat-shock response is mounted and stress-induced chaperones are synthesized, often to the exclusion of synthesis of other classes of proteins.

The heat-shock response

The heat-shock response is (almost) ubiquitous. Induction of one or more classes of stress-induced molecular chaperones (hsp's) in response to heat stress has been observed in a great number of species belonging to all major phylogenetic lineages (for review see Feder and Hofmann, 1999). Much as constitutively expressed chaperones are necessary in all cells under normal conditions for assisting in the folding and compartmentation of proteins during protein synthesis and maturation, heat-induced chaperones appear to be a nearly ubiquitous aspect of organisms' responses to heat stress. In only a few cases have investigations of heat stress failed to detect a heat-shock response. One instance, the first to be reported, involved a cold-adapted, stenothermal cnidarian, *Hydra oligactis* (Bosch et al, 1988). Unlike more eurythermal congeners of *Hydra*, *H. oligactis* failed to induce any size class of heat-shock protein following sublethal heat stress. As would be predicted by the inability of *H. oligactis* to mount a heat-shock response, this species disappears from waters in which it encounters heat stress. The mechanisms underlying the general failure of *H. oligactis* to synthesize any type of heat-shock protein are not completely understood. However, in the case of hsp70, this failure appeared to be due to an unstable mRNA for this protein, not the absence of the *hsp70* gene (Gellner et al., 1992).

A second example of an apparent absence of the heat-shock response was found in studies of cold-adapted, stenothermal Antarctic notothenioid fishes that never encounter temperatures above $0°C$ and die of heat death above $4°C$

(Somero and DeVries, 1967; Hofmann et al., 2000). In these extreme stenotherms, it appears that the heat-shock response has been lost during several million years of evolution in a cold, thermally stable environment. With the formation of the Drake Passage approximately 25 million years ago, the Southern Ocean surrounding the Antarctic continent was cut off from large-scale exchange with northern water masses, and water temperatures began falling. Temperatures gradually reached their current values near the freezing point of seawater about 14 million years ago. Much as these thermal conditions have favored the evolution of adaptations to extreme cold, for instance, highly efficient enzymes (figure 7.3) and antifreeze proteins and glycoproteins, they have allowed certain physiological traits to be lost. For instance, the high solubility of oxygen in near-freezing seawater may have reduced the need for hemoglobins, thus allowing icefishes of the family Channichthyidae to lose both circulating hemoglobin (Cocca et al., 1995) and, in many species, skeletal muscle and heart myoglobin (Sidell et al., 1997). The loss of the heat-shock response in the nototheniid fish *Trematomus bernacchii* likely reflects the absence of positive selection for this trait. The failure of *T. bernacchii* to synthesize any class of heat-shock protein indicates that either all hsp-encoding genes have been rendered dysfunctional or that some higher order regulatory system involved in activating expression of the hsp-encoding genes has been altered. The ability to synthesize constitutively expressed chaperones has of course been retained in this species. In summary, unlike the constitutively expressed protein chaperones needed for protein synthesis and compartmentation, heat-induced chaperones appear not to be essential for life. However, when organisms lack the heat-shock response, their range of thermal tolerance may be highly attenuated, and should they encounter habitat warming, their survival may be jeopardized.

Adaptive variation occurs in several properties of the heat-shock response. Although the heat-shock response probably occurs in greater than 99% of contemporary species, this response is not a single invariant program that involves triggering synthesis of the same set of proteins in all organisms in response to heat stress. Rather, several important characteristics of the heat-shock response are found to exhibit variation that reflects both the evolutionary histories of the species and the recent thermal conditions that individuals have faced (acclimatization and acclimation effects). The classes of hsp's induced in different species may vary considerably, for reasons that are not yet apparent. For example, whereas hsp104 may be the major heat-shock protein in yeast, hsp70 may be most strongly induced in most animals (Parsell et al., 1993). In multicellular species, tissue-specific patterns of hsp induction may occur (Dietz and Somero, 1993).

Variation among differently thermally adapted species is observed in several aspects of the thermal dependence of the induction process: (i) the temperatures at which hsp synthesis is first induced ("threshold induction temperatures", T_{on}), (ii) the temperatures at which maximal synthesis of hsp's occurs (T_{peak}), and (iii) the upper thermal limits of hsp synthesis (T_{off}). This type of temperature-adaptive variation is even found among closely related congeneric species that have evolved under different ranges of habitat (body) temperature. Furthermore, the heat-shock response exhibits a considerable degree of phenotypic plasticity in differently acclimated and differently acclimatized conspecifics, at least in terms of threshold induction temperature and temperature of maximal synthesis. There is, then, substantial adaptive variation in the heat-shock response, some of which appears genetically hard-wired, and some of which is modifiable in response to recent thermal history. Taken together, this variation may play critical roles in (i) fine-tuning an organism for the thermal conditions it encounters and (ii) setting biogeographic distribution patterns.

Before examining these types of variation in the heat-shock response and the potential roles this variation may play in setting thermal tolerance limits and biogeographic patterning, an important aspect of experimental design must be discussed. Each of the major characteristics of the heat-shock response listed in the previous paragraph involves interactions between temperature and time. The *intensity* of a heat shock is essentially the product of stress temperature multiplied by the rate at which heating occurs and the duration of exposure to this thermal stress:

$$\text{Intensity of heat stress} = [(\Delta\text{temperature})$$
$$\times \text{(rate of heating)}$$
$$\times \text{(duration of exposure)}]$$

One can dip a finger into boiling water without ill consequences, as long as the time of immersion is very short. In the context of environmental heat stress and induction of synthesis of heat-shock proteins, intensity of stress is a factor that must be measured or controlled very carefully if one set of experiments is to be compared meaningfully with another. For example, threshold induction temperatures (T_{on}) determined using a long period of heat stress might be lower than those determined when heat stress periods are relatively short. Because the intensities of heat stress are seldom the same in studies from different laboratories, care must be taken when comparing studies done by different investigators. Such caution is especially relevant when one seeks to determine how species adapted to different temperatures vary with respect to these major characteristics of the heat-shock response.

Congeneric marine snails of the genus Tegula: adaptive variation in the heat-shock response. Comparative studies of differently thermally adapted congeners have proven to be useful for elucidating evolutionary patterns in the heat-shock response, in much the way that congeners have been useful in studies of adaptation in protein structure and function. Congeners of intertidal invertebrates that occur along a vertical transect from the subtidal zone into the mid-to-high intertidal zone have proven to be especially suitable for this type of comparative study. Intertidal invertebrates that retain their vertical position during the tidal cycle experience alternating periods of immersion during high tide and emersion during low tide. These cyclical changes in exposure to water and air lead to considerable variation in body

temperature each day. During emersion body temperatures may increase rapidly, perhaps by as much as 20–25°C over 1–2 hour periods (Hofmann and Somero, 1995; Stillman and Somero, 1996; Tomanek and Somero, 1999). These high body temperatures may be maintained for several hours until return of high tide. In contrast, subtidal congeners may remain at relatively low and stable temperatures during the full tidal cycle.

Snails of the genus *Tegula* have provided an appropriate study system for comparing congeners with different vertical distributions. Congeners of *Tegula* have widely different latitudinal and vertical distribution patterns, and because of this, species vary in body temperature by at least 30–35°C. The heat-shock response was studied in four congeners of *Tegula* that are found in habitats that differ greatly in temperature (Tomanek and Somero, 1999). Two temperate zone, low-intertidal and subtidal species, *Tegula brunnea* and *Tegula montereyi*, encounter relatively low temperatures when immersed (approximately 10–18°C). Because *T. brunnea* and *T. montereyi* are rarely emersed, their body temperatures are unlikely to exceed 25°C except under rare circumstances, for instance, if individuals are stranded in the intertidal regions during an exceptionally low tide. In contrast, a temperate zone congener found in low- to mid-intertidal regions, *T. funebralis*, is exposed to air and to solar radiation for extended periods of time during low tides. Body temperatures as high as 32.5°C have been measured for this species. A fourth congener studied, *T. rugosa*, is found in the rocky intertidal region of the Gulf of California, where its body temperature is likely to rise to at least 40°C during prolonged periods of emersion on hot days.

To determine the values for T_{on}, T_{peak}, and T_{off} for these four species, isolated sections of gill tissue were exposed to a series of temperatures and then incubated in ^{35}S-methionine/^{35}S-cysteine to allow monitoring of patterns of protein synthesis. Newly synthesized proteins were separated by gel electrophoresis and visualized using autoradiography (figure 7.11). As illustrated for gills of 13°C-acclimated *T. funebralis*, strong induction of several hsp's

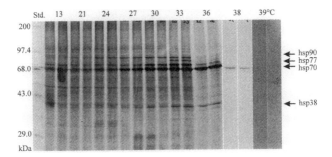

Figure 7.11. The effects of exposure temperature on protein synthetic patterns of isolated gill tissue from specimens of 13°C-acclimated *Tegula funebralis*. Autoradiographic images illustrate newly synthesized (^{35}S-labeled) proteins of several size classes (molecular mass standards are shown in the left lane). Two specimens from each temperature of incubation are shown. At temperatures above 24°C, synthesis of heat-shock proteins in the molecular mass ranges of 38, 70, 77, and 90 kDa is induced. Hsp synthesis becomes an increasingly large fraction of protein synthesis as exposure temperature increases, and by 38°C, only synthesis of hsp70 is observed. By 39°C, no protein synthesis takes place. (Figure modified after Tomanek and Somero, 1999.)

occurred. At temperatures above 24°C, synthesis of hsp38, hsp70, hsp77, and hsp90 commenced. For hsp70, the most strongly expressed hsp, T_{on} is 27°C, T_{peak} is 33°C, and T_{off} is 39°C. At the highest temperatures at which proteins were synthesized, strong preferential synthesis of hsp's is noted. At 38°C, the highest temperature at which *T. funebralis* gills can synthesize proteins, the only newly synthesized protein observed was hsp70. Digitizing of the autoradiograms permits a quantitative analysis of the synthetic patterns to be performed, and better allows T_{on}, T_{peak}, and T_{off} to be determined (figure 7.12).

To examine genetically based variation in the heat-shock responses of the four congeners, they were first acclimated to a common temperature (23°C) for one month. Then, synthesis of hsp's was studied by the method just described (figure 7.11). The heat-shock responses of the four 23°C-acclimated congeners (lower panels of figure 7.12) reflect their native habitat temperature conditions. For hsp70 and hsp38, T_{on}, T_{peak}, and T_{off} all exhibit the ranking: *T.brunnea* = *T.montereyi* < *T.funebralis* < *T.rugosa*. For some species, induction of hsp70 occurs at temperatures within the range of body temperatures expected in situ: T_{on} is near 27°C for *T. funebralis* and near 30°C for *T. rugosa*. Synthesis of hsp38 also is strongly induced at normal habitat tempera-

tures for *T. funebralis* and *T. rugosa*. Thus, for these two low-to-mid-intertidal species, induction of the heat-shock response is likely to be a frequent occurrence when low tides occur during sunny midday periods. For the two low-intertidal to subtidal species, *T. montereyi* and *T. brunnea*, induction of synthesis of hsp70 and hsp38 is not apt to occur except under circumstances in which specimens are left stranded at high vertical positions during low tide. These observations suggest that the costs of heat stress may differ substantially between intertidal species and subtidal species, and that even if differences in intrinsic stability exist among orthologous proteins of these species, these differences are not enough to compensate for the effects of environmental heat stress.

Temperatures of maximal synthesis of hsp70 and hsp38 also differ among species, in accordance with their adaptation temperatures. For the 23°C-acclimated specimens, T_{peak} for synthesis of hsp70 and hsp38 is near 30°C for *T. brunnea* and *T. montereyi*, 36°C for *T. funebralis*, and 38–40°C for *T. rugosa*. The upper temperatures (T_{off}) at which synthesis of hsp70, hsp38, and other proteins is fully curtailed show similar interspecific differences. For *T. brunnea* and *T. montereyi*, protein synthesis per se, not only hsp synthesis, is blocked at temperatures near 33°C, a temperature that their temperate zone congener *T. funebralis*

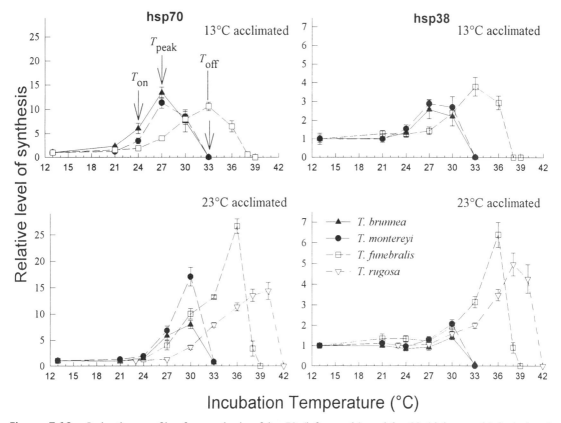

Figure 7.12. Induction profiles for synthesis of hsp70 (left panels) and hsp38 (right panels) in isolated gills of four species of snails belonging to the genus *Tegula*. Specimens were acclimated to either 13°C (upper panels) or 23°C (lower panels) for one month prior to the heat stress experiments. Amounts of newly synthesized hsp70 and hsp 38 were quantified by densitometric analysis of autoradiographs (see figure 7.11) and normalized to synthesis at the non-heat-stress temperature of 13°C. (Figure modified after Tomanek and Somero, 1999.)

may experience in its intertidal habitat on particularly hot days. *Tegula funebralis* continues to synthesize proteins up to approximately 38°C, although hsp70 is the only protein whose synthesis continues at this high temperature (figure 7.11). Protein synthesis by *T. rugosa* continues up to approximately 40°C. These data on thermal tolerance of protein synthesis suggest that temperature effects on this critical process may contribute to setting ectothermic species' distribution patterns. The acutely measured upper lethal temperatures of *T. brunnea* and *T. montereyi* are near 32–34°C, while that of *T. funebralis* is near 38–40°C (Tomanek and Somero, 1999).

The interspecific differences illustrated in figure 7.12 for synthesis of hsp70 and hsp38 by

snails acclimated to a common temperature of 23°C likely reflect either fixed genetic differences among the species or the influences of irreversible ontogenetic changes that, once established, cannot be reversed through acclimation (see Huey and Berrigan, 1996). However, two aspects of the heat-shock response, T_{on} and T_{peak}, do exhibit phenotypic plasticity among differently acclimated conspecifics (figure 7.12). For instance, for *T. brunnea* and *T. montereyi*, T_{on} and T_{peak} of hsp70 synthesis shifted to higher values as the acclimation temperature increased from 13 to 23°C. T_{peak} for hsp70 also shifted upwards in *T. funebralis*. However, the upper thermal limit for protein synthesis did not change with acclimation. This latter characteristic of the heat-shock response may be a genetically fixed characteristic of each species that cannot be modified even after several weeks of acclimation or as a result of seasonal acclimatization (Tomanek and Somero, 1999).

Timing and duration of the heat-shock response. The time required to initiate a heat-shock response and to complete the synthesis of hsp's varies among organisms for a variety of reasons related both to their phylogeny and to the severity of the heat stress they have encountered. Bacteria, with their capacities for rapid modulation of gene expression, may exhibit increased synthesis of hsp's within minutes after initiation of heat stress. In contrast, multicellular eukaryotes with slower kinetics of gene regulation and translation may be intrinsically slower in mounting the heat-shock response.

The severity of the heat stress imposed on an organism influences several characteristics of the heat-shock response that it is capable of mounting. In congeners of *Tegula*, the time required to initiate synthesis of hsp's, the maximal level of hsp synthesis, and the duration of synthesis reflect severity of heat stress (Tomanek and Somero, 2000; see also figure 7.13). Subjecting *T. funebralis* and *T. brunnea* to an identical heat-shock regimen, rapid heating under immersion in 30°C seawater for a period of 2.5 h, resulted in marked differences in the kinetics of their heat-shock responses. In *T. funebralis*, which commonly encounters body temperatures of 30°C, synthesis of heat-shock proteins was initiated rapidly, reached a maximal level within approximately one hour, and was completed within a few hours. In contrast, onset of synthesis of hsp's by *T. brunnea*, for which 30°C exposure is rare and near lethal, was delayed compared to *T. funebralis*. Furthermore, once its heat-shock response was activated, *T. brunnea* often exhibited higher levels of hsp synthesis and sustained these high levels of synthesis for relatively long periods of time compared to its congener. These data suggest that *T. funebralis* is capable of rapidly mounting a heat-shock response following exposure to heat stress during low tide, such that by the time of the following daytime low tide, it has accumulated the hsp's needed to

cope with heat stress. Its congener *T. brunnea* appears unable to initiate and complete a heat-shock response during a period of immersion between two low tides. Thus, *T. brunnea* appears poorly suited for coping with the heat stress that occurs in the intertidal zone. The delayed synthesis of hsp's in *T. brunnea* may reflect damage to the transcriptional or translational machinery that, while repairable, delays the onset of hsp production. Whatever the primary sites of thermal damage are, it is clear that *T. brunnea* suffers a greater degree of perturbation to its cellular machinery than does *T. funebralis* when immersed in 30°C water.

The rate of heating also may influence the kinetics and magnitude of the heat-shock response. When an organism is exposed to heating in air, body temperatures will rise much more slowly than when immersion in water is used for heat stress. For *T. funebralis*, no difference was noted in the rate and magnitude of hsp synthesis between heating in 30°C water and 30°C air, even though there was an approximately tenfold higher rate of heating in water (Tomanek and Somero, 2000). However, for *T. brunnea*, the slower rate of heating in 30°C air allowed the organism to more rapidly induce its heat-shock response.

Under natural field conditions, it appears that the heat-shock response may reach its highest levels only after the heat stress has been relieved and the organism is again able to function at optimal physiological temperatures. For instance, in the mussel *Mytilus trossulus*, synthesis of hsp70 reached maximal levels after approximately three hours of re-immersion following low tide (Hofmann and Somero, 1996a). Re-immersion of a gill-breathing species like *M. trossulus* not only restores a more equable body temperature, but also allows more effective exchange of oxygen and CO_2 and, therefore, a higher potential for aerobic generation of ATP. Synthesis and function of chaperones demands considerable energy, and under conditions of heat stress during emersion it may not be possible to produce or use hsp's at the high levels needed for ameliorating thermal damage.

Heat stress, protein damage, and biogeographic patterning. The finding that the

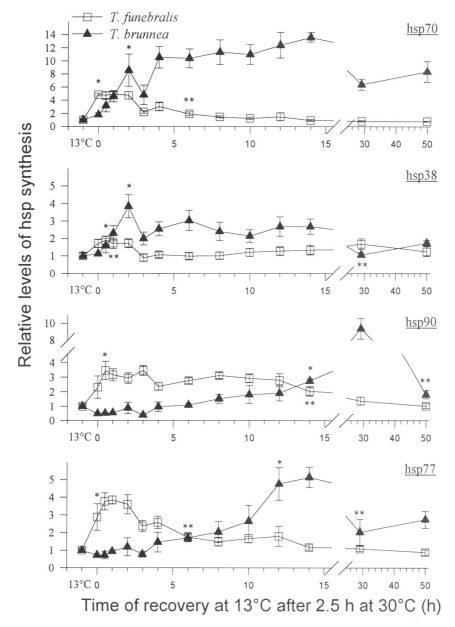

Figure 7.13. Patterns of synthesis of hsp70, hsp38, hsp90, and hsp77 in gill tissue from specimens of *Tegula funebralis* (mid-intertidal zone) and *Tegula brunnea* (subtidal) that had been exposed to 2.5 hours of heat shock at 30°C and then allowed to recover at the acclimation temperature, 13°C. At different times during recovery, gills were removed from the animals, placed into a medium containing ^{35}S methionine/cysteine, and allowed to synthesize proteins for 4 hours at 13°C. The first time at which a significant increase in hsp synthesis relative to control snails (held throughout at 13°C; data shown as initial (13°C) points on abscissa) occurred is indicated by a single asterisk. The time at which hsp synthesis returned to a value not significantly higher than the control value (13°C animals) is indicated by double asterisks. (Figure modified after Tomanek and Somero, 2000.)

heat-shock response is triggered at temperatures that lie well within the normal body temperature ranges of many ectotherms (Feder and Hofmann, 1999) has several important implications and consequences. Induction of the heat-shock response would appear to be a strong confirmation of the hypothesis that proteins are only marginally stable in the cell. Even though protein stability in vivo is difficult to measure, the fact that induction of heat-shock protein synthesis occurs at temperatures within the upper reaches of the normal range of body temperatures of many ectotherms is at least indirect evidence that thermal damage to proteins does occur under natural environmental conditions.

The thermal perturbation of protein structure that occurs under natural conditions appears to involve both reversible and irreversible denaturation. Although heat-shock proteins may be able to restore the native structures of reversibly unfolded proteins, proteins that have suffered irreversible damage must be removed from the cell through activities of proteolytic systems. One of the mechanisms for achieving proteolysis begins with covalent binding to irreversibly damaged proteins of a small, 76-residue protein termed *ubiquitin*, yielding ubiquitin conjugates (Hersko and Ciechanover, 1992). Ubiquitin serves as a tag that renders ubiquitin conjugates targets for proteolysis through nonlysosomal pathways. The higher the concentration of ubiquitin conjugates in a cell, the greater is the amount of nonlysosomal proteolysis. Significantly higher concentrations of ubiquitin conjugates were found in mussels (*Mytilus trossulus*) from high intertidal habitats (= warm-acclimatized specimens) than in mussels from subtidal sites (= cold-acclimatized specimens) (Hofmann and Somero, 1995). Thus, natural heat stress is severe enough to cause irreversible as well as reversible damage to proteins. Synthesis of ubiquitin conjugates, like synthesis of hsp's, occurred only after mussels were re-immersed during high tide (Hofmann and Somero, 1996a). Ubiquitination is an ATP-dependent process that may require the support of high levels of aerobic metabolism.

Thus, to cope with heat stress under natural conditions, organisms need to (i) restore structures of reversibly damaged proteins, by employing molecular chaperones—hsp's; (ii) ubiquitinate and then degrade irreversibly damaged proteins that cannot be rescued by hsp's; and (iii) replace these degraded proteins through new protein synthesis. These three requirements for maintaining protein homeostasis carry an important implication for the energy demands facing organisms that are subjected to heat stress. Synthesis of heat-shock proteins requires energy, as does the functioning of these proteins in the renaturation of heat-damaged proteins. Most classes of hsp's, in common with molecular chaperones in general, require ATP for their function. Chaperoning a single polypeptide may require dozens to hundreds of ATP molecules. Ubiquitin-mediated proteolysis also requires expenditure of energy (Hersko and Ciechanover, 1992). Substantial energy costs also may be entailed in synthesis of new proteins to replace those that were damaged irreversibly and removed by proteolysis. In sum, the events linked with heat damage to proteins may be an important component of the overall energy budget of an organism, and the ecological ramifications of thermal damage to proteins may be considerable. For instance, individuals of a sessile intertidal species that occur near the upper limits of the species' vertical distribution range, where emersion periods are greatest and heat stress is highest, may face limitations in energy budgets due to synergistic effects of reduced time for feeding and higher energy demands for coping with heat damage to its proteins. Thus, the effects of temperature on proteins may play an important role in establishing the upper distribution limits of intertidal species. More generally, the distribution limits of ectothermic organisms are apt to be constrained by temperature–protein interactions that lead to (i) perturbation of kinetic properties like K_m and k_{cat} and, thereby, to suboptimal metabolic function; (ii) damage to protein structure that leads to high energy costs and disruption of protein homeostasis; and (iii) ultimately the cessation of protein synthesis, whose thermal tolerance limits cannot be modified by acclimation.

Regulation of the heat-shock response: Cellular thermometers and control of transcription of heat shock genes

Regulation of synthesis of heat-shock proteins in response to thermal stress is a complex, multistep process that may differ substantially between prokaryotes and eukaryotes and among different families of heat-shock proteins. The initial event in all cases must be a sensing of heat-induced damage by some type of "cellular thermometer." This information then must be transduced, as rapidly as possible, to the up-regulation of synthesis of the specific classes of hsp's whose chaperoning activities are required to redress thermal damage to proteins. The steps in this regulatory cascade and the ways in which synthesis of different classes of hsp's are independently regulated are now understood in some detail, although several key questions remain unanswered. In particular, there is still debate as to the precise nature of the so-called "cellular thermometer," the event that triggers the regulatory cascade. Here, we will consider in detail but one model among several (see below) for how the regulatory cascade may operate. This model is based on regulation of hsp70 in eukaryotes (Craig and Gross, 1991; Morimoto, 1998; Morimoto and Santoro, 1998). An attractive element of this model is that it provides a linkage between thermal damage to proteins and activation of the *hsp70* gene, with hsp70 itself serving as a "thermometer" that senses and then helps to signal the need for its own synthesis.

This model for regulation of hsp70 synthesis involves several components: (i) preexisting pools of hsp70 and the co-chaperone Hdj-1 (= hsp40); (ii) a gene-regulatory protein termed *heat-shock factor 1* (HSF1), which is a transcriptional activator of the *hsp70* gene; and (iii) a gene regulatory element, the *heat-shock element* (HSE), multiple copies of which are located upstream of the coding region of the *hsp70* gene. Heat-shock factor 1 can bind to HSE as a trimer (figure 7.14). These are not likely to be the only players on the field, for additional pro-

teins are thought to play regulatory roles as well (see Morimoto, 1998; Morimoto and Santoro, 1998). For example, a second heat-shock protein, hsp90, also appears to affect the functional status of HSF1 (Ali et al., 1998). The components portrayed in figure 7.14 provide at least a minimal model for explaining how heat stress is transduced into increased expression of the *hsp70* gene.

Prior to heat shock, monomers of HSF1 are shown bound to hsp70. Hdj-1 (hsp40) and hsp90 also may bind to HSF1 under nonstressful conditions and, in concert with hsp70, block its gene-activating activity. In this hsp-bound form, HSF1 is not able to diffuse into the nucleus, bind as a trimer to HSE, and activate transcription of the *hsp70* gene. When heat shock occurs, the amount of non-native protein present in the cell rises. As hsp70 assumes its chaperoning function, it will increasingly be bound to non-native proteins rather than to HSF1. Unbound HSF1 is free to diffuse into the nucleus, trimerize, and bind to HSE, leading to activation of transcription of the *hsp70* gene. Heat-shock factor 1 may be active only when phosphorylated, so there is an additional level of control involving phosphorylation–dephosphorylation events. As translation of new hsp70 takes place, there may be sufficient build-up of this chaperone to satisfy the cell's needs for chaperoning activity and for fostering substantial rebinding of HSF1 to hsp70. Furthermore, free hsp70 may enter the nucleus, bind to HSF1 trimers associated with the HSE, and lead to inactivation of transcription through release of HSF1 from the HSE. Binding of hsp40 and hsp90 to HSF1 also is thought to have this effect. As a result of these processes, transcription of the *hsp70* gene is curtailed through an autoregulatory mechanism in which hsp70 contributes to regulation of its own concentration.

This model has received considerable experimental support, although it must still be viewed as an attractive hypothesis rather than a definitively established mechanism. The facts that different classes of hsp's are induced at different temperatures, and that induction of different hsp's follows different time courses (compare hsp70 and hsp90 in figure 7.13) suggest that a

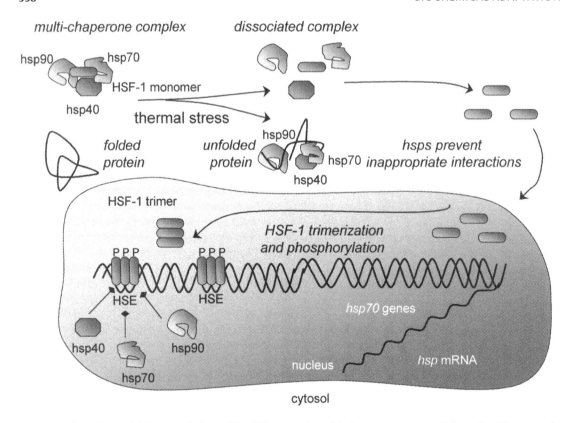

Figure 7.14. A model for regulation of hsp70 expression. Under nonstress conditions, hsp70 occurs in the cytoplasm in a multichaperone (hsp90 and hsp40) complex with which heat-shock factor 1 (HSF1) is associated (top). When heat stress is applied to the cell and unfolded proteins begin to appear, the complex comprising hsp70, hsp90, hsp40, and HSF1 dissociates. The three chaperones bind to unfolded proteins to prevent inappropriate aggregations and to assist in refolding to the native structure. The free monomers of HSF1 migrate into the nucleus and bind to the heat-shock element (HSE) as trimers. Phosphorylation of HSF1 at serine residues (P) activates the HSF1 trimers and leads to transcription of the *hsp70* gene. Translation of the hsp70 message leads to increased levels of hsp70. As levels of hsp70 rise and chaperoning activity is achieved, a build-up of free chaperones leads to an autoregulatory reduction in transcription of the *hsp70* gene. Binding of hsp70, hsp40, and hsp90 to HSF1 residing on the HSE blocks transcription and leads to dissociation of HSF1 from HSE. hsp70, hsp40, hsp90 and HSF1 diffuse into the cytoplasm and re-form the multichaperone complex shown at the top. (Figure modified after Morimoto and Santoro, 1998.)

"one model fits all" situation does not exist. There are, in fact, other mechanisms likely to be of importance in controlling the synthesis of heat-shock proteins. These include, but are not limited to, the following. First, heat-shock message may be preferentially translated at elevated (heat-shock) temperatures, such that synthesis of heat-shock proteins attains precedence over synthesis of other classes of proteins. The protein synthesis patterns at 36°C and 38°C in figure 7.11 are consistent with preferential translation of mRNA for hsp70. Although heat-shock messages typically appear to have very short half-lives, any pre-existing message for hsp's could be quickly incorporated into the translational apparatus under heat stress. Second, in yeast, trimerized HSF1 is bound to the HSE under non-heat-stress conditions (Craig and Gross, 1991), which shows that a single cellular thermometer model does not apply to all species. In yeast, regulation of HSF1 activity may be achieved by reversible phosphorylation of the bound HSF1. This could be a very rapid means for modulating expression of the *hsp70* gene. Third, the bacterial analog of the eukaryotic transcription factor HSF1, the 32 kDa transcriptional factor σ^{32}, may vary in concentration as cell temperature changes (Craig and Gross, 1991). σ^{32} has a very short half-life, and appears to be inactivated at low, rather than at high, temperatures. Regulation of concentrations of σ^{32} involves a set of chaperones, including the bacterial homolog of hsp70, DnaK, that inactivate σ^{32} and facilitate its degradation. This mechanism resembles the mechanism proposed in eukaryotic cells for regulation of hsp70 (figure 7.14) in that interactions between a chaperone and a transcription factor are pivotal in controlling the synthesis of the hsp in question. Fourth, synthesis of σ^{32} is mediated in part by a temperature-dependent conformational change in its mRNA (encoded by the *rpoH* gene in *E. coli*) (Morita et al., 1999; Storz, 1999). At low temperatures at which synthesis of σ^{32} is not observed, its mRNA occurs in a conformation that prevents it from binding to the ribosomes. Heat shock melts the region of RNA secondary structure that precludes ribosomal binding, and translation then can be initiated. Here, an RNA molecule appears to function as a "cellular thermometer." Fifth, increases in temperature may directly favor the trimerization and DNA binding of HSF1 (Zhong et al., 1998). At higher temperatures, hydrophobic interactions between leucine zippers on HSF1 monomers may form, leading to active trimers of the molecule. These responses of HSF1 to increases in temperature may allow it to perform a sensing role as a "cellular thermometer." Thus, there is no shortage of good candidates for "cellular thermometers." A variety of molecules, both RNAs and proteins, have temperature-dependent conformations that allow them to sense temperature changes. Here is another instance of the biological importance of the marginal stability of both nucleic acids and proteins. To date, it is not known if the conformational stabilities of these putative "cellular thermometers" vary among differently thermally adapted species, such that the set-points of the "thermometer" are in accord with the tempera-

tures at which a particular organism begins to experience heat stress.

It is apparent that the regulatory cascades involved in controlling levels of heat-shock proteins are complex. Regulation may involve a number of temperature-sensing ("thermometer") events and subsequent steps that govern transcription and translation. Together, these events provide tight control over the amounts of hsp's that accumulate in the cell. It is well established that too high a level of hsp's can be deleterious to cells. For instance, *Drosophila* that were genetically engineered to have additional copies of the gene encoding hsp70 were at a physiological disadvantage to wild-type flies under normothermic conditions (Feder, 1999; Krebs and Feder, 1997). Therefore, precise regulation of the heat-shock response is critical for coping with heat stress and for restoring normal conditions (lower levels of hsp's) when the damage from heat stress has been repaired. In this regard, it is interesting that severe, possibly lethal heat stress to the snail *Tegula brunnea* appears to switch on a strong heat-shock response that is not turned off, even 50 hours after cessation of heat stress (figure 7.13). This result could reflect the inability of hsp's to repair damage over this period, such that continued build-up of hsp's was necessary. Alternatively, this prolonged synthesis of hsp's could mean that the regulatory mechanisms that control production of hsp's have been damaged by heat, such that production of hsp's cannot be turned off when external heat stress is removed. One of the causes of thermal death, then, could be an uncontrolled—and highly deleterious—accumulation of hsp's as a result of heat damage to the regulatory controls of the heat-shock response. Because heat-shock proteins are often synthesized preferentially, a massive synthesis of hsp's could be linked with a severe down-regulation of production of other types of proteins, leading to disruption of protein homeostasis.

A final point concerning regulation of synthesis of hsp's concerns the fact that activities of chaperones often reflect a cooperative effort that involves two or more chaperones working in concert. Thus, more than one chaperone may need to have its concentration adjusted in response to heat stress, and interaction between the regulatory systems controlling synthesis of different classes of hsp's is likely to be important to ensure that the proper balance of different hsp's and co-chaperones is attained. This is an important fact, not only because it illustrates the complexities involved in the functioning and regulation of molecular chaperones, but also because it sounds a cautionary note for those wishing to study chaperones *in vitro* under conditions that simulate in-vivo function. As Ellis (1996a) has argued, putting the "bio" into the biochemistry of chaperone function is a major experimental challenge. In fact, this caveat applies not only in the context of chaperone–chaperone cooperativity, but also with respect to the influences of low-molecular-weight solutes on chaperone function.

Cooperation between molecular (protein) chaperones and low-molecular-mass stabilizers of proteins ("chemical chaperones")

As discussed earlier in this chapter and also in chapter 6, thermal stabilities of proteins in vivo are influenced by many constituents of the intracellular milieu, including low-molecular-mass protein stabilizers. The process of protein folding, whether during initial synthesis or following heat-induced unfolding, thus will be influenced not only by activities of protein chaperones, but also by the activities of low-molecular-mass organic solutes. In principle, heat stress could be ameliorated in part by accumulation of low-molecular-mass protein-stabilizing solutes that favor formation of the compact, folded state of proteins. Such "chemical chaperones" could complement the activities of protein chaperones.

An interesting illustration of the roles played by low-molecular-mass protein stabilizers in assisting cells to cope with heat stress is provided by work of Singer and Lindquist (1998a,b), who examined the complementary roles of the disaccharide trehalose and heat-shock proteins in recovery from thermal stress by the yeast *Saccharomyces cerevisiae*. Many types of yeast produce high concentrations of

trehalose when exposed to heat stress. As discussed in chapter 6, trehalose is a powerful stabilizer of proteins and membranes under stressful conditions, including those generated by heat and extreme desiccation, and it is utilized by a diverse array of organisms to cope with such stresses.

In *S. cerevisiae*, exposure to heat stress is followed by a rapid, yet transient production of high (approximately 0.5 M) concentrations of trehalose (Hottinger et al., 1987), which exert two favorable effects on proteins under conditions of heat stress in vivo. First, trehalose stabilizes the native structures of proteins, in keeping with its well-understood capacities as a protein stabilizer in vitro. Singer and Lindquist (1998a,b) were the first to demonstrate this capacity of trehalose in vivo. To do this, they used genetically engineered yeast cells that contained a heat-labile reporter protein, bacterial luciferase, whose activity could be monitored in vivo by measuring light emission. Heat-stressed mutant yeast lacking an ability to produce trehalose because of the deletion of a gene necessary for trehalose synthesis manifested only very low activities of luciferase. In contrast, wild-type cells with high concentrations of trehalose maintained high activities of the luciferase when subjected to heat stress.

Singer and Lindquist (1998a,b) also discovered a second critical function for trehalose in vivo: it prevented the aggregation of heat-denatured proteins. This second function of trehalose is of vital importance to the cell's ability to recover from heat stress, for it facilitates the abilities of protein chaperones to interact with, and restore, the native structures of heat-denatured proteins. Although heat-stressed yeast produce a heat-shock protein, hsp104, that is able to resolubilize aggregated proteins, preventing aggregation in the first place is likely to be to the cell's advantage.

In view of the favorable effects of trehalose on protein stability and prevention of aggregation, why is this solute rapidly removed from the cells after heat stress? Although the precise mechanisms involved are not clear, it is apparent that trehalose interferes with the subsequent refolding of heat-denatured proteins. Perhaps the nonaggregated, refolding-competent state of heat-damaged proteins that is stabilized by trehalose does not serve as an optimal substrate for protein chaperones. That is, if the partially denatured state of a protein is strongly stabilized by a chemical chaperone, then protein chaperones may find their activities reduced or blocked. In any event, trehalose must be removed from the cell before the complete refolding of denatured proteins can be accomplished by protein chaperones.

Trehalose is not the only organic solute to have these two effects—stabilization of native structure and prevention of aggregation—on proteins during heat stress. Singer and Lindquist (1998b) tested a variety of organic osmolytes known to accumulate to high concentrations in different organisms. Among these osmolytes, sucrose, maltose, glucose, and sorbitol were found to have favorable effects, but other sugars, for instance, mannitol, the amino acids proline, and the methylammonium solute glycine betaine were without effect. The highly specific patterns of osmolyte accumulation found in cells subjected to stress from temperature and other perturbants indicate that evolution of the "micromolecular" constituents of the intracellular milieu reflects a high degree of selectivity of appropriate solutes (see chapter 6).

Cold-shock effects on proteins and nucleic acids

When discussing effects of temperature on stabilities of macromolecules, it often is taken as axiomatic that heat stress represents a far greater challenge than stress resulting from exposure to low, but nonfreezing temperatures. Because increases in temperature lead to weakening of ionic interactions and hydrogen bonds and to an increase in the conformational entropy of a macromolecule, high temperature stress may seem to pose greater threats to macromolecular structure than does cold stress. Nonetheless, low temperatures also have negative consequences for macromolecular stability, and these effects appear to differ significantly between proteins and nucleic acids.

As mentioned earlier, proteins are subject to cold denaturation because they exhibit maximal stability at temperatures greater than $0°C$. The basis of this effect is the reduction in the stabilizing influence of hydrophobic interactions as temperature is reduced. Recall that the burial of hydrophobic side-chains in the folded protein is favored by entropy considerations (ΔS is positive), but that the enthalpy change associated with these burials is unfavorable (ΔH, too, is positive). Thus, as temperature decreases, there is less energy available to remove water from around hydrophobic groups in contact with the solvent. Furthermore, as temperature is reduced, the term $[-T\Delta S]$ takes on a smaller absolute value. For these reasons, the contribution of the hydrophobic effect to the net free energy of stabilization of a protein is reduced at low temperatures, and cold-induced unfolding of proteins (cold denaturation) may occur.

Nucleic acids present a very different structural problem at low temperatures. The base pairing that is responsible for stabilizing the secondary structures of nucleic acids is increasingly strengthened as temperature is reduced. Therefore, cold stress might tend to make the structures of nucleic acids too stable—they, too, must undergo conformational changes during activity—and, in addition, might lead to formation of abnormal secondary structural elements that are damaging to function. It is seen, then, that cold stress will negatively affect both protein and nucleic acid structures, but for quite different reasons: at low extremes of temperature, proteins become less stable and nucleic acids may become too stable.

Cold stress may induce synthesis of heat-shock (stress) proteins. Exposure of cells to cold shock may lead to the induction of one or more of the classes of molecular chaperones that also are induced by heat shock. This is strong evidence that low temperature, like high temperature, can lead to non-native protein structures in vivo and, therefore, to the requirement for enhanced chaperoning activity. Induction of cold-induced protein chaperones has been seen in bacteria (Salotra et al., 1995), in whole organism studies of ectothermic animals (Petersen et al., 1990; Yocum et al., 1991), and hypothermic mammals (Cullen and Sarge, 1997), and in human cells in culture (Liu et al., 1994). The extent of stress protein induction is generally proportional to the intensity of cold stress. Synthesis of cold-induced stress proteins may not occur during the actual period of cold stress, but only after the organism (or cell culture) is returned to higher temperatures. For instance, in *Drosophila*, transcription of the cold-shock genes does not occur until flies are returned to a normal environmental temperature after cold stress (Petersen et al., 1990). Low temperature suppression of transcription and translation may render the organism unable to repair cold-induced damage to its proteins until body temperature rises to a normal value. The impairment of transcription and translation by cold-shock is, in fact, a reflection of disruption of key nucleic acid structures needed for effecting these processes.

Chaperones are needed for nucleic acids as well as proteins.   The concept that the proper folding of macromolecules may depend on the activities of helper proteins—molecular chaperones—has recently been extended to nucleic acids, notably RNA. As pointed out above, the formation of secondary structures in nucleic acids is an exothermic process (ΔH is negative), and thus favored by reductions in temperature. If temperature decreases to very low values, nucleic acids may acquire too high a stability of native secondary structure to function well. Moreover, additional regions of secondary structure may form that disrupt normal functions such as transcription and translation.

To ameliorate these problems, cold-stressed cells, at least bacteria, may induce synthesis of *cold-shock proteins* (Csp's) that are thought to function in several capacities, including serving as RNA chaperones that prevent inappropriate secondary structures from forming (Graumann and Marahiel, 1998). Cold-shock proteins are a subset of a broader class of proteins, the *cold-induced proteins* (Cip's), which are synthesized at low temperatures. In *E. coli*, Cip's are encoded by genes belonging to a common gene regulatory system, the *cold-shock stimulon*, which is activated when temperature is

decreased. Cold-shock proteins, which may be the most strongly expressed Cip's, are low molecular weight (7.4 kDa) acidic proteins that have a characteristic sequence, the *cold-shock domain* (CSD), which is also found in a number of RNA-binding proteins of eukaryotes. Cold-shock proteins as such have not been found in eukaryotes. The bacterial Csp's are categorized on the basis of this specific sequence element, not in terms of whether they are induced by low temperature. Some Csp's are constitutively expressed and appear to be essential for normal housekeeping functions such as DNA recombination, transcription and translation (Jones et al., 1996). The study of Csp's thus shows a historical pattern parallel to that seen in the study of heat-shock proteins. Although the original discovery of each class of chaperone protein involved temperature shock, both hsp's and Csp's have turned out to be members of broader families of proteins, each of which plays important roles under normal, as well as under stressful conditions.

The RNA chaperoning activity of Csp's such as CspA (Jiang et al., 1997) and CsdA (Jones et al., 1996) involves relatively weak, nonspecific interactions between the CSD and single-stranded RNA (figure 7.15). It is thought that Csp's bind to RNA and prevent the RNA from forming intramolecular elements of double-stranded structure that interfere with the RNA's function. Thus, CsdA was shown to have a potent helix-destabilizing activity (Jones et al., 1996). The classes of RNA that may require chaperoning and the conditions of temperature under which this chaperoning is essential, remain to be fully determined. It is possible that tRNA, rRNA, and mRNA may require chaperoning. Inactive conformations of any of these classes of RNA could interfere with transcription or translation. Thus, cold block of protein synthesis could be due in large measure to alteration of native RNA structures. An example of this was seen in the effect of temperature on synthesis of σ^{32} during regulation of the heat-shock response in *E. coli* (Morita et al., 1999). Additional secondary structure in the mRNA for σ^{32} caused by reduced temperature led to a blockage of translation of the message.

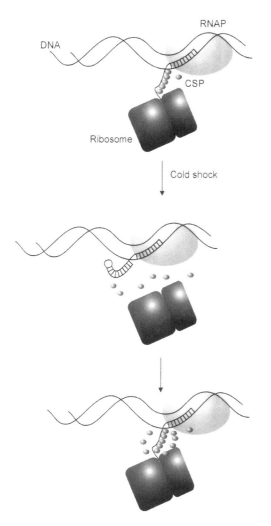

Figure 7.15. Functions of cold-shock proteins (Csp's) as RNA chaperones. The model shows how Csp's assist in coupling transcription to translation. Cold-shock proteins bind relatively weakly to nascent mRNA extending from the RNA polymerase complex (RNAP) and maintain the mRNA in a linear form that can be bound to ribosomes and translated into protein. Under nonstressful conditions, the weakly binding Csp's are present at adequate concentrations to perform this chaperoning function. However, during cold stress, the propensity for RNA to form secondary structures that block translation becomes greater. This necessitates that a higher level of Csp's be present in the cell, to ensure that chaperoning of mRNA is effective. (Figure modified after Graumann and Marahiel, 1998.)

Transcription may be especially prone to impairment by cold shock. During transcription, the newly transcribed mRNA must be kept in a linear configuration if binding to the ribosomes and subsequent translation is to occur. As shown in figure 7.15, Csp's, which bind only weakly to RNA as it is being transcribed by the RNA polymerase (RNAP) system, maintain this required linear structure and allow translation to occur. Any stress, for instance, low temperature, that disrupts the interactions between the nascent mRNA and the Csp's may lead to formation of base-pairing (secondary structure) in the mRNA, with concomitant blockage of translation. Although chaperoning of mRNA is likely to be important at normal cell growth temperatures, the activities of Csp's are apt to be especially critical at low temperatures, when intramolecular base pairing within the nascent mRNA becomes substantially stronger than the weak, nonspecific interactions between the CSD element and mRNA. To restore the necessary equilibrium, that is, the tendency for the mRNA to bind Csp's and retain a linear structure, elevated concentrations of Csp's are required.

Synthesis of increased concentrations of Csp's at low temperature appears to be achieved primarily by translational control processes, although up-regulation of transcription of *csp* mRNA also may take place (Graumann and Marahiel, 1998). Translational regulation has the benefit of being rapid and, under conditions of cold stress, it precludes difficulties that might arise from cold-induced blockage of transcription as a consequence of formation of secondary structure by nascent mRNA molecules. One of the primary steps in the regulation of csp synthesis involves turnover of *csp* mRNA. At normal cell temperatures, for instance at 37°C in *E. coli*, the half-life of the message for the major Csp, CspA, is extremely short. When cell temperature is lowered, *cspA* mRNA becomes more stable. The mRNAs for Cip's, including those for Csp's, are preferentially translated at low temperatures, a phenomenon that parallels the translation of hsp messages at high temperatures.

Regulation of the levels of Csp's also involves interactions between the protein and its message. The *cspA* mRNA has a long 5′ untranslated leader region (UTR) to which CspA can bind effectively. When the CspA–*cspA* mRNA complex is formed, the message is protected from degradation. However, when bound in this fashion, *cspA* mRNA is no longer active in translation. Thus, as [CspA] rises, the increase in complex formation between the protein and its mRNA leads to an automatic self-regulatory slowdown in its own synthesis (see chapter 2 for additional examples of this type of self-regulatory process). Complexes between CspA and RNA, including its own mRNA, also may influence turnover of the protein. Cold-shock proteins have an extremely low conformational stability, and they rapidly fold and unfold at physiological temperatures. However, in common with most proteins when they bind their appropriate ligand, Csp's are strongly stabilized in the presence of RNA. In summary, regulation of concentrations of Csp's is seen to depend on a complex suite of macromolecular interactions that affect both the activity and stability of the proteins and their mRNAs. As in the case of hsp's, the concentrations of Csp's manifest a strong reliance on autoregulatory processes.

The cold-shock domain: multifarious exploitation of an ancient structure. The cold-shock domain, which lies at the heart of interactions between Csp's and RNA, appears to be an ancient structure that likely was present in the ancestral cell that gave rise to contemporary organisms. Although the CSD has not been found in Archaea, in most bacteria and eukaryotes it is present in proteins having nucleic acid binding domains that interact with single-stranded DNA (ssDNA) and RNA. In some RNA binding proteins, for example, the Y-box proteins found in animals, the CSD confers sequence-specific RNA binding (Graumann and Marahiel, 1998). It will be intriguing to follow work on the evolution of this ancient protein domain, to discern how it has evolved to fulfill a number of functions in diverse proteins whose activities all are related to some type of nucleic acid binding. This domain may

represent a paradigm for further work on how a molecular system is recruited for diverse functions over long evolutionary periods.

Trigger factor: a cold-induced bacterial protein with multiple functions. Among the suite of proteins induced in *E. coli* by cold shock, one, *trigger factor* (TF), exhibits an impressive degree of multifunctionality (Kandror and Goldberg, 1997). Trigger factor is strongly induced during cold shock, and elevated concentrations of the protein greatly increase the viability of *E. coli* at low temperature. Studies of the functions of TF have revealed that the protein may facilitate several events that could be compromised at low temperatures. First, TF is a *peptidyl prolyl isomerase* (PPI). Isomerization of prolyl residues may be the rate-limiting step in protein folding, especially at low temperatures. Thus, elevated activities of TF could facilitate temperature-compensatory increases in rates of protein maturation. Second, TF interacts with the bacterial protein chaperone GroEL. These interactions increase GroEL's affinity for unfolded proteins. Trigger factor may thus be a "chaperone helper." Third, probably in conjunction with GroEL, TF can assist in enhancing the degradation of damaged proteins.

The discoveries of Csp's and trigger factor may represent the tip of a large iceberg. In view of the pervasive effects of low temperature on the structures of all classes of macromolecules, it is reasonable to conjecture that many more types of proteins will be discovered whose roles are to offset the effects of cold shock on the cell. Some of these molecules may be expressed constitutively and may be part of the normal machinery of the cell. For example, certain ribosomal proteins are thought to function as RNA chaperones, and if present in sufficient amounts, these proteins may allow the cell to cope with the effects of cold shock on the structures of certain classes of RNAs. In yeast, a constitutively expressed ribosomal protein has helicase activity, and mutation in the gene encoding the protein confers on the cells a cold-sensitive phenotype (Schmid and Linder, 1992). Perhaps the apparent absence of cold-induced RNA chaperones in eukaryotic cells is a reflection of the presence in these cells of constitutively expressed RNA chaperones that are present at adequate levels to perform the functions that, in bacteria, are the responsibility of cold-induced Csp's. Coping adaptively with environmental stress thus may involve a wide spectrum of mechanisms for ensuring that the right protein is available in the right amounts. At one extreme, simple prokaryotic cells with capacities for rapid production of new types of proteins may only induce a needed stress protein when the stress is imposed on the cell. More complex eukaryotic cells with longer time constants for transcription and translation may contain constitutive levels of stress proteins needed to cope with the day-in, day-out levels of stress that may be encountered, and reserve for more extreme levels of stress a "stress response" that leads to gene activation and up-regulation of stress protein synthesis.

Organic solutes may protect against cold stress as well as heat stress. The accumulation of protein-stabilizing organic solutes in cells grown at high temperatures may be an important mechanism for adapting to heat stress as shown, for example, by the build-up of trehalose in heat-stressed yeast cells and the occurrence of high levels of anionic solutes in certain thermophilic prokaryotes. Cold shock also may trigger the accumulation of solutes with stabilizing effects on macromolecules. For example, when subjected to low temperatures the bacterium *Listeria monocytogenes* takes up high concentrations of glycine betaine from the medium (Ko et al., 1994). Cells grown at 4°C and 30°C contained 310 mM and 65 mM glycine betaine, respectively. Despite the fact that reductions in temperature almost invariably retard rates of physiological processes, uptake of glycine betaine increased 15-fold when cultures were quickly cooled from 30°C and 7°C. Glycine betaine enhanced growth of cold-stressed cells, but not cells grown at 30°C. The mechanisms underlying enhancement of growth by glycine betaine at low temperatures are not known. However, in view of the fact that proteins are subject to cold denaturation as well as heat denaturation, glycine betaine's protective function may involve stabilization of quaternary and tertiary structures of proteins. Glycine betaine, as well as trehalose, may stabilize phospholipid membranes (Rudolph et al., 1986). The solute composition of the cellular water thus may be an important element of adaptation to low, as well as to high temperatures. A further illustration of the importance of the aqueous milieu in governing protein function in the face of varying temperatures is given by the phenomenon we discuss next: temperature-dependent variation in pH.

TEMPERATURE–pH INTERACTIONS: REGULATING PROTON ACTIVITY TO STABILIZE PHYSIOLOGICAL FUNCTION

pH Plays an Important Role in Diverse Physiological Processes

The proton, the smallest solute in the cellular water, illustrates particularly well the critical role of the aqueous milieu of the cell in governing macromolecular stability and function under both stable and variable thermal conditions. One of the ubiquitous features of cellular regulatory processes involves control of pH. No type of cell allows the proton activity within its cytoplasm to equilibrate with that of the external medium, whether the medium in question is the external environment or the extracellular fluids. Organelles, too, may maintain a steep proton gradient between the intra-organellar fluids, for instance, the mitochondrial matrix, and the cytoplasm.

The close regulation of intracellular pH (pH_i) noted in all types of cells is a reflection of the large array of processes whose activities are dependent on local pH_i or on proton gradients between the cell (or organelle) and the surrounding fluid. Many physiological processes are regulated by changes in pH_i in the range of one to a few tenths of a pH unit. Thus, it is critical for cells to maintain their pH_i at a value allowing sharp physiological responses to changes in pH_i. That is, if shifts in intracellular pH are to effectively "titrate" the activities of physiological processes, pH_i must be poised at a value near the pK values of the pH-sensitive processes. pH titration of physiological activity is common both in short-term regulation of metabolic flux and in longer term shifts in physiological function that include transitions between metabolically active and quiescent states. Changes in pH_i of muscle during vigorous bouts of contraction cause rapid shifts in glycolytic activity. Metabolic activation of eggs at fertilization is often correlated with a rise in pH_i of a few tenths of a pH unit (Busa and Nuccitelli, 1984). Entry into hibernation by small mammalian hibernators involves acidification of some organs in concert with a large-scale drop in their metabolic activity (McArthur et al., 1990). Quiescent cysts of the brine shrimp *Artemia* maintain an acidotic cytosol that dampens rates of overall metabolic flux and leads to strong specific inhibition of a variety of energy-demanding processes (Busa and Nuccitelli, 1984; Hand and Hardewig, 1996).

A common mechanism underlying many physiological responses to changes in pH_i is the influence of pH on protein structure and function. For example, pH-dependent shifts in the assembly state of trehalase, the enzyme responsible for fueling carbohydrate metabolism in the brine shrimp *Artemia*, may lead to inhibition of trehalose breakdown to glucose in quiescent embryos (Hand and Carpenter, 1986). Trehalase assembly state is strongly titrated between catalytically active and inactive forms over the range of pH values that characterizes transitions between active and quiescent states of the embryos. Thus, the supply of glucose to intermediary metabolism is curtailed and glucose stores (in the form of the glucose dimer, trehalose) are protected for use when development resumes.

Intracellular and Extracellular pH Vary with Temperature

Because of the importance of pH_i in regulating so many physiological processes, any changes in pH_i that occur as a result of changes in body temperature would seem likely to add another element of thermal stress to the system. Thus, one might predict a priori that the pH values of the blood (pH_B) and the cytosol would need to be closely conserved in the face of changes in body (cell) temperature if homeostasis is to be defended. This strategy of pH regulation, which involves defending a set pH at all temperatures, is referred to as *pHstat* regulation (Reeves, 1977). In fact, what is observed in diverse organisms, including unicellular species and complex metazoans, is that pH is *not* held at a stable value as temperature changes. Rather, the pH values of blood and cytosol vary with temperature in a highly regular manner: pH values fall with rising temperature, with an average rate of change of approximately -0.019 pH units per °C increase in temperature (figure 7.16). Note that the slope of the pH versus temperature relationship is temperature dependent: near 0°C, the slope is approximately -0.021 units $°C^{-1}$ and near 37°C the slope decreases to approximately -0.0147 units $°C^{-1}$.

A brief history of the notion of what constitutes a "normal" pH

The history of discovery of this relationship is an interesting story, one well told in a review by Cameron (1989). To students trained in the context of medical physiology, a pH value of 7.4, the pH value of blood at normal human body temperature, 37°C, is—or at least was in the past—presented as the "normal" pH value. In fact, a pH of 7.4 is a normal pH value for blood only near 37°C; at lower temperatures, a pH_B of 7.4 is acidic relative to the true physiological pH at that temperature (figure 7.16). In retrospect, this fact should have been obvious from an understanding of protein biochemistry. However, it took several decades for the temperature–pH relationship to be fully accepted and even longer for it to be understood mechanistically in terms of protein chemistry.

Early clues to the nature of the temperature–pH relationship and its tight link to protein biochemistry were, in fact, available in the first decades of the past century. As early as the 1920s, Austin et al. (1927) reported that the pH of blood of alligators decreased by about 0.018 pH unit with each degree Celsius rise in body temperature between 9°C and 35°C. In what proved to be a far-sighted interpretation of their data, Austin et al. conjectured that the observed change in pH with temperature was such as to stabilize the charge states of pro-

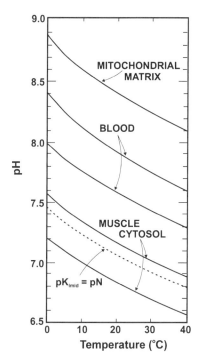

Figure 7.16. Temperature effects on the pH values of blood, cytoplasm, the mitochondrial matrix, the pK of the histidyl imidazole group (pK_{imid}) and the neutral pH of water (pN). Parallel lines shown for muscle cytosol and blood encompass the range of values that have been reported for these two variables.

Alphastat versus pHstat regulation of pH

Why is it advantageous to regulate pH in a temperature-dependent fashion, as shown in figure 7.16? The hypothesis of Austin et al. (1927) provides a partial answer to this question, an answer that has been elaborated in detail by Reeves, Rahn, Howell, and their colleagues (Rahn et al., 1975; Reeves, 1977). In essence, the temperature-dependent variation in pH_i and pH_B conserves the ionization states of proteins in all cellular compartments. The component of the protein that is pivotal in this relationship is the imidazole side-chain of histidine.

Histidine   Imidazole

Protonated and deprotonated states of the imidazole side-chain of histidine

Reeves (1977) has used the temperature dependent dissociation of the imidazole side-chain to develop the *alphastat model*, which focuses on conservation of alpha-imidazole (α_{imid}), the fractional dissociation of histidyl imidazole groups:

$$\text{alpha-imidazole } (\alpha_{imid}) = [\text{imidazole}]/$$
$$\{[\text{imidazole}] + [\text{imidazole}^+]\}$$

Under normal intracellular conditions of pH_i, α_{imid} is near 0.5. That is, at any instant, about half of the histidyl residues of proteins will be charged (protonated). This follows from the facts that (i) the pH_i of the cell is close to the pK of the imidazole group, and (ii) during changes in cell temperature, pH_i is regulated to maintain this similarity. As shown in figure 7.16, the slopes of the curves relating pH_i, pH_B, and pK_{imid} to temperature are essentially parallel.

teins in the face of temperature change. This path-breaking work was not followed by much additional study or theoretical analysis until the 1960s, when Robin (1962) and others began to reexamine temperature–pH relationships. It soon became apparent that both pH_B and pH_i varied regularly with temperature in diverse organisms, and that the pH of the cytosol was lower than the pH of blood or hemolymph. As techniques for accurately measuring pH_i improved, the number of instances in which temperature-dependent variation in pH_i was documented rapidly increased, and the "abnormal" temperature-dependent pH values found in poikilothermic organisms at last came to be appreciated as representing the normal physiological condition.

The pivotal significance of the imidazole group of histidine in biological pH relationships is principally due to one characteristic of imidazole chemistry: the histidyl imidazole group is the only amino acid side-chain with a pK value near physiological pH values. (This general statement, while correct, requires qualification. The local microenvironment of a side-chain that is capable of gaining or losing a proton can strongly affect the relevant pK value. For instance, the charge characteristics of the microenvironment around a glutamyl or aspartyl side-chain can significantly alter the pK of the COO^- group. Thus, proximity of one or more negative charges to a glutamyl or aspartyl side-chain may increase the pK of the equilibrium $COOH = COO^- + H^+$ by two to three pH units, and pK values may rise to levels close to pH_i in some cases.) Why is a pK value near pH_i so important? Proteins must be able to undergo reversible protonation, and histidyl residues represent the only raw material available for this function at biological pH values. (Here, for the moment, we beg some interesting questions: "Why did evolution select the pH values we find in contemporary organisms rather than a pH value much more acidic [or alkalotic]?" and "Were there other chemicals available to early cells that would have allowed fractional protonation at pH values consistent with life?") Many active sites of enzymes, including that of LDH, contain histidyl residues that are essential for binding of substrates (see figure 7.2). For this type of enzyme to be capable of working in both directions, for instance, from pyruvate to lactate and from lactate to pyruvate in the case of LDH, the histidyl residue (residue 193) involved in substrate binding must be neither fully protonated nor completely nonprotonated under conditions of cellular pH. Thus, for pyruvate to bind to the LDH active site, the histidyl residue must be protonated. For lactate to bind, it must enter a catalytic vacuole whose histidine-193 is not protonated. The decrease in pH_i that may accompany vigorous muscular activity facilitates anaerobic glycolysis by enhancing LDH's ability to bind pyruvate; K_m^{PYR} falls as pH decreases. With restoration of a higher pH_i following recovery from exercise, pyruvate binding is disfavored—more histidine-193s are unprotonated—and LDH then begins to convert the lactate produced through anaerobic glycolysis back into pyruvate, which can enter aerobic pathways of ATP production or be reconverted back to glucose and glycogen.

Because this kind of role for histidyl residues is present in diverse types of binding sites, two major benefits of alphastat regulation are evident (Somero, 1986). One benefit is that enzymatic activity can be responsive to changes in pH_i. Shifts in pH during activity or in concert with transition between life stages are able to effectively titrate the activities of enzymes, to ensure that their function occurs in the appropriate direction and at an appropriate level. A second and closely related benefit is the preservation of *reversibility* in enzymatic reactions, as seen in the pH effects on K_m values of LDH.

Alphastat regulation likewise conserves binding ability in the face of changes in body temperature. The conservation of K_m^{PYR} observed among differently adapted species and over wide ranges of temperature for eurythermal ectotherms (figure 7.7), is due to both intrinsic features of the protein, that is, to differences in amino acid sequence, and to temperature-dependent variation in pH. When K_m^{PYR} is determined under an alphastat pH regimen, the slope of the K_m^{PYR} versus temperature relationship is much less than that observed under pHstat conditions (Yancey and Somero, 1978).

Much as enzyme–substrate interactions may be governed by pH, so may the interactions between enzyme subunits and between enzymes and structural or contractile proteins. These relationships are shown in figure 7.17 for the glycolytic enzyme phosphofructokinase (PFK), which undergoes large shifts in subunit self-assembly equilibrium and in binding to actin when changes in pH occur. The assembly of subunits of PFK, a complex regulatory enzyme that is catalytically active only when present as a tetramer or multiple of tetramers, is highly dependent on the conditions of temperature and pH present in the medium (Bock and Frieden, 1974; Hand and Somero, 1983). As pH is reduced at constant temperature, the PFK tetramer may dissociate to dimers and monomers, leading to loss of enzymatic activity.

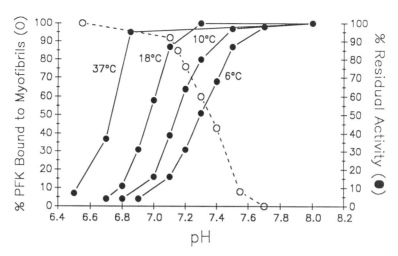

Figure 7.17. Effects of pH on binding of phosphofructokinase (PFK) to myofibrils (open symbols; dashed line) and interacting effects of pH and temperature on the self-assembly of PFK, as indexed by residual PFK activity (filled symbols; solid lines). Binding of PFK to myofibrils was measured using PFK-containing supernatants and myofibrillar preparations from white locomotory muscle of the teleost *Paralabrax nebulifer* (Roberts et al., 1998). PFK self-assembly was studied using purified enzyme from a mammal (*Spermophilus beecheyi*) (Hand and Somero, 1983). The percent residual PFK activity after incubation for 60 min under different combinations of pH and temperature provides an estimate of the fraction of PFK that remains as catalytically active tetramers or aggregates of tetramers. (Figure from Somero, 1997.)

The position of the activity versus pH titration curve shifts across the pH axis as temperature is changed: the lower the temperature at which the effects of pH are measured, the higher is the pH value at which activity begins to decrease. If the midpoint pH values of the titration curves shown in figure 7.17 are determined, it is found that the pH value yielding a 50% decrease in PFK activity decreases by about 0.015 pH unit $°C^{-1}$ rise in temperature, just as expected in alphastat regulation. It is evident that alphastat regulation is apt to play a major role in stabilizing PFK activity in the face of changes in body temperature. It also should be evident that in-vitro studies of PFK need to take into account pH-temperature relationships. Phosphofructokinase was long regarded as a "cold denaturing" enzyme because it tended to lose activity during low-temperature storage in many of the buffers typically used in biochemistry laboratories, for instance, phosphate-based buffers. Phosphate-based buffers are characterized by pK values that, unlike that of imidazole, are essentially

temperature-independent. Thus, chilling a solution of PFK in a pH 7.0 phosphate buffer may lead to the establishment in the buffer of an acidic and distinctly nonalphastat pH value, which is followed by dissociation of the enzyme's subunits and loss of catalytic activity.

One consequence of alphastat regulation for PFK function is analogous to that discussed above for LDH–substrate interactions: alphastat regulation ensures a high degree of reversibility of the process in question under physiological conditions of pH_i. The activity of PFK can be titrated as the pH_i of muscle cytosol changes. Falling pH_i during vigorous bursts of locomotion will lead, other things being equal (see below), to a decrease in PFK activity. Reducing PFK activity will slow down glycolytic flux and prevent excessive acidification of the muscle. There is another aspect to the PFK–pH story, however: as pH is reduced, the binding of PFK to the myofibrillar apparatus is increased (Roberts et al., 1988). Phosphofructokinase is the only glycolytic enzyme known to exhibit pH-dependent binding to actin. By binding to actin, to which the other glycolytic enzymes are known to bind as well, a glycolytic *metabolon* may be created, leading to a more effective transfer of substrates between the enzymes of this pathway and to a higher rate of glycolytic flux (see chapters 2 and 6).

Because changes in pH_i influence the self-assembly of PFK subunits and the tetramer's interaction with the contractile apparatus (filamentous actin), a complex pH dependence of PFK activity is likely. As a muscle becomes highly active and pH_i begins to fall, PFK will shift from a soluble to a bound state, as suggested by figure 7.17. Phosphofructokinase bound to the myofibrillar apparatus may be relatively resistant to dissociation by low pH (Roberts et al., 1988). This reversible binding may lead to an activation of glycolytic flux, at least for a period during which the further decrease in pH_i is not so severe as to lead to large-scale dissociation—and inactivation—of PFK. As vigorous muscle activity continues, PFK tetramers will increasingly dissociate, fewer tetramers will be available to bind to thin filaments, and PFK and glycolytic activities will decrease. Without titratable imidazole residues to mediate these pH effects, and without alphastat regulation to poise the system for titration by changes in pH, this type of regulation of glycolytic activity by pH would not be possible.

The benefits of alphastat regulation are reflected in evolution's selection of buffering substances

Within cells, the major buffering materials are histidyl-containing compounds, including most proteins and a family of histidine-containing dipeptide buffers: anserine (β-alanyl-L-1-methylhistidine), carnosine (β-alanyl-L-histidine), and ophidine (β-alanyl-L-3-methylhistidine). Free histidine generally is not found at high concentrations, even in strongly buffered tissues. Tissues in which a high capacity for proton generation exists, for example, locomotory muscle that is poised for a high level of anaerobic glycolysis, frequently contain large concentrations of one or more of the histidyl-

containing dipeptide buffers (Hochachka and Somero, 1984). The key feature of histidyl-containing buffers in the context of temperature effects is that these buffers vary their pK values with temperature according to the relationship shown for imidazole. Thus, buffering capacity is maintained as cell temperature varies.

The alpha-imidazole hypothesis is seen to provide a unifying explanation for many aspects of biological design, including (i) the frequent occurrence of histidyl groups in the catalytic centers, allosteric binding sites, and subunit interaction sites of enzymes, (ii) the use of dipeptide buffers to stabilize intracellular pH, and (iii) the regulatory strategies employed in adjusting pH values of the cellular fluids and the blood in the face of changes in temperature. The alpha-imidazole hypothesis emphasizes how the joint evolution of proteins and the medium in which they function leads to conservation of key physiological capacities.

The Importance of Being Ionized

Although the concept of alphastat regulation of pH provides an excellent conceptual framework within which to interpret biological pH regulatory mechanisms, we indicated above that an important question has gone begging up to this point: Why did the earliest cells "choose" a pH_i value near the pK of the imidazole group of histidine? Could not the same types of pH-mediated shifts in enzymatic activity, protein assembly states, and metabolic flux rates have been developed if either acidic amino acids (glutamate and aspartate) or basic amino acids (lysine and arginine) assumed the role played by histidine? The answer to the question, "Why histidine?," has been cast in a very creative manner by Davis (1958) and Rahn et al. (1975), who stressed the importance of maintaining a pH in the cell that ensures that most low-molecular-mass organic solutes remain ionized.

Davis' 1958 paper, "On the importance of being ionized," and subsequent extensions of his ideas by Rahn et al. (1975) focus on the broad physiological importance of keeping the metabolic intermediates of the cell in an ionized state. The central principle in their analyses involves the influence of charge state on the ease with which a solute can pass through a cellular membrane. In general, possession of charge reduces a solute's permeability. Thus, for the primordial cell, establishment of a pH_i value that facilitated ionization of most organic compounds can be understood as a means for keeping within the cell the organic molecules taken up from the environment or synthesized, using the limited repertoire of biosynthetic pathways present in these early cells. By selecting a pH value between 6 and 8, the majority of organic molecules in the cell would be ionized. Had a lower pH_i value been established, molecules such as carboxylic acids may have become protonated, that is, they would have lost their charge, and thus been able to more readily escape across the cell membrane. At higher pH values, other types of solutes, for instance, ammonium derivatives, may have lost their positive charge and, thus, been more able to escape from the cell. The fact that such a large fraction of metabolic intermediates are ionized at pH values between 6 and 8 supports the hypothesis that a pH regulatory system that targeted a pH_i within this range would have had a high selective advantage to the earliest cells. The "choice" of a pH_i in this range likely was coupled inexorably to the selection of histidine as the amino acid to be used in diverse biochemical processes in which a titratable side-chain was required. At least among the 20 amino acids found in contemporary proteins, histidine is unique in having a pK value in the pH range that ensures maximal ionization of metabolites.

MEMBRANE SYSTEMS AND ADAPTATION OF LIPIDS

Key Roles of Biological Membranes

Membrane-based processes generally are highly sensitive to changes in temperature. These sensitivities may be much greater than those exhibited by processes occurring in the aqueous phase of the cell, and because of this membranes may play vital roles in establishing organisms' thermal tolerance limits. Why are membrane-based processes so thermally sensitive? Commonly this sensitivity is due to the strong effects of temperature on the physical properties of membrane lipids, which account for about one-half of the mass of a membrane and have strong influences on the proteins they bathe. Adaptive modulation of the lipid milieu in which membrane proteins conduct their functions is a critical and ubiquitous aspect of adaptation to temperature. These adaptations bear certain similarities to the pH–temperature effects discussed above. In each case, an adaptive change in the milieu in which proteins carry out their tasks fosters retention of critical structural and functional traits of the proteins. Furthermore, these two types of extrinsic influences on protein structure and function are characteristic of adaptation to temperature by all taxa. Thus, as in the case of temperature–pH–protein relationships, we will find that organisms belonging to all domains of life tightly modulate the lipid compositions of their membranes to facilitate retention of physiological function in the face of different temperatures. However, even though the "goal" of adaptive changes in lipid systems is identical among all types of organisms, there are myriad ways in which this "goal" is achieved. The adaptive plasticity of organisms perhaps finds no better illustration than in the case of the types of compensatory alterations found in membranes from differently adapted or differently acclimatized/acclimated prokaryotic and eukaryotic organisms.

To appreciate the importance of temperature-adaptive changes in the compositions of biological membranes, notably in the types of lipids present in the membrane bilayer, it is instructive to review the diverse roles played by membranes. Membranes serve a wide range of essential functions, all of which are highly sensitive to changes in temperature, and each of which is a potential site of lethal damage by high- or low extremes of temperature. The most obvious and universal function of membranes is their role as *physical barriers* between (i) intracellular compartments, such as the cytoplasm and organelles; (ii) intra- and extracellular fluid compartments in multicellular organisms; and (iii) the organism and its external environment. Membranes prevent the free movement of water, small solutes, and macromolecules from taking place. Serious breaches in these membrane barriers, if not rapidly repaired, are almost certain to lead to cellular death. The "importance of being ionized" discussed above is but one indication of the significance of controlling movement of solutes between membrane-enclosed compartments of the cell or organism and between the organism and its environment.

Although serving as barriers in many different contexts, membranes also play major roles in *transport* by governing movements of specific molecules between different regions of the cell and between intra- and extracellular spaces. Movements of water through specific pores (via protein channels termed aquaporins), inorganic ions through specific channels such as that provided by the Na^+-K^+-adenosine triphosphatase (Na^+-K^+-ATPase), and proteins via specific mechanisms such as exocytosis are dependent on the integrity of membrane structure overall and on the provision of the appropriate lipid microenvironment for specific transport proteins. Conservation of tightly regulated transmembrane movement of substances ranging from water (Robertson and Hazel, 1999), to small ions, to macromolecules (Padrón et al., 2000) will be seen to be a critical aspect of adaptation to temperature.

Membranes also function in *bioenergetics*. The ability of eukaryotic cells to generate ATP aerobically is based on the presence of elaborate electron and proton transport systems in the inner membrane of the mitochondrion (chapter 2). One of the critical events in the bioenergetic functions of membranes is the establishment of proton gradients and the exploitation of the potential energy in these gradients to drive the endergonic production of ATP. The potential energy stored in the ion gradients that are established by membrane pumps like the Na^+-K^+-ATPase can also be used to drive endergonic transport processes, for instance, the uptake into the cell of dissolved organic molecules like free amino acids, using the energy provided by dissipation of a sodium ion gradient. Ion gradients and their dissipation also play major roles in *thermoregu-*

lation. Uncoupling of proton entry into the mitochondrial matrix from generation of ATP by the F_1-ATPase releases vast amounts of heat that can be used to warm the organism. As discussed later in this chapter, a wide variety of organisms—animals and plants—appear to "waste" the potential energy of mitochondrial proton gradients to warm themselves. Transmembrane ion flux involving Na^+ and K^+ movements driven by the Na^+-K^+-ATPase also may be important in the thermoregulatory strategies of birds and mammals. These endotherms are hypothesized to generate a substantial fraction of the heat they require for thermoregulation through splitting ATP during Na^+ and K^+ transport across the plasma membrane (see chapter 2).

Membranes also are of critical importance in *cellular signaling processes*. Binding of hormones to the external surface of a membrane leads to generation of signals that activate enzymes or regulate the expression of genes. In certain types of signaling processes, membrane lipids serve as the raw material for fabricating signaling molecules, as in the case of lipid-derived second messenger compounds like inositol 1,4,5-trisphosphate (IP_3) and diacylglycerol. Like other membrane-based activities, these important integrative mechanisms stand to be severely compromised by temperature-induced alterations in membrane structure.

Neural activity, which involves transmembrane ion fluxes and the release and uptake of chemical transmitters at synapses, is a highly important membrane-based function and a primary site of thermal perturbation in animals. Both axonal conduction and, especially, synaptic transmission may be involved in setting thermal tolerance limits.

The sensitivities to temperature of all of these membrane-localized functions arise from the complex effects that temperature has on both the protein and lipid components of the membrane. Likely of greatest importance, however, are the effects of thermally induced changes in the physical states of lipids on the functions of proteins. Many aspects of thermal perturbation of membrane function—as well as key elements of the adaptive changes that occur in membrane lipids in response to change in temperature—

reflect the pivotal role that the lipid microenvironment of a membrane protein plays in supporting the protein's function. As in the case of osmolyte–protein and proton–protein relationships, adaptation of membrane-based processes is seen to depend very strongly on the establishment, through complex regulatory mechanisms, of a fit milieu for protein function.

The Composition of Membranes: General Characteristics and Fine-Scale Heterogeneity

In order to understand (i) why lipid-containing structures are so sensitive to temperature, (ii) why proteins are so affected by alterations in the physical state of the membrane, and (iii) what types of raw material are present for adaptive modifications of membranes, it is necessary to review the fundamental constituents and organization of cellular membranes. The typical membrane surrounding most types of eukaryotic and prokaryotic cells or an organelle is a lipid bilayer on which and in which are found a wide variety of proteins (figure 7.18). In many membranes, proteins and lipids are present in approximately equal amounts in terms of contributions to total mass. It follows from this fact that, on average, proteins may be separated from each other by only a few lipid molecules. However, as discussed below, neither proteins nor specific classes of lipid are distributed randomly in the membrane. Rather, membranes are highly structured at a fine-scale level such that proteins serving a common function are organized together, and lipids of different types are thought to be organized into various domains associated with the specific types of functions they help to support.

Proteins that intercalate into the membrane—and many proteins involved in transmembrane transport and signaling have several membrane-spanning domains—are termed *integral* or *intrinsic* proteins. The anchoring of integral proteins may involve hydrophobic interactions with the nonpolar core of the bilayer and polar and charged interactions with groups on the inner or outer surfaces of the membrane. Proteins that are attached to the surface of the membrane and do not penetrate into the core of the bilayer are called *peripheral* or *extrinsic* proteins. They often can be removed by treating the membrane with buffers of high ionic strength, whereas integral proteins may require extraction with detergents to free them of lipids.

The lipid bilayer is stabilized by the same types of forces discussed in the context of protein structure, forces that derive in considerable measure from the different propensities of distinct regions of membrane lipids and proteins to interact with water. Lipids commonly are amphipathic, having some regions that avoid water and others that interact well with water. The hydrophobic effect is responsible for the distribution of the nonpolar acyl chains of the phospholipids within the internal core of the bilayer, away from water (figures 7.18 and 17.9). The polar (e.g., ethanolamine) or charged (e.g., choline) headgroups (figure 7.19) face the aqueous phase on either side of the membrane. Cholesterol is also amphipathic and intercalates into the nonpolar bilayer while retaining interactions with the polar headgroup region. The steroid moiety is buried within, and parallel with, the acyl chains and the 3-β-hydroxyl group lies near the ester carbonyl linkage of the phospholipids (Robertson and Hazel, 1997).

This general "textbook" picture of membrane structure, although correct overall for most bilayer membranes, misrepresents or obscures two extremely important aspects of membrane structure: dynamism and heterogeneity. Much as a static image of a protein obtained through X-ray diffraction fails to portray the dynamic nature of protein structural fluctuations—such models tell us a lot about the enthalpy of the system but little about its entropy—the drawing of membrane structure shown in figure 7.18 fails to portray the types of movements that characterize the constituents of membranes. Thus, rather than remaining static on or within the bilayer, proteins may move laterally, along the plane of the membrane. Such movements of proteins may be necessary for signal transduction and other important physiological functions. In addition, the lipid molecules are in rapid thermal motion, and the extent of this motion determines the lateral

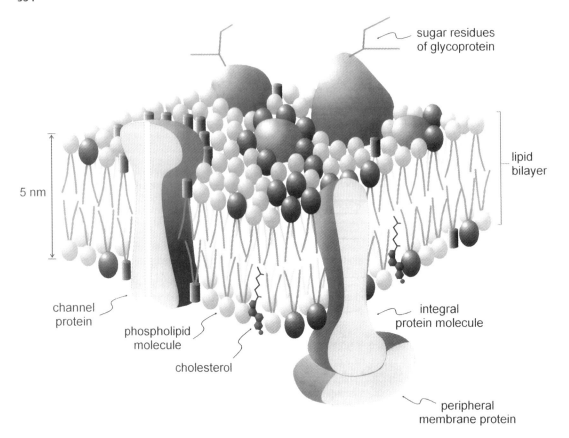

sugar residues
of glycoprotein

lipid
bilayer

5 nm

channel
protein

phospholipid
molecule

cholesterol

integral
protein molecule

peripheral
membrane protein

Figure 7.18. A cartoon of a bilayer membrane, e.g., a plasma membrane, illustrating the principal components of the membrane and their organization. Proteins that extend through the bilayer are termed integral membrane proteins. Proteins held to the surface of the membrane are called peripheral proteins. Proteins may have sugar residues of varying chain-length attached to them. Heterogeneity of lipid composition is indicated for headgroups (lipid class) by differently shaped and shaded headgroups; acyl chain structures (lipid species) also vary widely. Two molecules of cholesterol insert into the inner leaflet of the membrane. More than 200 individual types of lipids may be present in a single membrane, and their organization may be nonrandom, as shown by the preferential clustering of different lipid classes around the integral membrane proteins. However, lipid clustering around proteins and, in general, lipid position in membranes is dynamic. Lipids may move rapidly in the plane of the membrane (lateral diffusion) and, at a much slower rate, they may "flip-flop" between hemilayers (transverse diffusion). Proteins tend not to undergo transverse diffusion, so they maintain their asymmetrical distributions in and on the membrane.

movements of lipids, the "flip-flopping" of lipids between the inner and outer leaflets of the bilayer, and the physical state (phase and static order; see below) of the membrane. The thermal movements of acyl chains are of particular importance in establishing what is defined below as the "physical state" of the membrane (Hazel, 1995). Rotations about carbon–carbon single bonds (gauche rotamers) occur along the length of the acyl chain, leading to a relatively high degree of disorder in the bilayer core. This motion is not uniform along the full length of an acyl chain, however. There is some constraint on movement for the first 8–10 carbon atoms of the chain. As discussed below (see figure 7.20), changes in temperature not only alter the rates of C–C rotations, but also lead to shifts in the phase state of the membrane. These dynamic aspects of membrane structure are key to membrane function and to the sensitivities of membranes to changes in temperature. Both the lipid and protein moieties of

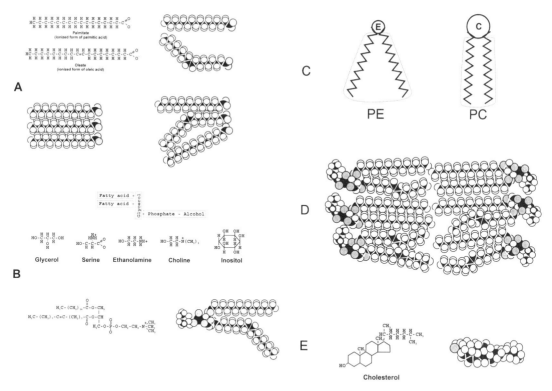

Figure 7.19. Structures of lipids. (A) (Top) Chemical structures (left) and space-filling models (right) of the ionized forms of two fatty acids: palmitic acid (16 carbons, no double bonds, melting temperature 63°C), and oleic acid (18 carbons, one *cis* double bond, melting temperature 16°C). (Bottom) The effect of addition of a single *cis* double bond on the geometry of lipids. Shown on the left are three molecules of stearic acid (18 carbons, no double bonds, melting temperature 69.6°C) that pack tightly because of their linear geometries. Shown on the right is the effect of adding a single molecule of oleic acid on membrane geometry. (B) Structures of phosphoglycerides. (Top) general structure of phosphoglycerides. (Middle) Glycerol and the common head groups of phosphoglycerides (determinants of phosphoglyceride class). (Bottom) Chemical structure and space-filling model of one species of phosphatidylcholine (PC). (C) Cartoon illustrating the different geometries of phosphatidylethanolamine (PE) and phosphatidylcholine (PC). (D) Space-filling model of a cross section through a highly fluid phospholipid bilayer. (E) Cholesterol: (left) chemical structure; (right) space-filling model.

the membrane occur in broad ensembles of configurational and positional states, a fact that static views of the membrane tend to obscure.

A second aspect of membrane structure that often is not manifested adequately in simple diagrams of membranes is the high degree of *heterogeneity in lipid composition* and lipid *domain organization* found in most membranes. Membranes contain a large number of different lipids and, despite the thermal motion in the membrane, these lipids are not arrayed in a random or chaotic fashion. Figure 7.19 illustrates the basis of the heterogeneity in lipid composi-

tion of membranes. Variation in structure arises from three primary sources: (1) different types of lipids, including phospholipids and sterols like cholesterol, (2) different headgroups in phospholipids (lipid *classes*), and (3) widely varying acyl chain composition of phospholipids (lipid *species*). Among phospholipids, an enormous number of structural permutations are possible, and cells exploit this potential to provide a wide range of specific lipid domains for different membrane proteins and for adapting membranes to environmental change. In a single bilayer, it is estimated that hundreds of

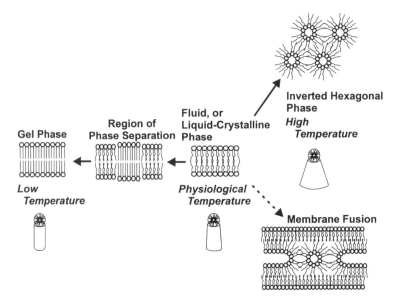

Figure 7.20. Effects of temperature on *phase* and *static order* of the membrane bilayer. Reductions in temperature from the physiological temperature of the organism (cell), that is, temperatures near those of adaptation or acclimation, lead to formation of gel-phase regions, which may separate from lipids that remain in the liquid-crystalline phase, the phase characteristic of most of the bilayer at physiological temperatures. At sufficiently low temperatures, the bulk of the membrane phospholipids enter the gel phase.

As temperature is raised above physiological temperatures, the propensity for lipids to form the inverted hexagonal (H_{II}) phase is increased, in part because the geometry of the acyl chains changes, with the lipid assuming a more "fanned-out" configuration (see the three cartoons of lipid molecules shown under "low temperature," "physiological temperature," and "high temperature"). Inverted hexagonal phase structures may be important under physiological conditions, for instance, during exocytosis. Thus, some capacity for forming H_{II} phase structures must be maintained. (Figure modified after Hazel, 1995.)

different phospholipid species are present. The inner and outer leaflets of a bilayer may differ in phospholipid composition. With changing temperature, each of the primary sources of variation in lipid composition is tapped to alter membrane composition: cholesterol content, ratios of different lipid classes, and acyl chain compositions of phospholipids all vary extensively—and adaptively—as discussed below.

The complex suite of membrane lipids would seem to create a potential for localized variation in lipid composition around specific membrane proteins. The roles played by such lipid domains are an area of active research (Williams, 1998). In view of the dynamic nature of membrane structure, however, it is extremely difficult experimentally to isolate and characterize small regions of the bilayer. Despite these difficulties, investigators of fine-scale membrane

structure are beginning to draw a new picture of the organization of membrane lipids. In essence, the complex mixture of phospholipid classes and species is not distributed randomly in the bilayer. Rather, specific types of lipids are organized into small structural units—domains—which are likely to provide the appropriate lipid microenvironment for specific types of membrane proteins. The needs for such protein-specific domains are not hard to envision. The three-dimensional configurations of proteins differ, and to satisfactorily incorporate ("pack") a protein into the bilayer, lipids of different geometries may be required. Also of importance is the need to provide for each membrane protein the appropriate microenvironment within which the changes in conformation or position required for function can occur. For example, a highly ordered or rigid lipid microenvironment might inhibit protein conformational changes and interrupt the reversible assembly of multiprotein complexes. Thus, as in the case of our analysis of protein structure–function relationships, we can envision a scenario for membrane proteins in which the appropriate balance between flexibility and rigidity of the lipids surrounding the protein plays a key role in governing protein function. As seen in so many contexts of adaptation to the environment, intrinsic properties of proteins and adaptive change in extrinsic factors that affect proteins play important complementary roles.

Homeophasic Adaptation: The Dynamic Phase Behavior Model

It is important to begin the analysis of temperature-adaptive changes in membranes with an attempt to define the fundamental aspects of membranes that demand close conservation under all thermal conditions, in most, if not all, types of membranes. In view of the multiple functions of membranes and the complexity of membrane structure, it might seem a daunting challenge to identify those features of membranes that are most sensitive to thermal perturbation and, thus, serve as focal points of adaptive change. However, two primary aspects of membrane structure stand out as being especially important as targets for conservation during adaptation to temperature: *membrane phase* and *membrane static order* ("viscosity" or "fluidity"). The phase structure and the static order of the bilayer influence virtually all of the functional properties of membranes. Thus, most of the alterations in membrane composition noted during adaptation to temperature, whether comparisons involve differently adapted species or differently acclimatized (or acclimated) conspecifics, can be interpreted in terms of defending these two traits.

Temperature has strong effects on the phase of the bilayer

Figure 7.20 illustrates how increases and decreases in temperature affect the phase structure of the membrane bilayer. At physiological temperatures, that is, at temperatures near the adaptation or acclimation temperature, the bilayer exists in what is commonly termed a "liquid-crystalline" or "fluid" phase (Hazel, 1995). The expression "liquid-crystalline" denotes a balance between flexibility and order in the membrane lipids. This balance is temperature sensitive: as cell temperature is acutely decreased, the order of the membrane lipids increases. Motion of acyl chains is reduced and they begin to align closely and pack more tightly within the bilayer, allowing stronger van der Waals interactions. At a sufficiently low temperature, the *phase transition temperature* (T_m), regions of the bilayer enter what is termed a *gel phase*. Lowering temperature does not lead to a quantitative conversion of the fluid-phase bilayer to a gel phase because of the heterogeneity of lipids present in the membrane. Thus, over a certain range of temperatures, fluid- and gel-phase regions may coexist in the membrane; this is referred to as *phase separation* (Hazel, 1995). In the gel-phase regions, the functional properties of the membrane may be severely impaired. During gelation, the distribution of different species of phospholipid may shift, leading to localized aggregations of certain types of lipids in highly viscous aggregates. Integral membrane proteins tend to be excluded from gel-phase lipid clusters, so these proteins may form nonfunctional aggregates when gelation commences. Lateral movement of membrane proteins may be restricted, leading to a reduction in activity of functions that rely on protein diffusion. Formation of gel-phase regions may create packing defects in the membrane at junctions between fluid- and gel-phase zones, and these may cause breaches in the permeability barriers of the membrane that lead to uncontrolled fluxes of water and solutes. The transition from a liquid-crystalline phase to a gel phase at low temperatures thus presents a serious threat to cellular survival.

When temperature is raised, the membrane bilayer not only becomes increasingly fluid due to enhanced motions of acyl chain, but it also tends to shift increasingly towards forming lipid aggregates in the *inverted hexagonal phase* (*hexagonal II, H_{II}, phase*) (Hazel, 1995). The temperature at which this type of phase change occurs is termed T_h. The tendency for phospholipids to enter the hexagonal II phase is due to the effect of increasing temperature on the geometry of individual phospholipid molecules, as shown in figure 7.20. As temperature is increased, the increased mobility of acyl chains causes them to fan out and assume a more conical configuration. Packing of conically shaped lipids in the bilayer is more difficult than incorporating relatively cylindrical lipids. In fact, conically shaped phospholipids can only be incorporated into a bilayer if substantial amounts of cylindrically shaped lipids also are present. As the ratio of these two geometrical classes of lipid changes with rising temperature, the propensity for hexagonal phase aggregates to form increases. As they do, bilayer structure is disrupted and the barrier properties of the bilayer are destroyed.

Phospholipid composition is adjusted to maintain proper phase structure

The adaptations that thwart inappropriate phase changes have been presented as theories of *homeophasic adaptation* (McElhaney, 1984) and *dynamic phase behavior* (Hazel, 1995). In essence, both theories stress the same primary points: the lipid composition of the bilayer must be modified in the face of temperature change to conserve the appropriate phase structure. The liquid-crystalline phase must be conserved at low temperatures. At higher temperatures the propensity to form the hexagonal II phase must not become too great. Thus, T_m and T_h must be adjusted during adaptation.

The dynamic phase behavior model of Hazel emphasizes that the membrane must remain suitably poised between propensities for forming both bilayer (lamellar) and hexagonal II structures. Although excessive formation of hexagonal phases at high temperatures is disruptive of cellular function—and potentially of lethal consequence to the cell—under normal conditions cellular membranes must possess domains in which hexagonal II structures can be assembled. These structures are essential components of such normal membrane functions as membrane fusion during exo- and endocytosis and membrane trafficking. Hexagonal II phases are also important in regulating the activities of certain membrane-localized enzymes, for instance, protein kinase C, phospholipase A_2, phospholipase C, Mg^{2+} ATPase, and ubiquinone-cytochrome c reductase (see Williams, 1998, for review). Loss of ability to form hexagonal structures thus could be as damaging to the cell as having too high a tendency for phospholipids to shift from lamellar to hexagonal phases.

The dynamic phase behavior model stresses that the ratio of conically shaped and cylindrically shaped lipids must be closely regulated so as to permit the formation of physiologically required hexagonal II phases, yet to prevent unregulated formation of membrane-disruptive hexagonal structures. The primary mechanism by which cells regulate the hexagonal II forming propensities of membrane phospholipids is quite simple and relies on the differences among headgroups in fostering cylindrical versus conical orientations of acyl chains. Phosphatidyl choline (PC), with its bulky and charged headgroup (figure 7.19), favors the cylindrical form of acyl chain orientation. Phosphatidyl ethanolamine (PE) favors the conical geometry required for hexagonal II structures to form. As would be predicted from these facts, the ratio of PE to PC in cellular membranes exhibits a strong dependence on temperature: the more warm-adapted the animal, the lower is the PE:PC ratio, that is, the lower the inherent tendency of the membrane to form hexagonal II phases (Hazel, 1995). The tendency for acyl chains to fan out into a conical configuration as temperature rises is thus offset by a shift towards a class of phospholipid, phosphatidyl choline, which favors the cylindrical geometry needed for a stable lamellar phase.

Differences in the PE:PC ratio are observed among differently adapted animals and between differently acclimated/acclimatized conspecifics (Hazel, 1995), as discussed in more detail below. An analogous type of homeophasic adaptation is found in higher plants. The ratio of monoglucosyldiglycerides (MGDG) (bilayer-stabilizing) to diglucosyldiglycerides (DGDG) (bilayer-destabilizing) increases with adaptation temperature (Hazel, 1995).

Homeoviscous Adaptation: Conservation of Static Order

What is meant by the "physical state" of the bilayer?

The earliest general model of adaptation to temperature in membrane lipids focused on the "physical state" ("static order" or "viscosity" [= 1/"fluidity"]) of the bilayer. The finding that the physical state of membrane lipids from *Escherichia coli* cultured at different temperatures was similar at the different growth temperatures led to the *homeoviscous adaptation hypothesis*, which states that lipid composition is modified during thermal acclimation to facilitate retention of a relatively stable membrane physical state (Sinensky, 1974). At the outset of any discussion of homeoviscous adaptation, it is important to examine carefully what is meant by "physical state" (or the related terms "static order," "viscosity," and "fluidity"). In such an analysis, one must also consider the physical methods that are used to make such measurements—and the limitations of these techniques.

By "physical state," lipid biophysicists refer to aspects of the bilayer that reflect the *freedom of motion* and the *extent of motion* of lipids, especially the acyl chains of phospholipids. When motions of acyl chains are relatively unconstrained, they will undergo more rapid motion and the region of motion will also be larger. The fanning out of acyl chains from cylindrical to conical configurations as temperature is increased can be viewed in the latter context. These physical states of membrane lipids are commonly measured by techniques that quantify the freedom of movement of some type of probe molecule that has been added to the membrane. In the most general of terms, the freedom of movement of a probe that intercalates into a membrane will be a direct reflection of the degree to which the membrane hinders the rate and extent of motion of the probe. One commonly used probe is 1,6-diphenyl-1,3,5-hexatriene (DPH). This probe is fluorescent, and when excited by polarized light, it will subsequently emit light of the same state of polarization. If probe movement is extensive during the period between excitation and emission, the

polarization signal will be relatively low. Thus, the intensity of fluorescence emission of polarized light, commonly expressed as *fluorescence anisotropy*, can provide a quantitative estimate of the physical state of the membrane. Fluorescence anisotropy, r, is related to the polarization intensity (P) by the equation:

$$r = 2P/(3 - P)$$

While useful in providing an overall picture of membrane physical state, measurements of fluorescence anisotropy have strict limitations. The most obvious of these limitations has to do with the scale of resolution that can be obtained. Probes such as DPH or *trans*-parinaric acid provide estimates only of bulk (globally averaged) physical state, not of the physical states of individual domains of lipids surrounding specific proteins. For this reason, it is not surprising that the effects of temperature on specific membrane-localized proteins may not reflect thermal effects on fluorescence anisotropy of the membrane at large (see Hazel, 1995; Williams, 1998). Another uncertainly about molecular probes like DPH and *trans*-parinaric acid concerns whether the fluorescence anisotropy effects arise primarily from the distance over which the probe moves (amplitude of movement) or the rate of probe movement. Studies by Behan-Martin et al. (1993), which used sophisticated, time-resolved fluorescence spectroscopy, suggest that the amplitude, rather than the rate of probe movement, is what is primarily subject to adaptive change.

Homeoviscous adaptation is extensive, although not always complete

Despite these limitations in the ability of fluorescence anisotropy to quantify physiologically relevant changes in membrane physical state, use of this technique in comparative studies of differently adapted (-acclimated) organisms has revealed a remarkably consistent relationship between the thermal history of the organism and membrane physical state. Figure 7.21 illustrates the relationships between fluorescence anisotropy (DPH) and measurement

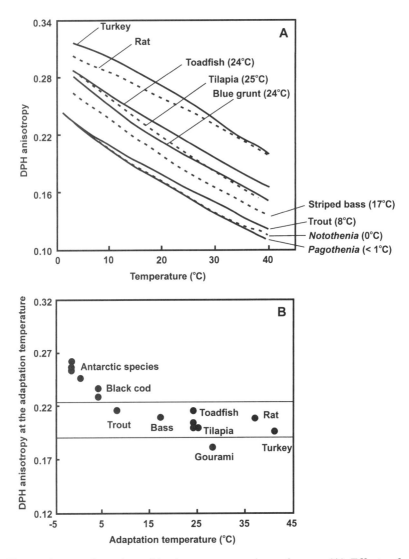

Figure 7.21. Homeoviscous adaptation of brain synaptosomal membranes. (A) Effects of measurement temperature on the physical states of synaptosomal membranes of differently adapted vertebrates, as determined by fluorescence anisotropy using 1,6-diphenyl-1,3,5-hexatriene (DPH) as the probe. (B) DPH anisotropy at each species' adaptation temperature. The horizontal lines enclose species where essentially complete homeoviscous adaptation was found. (Figure modified after Logue et al., 2000.)

temperature for brain synaptosomal membranes (synaptosomes) isolated from vertebrates whose body temperature ranged from approximately −1.9°C (Antarctic notothenioid fishes: *Pagothenia borchgrevinki, Trematomus bernacchii, Dissostichus mawsoni,* and *Notothenia neglecta,* and an Antarctic zoarcid (eelpout): *Lycodichthys dearborni*) to 39°C (turkey) (Logue et al., 2000; also see Behan-Martin et al., 1993; Gracey et al., 1996). When fluor-escence anisotropy values for any single temperature of measurement are compared, there is seen to be a regular increase in fluorescence anisotropy with increasing adaptation temperature (upper panel). Thus, the inherent static order of the synaptosomal membranes is greatest in the most warm-adapted species and lowest in Antarctic fishes. When anisotropy values at the adaptation temperatures of the species are plotted (figure 7.21, lower panel), a high degree of compensation to temperature, i.e., a pronounced homeoviscous adaptation, is manifested. Antarctic fishes and a cold-temperate notothenioid, the New Zealand black cod (*Notothenia angustata*), have higher degrees of static order than the other species, at normal body temperatures, and membranes of pearl gourami fish (*Trichogaster leeri*) have a slightly lower degree of order. Nonetheless, there is a high degree of homeoviscous adaptation among these differently adapted species. The pattern seen in these experiments done with DPH as the fluorescent probe may actually under estimate the full extent of homeoviscous adaptation. Studies by Behan-Martin et al. (1993) showed that measurements made with *trans*-parinaric acid showed a higher degree of homeoviscous adaptation than found in experiments using DPH. *Trans*-parinaric acid may provide a more realistic estimate of bulk membrane order because, unlike DPH, it is more apt to partition into the membrane in a way that parallels the orientation of phospholipid molecules in the bilayer (Behan-Martin et al., 1993).

The incomplete extent of homeoviscous adaptation seen for some species when DPH was used as the probe of membrane physical state reflects a common observation: the completeness or "efficacy" of homeoviscous adaptation is often less than one 100%. *Homeoviscous efficacy* is defined as the ratio of the difference in measurement temperature required to produce identical polarization (anisotropy) values to the actual difference in body temperatures between the organisms under study. In interspecific comparisons, homeoviscous efficacy ranges between approximately 0.7 and 1.0, whereas in intraspecific comparisons, efficacies are generally lower, commonly between 0.2 and 0.5 (for review, see Hazel, 1995). Based on the observed differences in homeoviscous efficacy between probes (Behan-Martin et al., 1993), some of the incomplete homeoviscous adaptation found using DPH could be an artifact of the probe itself. And, to return to the caveat made earlier, homeoviscous efficacy in local lipid domains near specific proteins cannot be unambiguously determined from such bulk measurements.

Homeoviscous efficacy varies widely among membranes. As a general rule, membranes with complex functions, such as mitochondrial membranes, exhibit a higher degree of homeoviscous efficacy than membranes with fewer functions, e.g., myelin (Hazel, 1995). It is possible that a membrane with diverse functions supported by diverse types of proteins will require elaborate restructuring of numerous lipid domains, if function is to be conserved as temperature changes. To the extent that the different functions of membranes can be grouped according to "importance," barrier functions may be less demanding of homeoviscous adaptation than functions such as signaling, transport, and ATP generation, all of which may depend on a closely regulated physical state for the domains surrounding the relevant proteins.

Homeophasic and Homeoviscous Adaptation: Correlations with Biochemical, Physiological, and Behavioral Functions

If homeophasic and homeoviscous adaptations are critical in responding to changes in cell temperature, and if physical measurements using probes like DPH and *trans*-parinaric acid do provide adequate estimates of physiologically relevant changes in membrane physical state, then strong correlations should be observed between lipid physical state, on the one hand, and biochemical, physiological, and behavioral traits, on the other. Although there are instances in which a change in bulk membrane fluidity is not reflected in a change in a specific membrane-localized function (see Williams, 1998), the many correlations found between shifts in fluorescence anisotropy and function argue convincingly for causal relationships between membrane physical state and function that are important in adaptation to temperature. The correlations between shifts in PE:PC ratios and function likewise suggest widespread roles for homeophasic modifications of membranes. These correlations have been found in studies of various levels of biological organization, ranging from individual proteins to behavior of whole organisms.

Effects of membrane order on enzymatic activity and stability

The extent to which the functional and structural properties of proteins are influenced by the balance between stabilizing and destabilizing forces in the protein's microenvironment is well illustrated by membrane-localized proteins, whose activities are influenced by the domain of lipid molecules that surround them. Many membrane proteins require lipids, in some cases specific types of lipids, to be active. Most proteins that intercalate into the bilayer are likely to be influenced by the specific physical properties of the lipid domain with which they are in close contact. Variation in the order of the lipid domain around an enzymatic protein can have a strong influence on catalytic activity due to what are termed "viscotropic effects." This expression refers to the influences that alterations in the lipid microenvironment of a protein have on the energy changes that accompany functionally essential conformational changes of the protein. A relatively viscous lipid microenvironment may increase the amount of energy that is needed to allow the protein to displace vicinal lipids during changes in conformation.

As shown in figure 7.22(A), increases in membrane static order caused by supplementing the growth medium of Chinese hamster ovary cells with cholesterol led to regular decreases in the specific activity of the Na^+-K^+-ATPase (Sinensky et al., 1979). Presumably, the increased viscosity of the domain of lipids adjacent to the enzyme hindered the conformational changes required for ion transport, leading to reductions in enzymatic activity.

Viscotropic effects in cells cultured at a single temperature may be indicative of effects that result from immediate temperature-dependent changes in lipid order and from subsequent adaptive alterations in lipid composition. Acute decreases in temperature increase static order and thereby increase resistance to conformational movements; however, the compensatory decrease in intrinsic membrane order in cold-adapted or cold-acclimatized organisms (figure 7.21) resulting from changes in composi-

tion of the bilayer would alleviate this inhibition. Modifications in lipid domains around the proteins may be responsible for the temperature compensation of rates of activity of membrane-localized proteins. Increases in specific activity of cytochrome c oxidase in mitochondria of cold-acclimated goldfish (Wodtke, 1981) and of Na^+-K^+-ATPase in erythrocytes of cold-acclimated trout (Raynard and Cossins, 1991) were not linked with changes in enzyme concentration. Rather, alterations in lipid microenvir-

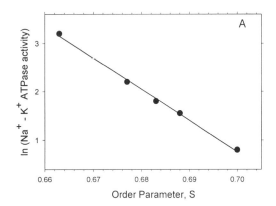

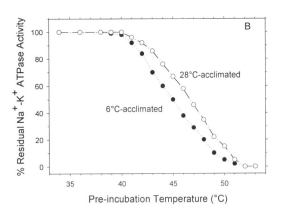

Figure 7.22. Effects of lipid microenvironments on physiological functions. (A) Effects of changes in membrane order (Order parameter, S) generated by alterations in cholesterol content on the activity of Na^+-K^+-ATPase of Chinese hamster ovary cells (after Sinensky et al., 1979). (B) Resistance to heat denaturation of Na^+-K^+-ATPase in gills of differently acclimated goldfish. Membranes were pre-incubated for 15 min at a series of temperatures prior to measurement of Na^+-K^+-ATPase at 25°C. (After Cossins et al., 1981.)

onments of the enzymes were proposed to have led to enhancement of catalytic activity.

The effects of membrane order on enzymatic activity observed for the Na^+-K^+-ATPase of hamster ovary cells mirror effects noted for a wide range of membrane-localized proteins involved in enzymatic activity, transport, and cellular signaling. There is a general tendency for proteins to exhibit increased activity as the order of their lipid microenvironment decreases, albeit there is a limit to this relationship at extremes of temperature where membranes undergo phase changes that disrupt function of membrane-localized proteins.

Viscotropic effects on protein function may be linked to changes in protein stability. As demonstrated in the context of solute effects on the activity and thermal stability of enzymes (chapter 6), a microenvironment that enhances the activity of a protein may reduce its stability, and vice versa. In the case of viscotropic effects, a similar relationship is likely. Figure 7.22(B) shows how the thermal stability of the Na^+-K^+-ATPase of goldfish gill rises with increased acclimation temperature (Cossins et al., 1981). Although it is not known if the gill membranes of the 6°C and 28°C fish used in these experiments differed in static order, it is reasonable to assume that this was the case, and that at any given test temperature the more viscous microenvironment of the enzyme from the 28°C-acclimated fish inhibited unfolding of the protein at elevated temperatures.

The effects that lipid composition has on the activities of membrane-localized proteins might suggest that temperature compensation of metabolism could be achieved through incorporating into membranes of cold-adapted organisms extremely fluid lipids, which would allow conformation changes of enzymes to occur with relatively low energy barriers. However, compensation of metabolic rates to temperature does not seem to exploit alterations in membrane lipid composition. Homeoviscous and homeophasic adaptations seem targeted to restore the status quo of the membrane's physical state, rather than to serve as mechanisms for offsetting the Q_{10} effects of temperature on rate processes. For instance, it does not appear that organisms adapting to low temperatures

generate hyperfluid, ultralow viscosity membranes in order to provide a lipid milieu in which their membrane-localized enzymes can work at exceptionally high, that is to say, temperature-compensated, rates. What might be gained by this strategy in terms of rates of enzymatic activity is likely to be more than offset by impairments in other roles of membranes, such as barrier functions.

Temperature effects on mitochondrial respiration and membrane order

Mitochondrial membranes exhibit a high degree of homeoviscous adaptation, which may be a reflection of the large number of key membrane-localized functions performed by this organelle (Hazel, 1995). Alterations in physical properties of mitochondrial membranes are correlated with changes in the responses of oxygen consumption rates to rising temperature. Most notably, adaptive shifts are found in the temperatures at which mitochondrial respiration is heat-inactivated. The relationship between acclimation or adaptation temperature and thermal resistance of mitochondrial respiration is seen especially clearly when respiration rates are graphed on Arrhenius axes (figure 7.23, upper panel). As temperature of measurement is increased, the rate of respiration initially rises linearly with temperature. However, at some high temperature, termed the Arrhenius break temperature (ABT), a discontinuity ("break") in the sign of the slope of the Arrhenius plot is observed. Thus, at temperatures above the ABT, the rate of respiration drops with rising temperature, likely as a consequence of irreversible heat damage to the mitochondria.

Among differently adapted species of fishes and invertebrates, the ABT of mitochondrial respiration varies regularly with adaptation temperature (figure 7.23, lower panel). The animals that were compared included deep-sea invertebrates from both warm (hydrothermal vent) and cold habitats plus several shallow occurring marine invertebrates and fishes adapted to widely different temperatures, including the Antarctic fish *Trematomus bernacchii* (boxed + symbol; Dahlhoff et al., 1991; Weinstein and Somero, 1998). Also

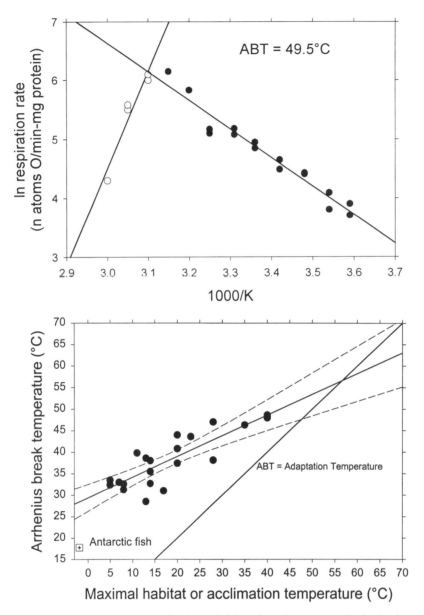

Figure 7.23. Effects of temperature on mitochondrial function. (Upper panel). Arrhenius plot illustrating the slope discontinuity ("break") that commonly occurs at a high temperature of measurement, the Arrhenius break temperature (ABT). Data are for mitochondria of the hydrothermal vent tubeworm *Riftia pachyptila* (after Dahlhoff et al., 1991). (Lower panel) Arrhenius break temperatures for mitochondrial respiration of diverse invertebrates and fishes. The open square is for mitochondrial respiration of the Antarctic nototheniid fish *Trematomus bernacchii* and is not included in the regression analysis. A line of identify (ABT = adaptation temperature) is also shown (see text for analysis). (Data from Dahlhoff and Somero, 1993b; Dahlhoff et al., 1991; Weinstein and Somero, 1998.)

show on this figure is a line of identity, where ABT = adaptation temperature. Two characteristics of this line of identity raise interesting issues concerning thermal tolerance relationships of animals. First, the vertical distance between the ABT regression line for the 20 species and the line of identity decreases with rising adaptation or acclimation temperature. Thus, the more warm-adapted is the species, the closer is the ABT of mitochondrial respiration and, by extension, the organism's upper lethal temperature, to its adaptation temperature. We revisit this correlation in a later section of this chapter: "Thermal optima and thermal tolerance limits." Second, the intersection of these two lines at approximately 55°C–60°C has implications concerning the upper thermal limits for animals (and, perhaps, for eukaryotes in general). One interpretation that might be given to the temperature of intersection is that mitochondria of animals would be unable to adapt to temperatures above 55°C–60°C. In fact, these temperatures match closely the highest body temperatures estimated for animals. Among the most thermophilic of animals are desert ants of the genus *Cataglyphis*, which forage at temperatures above 50°C (Gehring and Wehner, 1995). Critical thermal maxima for two species, *C. bicolor* and *C. bombycina*, are 54°C and 55°C, respectively. To our knowledge, these are the highest thermal tolerance limits estimated for any animal, at least for any terrestrial species. Even higher tolerance limits have been suggested for certain deep-sea animals. Cary et al. (1998) presented evidence that a deep-sea hydrothermal vent polychaete worm (*Alvinella pompejana*) encountered water temperatures within its tube that briefly spiked above 80°C and remained just above 60°C for periods of over an hour. It is not known, however, if the worm's body temperature equilibrated with the high temperatures of the water flowing through the tube. The worms appear to remain in their tubes during prolonged exposure to water near 60°C, but because they are mobile they may abandon their tubes when bursts of lethally hot water flow through them. The ABTs given in figure 7.23 for the two alvinellid worms *Alvinella pompejana* and *Alvinella caudata*, 48.6°

C and 48.0°C, respectively, are plotted for habitat (body) temperatures near 40°C, in accord with earlier estimates of the two species' habitat temperatures (See Dahlhoff et al., 1991, for discussion). While we tentatively regard these species as being adapted to temperatures closer to 40°C than to 60°C, a caveat must be raised concerning the measurement of membrane-based processes at nonphysiological pressures. The ABT values for the alvinellids, like those of the other species studied, were determined at one atmosphere pressure. However, elevated pressure offsets some of the effects of high temperature on diverse membrane-associated structures and processes (see Macdonald, 1984). This pressure-temperature interaction raises the possibility that the high pressures of hydrothermal vent habitats (approximately 250 atmospheres in this case) might confer enhanced stability on membrane-based structures like mitochondrial membranes, allowing them to function at temperatures in excess of 50°C. Studies of temperature–pressure interactions on mitochondria of hydrothermal vent species are thus warranted to help resolve this issue about the upper temperature limits of animal life. In addition, studies of temperatures at which failure of other classes of membranes occurs could reveal whether eukaryotic membranes in general are limited to temperatures below approximately 55°C–60°C.

Individual mitochondrial enzymes such as the lipid-requiring enzyme cytochrome C oxidase exhibit interspecific variation in ABTs similar to that seen for mitochondrial oxygen consumption (O'Brien et al., 1991; Dahlhoff and Somero, 1993b). Thus, the impairment of mitochondrial respiration at high temperatures may be due to loss of activity of enzymes in ATP-generating pathways.

Parenthetically, it should be noted that mitochondrial respiration rates normalized to mitochondrial protein content do not exhibit a significant degree of compensation to temperature (see Johnston et al., 1994). For mitochondria, then, changes in membrane physical state linked to homeophasic and homeoviscous adaptation do not appear linked to temperature-compensatory changes in specific activities of enzymes.

Comparisons of differently acclimated congeneric abalone (genus *Haliotis*) have revealed similarities between interspecific and intraspecific responses to exposure temperature (figure 7.24) (Dahlhoff and Somero, 1993b). Acclimation of conspecifics has been shown to lead to shifts in ABT and to changes in membrane static order, as indexed by fluorescence anisotropy using DPH. A cold stenothermal species, *Haliotis kamtschatkana* (pinto abalone), that tolerates temperatures of 4°C–14°C, showed acclimation-dependent changes in ABT and membrane order (fluorescence polarization) between 4°C and 10°C. Between 10°C and 14°C, no additional change in either trait was found. In contrast, a more warm-adapted and eurythermal species, *Haliotis fulgens* (green abalone), which tolerates temperatures from 14°C–27°C, adjusted ABT and order over a wider range of temperatures. The homeoviscous efficacy observed in DPH polarization was approximately 90%, in agreement with other studies showing high efficacy in mitochondrial membranes (Hazel, 1995). Although ABT and membrane order were correlated, the correlation was not perfect. For instance, the increase in polarization intensity (order) observed for mitochondria of the green abalone between 22°C and 26°C did not correlate with a regular increase in ABT over that interval. It is possible that measurements of bulk fluidity obtained with DPH polarization mask the effects of temperature on the local domains of lipids that are of primary importance in setting the ABT.

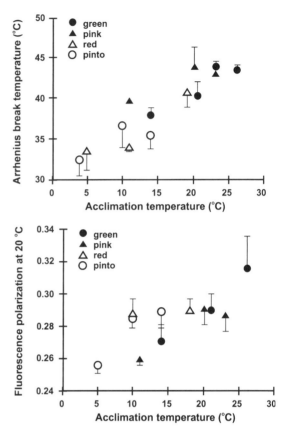

Figure 7.24. Mitochondrial respiration and membrane fluidity in differently acclimated congeners of abalone (genus *Haliotis*). (Top panel) Arrhenius break temperatures for mitochondrial respiration. Note: overlapping data points (pinto at 5°C; red and green at 20°C) have been offset by 1°C for clarity. (Bottom panel) Fluidity of mitochondrial membranes as estimated from the fluorescence polarization of DPH. Note: 20°C points have been offset for clarity. (Data from Dahlhoff and Somero, 1993b.)

Correlated changes in behavior and synaptosomal structure

Adaptation of the nervous system to temperature is likely to play a major role in governing the thermal tolerance ranges and thermal optima of animals (Cossins and Bowler, 1987). Conduction along axons and, particularly, transmission of signals at synapses are strongly affected by temperature. It is probable, therefore, that alterations in the properties of neural membranes will be found to correlate closely with changes in the thermal sensitivity of behavior. The nearly perfect homeoviscous adaptation of brain synaptosomes from differently adapted vertebrates (figure 7.21) supports this prediction, but correlations between this type of biophysical change and alterations in behavior would greatly strengthen the case.

One of the best demonstrations of this type of correlation remains the 1977 study by Cossins et al. in which cross-acclimation of goldfish (*Carassius auratus*) was studied (figure 7.25). Goldfish were acclimated initially to either 5°C or 25°C and then transferred to the opposite temperature and reacclimated for sev-

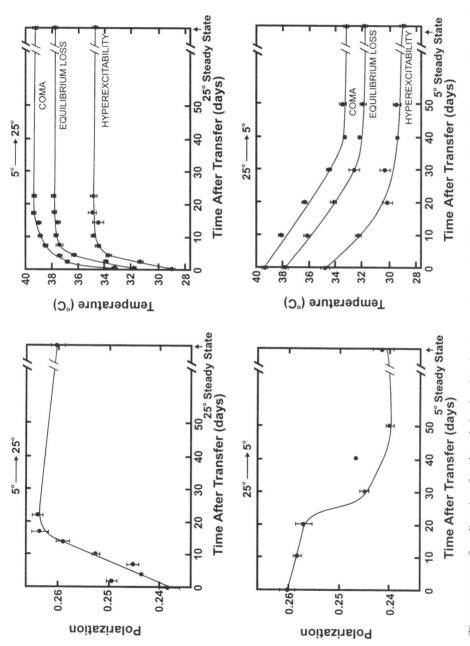

Figure 7.25. Time courses of acclimation for three behavioral traits (temperatures at which coma, loss of equilibrium, and hyperexcitability occurred) and synaptosomal fluidity in goldfish (*Carassius auratus*). Fish were first acclimated to either 5°C or 25°C and then transferred to the alternate temperature. (Modified after Cossins et al., 1977.)

367

eral weeks. During this acclimation period, three behavioral characteristics, coma, equilibrium loss, and hyperexcitability, were monitored as functions of acute temperature of exposure. Synaptosomes were isolated from brain and their physical state was indexed by measuring fluorescence polarization of DPH.

The data from this study revealed several important relationships. First, the three behavioral traits exhibited pronounced acclimation to temperature, which occurred with similar time courses. Second, the rate of acclimation was substantially faster at 25°C than at 5°C. This difference in kinetics of acclimation is probably a manifestation of Q_{10} effects on the biochemical processes that were responsible for effecting adaptive change. Third, DPH fluorescence polarization changed during reacclimation to reestablish the original fluidity of the synaptosomal membranes. That is, there was virtually complete homeoviscous adaptation. Fourth, the time courses of acclimation in the three behavioral traits agreed fairly well with the time course of change in membrane fluidity.

The similar time courses of the responses in behavior and membrane fluidity do not, or course, prove a cause–effect relationship. However, the correlation is striking, and is certainly suggestive of a mechanistic link between whole organism and molecular-level effects.

Mechanisms for Modifying Phase Transition Temperatures (T_m and T_h) and Localized Order in the Bilayer

Substantial raw material is present for modifying membrane structure

Cells can draw on a large number of types of raw material to modify the functional properties of membranes in temperature-adaptive manners. In the most general of terms, there are two fundamental ways in which phase transition temperatures and localized order can be altered. These are: (1) *intrinsic* changes in the lipid composition of the membrane, notably in lipid class, molecular species, and cholesterol content, and (2) *extrinsic* changes, alterations in the solution bathing the inner and outer surfaces of the bilayer. The latter changes include

shifts in pH and in organic solute composition. These two basic routes for adaptive change are the same as the options available to cells for adjusting the temperature-sensitivities of proteins, as discussed above and detailed further in chapter 6. However, there is one essential distinction between the intrinsic changes characteristic of proteins and those observed for lipids. Proteins are gene products, so alterations in protein structure, other than post-translational modifications and altered expressions of isoform-encoding genes, are not possible. Lipids are *reaction products*, and because of the wide variety of types of enzymes available to synthesize different types of lipids, the diversity of raw material available for altering the intrinsic properties of membrane lipids is enormous.

Although there is increasing evidence that the milieu surrounding a membrane can have pronounced influences on its properties, most studies of temperature adaptation to date have focused on the intrinsic properties of membranes. Despite wide variation among species in the precise types of lipid adjustments that are made and in the kinetics of these adaptive changes, some broadly applicable generalizations can be made about the exploitation of intrinsic changes in lipid composition for adapting membrane function to temperature.

Changes in headgroup composition: lipid class. A commonly observed change in lipid composition during thermal acclimation is a shift in the relative amounts of different classes of lipids present in a membrane. Cold acclimation frequently leads to an increase in phosphatidylethanolamine (PE) and a decrease in phosphatidylcholine (PC). Thus, the PC/PE ratio falls, as shown for phospholipids isolated from gills of rainbow trout (*Oncorhynchus mykiss*) acclimated initially to either 5°C or 20°C and, then, transferred to the reciprocal temperature (figure 7.26; Hazel and Carpenter, 1985). The PC/PE ratio falls rapidly in the trout transferred to 5°C, and rises even more quickly in the trout transferred to 20°C. Note, however, that the PC/PE ratios did not reach stable plateau values during the 28-day acclimation period. Rather, after the initial rise (20°C) or fall

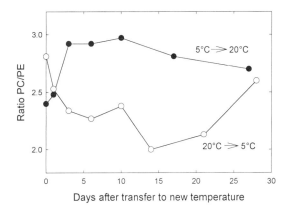

Figure 7.26. Temperature acclimation and phospholipid class. Changes in the ratio of phosphatidylcholine (PC) to phosphatidylethanolamine (PE) in membranes of gill cells isolated from rainbow trout acclimating to 5°C and 25°C (Hazel and Carpenter, 1985.)

(5°C) in PC/PE ratio, the ratio tended to equalize between the two acclimation groups, as time progressed. The kinetics of the change in PC/PE ratio reflect a not uncommon aspect of membrane acclimation to temperature: different types of changes in intrinsic properties mark different stages of the acclimatory response. These time-dependent changes in lipid composition may be a reflection of the speed with which different types of mechanisms for modifying lipid composition can be recruited. Changes in headgroup may occur relatively quickly compared to other types of changes. In renal membranes isolated from trout subjected to transfer from 20°C to 5°C, the PC/PE ratio decreased by approximately 50% over eight hours (Hazel and Landrey, 1988). Rapid shifts in the PC/PE ratio may be important in acclimatization to diurnal temperature changes (Carey and Hazel, 1989). Sonoran desert cyprinid fishes encounter wide variation in stream temperature during the course of the day. Fish acclimatized to midday heat (approximately 34°C) had about 3% PE in their phospholipids; fish taken from cooler waters at night (∼ 21–26°C) had a PE content of 12%.

The change in PC/PE ratio can be rationalized partially in terms of the geometrical properties of these lipids. As discussed above (see

figure 7.19), lipids with a PE headgroup tend to form a more conical structure than PC-containing lipids, which assume a more cylindrical geometry. According to the dynamic phase behavior model of Hazel (1995), the incorporation of an appropriate mixture of PC- and PE-containing lipids helps to poise the membrane properly in terms of its propensity for forming hexagonal phases (H_{II}), which are important for the function of certain enzymes, for regulating permeability, and for allowing exo- and endocytosis (see Hazel and Williams, 1990). Padrón et al. (2000) have shown that rates of endocytosis by hepatocytes from rainbow trout acclimated to 5°C and 20°C exhibited essentially complete (95%) temperature compensation. However, they also observed an eightfold higher rate of endocytosis in rat hepatocytes at 37°C than in fish hepatocytes, measured at their acclimation temperatures. Thus, in keeping with other membrane-localized rate processes (see the discussion of mechanisms of endothermy presented later in this chapter), ectotherms and endothermic homeotherms show large differences in rates at physiological temperatures.

Shifts in the PC/PE ratio may have effects on the local order of the bilayer as well as on H_{II} phase behavior. At first glance, it would seem that PE would be an inappropriate choice for incorporation at relatively high levels in membranes of cold-adapted organisms. Because the size of the PE headgroup is less than that of PC (figure 7.19) and because PE is less hydrated than PC, PE-containing lipids can pack together more closely. This closer packing tends to increase the van der Waals interactions among acyl chains, favoring an increase in the gel-to-fluid phase transition temperature. However, offsetting this order-generating effect of PE is the occurrence in PE-containing lipids of relatively higher contents of unsaturated acyl chains (Hazel and Williams, 1990). The decrease in order caused by the *cis* double bonds of these chains offsets the effects of size and hydration of PE.

How the rapid changes in PC/PE ratio that have been observed in some studies of thermal acclimation are brought about is not known in great detail. Studies of synthesis of PE and PC in trout hepatocytes (see Hazel, 1990) have shown that the Q_{10} values for synthesis of these headgroups are different. The Q_{10} for PC synthesis was 2.98, whereas that for PE was only 1.80. It is conceivable, therefore, that an acute drop in temperature could directly lead to a shift in the balance between PC and PE synthesis. The methylating enzymes that convert PE to PC also may be regulated in a temperature-compensatory manner (Chapelle et al., 1982). The fact that reversible methylation of PE plays a role in rapid signal transduction events (see Hirata and Axelrod, 1980) suggests that the enzymatic potential for shifting the PC/PE ratio may be generally present in plasma membranes. Thus, temperature-dependent regulation of these enzymes could contribute to rapid acclimation/acclimatization of membrane function.

Changes in acyl chain composition: molecular species. The intrinsic change in membrane lipid properties that has received the greatest attention is the shift in phospholipid molecular species, that is, in acyl chain composition and positioning of acyl chains on the glycerol backbone, that accompanies acclimation or acclimatization. Adaptation in molecular species involves five different types of changes: (1) acyl chain length, (2) content of double bonds, (3) positions of the double bond(s) along the acyl chain, (4) *cis* versus *trans* configurations of double bonds, and (5) the position of a specific acyl chain on the glycerol backbone. These diverse avenues for altering molecular species compositions of phospholipids provide a large number of alternatives for adaptation that may have different time courses and, therefore, be recruited at different stages of membrane adaptation.

One of the commonest relationships noted in adaptation of membranes to temperature is a decrease in acyl chain saturation during acclimation to reduced temperature. Hazel (1988) has reviewed changes in molecular species composition during acclimation in bacteria, plants, and animals. As a broad generalization, a decrease in acclimation temperature of 20°C is accompanied by a decrease of approximately 19% in the percentage of fully saturated acyl

chains. This change can be quantified by the *unsaturation ratio*, the ratio of unsaturated to saturated acyl chains. The 19% shift in composition mentioned above translates into to a 1.4-fold rise in unsaturation ratio. Different types of membranes show different amounts of change in the unsaturation ratio during thermal acclimation. For example, mitochondrial membranes exhibit a greater compensatory shift in unsaturation ratio than microsomal or synaptosomal membranes (Hazel and Williams, 1990). This is in keeping with the high degree of homeoviscous efficacy ($\sim 90\%$) characteristic of differently adapted mitochondrial membranes (Dahlhoff and Somero, 1993b).

Changes in the unsaturation ratio per se during thermal acclimation belie the full complexity of the underlying events taking place in the membrane's intrinsic properties. For instance, the type of double bond that is formed can have a strong effect on the order of the membrane. The prevalent double bond found in the lipid acyl chains of most types of organisms is the *cis* double bond (see figure 7.19). These bonds create a "kink" in an acyl chain, which reduces the chain's potential for interaction with other acyl chains. In contrast, *trans* double bonds, which occur in some bacteria and plastids, do not induce this kink in geometry and, for this reason, have a less disordering effect on the bilayer than *cis* double bonds.

The magnitude of the functional consequences of altering numbers and types of double bonds is suggested by the melting temperature of pure lipids. The melting temperature of stearic acid (octadecanoic acid: 18 carbons and no double bonds) is 69°C, that of elaidic acid (*trans*-delta9-octadecenoic acid) is 45°C, and that of oleic acid (*cis*-delta9-octadecenoic acid) is 12°C. These data not only show how strongly the addition of a single double bond affects acyl chain order, but also how much the nature (*cis* versus *trans*) of the double bond contributes to the reduction in order. Conversion between *cis* and *trans* configurations of double bonds is catalyzed by specific isomerase enzymes. Changes in the activities of these enzymes could provide a very rapid and effective mechanism for adapting the physical order of the membrane. The prevalence of these isomerases and their function in adapting membrane properties to temperature remain relatively unexplored.

Another subtlety in double bond chemistry that is important in determining the effects of double bonds on membrane structure is the position within the acyl chain at which double bonds are found. The introduction of a double bond near the center of the acyl chain, for instance at position 9 in the formation of oleic acid from stearic acid, has the largest effect on acyl chain order. Long-chain polyunsaturates with multiple double bonds have disordering influences that are highest near the membrane interior (Hazel et al., 1992). Cold acclimation is frequently characterized by the incorporation into phospholipids of long-chain polyunsaturates such as docosahexanoic (DHA) acid, a 22-carbon acid with six double bonds.

Although long-chain polyunsaturates appear to play important roles in determining membrane order, it is the introduction of the first double bond into an acyl chain that has by far the largest effect on order. For this reason, the *unsaturation ratio* (the fraction of acyl chains having one or more double bonds) is a better index of adaptation of membrane order than is the *unsaturation index*, the average number of double bonds per acyl chain (Cossins and Lee, 1985). The recruitment of monoenes (single double bond) and polyunsaturates into phospholipids is not uniform among different lipid classes, a further indication of the complex fine-tuning that occurs in membranes during adaptation. In PE-containing lipids, monoenes show larger changes relative to polyunsaturates; in PC lipids, the opposite trend is found (Gracey et al., 1996).

Another subtlety of molecular species adaptation involves the position on the glycerol backbone to which an acyl chain is esterified. The *sn*-1 acyl chain, the chain attached to the first carbon on the glycerol moiety, is oriented more or less perpendicularly to the surface of the membrane throughout its length. In contrast, for the acyl chain attached to the *sn*-2 position, the middle position of glycerol, the first –CH$_2$– group lies parallel to the membrane surface. Thus, the locations in the bilayer of

double bonds in identical acyl chains at the *sn*-1 and *sn*-2 positions will be different, as will the effects of the double bonds on membrane static order. Because of these positional effects, lipids with identical acyl chains may have different physical properties. In theory, then, minor temperature-adaptive modification of phospholipids may not require changes in acyl chain composition, but only shifts in chain position. However, these positional rearrangements probably contribute only modestly to temperature-compensatory adjustments in static order.

The primary mechanisms involved in altering molecular species composition do, in fact, entail substantial restructuring of the types of acyl chains in phospholipids. Here as elsewhere in adaptation of intrinsic properties of membranes, a number of options are open (Hazel and Williams, 1990). There may be shifts in the pools of free fatty acids upon which the phospholipid synthesizing systems of the cell can draw. In addition to de novo synthesis of new molecular species (and new lipid classes), there may be remodeling of existing phospholipids by what is termed "acyl chain reshuffling." Here, a battery of membrane-localized enzymes removes one type of acyl chain and replaces it with another, through the deacylation/reacylation cycle. Phospholipases clip off an acyl chain, generating a lysophospholipid, and a lysophospholipid acyltransferase then replaces the excised acyl chain with a more appropriate one, for instance, one with a double bond. Because both classes of enzyme are membrane-localized, their activities may be highly dependent on temperature, that is, on membrane static order and phase. There is some evidence that enzymes in the deacylation/reacylation cycle possess temperature-dependent substrate specificities, such that at low temperatures unsaturated acyl chains become the preferred substrate for incorporation into phospholipids (Farkas and Roy, 1989).

The provision of an appropriate fatty acid pool for use in synthesis of phospholipids involves a complex mixture of dietary and biosynthetic effects. To at least some extent, "one is what one eats" applies in the context of adaptation of lipid-containing structures, a point

that will become clear below when prehiberna-
tion food choices are considered. Most of the
regulation of the fatty acid pools of cells
involves biosynthetic processes, however.
These reactions lead to the accumulation, at
least in the short term, of a balanced set of
fatty acids that, when esterified into phospholipids, have the appropriate effects on membrane
phase and order. The regulated synthesis of
fatty acids in response to changes in temperature frequently involves the activities of *desa-
turases*, enzymes that introduce double bonds
into saturated fatty acids. The activities of desa-
turases increase in the cold and decrease in the
heat, often very quickly in the case of unicellular species. In the bacterium *Bacillus megater-
ium*, strong induction of desaturase activity
occurred as a rapid response to a drop in culture temperature (Fujii and Fulco, 1977). When
cells were transferred to a high temperature,
induction was suppressed and the desaturase,
now no longer advantageous to the cell, was
rapidly removed by apparent heat inactivation.
In animals, induction of desaturase activity
occurs more slowly, and appears to involve a
combination of activation of preexisting, inactive desaturase molecules and new synthesis (as
gauged by rising levels of mRNA for desa-
turases) (Gracey et al., 1996).

The pool of fatty acids remaining unesteri-
fied in the cell may belie the amount of change
in molecular species composition that has taken
place in a membrane (Hazel and Livermore,
1990). As the appropriate fatty acids are generated, they may be withdrawn rapidly from the
fatty acid pool and incorporated into membranes. Thus, the full extent to which phospholipid composition has been altered may not be
evident from the fatty acids that remain in the
cytoplasmic pool.

One of the best studies to date of the complex changes that occur in molecular species
composition during homeoviscous adaptation
is by Logue et al. (2000), who performed
detailed lipid analyses of the synaptosomal preparations used to generate the data presented in
figure 7.21. The interspecific differences in percent saturation of acyl chains in phosphatidylethanolamine and phosphatidylcholine lipids
account in large measure for the differences

observed among species in anisotropy of DPH
fluorescence (figure 7.27). Thus, with increasing
cold adaptation, there is a highly regular
increase in the percentage of unsaturated phospholipids in both PC and PE. Underlying these
broad trends are further important differences
in lipid structure. For PC, polyunsaturated
fatty acids (PUFAs) showed large increases in
cold-adapted species: in turkey and rat, PUFAs
accounted for only 7–8% of fatty acids in PC,
whereas in Antarctic fish, they represented 35%
of the acyl chains. In contrast to PUFAs,
monounsaturated fatty acids (MUFAs) varied
little among species. Phosphatidylethanolamine
showed different adaptive variation from PC.
For PE, there were large differences in
MUFAs: values ranged from 5–10% in warm-
adapted species to 25–30% in Antarctic fishes.
Conversely, PUFAs varied little with respect to
adaptation temperature.

The position of fatty acid changes on the
glycerol backbone differed between PC and
PE. Polyunsaturated fatty acids tend to occur
at the *sn*-2 position, and saturates and MUFAs
preferentially occur at the *sn*-1 position.
Consequently, in PC, the adaptive changes

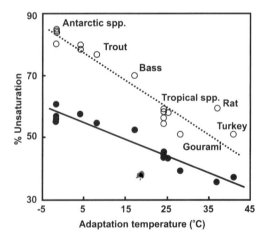

Figure 7.27. The relationship between adaptation
temperature and percentage of unsaturated acyl
chains in synaptosomal phospholipids of differently
thermally adapted vertebrates. Each symbol represents a different species. Open symbols denote
phosphatidylethanolamine; filled symbols denote
phosphatidylcholine. (Figure modified after Logue
et al., 2000.)

were concentrated at the *sn*-2 position, whereas for PE, changes were most marked at the *sn*-1 position. The dominance of changes at the *sn*-1 position in PE may reflect the fact that, even in synaptosomes of warm-adapted species like mammals, a PUFA (22:6*n*3) is present at the *sn*-2 position. (Note: 22:6*n*3 denotes a 22 carbon acyl chain having total of six double bonds, the first of which lies three carbons in from the terminal methyl group.) This PUFA tends to keep PE in its conical configuration. However, by having a highly unsaturated acyl chain at this position, increasing unsaturation at the *sn*-2 position during adaptation to low temperatures is precluded (see Logue et al., 2000). Thus, in PE, changes in acyl chain saturation are focused on the *sn*-1 position.

The dominance of changes at the *sn*-2 position in PC may reflect the importance of viscotropic relationships. It has been proposed that a high degree of unsaturation at this position could contribute to the abilities of membrane-spanning proteins to undergo conformational changes (Litman and Mitchell, 1996).

In summary, changes in molecular species composition are complex and reflect the wide variety of ways in which the physical state of the membrane can be adjusted to conserve membrane properties.

Changes in cholesterol content. A third type of intrinsic change involves alteration in the amount of cholesterol in a membrane (Robertson and Hazel, 1997). Cholesterol can be incorporated into a membrane up to an approximately one-to-one ratio with phospholipids. Most membrane-localized cholesterol is found in the plasma membrane. Cholesterol is an amphipathic molecule, that is, different regions of the molecule have affinities for either polar or nonpolar environments (figure 7.19). In a membrane, the flexible alkyl tip of the molecule penetrates into the bilayer; the 3-β-hydroxyl group remains near the surface of the membrane, near the ester linkages between the acyl chains and the glycerol moiety.

The effects of cholesterol are varied and would seem to provide a number of adaptive possibilities for modulating the properties of membranes in temperature-compensatory man-

ners. The order of acyl chains near cholesterol is increased, which leads to a number of physical effects: increased membrane thickness, reduced membrane surface area, and reduced membrane compressibility. Cholesterol disrupts the packing of gel phases and broadens or even eliminates the gel/fluid phase transition noted at reduced temperatures. Thus, cholesterol tends to stabilize the fluid phase of a membrane. However, cholesterol has only small effects on the rotational diffusion of membrane constituents and it tends to preserve microscale order or viscosity. Cholesterol is thought to help maintain "rafts" of sphingolipids (lipids built on the long-chain amino alcohol sphingosine rather than the three-carbon alcohol glycerol) in a functional state (Simons and Ikonen, 2000). Because the hydroxyl-containing end of the cholesterol molecule remains near the membrane surface, the addition of cholesterol to a membrane acts to separate the headgroups and allow water to penetrate farther into the membrane.

Available data on differently acclimated organisms illustrate the roles that cholesterol plays in adaptation to temperature. Robertson and Hazel (1995) demonstrated a positive correlation between membrane cholesterol content, as indexed by the cholesterol to phospholipid ratio, and acclimation temperature in rainbow trout. An increased cholesterol/phospholipid ratio was found in all tissues studied, although differences in the ratio were noted among tissues. Because the amount of *change* in this ratio varied among tissues as well, different types of adaptive processes may characterize each type of membrane. Different classes of membrane-localized proteins, with varied requirements for specific lipid domains, may distinguish different types of membranes. These authors proposed that the higher relative amounts of cholesterol in the membranes of warm (20°C) acclimated trout, regardless of the magnitude of the effect that occurred, achieved membrane stabilization in the face of the loss of static order that would occur at high temperature. The observation that cholesterol content is lower in ectotherms like trout relative to endothermic homeotherms like birds and mammals further supports a role for cholesterol in stabilizing membrane function at high temperatures (Robertson and Hazel, 1997). The stabilizing effects of cholesterol are suggested by the data in figure 7.22(A), which show how cholesterol-induced ordering reduces activity of the Na^+-K^+-ATPase, and by the observation that supplementation with cholesterol of preparations of purified phospholipids from trout led to a large increase in static order, as quantified by polarization of DPH (Robertson and Hazel, 1995). In the latter experiment, cholesterol-free phospholipids from 5°C-acclimated trout were supplemented with levels of cholesterol representative of those measured in 20°C trout, approximately 20 mol%. Addition of this level of cholesterol increased the order of the phospholipids significantly and led to identical values of DPH polarization at 5°C for the cholesterol-free phospholipids and at 20°C for the cholesterol-supplemented phospholipids.

In summary, cholesterol appears to play an important role in modifying membranes, at least the plasma membranes of animal cells, in temperature-compensatory manners. The significance of cholesterol in adaptation to temperature by animals raises several interesting evolutionary questions. Do the many taxa that lack cholesterol employ other types of molecules to achieve the sorts of adaptations effected by cholesterol in animal cells? In view of the requirement for molecular oxygen for the synthesis of cholesterol, did the earliest cells, which evolved in the near absence of molecular oxygen, develop oxygen-independent synthetic pathways for producing lipids with cholesterol-like effects?

Cholesterol substitutes and evolution of biosynthetic pathways leading to cholesterol. In their review of cholesterol effects on membranes, Robertson and Hazel (1997) outline a broad evolutionary picture in which the origins and the functional roles of cholesterol substitutes and bilayer-spanning membrane stabilizers in bacteria, Archaea, and plants are presented. Figure 7.28 portrays the types of molecules that serve as membrane stabilizers in these different taxa: *rigid hemilayer inserts*, which have a cholesterol-like chemistry and membrane localization; *rigid bilayer inserts*, which extend across the bilayer; and *rigid* and *nonrigid bilayer spanners* that are proposed to firmly reinforce bilayer structure and serve to defend membrane integrity against extremes of stress.

In bacteria, a family of molecules with a striking chemical similarity to cholesterol, the *hopanoids*, insert into the membrane hemilayer and stabilize membrane structure (figure 7.28: bacteriohopanetetrol). The effects of these prokaryotic cholesterol analogs are similar to those of cholesterol: they broaden the gel–fluid phase transition, condense the bilayer, and reduce bilayer permeability. Contents of hopanoids in bacterial membranes may rise with acclimation temperature (Poralla et al., 1984).

Both prokaryotes and eukaryotes may contain non-polar compounds that insert into both hemilayers (e.g., the carotenoid compounds corynexanthin and spirilloxanthin; figure 7.28). If polar groups are present at each end of the molecule, the molecule may span the entire bilayer (e.g., bis-phytanol; figure 7.28). Bilayer-spanning carotenoids are thought to be extremely effective in stabilizing the integrity of the bilayer, as suggested by their occurrence in extremophiles like halophilic members of the Archaea (see next section).

The evolution and phylogenetic distributions of cholesterol and analogous polyterpenoids such as carotenoids are proposed to reflect the availability of atmospheric oxygen at the time of origin of these compounds (see Ourisson et al., 1987). Tetraterpenoids like carotenoids, whose synthesis does not depend on oxygen, are viewed in this context as "primitive" membrane stabilizers. Addition of a proton-catalyzed cyclization reaction to convert squalene into polycyclic triterpenoids like the hopanoids represents a further development of this biochemistry, yet one that remains independent of molecular oxygen. Oxygen-dependent biosynthesis of cholesterol follows a different pathway from that which generates hopanoids. The absence of cholesterol in prokaryotes is viewed as a reflection of the origin of these organisms prior to the advent of green plant (oxygenic) photosynthesis.

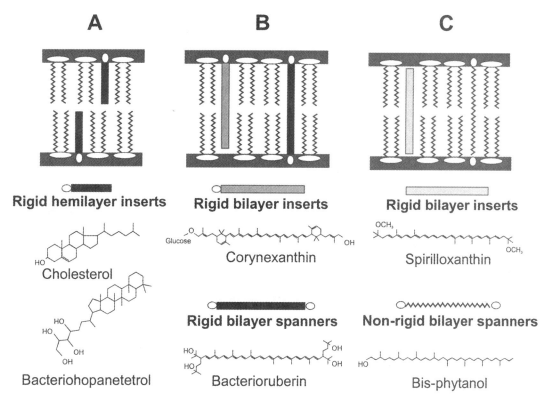

A **B** **C**

Rigid hemilayer inserts   Rigid bilayer inserts   Rigid bilayer inserts

Cholesterol   Corynexanthin   Spirilloxanthin

Bacteriohopanetetrol   Rigid bilayer spanners   Non-rigid bilayer spanners

Bacterioruberin   Bis-phytanol

Figure 7.28. Structures and functions of membrane stabilizing molecules ("inserts"). (A) Rigid hemilayer inserts. Amphipathic rigid inserts are thought to enhance membrane order by intercalating into one of the two hemilayers and interacting with other lipid components in a way that stabilizes membrane order. In eukaryotes, cholesterol may serve this function; in bacteria, bacteriohopanoids (bacteriohopanetetrol is shown) perform this function. (B) Rigid amphipathic bilayer inserts (corynexanthin) and rigid bilayer spanners (bacterioruberin), and (C) rigid hydrophobic bilayer inserts (spirilloxanthin) and nonrigid bilayer spanners (bis-phytanol). These molecules may exert their stabilizing influences by extending across the bilayer. (Figure modified after Robertson and Hazel, 1997.)

The "tough" membranes of extremophilic Archaea and Bacteria

Extremophiles, loosely defined as members of the domains Archaea and Bacteria that are tolerant of extremes of temperature, salinity, pressure, and acidity (for reviews, see Horikoshi and Grant, 1998), usually are characterized by membrane components that add an additional degree of "toughness" to the integrity of the membrane. Above, we mentioned that long-chain carotenoids that intercalate into the membrane and may span the bilayer confer a high level of stability to the membrane. There are other unusual components of the membranes of extremophiles that also may serve this type of function. In the

Archaea, the nonpolar chains of membrane lipids are fully saturated isopranoid alcohols, which are of two characteristic chain lengths, C_{20} and C_{40}. In effect, the C_{40} alcohol is a head-to-head condensation product of two C_{20} alcohols. These alcohols are attached to glycerol through ether linkages instead of through the ester linkages common in phospholipids. If the two isopranoid alcohol chains are linked to only a single molecule of glycerol, a phytanyl glycerol diether is formed. These lipids can contribute to bilayer formation like the phospholipids discussed earlier. If two C_{40} alcohols are attached to two glycerols, one at each end of the C_{40} chains, the resulting lipid is a di(biphytanyl) diglycerol tetraether (figure 7.29). These lipids are long enough to span the

A

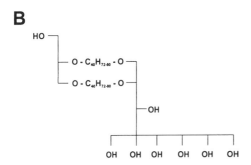

B

Figure 7.29. Structures of some membrane lipids found in the Archaea. These lipids are able to form stable monolayers. (A) A tetraether lipid, diphytanylglycosylglycerol. (B) A tetraether lipid of an extreme thermoacidophile, *Sulfolobus sulfataricus*. $C_{40}H_{72-80}$ denotes the two biphytanyl chains (including 0 to 3 cyclopentanes). In thermophilic members of the Archaea, the ratio of tetraether lipids to diether lipids rises with increasing temperature. (Figure modified after Hazel and Williams, 1990.)

bilayer, and they are regarded as an extremely effective tool for stabilizing membranes of extremophiles (hyperthermophiles) at high temperature. Membranes rich in these tetra-ethers are not likely to undergo bilayer separation at extremes of temperature, for example.

As the foregoing analysis suggests, the Archaea play by somewhat different rules from those used by other types of organisms in adjusting the physical properties of their membranes to cope with high temperatures. Lipid saturation is not varied; under all thermal conditions, the isopranoid alcohols lack double bonds. Instead, the ratio of tetraethers to diethers, that is, the ratio of membrane-spanning to bilayer-forming lipids, is modulated. In general, the ratio of tetraethers to diethers rises with adaptation temperature, reaching high values in hyperthermophilic species capable of growth near 100°C. Note that, although archaeal membranes remain intact at temperature exceeding 100°C, maintaining a transmembrane proton gradient may not be possible and a sodium gradient may serve to drive ATP synthesis.

Another remarkable feature of the cell membranes of hyperthermophilic archaea is their ability to maintain a liquid-crystalline state over extremely wide ranges of temperature (Horikoshi and Grant, 1998). The exact biophysical basis for this impressive degree of eurythermy is not fully understood, albeit the unusual membrane-spanning tetraether lipids could play a role.

Extremophilic bacteria employ mechanisms analogous to those used by thermophilic members of the Archaea. In some anaerobic thermophilic bacteria, C_{30} dicarboxylic acids may provide 10–20% of the acyl chains of membrane lipids (Langworthy and Pond, 1986). These acyl chains may be esterified to a glycerol molecule at each end of the C_{30} chain to form a membrane-spanning lipid with a high ability to stabilize the membrane against thermal perturbation.

It is revealing to contrast the adaptations noted in proteins and in lipids among the hyperthermophiles. Proteins of these extremophiles look surprisingly similar to those of mesophiles and psychrophiles. Proteins, as gene products, can vary little in their basic chemical composition. There are only 20 common amino acids, and even though covalent modifications of many sorts are possible, the adaptation to high temperature observed in proteins of hyperthermophiles represents fine-tuning of stability using rules held in common with mesophilic and psychrophilic organisms. In contrast, because lipids are reaction products whose properties are subject to extremely wide variation through a diverse set of biosynthetic pathways, the emergence and use of unique forms of lipids in Archaea and bacteria is not surprising.

"You are what you eat": Adaptive changes in depot lipids in mammalian hibernators

Up to this point in the treatment of lipid-containing systems we have focused exclusively on the lipids of cellular membranes and have shown how adaptive variations in lipid composition conserve function in the face of temperature change. What, if any, types of adaptation to temperature occur in lipids that merely serve as energy stores? The depot lipids held in adipocytes as energy reserves are primarily triacylglycerides, and because they are not linked to membrane function they might seem less likely than membrane phospholipids or cholesterol to exhibit temperature-adaptive change. However, depot lipids can only be mobilized if they are in a fluid state, a fact that presents a potential problem for small mammalian hibernators that may allow their body temperatures to fall as low as $-1.9°C$ in the case of Arctic ground squirrels (Barnes, 1989). Depot lipids of normothermic mammals have melting temperatures as much as $30°C$ higher than this, so if lipids are to be accessed during hibernation or the early stages of arousal, it is likely that some type of compensatory change in lipid composition must take place.

Frank (1991, 1992) has shown that squirrels (*Spermophilus beldingi*) capable of hibernation contain lipids with melting temperatures approximately $25°C$ lower than those of normothermic mammals. He hypothesized that the animals selectively fed on plants containing high levels of polyunsaturated fatty acids, and that the composition of the resulting depot

lipids was determined in large measure by the lipid composition of the diet. This hypothesis was examined in laboratory studies in which another species, *Spermophilus lateralis*, was offered diets that contained varying percentages of polyunsaturated fatty acids. Consistent with his hypothesis, Frank (1992) found that the composition of the depot lipids closely mirrored that of the dietary lipids. Moreover, compared to squirrels fed diets with relatively low levels of polyunsaturated lipids, animals fed diets with high levels of polyunsaturated fatty acids were more likely to enter into hibernation, to have lower body temperature set points during hibernation, and to survive hibernation better.

A somewhat analogous phenomenon was observed in lizards (*Tiliqua rugosa*) fed diets with varying contents of polyunsaturated fatty acids (Geiser et al., 1992). Specimens fed diets high in polyunsaturated fatty acids selected cooler environments, that is, lower body temperatures, than lizards fed diets with lower levels of polyunsaturated fatty acids. The most intriguing finding of this study is the suggestion that selection of habitat (body) temperature by ectotherms might be determined in part by the types of lipids available in their diets. There is clear evidence in mammals that the lipid composition of the diet influences the species of phospholipid found in membranes (Neelands and Clandinin, 1983), so dietary influences on the thermal properties of membranes of ectotherms may be important in thermal physiology.

Extrinsic Effects on Membrane Physical State

In view of how effectively the physical properties of membranes can be regulated by changing lipid composition—headgroups, types and positions of acyl chains, and cholesterol content—it might seem reasonable to conclude that adaptation to temperature can be achieved strictly through these intrinsic compositional changes, without any role being played by the medium surrounding the membrane. So many reaction products can be generated by the biosynthetic systems responsible for building a cell's suite of lipids that no assistance from extrinsic factors may seem to be required. In the case of proteins, it is abundantly clear that alterations in the solute composition and pH of the medium bathing aqueous-phase proteins play a major role in establishing their stabilities and functional properties. And, for proteins embedded in a lipid bilayer, alterations in lipid composition cause large changes in function, as discussed above. However, what role, if any, does the milieu in which a membrane resides play in adaptively modifying its physical state?

A closer look at the properties of the bilayer shows that certain characteristics of the solution bathing a membrane are likely to influence its physical state and, thereby, affect its sensitivity to temperature. Although these extrinsic effects remain much less studied than effects involving changes in lipid composition, there is increasing evidence that temperature-dependent changes in the intra- and extracellular fluids affect membranes as well as cytosolic proteins.

Effects of pH

The phase state and the fluidity of membranes are sensitive to changes in pH (Hazel et al., 1992). It thus is pertinent to examine how the changes in pH that accompany shifts in body temperature (figure 7.16) affect the physical properties of membranes. Hazel et al. (1992) showed that the sensitivity to temperature of fluorescence anisotropy of plasma membranes from 20°C-acclimated rainbow trout differed between imidazole and phosphate buffers (figure 7.30). The imidazole buffer established a temperature-dependent pH similar to that shown in figure 7.16. The pH of a phosphate buffered solution is only minimally temperature-dependent because the pK of phosphate varies by only about 0.001 pH unit per degree Celsius change in temperature. In the imidazole buffer approximately 40% of the compensation of fluidity for change in temperature could be attributed to the temperature-dependent pH of the buffer.

What underlies the effect of pH on membrane fluidity and phase state? The effect of an alphastat pH regimen on membrane phospholipids differs fundamentally from the influence that alphastat regulation has on protein

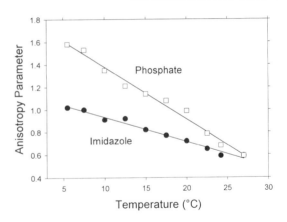

Figure 7.30. Effects of pH regimen on the temperature-dependence of membrane fluidity, as indexed by fluorescence anisotropy. (Figure modified after Hazel et al., 1992.)

histidyl groups. Alphastat regulation stabilizes the dissociation state of the imidazole groups of histidyl residues—this, in fact, is how alphastat regulation is defined—whereas this pattern of pH regulation will lead to *increases in net charge of phosphate groups as temperature falls*. As the pH of the solution bathing the membrane rises with falling temperature under alphastat conditions, the extent of dissociation of the phosphate groups of phospholipids increases. This increase in charge has important effects on the physical state of the membrane. The higher the level of charge on the phosphate groups, the greater is their water-binding ability. Thus, as the hydration state of phosphate groups increases, the effective volume of the headgroup increases. This, in turn, favors dispersal of the phospholipids in the plane of the membrane, with a concomitant increase in mobilities of their acyl chains. Thus, the increase in charge of phospholipids with falling temperature under alphastat regulation favors a higher level of fluidity and stabilizes the potential for forming hexagonal II phases. Conversely, as pH decreases with rising body temperature, membrane phospholipids become less ionized, so they tend to pack more tightly, leading again to temperature compensation in fluidity and propensity for formation of hexagonal II phases.

Although the data given in figure 7.30 support the hypothesis that adaptive changes in membrane physical properties may be established in part by alterations in the milieu surrounding the membrane, caveats must be raised. The differences in the response of fluorescence anisotropy to changing temperature noted between imidazole and phosphate buffers for membranes from 20°C-acclimated trout were not observed in membranes from trout held at 5°C (Hazel et al., 1992). Because shifts in phospholipid composition occur during thermal acclimation, it appears probable that the lipid composition of a membrane may help to determine the response of the membrane's physical state to changes in pH. Additional studies of pH effects, including those of buffer-specific influences, on membranes are needed to more fully elucidate this potentially important aspect of adaptation.

Inorganic and organic osmolytes

The discovery that the responses of membrane physical state to changing temperature can be influenced by the species of buffer used raises the general issue of how other small solutes in the membrane's local microenvironment might influence fluidity and phase state. Inorganic cations may bind to charged headgroups, neutralizing their charge and, thereby, affecting their hydration states. Organic osmolytes also may have important roles to play in stabilizing membranes in the face of thermal stress (see Tsvetkova and Quinn, 1994). It is known that trehalose, an organic solute that is accumulated in yeast during heat stress (Singer and Lindquist, 1998a) and in many organisms under conditions of low temperature or desiccation stress, is a stabilizer of the phase state of membranes (Crowe and Crowe, 1992). It may be revealing to examine trehalose and other organic osmolytes that interact with and stabilize membrane structure in the context of adaptation of membranes to temperature change. In fact, inclusion of a biologically realistic solute mixture in the in-vitro media used to study membranes may be necessary if the properties of the membranes in vivo are to be discerned.

Physical states of lipids: some final thoughts

Study of influences of temperature on the physical states of lipids has a long history. One of the earliest studies of thermal acclimation was an investigation, published in 1901, of changes in subcutaneous lipids in pigs that either were provided with insulating clothing or left naked in the cold Swedish winter (Henriques and Hansen, 1901). The subcutaneous fats of the clothed pigs had higher melting temperatures than those of the naked pigs—the first hint of homeoviscous adaptation.

Close modulation of the physical states of lipids is important in a variety of other contexts. Lipids play major roles as buoyancy-regulating devices in which temperature-induced alterations in lipid density play important functions in setting the overall buoyancy of the organism (e.g., the spermaceti organ of sperm whales; see Clarke, 1979). Cuticular lipids function as important barriers to water movement in terrestrial arthropods (Gibbs, 1998; Hadley, 1981), and the chemical compositions and physical states of these lipids manifest temperature responses comparable in many ways to those observed for membrane lipids.

In all instances in which temperature-lipid effects are observed, a consistent principle—one observed as well in studies of temperature-protein interactions—is noted: some degree of *metastability of structure* is a requisite for biological function. Lipids, like proteins, manifest a balancing act, one in which structures are favored that are neither too stable nor too labile. This fine balance is found to depend on the intrinsic properties of the large molecules (lipids and proteins) and on the influences of numerous extrinsic factors (protons, water, inorganic ions, and organic osmolytes) that affect molecular stability. Adaptation often represents a "communal effort" by the largest and smallest entities of the cell, and this joint effort involving intrinsic and extrinsic factors is observed during multigenerational evolutionary processes as well as during phenotypic acclimatizations and acclimations.

REGULATION OF BODY TEMPERATURE: ENDOTHERMY AND HOMEOTHERMY

Costs and Benefits of—and Access to— Endothermic Homeothermy

Endothermy and homeothermy are not the same thing

At the outset of this discussion of regulation of body temperature, it is important to review— and contrast—endothermy and homeothermy. These terms refer to two distinct types of thermal relationships and apply to organisms belonging to many taxa of plants and animals, not just to mammals and birds. *Homeotherms* are organisms that succeed in regulating their body temperatures within a narrow range, using a variety of mechanisms. Stabilization of body temperature may be achieved through: (1) *behavior*, such as selection of a stable thermal microclimate, basking in the sun to stay warm, seeking shade during hot periods, clustering together during cold stress, or undergoing seasonal migrations; (2) *insulation*, such as fur and feathers or layers of subcutaneous lipids; (3) *coloration*, such that heat energy is either absorbed or reflected, depending upon the heat budget of the organism; (4) *regulation of heat loss by changing circulatory flow*, as seen in numerous organisms, ranging from diving mammals that use the flipper as a radiator to exhaust excess heat to sphinx moths that radiate through their abdomens the heat produced in the thoracic flight muscles; and (5) *controlling the amount of heat produced by cells*, a response that is surprisingly widespread among organisms. Homeothermy does not necessarily imply a high body temperature, although the most familiar homeotherms, birds and mammals, which are endothermic homeotherms, usually have core temperatures between 35 and 40°C.

Endotherms are organisms that are capable of regulating the amount of heat produced in catabolic processes in order to enable the body, or regions thereof, to have an elevated temperature. When an organism with a large capacity for heat generation also has access to one or more of the other mechanisms known to foster homeothermy, notably, tight regulation of heat lost to the environment across the body surface, then the species may be a highly effective *endothermic homeotherm*. At the extreme, the capacities for generating heat and controlling its exchange with the environment may support *whole-body (systemic) endothermic homeothermy*. In many cases, however, especially in aquatic species, *regional endothermic homeothermy* represents the limit to what metabolic, circulatory, and behavioral adaptations can accomplish in the face of physical constraints inherent in the organism or in the environment.

It may seem to stretch the conventional definition of endothermy to include among the regional endotherms species that heat up specific structures for short periods of time, for instance, plants with heated floral regions that emit volatile, insect-attracting pheromones, to ensure pollination. However, we will consider the spatially and temporally restricted endothermic capacities of these species because, at the molecular level, these organisms exploit some of the same strategies for heat generation that are found in systemic endothermic homeotherms like birds and mammals. In fact, the heat-generating strategies of diverse animals and plants are fabricated using a relatively small number of types of starting raw material. Typically, the material from which endothermic machinery has evolved comprises biochemical reaction systems whose original functions were not the production of heat, but rather the accomplishment of some other important task, such as locomotion, ATP production, ion transport, or defense against the production of reactive oxygen species (ROS). Evolutionary modification of these biochemical systems to enable them to "waste" energy in large-scale production of heat represents acquisition of a derived, secondary function in all cases.

Endothermic homeothermy: A cost–benefit analysis

The benefits of being an endothermic homeotherm, especially one with systemic regulation of body temperature, are readily apparent. By maintaining a stable body temperature, an organism is freed from the effects of the Q_{10} relationship (the "tyranny of the Arrhenius equation," to quote the physiologist Joseph Barcroft), so that changes in ambient temperature do not inevitably lead to rapid changes in the rates of metabolic processes. Thus freed from conformity with ambient temperature, endothermic homeotherms can select their habitats using criteria other than environmental temperature, which is an exceedingly important advantage in many contexts. For instance, small endothermic homeotherms may be capable of exploiting a habitat nocturnally, at times when large ectothermic predators are inactive due to low nighttime temperatures. Moreover, endothermic homeotherms may be able to move between habitats with markedly different temperatures. Diving mammals may bask in full sun on land and then dive for prolonged periods in water only slightly above freezing. Because most endothermic homeotherms have relatively high body temperatures relative to ambient temperature, that is, relative to the body temperatures of most ectotherms, they are able to take advantage of the Q_{10} effect and obtain more activity per enzyme molecule per unit time than low-body-temperature species. Even though k_{cat} values for orthologous enzymes of mammals and birds may be lower than those of orthologs from cold-adapted ectotherms when orthologs are compared at a common temperature of measurement (figure 7.3), at the higher body temperature of mammals and birds, enzymatic reaction rates per enzyme molecule will exceed those for enzymes of cold-adapted ectotherm at their low body temperature. The higher metabolic rates that can be sustained by endothermic homeotherms may greatly increase locomotory performance, allowing for more effective predation and escape from predators and for abilities to move rapidly over wide distances in selecting advantageous habitats. Of particular importance is the ability to maintain a stable level of neural function in the face of changing ambient temperature. This allows neuromuscular coordination, sensory perception, and processing of neural inputs to occur at stable rates regardless of ambient temperature. The impor-

tance of stabilizing membrane-based neural activity should be apparent from the discussion of adaptation of membrane systems, and is reflected in the occurrence of specific heater organs in fishes that warm the eye and brain (see below; Block, 1991).

Access to endothermic homeothermy

Why, then, are endothermic homeotherms the exception rather than the rule among animals? There are certain basic physical constraints to developing endothermic homeothermy. One is body size. Heat flux is determined substantially by surface to volume ratio, so very small organisms, even ones with high mass-specific respiration rates, are unlikely to be able to maintain high enough rates of energy turnover to offset the rate at which they lose heat to the environment. The smallest endothermic homeotherms, organisms like shrews and small hummingbirds, must maintain enormous mass-specific metabolic rates in order to regulate their body temperatures near 37–40°C. Small endothermic homeotherms have some of the highest mass-specific metabolic rates known, rates which may approach the upper limit of what is possible due to physiological and anatomical constraints (Suarez, 1998). Thus, there appear to be strict limits to the amount of heat-generating capacity that can be packaged within an organ designed to do work. For instance, there are limits to the fraction of total tissue volume that can be occupied by mitochondria in muscle tissues. A different engineering situation applies, of course, for the limited number of organs and tissues whose function is strictly heat generation, as discussed later in the context of brown adipose tissue of mammals and heater organs of fish. The rate at which heat-generating structures can be supplied with metabolic fuels and purged of metabolic end-products likewise may face limitations (Suarez, 1998).

Another physical constraint to endothermic homeothermy is the rate of heat loss during respiratory gas exchange, especially in water. The oxygen concentration in water is only about one-fortieth that of air, but water's heat capacity exceeds that of air by approximately

3,000-fold. Thus, across a fish's gill, the diffusion of heat occurs about 50 times more rapidly than diffusion of oxygen or CO_2 (see Block, 1991, for a detailed account of heat retention in aquatic species). Heat lost during aerial respiration also may be substantial, and airbreathing endothermic homeotherms often employ adaptations for restricting ventilatory loss of heat (and water).

In addition to these challenging physical constraints, the demands for food that an endothermic homeotherm faces are substantially greater than those for an ectotherm of the same body mass. At the same body temperature, on a unit mass basis, similar-sized endotherms and ectotherms differ in oxygen consumption on average by at least four- to fivefold (see Brand et al., 1991). It is obvious that many ectothermic species may not have access to enough food, at all times, to make it possible, even in principle, for them to become endothermic homeotherms. An ecosystem in which all animals are endothermic homeotherms is probably impossible.

Ectothermy has many advantages

Despite some of its limitations, ectothermy is seen to have certain major advantages over endothermic homeothermy. Ectothermy allows a less energetically costly mode of living due to the four- to fivefold lower energy demands per unit mass relative to a similar-sized bird or mammal. One beneficial consequence of reduced energy demands is decreased foraging times. These may significantly reduce dangers of predation and, as well, they further reduce the cost of living because locomotory activity commonly requires the largest single share of an animal's ATP turnover, whether it is an ectotherm or endotherm. Minimization of energy costs associated with regulating body temperature and foraging tends to maximize the fraction of the energy consumed that can be directed towards growth and reproduction. Many ectotherms are highly fecund and grow to reproductive size rapidly. Finally, the small sizes that ectothermic animals can attain allow them access to niches unavailable to endothermic homeotherms. Because of the numerous

physical and biological limitations to endothermic homeothermy and the many advantages of ectothermy, more than 99.9% of the species in the biosphere are strictly ectothermic.

Basic Principles of Biological Heat Generation

Heat is a normal by-product of metabolism

The laws of thermodynamics tell us that no chemical process can be 100% efficient in trapping in new covalent bonds the free energy released during an exergonic chemical reaction. Of particular relevance for metabolic heat production is the efficiency with which the energy released during catabolism of foodstuff molecules is trapped in the synthesis of ATP, the cell's "energy currency" compound. Current estimates suggest that only about 38% of the energy released during catabolism of glucose is trapped in ATP (Streyer, 1988). The fact that over 60% of the energy released during catabolism may appear as heat suggests that development of effective mechanisms for heat generation are likely to involve one of two strategies: (1) *increasing metabolic flux*, to capitalize on the inherent thermodynamic inefficiency of metabolism, or (2) *reducing the efficiency of free energy capture even further*, such that most or all energy released during catabolic reactions is converted to heat, rather than being used to perform work such as ATP synthesis. The varied mechanisms that animals and plants have evolved to exploit these two routes to endothermy reveal several fascinating examples of how preexisting physiological systems can be modified for a new function.

Endothermy could, in principle, simply involve "doing more of the same thing," biochemically and physiologically. For instance, cold stress could lead to increased locomotory activity to exploit the high ATPase activity of the contractile machinery. For most vertebrates, by far the largest source of ATP turnover and, therefore, of heat generation, is in locomotory activity. Endothermy based on high levels of locomotory activity is characteristic of some animals, notably the continuously swimming tunas who use the heat generated by the swimming musculature to effect endothermic homeothermy in part of the muscle mass and in other organs (Block, 1991).

Modulating for purposes of heat generation the rates of activity of physiological processes whose principal functions are not the production of heat is not an optimal strategy in most cases, however. The needs for heat generation are not likely to correlate strongly with the demands for activity of the physiological process in question. For instance, it may behoove a small endothermic homeotherm to remain quiet to avoid predators; moving about simply to keep warm could be a fatal strategy. The challenge for an endotherm, then, is to find mechanisms that can be used *exclusively* for heat generation, so that body temperature can be regulated without negatively impacting other physiological processes or creating behavioral trade-offs of the sort just mentioned. Large-scale heat production not linked to physiological work, especially locomotory effort, is what is required.

Endothermy is based on relatively small sets of "engineering principles" and biochemical "raw material"

In light of the diverse array of taxa—mammals, birds, fishes, insects, and plants—in which either systemic or regional endothermy is found, one might expect that an extremely varied set of strategies for generating heat would be exploited. However, as mentioned earlier, only a rather small set of "engineering principles" and biochemical processes are exploited in endothermic animals and plants. There are essentially only two basic strategies used by endotherms for generating large amounts of heat *strictly for purposes of thermal regulation.* First, energy that normally would be used to synthesize ATP in mitochondrial electron transport is redirected towards heat generation, away from coupled production of ATP. Second, the energy that is temporarily stored in ATP is rapidly converted to heat by ATP-consuming processes that typically lead to no net biological work, but only to heat production. Each of these basic strategies involves modification of preexisting, work-supporting biochemical pathways. The primary modifications required for converting these pathways to effective endothermic mechanisms include: (i) supply of large amounts of substrate and oxygen for ATP-generating systems, whether or not the systems remain coupled to ATP production during heat generation, (ii) creation of short-circuits within ATP-synthesizing pathways to allow production of heat rather than of ATP, and, (iii) the addition to systems where coupled ATP production continues of ATP-utilizing reactions that allow rapid regeneration of ADP and P_i.

Brown Adipose Tissue: Uncoupling Synthesis of ATP from Mitochondrial Electron Transport

Brown adipose tissue: a mammalian invention that exploits ancient "raw material"

If evolutionary processes could be given the proverbial "clean sheet of paper" to engineer the most effective system for generating large amounts of heat precisely as needed for short-term and long-term regulation of body temperature, it is difficult to imagine that they would produce a better solution to the problem than that exemplified by brown adipose tissue (BAT). Brown adipose tissue is a strictly mammalian invention; attempts to find heat-generating organs like BAT in birds and other nonmammalian vertebrates have been unsuccessful. However, as discussed below, fundamental aspects of BAT-like biochemistry may be widespread among eukaryotes, so certain species that lack a specialized heat-generating organ like BAT nonetheless may be able to exploit some of the biochemical mechanisms used in heat generation by BAT.

Brown adipose tissue is most prevalent in neonatal mammals, but it is now thought to persist in many adult forms as well, including adult humans (for review, see Ricquier and Bouillaud, 2000). Small mammals such as rodents rely heavily on BAT thermogenesis as adults. The high surface-to-volume ratios of small mammals appear to favor the persistence of this mode of heat generation throughout life.

Larger mammals, with their lower surface-to-volume ratios, appear to sustain endothermic homeothermy with, at most, minimal contributions from BAT. Brown adipose tissue also plays a vital role in hibernators (Boyer and Barnes, 1999). Small hibernating mammals like squirrels rely strongly on BAT for rapid rewarming after a bout of hibernation. The localization of BAT seems well suited to effect rapid warming; BAT deposits are found in interscapular, perirenal, thoracic, and neck muscle sites, areas where heat production would facilitate warming of blood serving critical organs.

Structurally, BAT is characterized by a high density of storage lipids (triacylglycerides) and a massive concentration of mitochondria with highly proliferated inner membranes, which enhance the level of electron transport activity in the organelle. The brown color of BAT is due to the respiratory pigments found in these abundant mitochondria. White adipose tissue (WAT), which is the primary lipid storage tissue in animals and which is probably nonthermogenic, is relatively low in mitochondrial density and, hence, lacks the dark color of BAT. Brown adipose cells have been found dispersed in WAT, but their role in thermogenesis is not established (Lowell and Spiegelman, 2000). Brown adipose tissue is richly supplied with blood vessels, and flow of oxygenated blood into this tissue is closely regulated in concert with the body's need for this supplementary source of heat. The circulatory flow through BAT is such as to ensure rapid transfer of heat into large blood vessels that supply critical organs such as the brain.

Physiologically and biochemically, BAT is characterized by a suite of neural, hormonal, and genetic regulatory circuits that are responsive to the mammal's thermal status, plus one novel and pivotal adaptation in the mitochondrial inner membrane: the insertion of an *uncoupling protein* that mediates a net influx of protons that is not linked to ATP generation. The regulatory circuitry, described later, functions to control the quantities and activity of uncoupling protein and to provide sufficient fatty acids used for catabolism and for serving as proton transport vehicles. Prolonged activation of the regulatory circuitry also leads to proliferation of mitochondria and BAT.

In mammals, uncoupling proteins occur in at least three isoforms, all of which are members of a broad family of mitochondrial carrier proteins (Ricquier and Bouillaud, 2000). Uncoupling protein-1 (UCP1; formerly termed "thermogenin") is found exclusively in BAT. Uncoupling protein-2 (UCP2) is widely expressed among tissues, and has been identified in brain, heart, liver, intestine, lung, spleen, kidney, testis, uterus, WAT, and BAT. Uncoupling protein-3 (UCP3) appears to be expressed only in muscle and BAT. All three UCP isoforms comprise 306–308 amino acid residues and have six transmembrane domains. Uncoupling proteins 2 and 3 are 75% identical in sequence. They share a lower sequence identity, approximately 60%, with UCP1. The roles of UCP2 and UCP3 in thermogenesis are controversial (see Echtay *et al.*, 2000; Ricquier and Bouillaud, 2000), so the discussion to follow focuses chiefly on UCP1, whose thermogenic function is unequivocal.

Short-circuiting ATP synthesis to generate heat: the role of fatty acid transport and UCP1

At the core of the heat-generating mechanism in BAT is a vehicle for conducting protons across the inner mitochondrial membrane into the mitochondrial matrix that bypasses the F_1F_0 ATPase (ATP synthase) channel where proton influx normally is coupled to synthesis of ATP (figure 7.31). Dissipation of the mitochondrial proton electrochemical gradient ($\Delta\mu H^+$) is proposed to involve a novel mechanism in which free fatty acids (FFAs) serve as protonophores (proton carriers). Although the mechanism by which uncoupled proton flux occurs remains under debate, it appears probable that protons do not move through UCP1 itself. Rather, they are bound to carboxylate groups of free fatty acids that can readily pass through the inner mitochondrial membrane. This mechanism for dissipation of the proton gradient involves a "revolving door" process using free fatty acids in both protonated (electroneutral: FFA-H) and deprotonated (anionic: FFA$^-$) forms. In

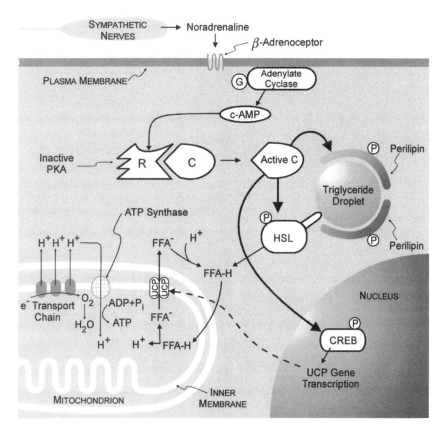

Figure 7.31. The pathways involved in the thermogenic function of brown adipose tissue (BAT) and the regulatory mechanisms for governing BAT activity. Brown adipose tissue metabolism is fueled by free fatty acids (FFAs) released from triglyceride droplets through activity of a hormone-sensitive lipase enzyme (HSL). Hormone-sensitive lipase enzyme is activated by phosphorylation (P) catalyzed by the catalytic subunit (C) of protein kinase A (PKA). Protein kinase A also phosphorylates a protein called perilipin that may help to control access of HSL to the triglyceride droplet. Activation of PKA requires dissociation of the regulatory subunit (R) from the catalytic subunit (the holoenzyme comprises two R and two C subunits; only one subunit of each type is shown). Dissociation of the catalytic and regulatory subunits follows binding to the regulatory subunit of cyclic AMP (cAMP). CyclicAMP is produced from ATP by an adenylate cyclase enzyme localized on the inner surface of the plasma membrane. The adenylate cyclase is activated by the β-adrenoceptor when noradrenaline is bound to the receptor. Noradrenaline is released from the endings of sympathetic nerves that connect BAT to the hypothalamus.

Free fatty acids serve two functions in BAT: (i) fuels for oxidative metabolism and electron transport, which drives protons out across the inner mitochondrial membrane, and (ii) protonophores, which carry protons back through the inner membrane without coupling proton movement to ATP synthesis. The uncoupling of proton movement through the inner membrane of the mitochondrion from ATP synthesis by the ATP synthase is conjectured to involve transmembrane movement of neutral (protonated) FFA (FFA-H) into the matrix of the mitochondrion. There, FFA-H dissociates to FFA^- and H^+. The FFA^- exits the matrix through a channel provided by uncoupling protein-1 (UCP). In the extramitochondrial space, which is highly acidic relative to the matrix, FFA^- is protonated and then able to reenter the matrix and carry another proton through the membrane.

Hormonal activation of BAT leads to a high degree of heat generation within seconds to minutes. Longer-term stimulation leads to hormonally mediated increases in gene expression. Protein kinase A phosphorylates a gene regulatory protein, cAMP-response-element-binding protein (CREB), which increases expression of the gene encoding UCP1. Stimulation by thyroid hormones (not shown) also elevates levels of UCP1. (Figure modified after Lowell, 1996, and Ricquier and Bouillaud, 2000.)

the relatively acidic medium outside of the inner mitochondria membrane, into which lipid-fueled electron transport pumps protons, free fatty acids become protonated (neutralized). As neutral molecules (FFA-H), fatty acids readily cross the inner mitochondrial membrane and enter the matrix. Within the matrix, where the pH is relatively alkaline, the FFA-H molecules dissociate to form fatty acid anions (FFA$^-$) and protons. As protons continue to be pumped out of the matrix during electron transport, electroneutrality is maintained by exit of FFA$^-$ anions through the uncoupling protein channel in the inner mitochondrial membrane. In the extramitochondrial space, FFA$^-$ and H$^+$ associate to form FFA-H, and another cycle of proton entry into the matrix can commence. Free fatty acids thus are seen to play two essential roles in thermogenesis: they serve as metabolic substrates for electron transport activity and, as protonophores, they mediate uncoupled entry for protons. Thus, catabolism of free fatty acids in BAT leads to the production of CO_2, H_2O, and heat, but to no synthesis of ATP, because free fatty acids (FFA-H) rather than the ATP synthase channel are used to dissipate $\Delta\mu H^+$.

Regulation of BAT activity involves a complex hierarchy of regulatory mechanisms

Several aspects of BAT function are seen to dictate that thermogenesis in this organ be very closely regulated. When thermogenesis is required, BAT must be subject to rapid activation, but it must attain a graded level of thermogenic activity that is consistent with the degree of cold stress the animal is experiencing. When not required in thermogenesis, BAT must be kept switched off. The enormous heat-generating capacity of BAT could pose a threat to survival if BAT's activity were not reduced when thermally equable conditions are reestablished. Unregulated heat production by BAT might quickly raise the body temperature to a lethal level. Energy conservation is another important factor underlying the need to control BAT's activity and mass; BAT is ultimately wasteful of energy-rich substrates. Triglycerides shunted into BAT for heat generation could instead serve as an important

energy storage depot for the organism, were they to be deposited in WAT. The mass of BAT is costly to maintain, so over longer time courses of thermal adaptation, for instance, during seasonal temperature cycles, it may be advantageous to change the amount of BAT present in the body.

Because of the need to regulate closely the activity and amount of BAT, a diverse set of regulatory mechanisms achieves both rapid regulation of existing BAT machinery and longer-term adjustment in the amount of BAT that is present (figure 7.31; Lowell, 1996; Lowell and Spiegelman, 2000). Short-term regulation is effected by several mechanisms. Purine nucleotides (ADP, ATP, GDP, and GTP) are negative modulators of the activity of UCP1 and can rapidly (within seconds) change the rate of thermogenesis. The activity of UCP1 also is modulated by the level of oxidized (but not reduced) coenzyme Q (ubiquinone) that is present (Echtay et al., 2000). The supply of free fatty acids for catabolism and proton shunting also plays a key role in short-term regulation of BAT's activity. Free fatty acids stimulate UCP1 activity, through providing the vehicle needed for uncoupled proton translocation, and activate respiration in BAT. The generation of free fatty acids is mediated by hormonally controlled degradation of triacylglyceride droplets within BAT. When the temperature-regulating center in the hypothalamus detects a reduction in body temperature, sympathetic nerves innervating BAT release noradrenaline, which then binds to hormone receptors in the plasma membrane of BAT cells. Signal transduction involves a G-protein-linked adenylate cyclase that produces cyclic AMP (cAMP). The function of cAMP in the regulatory cascade is the activation of protein kinase-A (PKA). When inactive, PKA is a tetrameric enzyme comprising two regulatory (R) subunits and two catalytic (C) subunits. Cyclic AMP binds to the R-subunits of PKA, which causes them to dissociate from the two C-subunits. When released from the R-subunits, the two C-subunits dissociate to catalytically active monomers that are competent to phosphorylate their target proteins.

Activated PKA plays at least three roles, each of which involves phosphorylation of a specific type of regulatory protein (Himms-Hagen, 1990; Lowell, 1996). First, PKA phosphorylates and thereby activates a hormone sensitive lipase (HSL) that hydrolyzes triacylglycerides to free fatty acids. Second, PKA phosphorylates a protein termed perilipin, which is found on the surface of triacylglyceride droplets in both BAT and white adipose tissue. It is hypothesized (Lowell, 1996) that perilipin modulates access of HSL to triacylglycerides. Phosphorylated perilipin may allow increased hydrolytic attack by HSL on its substrate. Third, PKA phosphorylates a gene regulatory protein, cAMP-response-element-binding protein (CREB), which enhances the transcription of the gene encoding UCP1. This latter regulatory event is part of the enhanced biogenesis of BAT that occurs in response to hormonal signaling. Intracellular levels of triiodothyronine are also elevated in response to prolonged cold stress, and this hormonal change also increases transcription of the *Ucp1* gene. Unlike the gene encoding UCP1, the genes encoding UCP2 and UCP3 are not known to be up-regulated by low temperature (Ricquier and Bouillaud, 2000). Lastly, correlated with up-regulation of UCP1 is down-regulation of the F_1F_0 ATPase, leading to an increased propensity for proton entry into the matrix to be unlinked to synthesis of ATP. This hierarchical network of regulatory mechanisms allows the activity of BAT to be rapidly modulated in the face of short-term demands for varying amounts of heat generation. Regulatory schemes that involve hormonal signaling enable the total amount of BAT to be altered in response to environmental and physiological conditions (see Himms-Hagen, 1990; Lowell, 1996).

pH may help to modulate BAT activity in small mammalian hibernators

There is one further aspect of regulation of BAT activity that merits discussion, the role that shifts in pH may play in governing BAT thermogenesis in hibernators (Malan and Mioskowski, 1988). GDP is a potent inhibitor of UCP1 activity, and its binding to the protein is strongly affected by pH. Reductions in pH through the physiological pH range stabilize the GDP–UCP1 complex and inhibit thermogenesis. When alphastat pH regulation is present, binding of GDP to UCP1 is temperature-independent, so reduced body temperature will not affect thermogenesis insofar as the regulatory effects of GDP are concerned. However, when decreases in body temperature are not paired with the rise in pH associated with alphastat regulation, the acidification that occurs will enhance GDP binding to UCP1 and reduce or curtail BAT thermogenesis. Because small mammalian hibernators frequently undergo respiratory acidosis during entry into hibernation, leading to retention of excess CO_2 and a concomitant fall in pH, GDP binding to UCP1 may increase and lead to a curtailment of heat generation by BAT. During arousal, hyperventilation leading to removal of CO_2 and, thus, to an increase in pH back to the alphastat value, will reverse the inhibition of BAT activity and allow thermogenesis. Small mammalian hibernators like squirrels and hamsters thus may use divergence from alphastat regulation to modulate thermogenesis as well as the activities of pH-sensitive enzymes like phosphofructokinase (Hand and Somero, 1983).

Evolutionary origin of uncoupling proteins

The UCPs belong to an ancient and broad superfamily of mitochondrial transporter proteins, one that includes the ATP/ADP carrier and the phosphate carrier among others, all of which appear to have arisen from a common gene that encoded an ancestral transporter having approximately 100 residues (Fleury et al., 1997). Uncoupling protein-1, as its name implies, was the first uncoupling protein to be discovered. Initially, UCP1 was regarded as a recent mammalian invention, a novel type of protein having a unique function and a unique localization, the inner membrane of BAT mitochondria. With the discovery of UCP2 and UCP3 in a variety of mammalian cell types and the identification of UCP homologs in plants (Laloi et al., 1997) and protozoans (see Ricquier and Bouillaud, 2000, for an evolutionary tree for UCPs and other mitochondrial carriers) it has become clear that uncoupling proteins are not unique to BAT, and may play roles in addition to thermogenesis.

Current hypotheses about the evolution of UCPs suggest that functions other than thermogenesis may have provided the initial selective advantages of this class of proteins. For example, uncoupling proteins may reduce the rate at which reactive oxygen species (ROS) like superoxide are produced (Ricquier and Bouillaud, 2000). By increasing the rate of electron transfer to molecular oxygen, uncoupling proteins prevent electrons from backing-up in the electron transport chain. Uncoupling proteins thereby reduce the lifetimes of ROS-generating centers in the electron transport chain, notably, reduced coenzyme Q (CoQ^{-}), which is a powerful one-electron donor to oxygen and, therefore, a highly potent superoxide (O_2^{-}) generator. One scenario, therefore, for the development of uncoupling proteins from an ancestral mitochondrial transmembrane carrier protein envisions the need, early in the evolution of eukaryotic cells, to provide means for reducing the rate of ROS production. Subsequently, one or more of these uncoupling proteins assumed a role in thermogenesis, probably through gaining the correct regulatory sensitivities to allow its activity to be modulated in concert with the needs for heat generation. Another scenario for the origin of uncoupling proteins suggests that they may have arisen to allow decoupling of NADH oxidation from ATP synthesis, when this is advantageous to the cell, for instance, during synthesis of fatty acids from glucose (Ricquier and Bouillaud, 2000). Whatever the initial selective advantages of uncoupling proteins were, it is apparent that the appearance in mammals of a thermogenic UCP is a recent invention fabricated from raw material that appeared early in the evolution of eukaryotic cells.

The roles of UCP2 and UCP3 remain controversial (Lowell and Spiegelman, 2000; Ricquier and Bouillaud, 2000). If UCP2 and UCP3 function effectively as protonophores, they could play several metabolically important roles, including the so-called "primitive" uncoupling functions of reducing production

of ROS and of maintaining the NADH/NAD ratio at physiologically appropriate levels.

Uncoupling proteins are also conjectured to play roles in regulating body weight (see review by Lowell and Spiegelman, 2000). Uncoupling proteins could be modulated such that their activities rise when a high caloric load is imposed on the organism, which would lead to homeostasis of body weight and composition. Diet-induced thermogenesis (DIT) is common in mammals, especially when the diet is rich in lipids and low in proteins. To gain sufficient amounts of amino acids to support protein synthesis, the organism may have to consume many more calories (as lipid) than needed for maintenance of body mass and lipid stores. Therefore, a diet high in lipid and low in protein may lead to "wastage" of energy in order to avoid obesity during acquisition of sufficient levels of amino acids. The hormone *leptin*, which is produced in adipocytes of WAT, is a signal to the hypothalamus that lipid stores are sufficient and that intake of lipid can be reduced. Leptin also activates metabolism in BAT through increasing sympathetic nerve signaling to the tissue. However, despite clear evidence that UCP1 is involved in DIT, there remains uncertainty about the roles of UCP2 and UCP3 in this homeostatic process. Dietary studies have provided conflicting evidence on this issue. However, some studies have shown clear linkages between diet and expression of UCP2. When mice were fed a high-fat diet, the expression of the *Ucp2* gene was up-regulated in WAT (Fleury et al., 1997). Thus, in addition to functioning in maintenance of the appropriate thermal equilibrium, one or more of the uncoupling proteins in mammals may serve the additional role of maintaining the correct equilibrium body weight.

Thermogenesis and Regional Endothermy in Plants: UCPs and Alternative Oxidase Systems

How good are plants at heat generation and how does endothermy benefit them?

In light of the constraints that animals face in developing endothermic homeothermy, it may be surprising to learn that certain types of plants are capable of generating a substantial amount of heat that is used to maintain an impressive degree of endothermic homeothermy in specific structures, notably reproductive organs. Biologists with an animal bias to their perspective may be especially surprised to learn that the oxygen consumption rates of flowering structures of lilies of the genus *Arum* can be as high as those of hummingbirds in flight, that is to say, as high as those of the most active endothermic homeothermic animals (Raskin et al., 1987). The initial observation of warm-bodied plants appears to have been made by Lamarck as early as 1778, so regional endothermy in plants has been appreciated by biologists for over two centuries. What have required considerable time to elucidate are the benefits of this heat-generating capacity and the biochemical mechanisms that support this ability.

Several advantages of regional endothermy in plants have been proposed. These include certain benefits held in common with endothermic animals, for instance, avoidance of freezing at low temperatures and the stabilization of metabolic processes in the face of changing ambient temperature. Other benefits of endothermy are unique to flowering plants: enhanced production and volatilization of insect-attracting chemicals and the provision of warm pollination chambers that enhance the likelihood that insect pollinators will be able to carry out this function effectively (Seymour and Schultze-Motel, 1996). Many insect-attractant substances are volatile organic molecules whose synthesis is likely to have a Q_{10} near 2, and whose dispersion into the atmosphere is also likely to be temperature-dependent. Thus, heated flowers that generate and release large amounts of insect attractants may increase the likelihood that a plant is successful in reproduction. Provision of a warm pollination chamber in the flowering structure also can enhance reproductive success. Many flying insects require thoracic temperatures of 30°C or higher to initiate flight. Thus, a warm chamber in which these insects could gain (or shed) pollen and maintain thoracic temperatures permissive of flight could be to the mutual advantage of plant and insect. Beetles trapped overnight in a warm pollination chamber were observed to feed and copulate, so flowering plants that can maintain elevated temperatures even on cool nights may provide especially favorable microhabitats for their insect partners.

Some plants, for example the sacred lotus, *Nelumbo nucifera*, are able to achieve a high degree of regional endothermic homeothermy by modulating metabolic heat production as ambient temperature changes (Seymour and Schultze-Motel, 1996). Lotus flowers maintained a temperature of 30–35°C in the face of air temperatures ranging between 10°C and 30°C, for a period of 2–4 days. Oxygen consumption rate of the flowers varied inversely with ambient temperature. The metabolic systems responsible for heat production have not been characterized in the lotus, but studies of other flowering plants are consistent with the occurrence of at least two types of thermogenic processes in vascular plants.

Mechanisms of thermogenesis in plants

In common with animals, uncoupling proteins in the inner mitochondrial membrane may serve as heat generators in some plants. An uncoupling protein exhibiting strong homology to UCP1 and UCP2 has been identified in the potato (*Solanum tuberosum*) (Laloi et al., 1997). Its sequence is 44% and 47% identical to UCP1 and UCP2, respectively. This UCP, termed StUCP, appears to be present in all tissues of the plant, and is strongly induced by exposure to cold temperatures (4°C for 1–2 days). The role played by StUCP in protecting the plant from cold injury remains to be shown, but the presence of this potential heat-generating mechanism could be important in preventing damage at low temperatures.

The thermogenic mechanism best understood in plants is a cyanide-insensitive nonphosphorylating electron transport pathway that is found only in plant mitochondria (Raskin et al., 1987). This pathway is distinct from the electron transport pathway involved in mitochondrial ATP production, and is under the control of *calorigens*, molecules that can lead to a strong activation of this pathway. In lilies of the genus *Arum*, the calorigen responsible for the massive rise in heat production during reproduction is 2-hydroxybenzoic acid, known commonly as salicylic acid, and a close relative of aspirin. Salicylic acid is synthesized and transported to the flowering structures in a photoperiod-dependent manner, which allows the triggering of heat generation to occur when the plant is reproductively mature.

In summary, some plants, like certain endothermic animals, possess thermogenic pathways whereby the energy released in oxidation of reduced organic substrates can be directly and quantitatively released as heat, without ATP being formed as an intermediate. These highly efficient thermogenic pathways involve electron transport systems that can operate at extremely high rates. And, because thermogenesis is based on aerobic pathways, the metabolic end-products formed are relatively nontoxic ($H_2O + CO_2$). The thermogenic pathways involving uncoupling proteins appear to be widespread among taxa, and to represent evolutionary exploitation of "raw material" common to all mitochondria, namely proteins of the inner mitochondrial membrane that are involved in a diverse array of transmembrane transport processes. Through the processes of gene duplication and subsequent sequence divergence, variants of these transport proteins have arisen that have lost their original functions and have gained new abilities: "wasting" of metabolic energy to allow (i) reductions in ROS production, (ii) more effective metabolic regulation (e.g., from maintaining NADH/ NAD ratios), (iii) modulation of body mass, and, (iv) effective endothermic control of body temperature.

Endothermy Fueled by High Rates of ATP Turnover

Multiple means exist for "wasting" metabolic energy

Thermogenic systems based on uncoupling proteins or on the alternative electron transport pathways found in mitochondria of certain plants represent what in many ways is the simplest and most direct way for generating heat: decouple catabolism from work so that all energy released during oxidation of reduced organic molecules can be directly dissipated as heat. In principle, complete "wasting" of metabolic energy also could be achieved if cells were able to couple synthesis of ATP with rapid and quantitative hydrolysis of ATP in some type(s) of work. In a thermogenic system of this type, *ATP turnover rates* are the pivotal factor in setting rates of heat production. This second approach to heat generation is, in fact, a common strategy of thermogenesis in numerous taxa. It is employed to support highly effective regional endothermy in diverse ectotherms, it can support both systemic and regional endothermy in birds and mammals, and it may have played an important role in the initial evolutionary development of systemic endothermic homeothermy in the reptilian ancestors of mammals.

Requirements for endothermy based on enhanced turnover of ATP

There are certain types of "raw material" that are needed to fabricate thermogenic systems that rely on massive turnover of ATP. On the supply side of the equation, the generation of large amounts of ATP to support thermogenesis is likely to require a rich supply of mitochondria because, in the absence of aerobic metabolism, only a minor fraction of the bond energies in foodstuffs can be released through anaerobic pathways, which fail fully to convert the foodstuff in question to CO_2 and H_2O (chapters 2 and 3). Coupled to a high oxidative capacity in mitochondria is the requirement for supplying large amounts of oxygen and removing CO_2. Thus, circulatory adaptations are likely to be important components of heat-generating mechanisms. On the ATP-consuming side of the equation, it is essential to link ATP production to some type of ATP-requiring work mechanism whose activity can be scaled up sufficiently to allow rates of ATP turnover that are consistent with thermogenic demands.

There are several obvious candidates for this latter function. For many animals, and certainly for virtually all vertebrates, the largest share of

ATP turnover is associated with locomotory activity. Splitting of ATP by the actomyosin ATPase of the contractile apparatus, and using ATP to drive ion transport within muscle, notably, the resequestration of calcium ions into the sarcoplasmic reticulum (SR), are two pathways by which large amounts of heat could be generated. In isometric contraction, calcium ion pumping in muscle may require from about one-quarter to one-third of ATP turnover, and in sustained (tetanic) contraction, 40–60% of ATP produced may be used by the Ca^{2+} ATPase (calsequestrin) (Block, 1987, 1991). In resting cells, maintenance of transmembrane ion gradients, for instance, those for Na^+ and K^+, may represent one of the costliest homeostatic processes. It is estimated that up to one-quarter of ATP turnover in a typical resting cell may be linked to the Na^+-K^+-ATPase (chapter 2; Hulbert and Else, 1990). Therefore, in most animals, three highly promising schemes exist for producing large amounts of heat through ATP-consuming work: (i) contraction of actomyosin filaments, (ii) transport of Ca^{2+}, and (iii) transmembrane movements of Na^+ and K^+.

Shivering thermogenesis: using the actomyosin ATPase system while remaining stationary

In birds and mammals facing cold stress, shivering is a common strategy for achieving systemic endothermic homeothermy. Sympathetic neural stimulation activates the actomyosin ATPases of locomotory muscle, but this activation does not lead to the type of coordinated contraction that supports locomotion. Shivering thermogenesis exploits the large muscle mass present in a bird or a mammal. However, shivering carries with it the liability that heat generation and locomotory activity may work at cross purposes: stationary heat generation by shivering precludes locomotory activity. The latter activity, if it occurs at a relatively slow pace, may not provide sufficient heat for keeping the body warm. Thus, shivering thermogenesis is apt to be a short-term solution to the problem of cold stress. Longer-term, more effective solutions to the problem must involve mechanisms that allow a high rate of heat generation without creating a concomitant handicap in locomotory function.

Nonshivering thermogenesis in mammals and birds

During prolonged exposure to cold, shivering thermogenesis gives way to nonshivering thermogenesis (NST). The complete set of processes exploited to elevate production of heat in NST is only partially understood. The mechanisms used involve processes in addition to those localized in BAT, the major site of NST in small mammals but a tissue absent in birds. One of the potentially important sites of heat generation is muscle. Again, because of its large contribution to body mass and its high levels of ATPases associated with contractile work and ion pumping, muscle would appear to be a rich source of "raw material" for heat generation. Although the fractional contribution of skeletal muscle to NST remains unclear (see Block, 1994, for review), there are several lines of evidence pointing to an important contribution by this tissue.

Cold acclimation of mammals is marked by increased ion permeability of membranes in a number of tissues (Chaffee and Roberts, 1971). As discussed below in the context of the origin of endothermic homeothermy in mammals, increased ion permeability sets up the potential for increased heat generation through ion-pumping futile cycles. In skeletal muscle, increased ion permeability may be linked with elevated levels of FFA to greatly increase heat production. A possible mechanism is as follows. The increased activity of the sympathetic nervous system at low temperatures leads to increased activity of lipases, as discussed for BAT regulation. The higher levels of FFA produced by the lipases could have at least two major thermogenic effects in skeletal muscle. First, as substrates for energy metabolism, rising FFA concentrations could boost oxidative metabolism and, thereby, increase heat production. Second, FFAs may bind to the calcium release channel in the SR membrane and increase permeability of the membrane to Ca^{2+}. Elevated levels of Ca^{2+} would stimulate mitochondrial metabolism and create a need for increased ATP turnover to restore the Ca^{2+} to the SR. Heat generation involving elevated flux of Ca^{2+} is conjectured to play an important role in skeletal muscle of cold-acclimated mammals and birds. During cold acclimation in birds, Ca^{2+} ATPase and ryanodine-receptor (calcium channel) contents increase in muscle, favoring heat generation through this type of Ca^{2+} cycling (Dumonteil et al., 1995).

Calcium cycling is a two-edged sword in the context of thermogenesis, however, for it may also be the basic cause of a pathological process in mammals termed *malignant hyperthermia* (MH) (Denborough, 1998). Malignant hyperthermia involves an extremely large increase in muscle heat production under certain types of stresses, for instance, exposure to certain anesthetics during surgery. The molecular basis of MH is a faulty SR calcium release channel. Mutant forms of the channel allow a pathologically high rate of Ca^{2+} entry into the cytoplasm, with concomitant splitting of ATP during resequestration of Ca^{2+}. A single point mutation responsible for this effect has been identified in the porcine calcium release channel. A cysteine replaces an arginine as the result of a single base change at position 1843 in the nucleotide sequence (Fujii et al., 1991).

The exploitation of the heat-generating capacity of calcium ion cycling in muscle by cold-acclimated mammals and birds may reflect a primitive temperature-acclimation pathway already present in ectotherms, that is, a pathway that is hard-wired into the vertebrate genome, according to Block (1994). She points out that cold acclimation of ectothermic vertebrates may lead to increased mitochondrial content and to elevated SR volume in muscles, that is, to higher capacities for aerobic ATP production and for ATP usage, in the transport of Ca^{2+}. These two physiological changes are viewed as temperature-compensatory mechanisms for facilitating a stable rate of muscle function at reduced temperature in ectotherms such as fishes. In birds and mammals, which sustain a stable and high body temperature in the cold, these same changes would be temperature-compensatory in an entirely different sense: maintaining a stable

core temperature during cold stress by operating calcium cycling reactions at higher rates than under normothermic conditions. Thus, the same changes that lead to stabilization of rates of contraction and ATP turnover in muscle in differently acclimated ectotherms promote large increases in ATP turnover rates in birds and mammals, with a concomitant stabilization of body temperature. Sustaining high ATP turnover in endotherms may depend on continuing up-regulation of heat-generating reactions such as Ca^{2+} cycling by sympathetic stimulation or hormones such as thyroid hormones.

In summary, in most vertebrates, skeletal (locomotory) muscle offers a substantial potential for heat generation because of its large percentage contribution to body mass and its high ATPase activities. Exploitation of this potential for heat generation contributes significantly to regional and systemic endothermy—and, in the case of MH, excessive production of heat through one of the same pathways used for endothermy leads to a pathologically high level of heat production. The molecular and biochemical factors responsible for generating heat and the physiological regulators instrumental in controlling the rate of heat production are, of course, but a part of the story: the heat produced within the body must be retained—or removed—as thermal regulatory demands change.

Endothermy in tunas and lamnid sharks: Integration of heat generation and heat loss

The development of endothermy in fishes faces extreme challenges for reasons discussed earlier, notably, the high thermal conductivity of water and the rapid loss of heat across the gills during exchange of gases. Thus, it is not surprising that only 27 species of fish (or approximately 0.1% of all fishes) are currently known to be able to achieve endothermic control of substantial fractions of their bodies. These 27 species are tuna and lamnid sharks, which are large and actively swimming fish capable of generating high amounts of heat through locomotory activity. Even in these species, however, endothermic homeothermy is restricted to only certain tissues and organs: locomotory muscle, the viscera, the eyes, and the brain (Block, 1994). The abilities of these fishes to attain endothermic control of body temperature is based on several factors: (i) their large size, which leads to a high degree of thermal inertia (favorable surface-to-volume ratio for retention of heat); (ii) their high aerobic metabolism in white locomotory musculature (heat-generating capacities in red muscle of tuna appear to be no higher than in their similar-sized ectothermic relatives) (Block, 1991); (iii) the internalized location of the red muscle mass used to power steady-state swimming; and (iv) the interposition in the circulatory system of heat exchangers that allow heat generated in the muscles to be transferred from the venous circulation into the arterial circulation.

These traits have received most study in tunas, a group of fishes noted for continuous swimming and for major anatomical differences from other fishes. Of particular importance in the anatomical organization of tunas is the internalization of red muscle, an anatomical feature that appears critical for allowing endothermy to develop. In most fishes, the red muscle is located superficially, where it would be difficult, if not impossible, to prevent loss of metabolically generated heat to the environment. The internalization of the red muscle mass in tunas isolates this tissue from close contact with seawater. There is also an effective isolation from the medium of the circulatory system within red muscle: countercurrent exchangers interspersed between red muscle and the arterial circulation supplying the tissue allow much of the heat produced in red muscle to be retained, rather than lost to the environment.

The anatomical organization of countercurrent heat exchangers in tunas reflects the same engineering principles found in other countercurrent exchangers, such as the heat exchangers found in legs of sea birds and seals and in the eye and brain heaters of billfishes (see figure 7.32, upper panel), and the gas exchangers found in the gas gland of the teleost swim bladder. Close juxtaposition of fine arteries and veins allows outwardly flowing blood to transfer heat (or oxygen, in the case of the swim bladder) into the in-flowing circulation. In

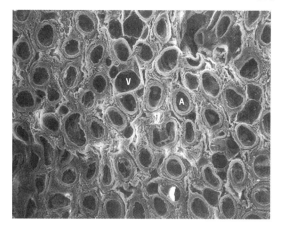

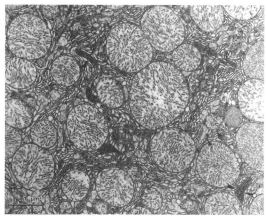

Figure 7.32. Electron micrographs of the heat exchanger and a cranial heater organ cell of the blue marlin (*Makaira nigricans*). (Upper panel) A scanning electron micrograph of the heat exchanger located at the base of the heater organ. Note the close juxtaposition of arteries (A) and veins (V). (Figure from Block, 1991, with permission.) (Lower panel) Transmission electron micrograph of a heater organ cell. Note the lack of contractile filaments in this highly modified muscle cell. The cell is tightly packed with mitochondria and sarcoplasmic reticulum (arrows). (Photograph courtesy of Dr. Barbara A. Block.)

endothermic fishes, countercurrent heat exchangers have thick walls, which preclude transvessel movement of oxygen while allowing effective transfer of heat. Heat exchangers also lead to elevated temperatures in the viscera and brain. The heat used to warm the latter two regions is only partially formed in these organs; some of the heat is supplied from blood warmed in parts of the red muscle circulation.

The critical roles played by red muscle placement and countercurrent heat exchangers for restricting loss of heat in endothermic fishes is further manifested through comparing other large, fast-swimming fishes that, despite many other similarities to tunas and lamnid sharks, lack these two particular anatomical adaptations. In these fishes, only limited regional endothermy is present, and the heat-generating mechanisms used for this function represent a reengineering of muscle biochemistry rather than trapping of heat generated by excitation–contractile coupling.

Cranial Heater Organs in Fish: Excitation–Thermogenic Coupling

Cranial heaters: distribution and relationship to thermal niche

The advantages gained by tunas from having warmed brains and eyes would apply even if these fishes did not succeed in effecting endothermic homeothermy in other regions of their bodies. The ability to shield the visual sense and the capacity to processes neural information from the effects of fluctuating temperatures has enormous significance in terms of establishing the breadth of a fish's thermal niche. These advantages also are apparent in a restricted group of fish comprising 10 known species in which cranial heaters allow regional endothermic homeothermy of the brain and eye.

These 10 species include a single representative of the family Scombridae, the butterfly mackerel *Gasterochisma melampus*, and nine species of billfishes belonging to the families Xiphiidae (swordfish) and Istiophoridae (marlins) (see Block, 1991, 1994, for reviews). These species include the swordfish *Xiphias gladius*, which ranges from the surface to depths of over 600 m and, over this depth range, encounters changes in water temperature of up to approximately 19°C (Carey, 1990). Despite these large changes in ambient temperature, the temperature of the cranial region of the fish remains remarkably stable and may exceed ambient temperatures by up to 10–15°C. In a telemetric study by Frank G. Carey, cranial

temperature remained at 28°C ± 1°C for 36 h as the fish moved between waters having temperatures between 13°C and 17°C (Carey, 1990). The ability to move into cold, deep waters enables such regionally endothermic fishes to feed successfully on deep-living prey like squids. The extent of development of the cranial heater organ in fact reflects the absolute temperatures of a species' thermal niche, with cold-dwelling species having a larger amount of heat-generating tissue and, within this tissue, a higher mass-specific ability to produce heat. Cranial heater organs, which are hypothesized to have evolved before the more extensive mechanisms of endothermy appeared in tunas, are seen to have an advantage over the latter mechanisms in that eye and brain temperatures can be regulated independently of the level of locomotory activity.

Anatomical properties of cranial heaters

The cranial heaters found in swordfish, marlins, and the butterfly mackerel represent the extreme to which skeletal muscle can be modified to function as a site of heat production. These highly modified extraocular muscles insert on the eyeball and control its movements. It is noteworthy that different extraocular muscles have evolved a heat generation function in billfishes (*superior rectus* muscle) and the butterfly mackerel (*lateral rectus* muscle), illustrating the separate evolutionary origin of these highly convergent systems. The cellular and biochemical properties of these organs in billfishes and the butterfly mackerel, at least insofar as these are understood, are very similar despite the independent evolutionary origins of the organs.

As the ocular muscle enters the orbit, its appearance changes dramatically. Most of the muscle cytoplasm is lost, contractile proteins largely disappear, and mitochondrial abundance increases dramatically, to assume up to about two-thirds of cell volume. Another striking feature of heater organ cells is the development of an elaborate membrane "wrapping" around the mitochondria (figure 7.32). This extensively developed membrane system is derived from the sarcoplasmic reticular membranes. The high densities of ion pumps in the

SR provide a key element of the thermogenic mechanism, as discussed below.

Before examining the biochemical mechanisms responsible for heat generation and its regulation, the circulatory anatomy of the heater organ bears mention. The pathway taken by the carotid artery, as it runs towards the brain and eye, allows most of the blood entering the cranial region to be shunted through the heater organ. There, a vascular heat exchanger termed a *rete mirabile* ("wonderful net") allows the inflowing, cool arterial blood to come into intimate contact with the out-flowing warmed, venous blood moving toward the gills (figure 7.32). The close juxtaposition of small blood vessels in the rete mirabile allows effective transfer of heat to the arterial blood and, therefore, a high degree of heat retention in the heater organ. A similar rete mirabile is used to retain heat in the locomotory muscle. To complement the heat-retaining abilities of the countercurrent heat exchanger of the heater organ, the organ is surrounded by is a thick layer of insulative lipid.

Biochemical properties of cranial heater organs

Cranial heaters are the only organs in animals besides BAT that are known to have as their sole function the generation of heat. However, the heat-generating principles of these two types of organs are significantly different, as are their ontogenies. In cranial heater organs, unlike BAT, mitochondrial ATP production is highly coupled, and large amounts of ATP are produced as carbohydrate and lipid substrates are catabolized. There is no evidence for the involvement of uncoupling proteins in the thermogenic processes of mitochondria of cranial heater organs. The challenge facing these organs, then, is to harness some type(s) of ATP utilizing reaction(s) to hydrolyze this mitochondrially generated ATP, in order to allow a sustained high level of energy metabolism and heat output, estimated at up to 250 W kg^{-1} (Block, 1994).

The mechanisms present in cranial heater organs for maintaining an extremely high rate of ATP turnover are now understood in fair detail. Block (1994) terms these mechanisms *excitation–thermogenic coupling* (as opposed to the typical excitation–contractile coupling found in skeletal muscle). Central to these mechanisms is calcium ion, whose concentration may help to modulate the rate of ATP production by mitochondria as well as govern the splitting of ATP by the dominant ATPase of the organ, the Ca^{2+} ATPase *calsequestrin*. This calcium pump is the rate-limiting enzyme for Ca^{2+} sequestration in the SR, and an enzyme that is present in extremely high concentrations in the membranes surrounding the mitochondria (figure 7.33). The isoform of calsequestrin present in the heater organ is the one normally found in fast-twitch muscles. Another biochemical adaptation of heater organ cells is the absence in their cytoplasm of large amounts of two calcium-binding proteins, parvalbumin and troponin-C, which normally are abundant in muscle and bind calcium released from the SR membrane. The absence of these two proteins in the heater organ ensures that the Ca^{2+} released into the cytoplasm remains free and thereby able to stimulate ATP production and ATP consumption.

The conjectured overall mechanism for promoting a high rate of ATP turnover is complex and may involve a number of initial stimuli (see Block, 1994). Stimuli for increased ATP turnover may include activity of the sympathetic nervous system, hormone signals, or direct electrical stimuli reaching the heater organ from adjacent regions of the ocular muscle that maintain contractile activity. All of these stimuli may trigger release of Ca^{2+} from stores within the SR membranes. Release of Ca^{2+} leads to two major effects on ATP turnover: stimulation of mitochondrial respiration and hydrolysis of ATP by calsequestrin, as Ca^{2+} is returned to the SR. Calcium ion is known to stimulate certain dehydrogenase enzymes localized within the mitochondrial matrix. This stimulation leads directly to higher levels of NADH and, therefore, to increased flux through the electron transport chain. And, because of tight coupling of transmembrane flux of protons and ATP synthesis, stimulation by Ca^{2+} quickly leads to a rise in ATP supply. A large fraction of this ATP is used by calsequestrin to pump Ca^{2+} out

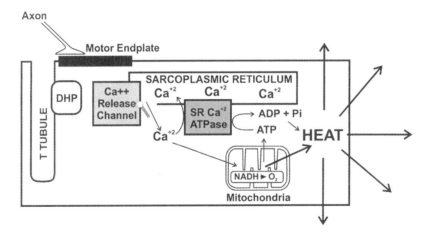

Figure 7.33. Proposed mechanism for excitation–thermogenic coupling in the ocular heater organ of swordfish. Neural stimulation mediated through the T tubule voltage sensor (the dihydropyridine [DHP] receptor) may lead to opening of the Ca^{2+} release channel. Large amounts of Ca^{2+} pass from the SR into the sarcoplasm. Ca^{2+} entering the mitochondria may stimulate ATP synthesis. Much of the ATP produced is used by the SR Ca^{2+} ATPase (calsequestrin) to pump Ca^{2+} back into the SR. This cycling of Ca^{2+} between the SR and sarcoplasm represents a futile cycle. See text for additional details. (Modified after Block, 1991.)

of the cytosol, back into the space within the SR membrane—from which it can again leak to enhance ATP turnover. The cycling of Ca^{2+} in this manner represents what is termed a *futile cycle*; it is the act of Sisyphus being carried out at the molecular level. However, while "futile" in terms of accomplishing net work, this cycling of Ca^{2+} achieves a highly important function: warming of two critical components of the fish's body. Even if systemic endothermic homeothermy cannot be achieved, the localized maintenance of elevated organ temperatures may be of enormous selective advantage to fishes in terms of habitat access and stability of function of key organs involved in sensing and information processing.

Ion Flux and the Origin of Systemic Endothermy in Mammals

Ultimate and proximate causes of endothermy

Mammals and birds are the only groups of animals having a capacity for effective systemic endothermic homeothermy. The origin of this important capacity has long intrigued physiol-

ogists, for two principal reasons—the "why" and the "how" of the evolutionary process that has led to this unique ability. Much debate surrounds the issue of *ultimate* cause: Why, in terms of initial selective advantage, did this capacity arise? The second question concerns *proximate* cause—"how": What cellular mechanisms were harnessed to provide the heat needed for control of body temperature? (Note: an excellent discussion of ultimate and proximate cause is found in Mayr, 1982, pp. 67–71.) Although the issue of ultimate cause remains unsettled, there has been considerable experimentation during the past two decades to determine systemic endothermy's proximate causes. Thus, even though the issue of "why" remains conjectural, for reasons discussed at the conclusion of this section, the "hows" are becoming clear thanks to insightful comparative studies of cellular mechanisms of heat generation.

The analysis that follows begins with a consideration of the proximate causes of systemic endothermy, an issue that can be approached by asking, "How does an ectothermic vertebrate like a reptile differ from a mammal in terms of mechanisms for supporting endothermic homeothermy?" Recent studies point in the direction of a unifying concept, one involving exploitation of two primitive futile cycles that are present in most eukaryotic cells and which in mammals and birds have been amplified to provide a high capacity for heat production. Moreover, certain of the data obtained in these analyses of thermogenic capacity also shed light on the differences in mass-specific metabolic rate (*allometric scaling of metabolism*) found among animals of different body mass. Thus, the development of endothermic homeothermy in mammals will be examined with a dual focus. First, we will consider the initial evolutionary fabrication of an elevated heat-generating capacity in cells of ancestral mammals, an event that may or may not have been initially selected for on the basis of its beneficial effects on body temperature regulation. Second, we will examine the variation (scaling) of mass-specific metabolic rate, a relationship that may be an important contributor to, yet not a primary adaptation for, allowing mammals of widely different sizes to maintain stable, high body temperatures.

Physiological differences between mammals and reptiles of a common size and body temperature

Endothermic homeotherms are characterized by high mass-specific rates of oxygen consumption relative to similar-sized ectotherms. This difference can be shown by examining the allometric scaling relationship between rate of oxygen consumption (M) and body mass (W). For ectothermic and endothermic animals, whole animal oxygen consumption rate is proportional to total body mass raised to approximately the 0.75 power:

$$M = aW^{0.75}$$

The differences in metabolic rate between ectotherms and endotherms thus are due to the preexponential term a, which is approximately four- to fivefold higher in birds and mammals relative to reptiles. On a mass-specific basis (for instance, oxygen consumption per gram wet mass) the mass exponent is near

−0.25. Thus, to a first approximation, questions about the origins and mechanisms of endothermy can be reduced to questions about the underlying determinants of *a* in the allometric equation given above.

To conduct such an analysis in a logically correct manner, considerable attention must be given to selecting appropriate reptiles and mammals for comparative investigation. Because the rate at which an organism consumes oxygen is strongly affected by both body mass and temperature (Q_{10} effects), the reptiles and mammals to be compared must be of similar size and, under normal habitat conditions, have similar core body temperatures. With the playing field thus leveled, it may be possible to determine quite precisely how the magnitude of the a term is established through alterations in physiological and biochemical systems.

Among the studies in which mammals and reptiles have been compared metabolically in an effort to explain the four- to fivefold higher oxygen consumption rates of the former species, the work of Hulbert, Else, Brand, and colleagues has provided especially useful data, in part because of their appropriate choice of experimental subjects (Brand et al., 1991; Else and Hulbert, 1985; Hulbert and Else, 1989, 2000). Comparisons of the bearded dragon, *Amphibolurus vitticeps*, with the rat *Rattus norvegicus,* species that have similar body masses and core temperatures, revealed that the mass-specific rate of whole organism oxygen consumption of the rat was about sevenfold higher than that of the lizard, and rates of oxygen consumption by isolated hepatocytes were fourfold higher for the rat (Brand et al., 1991) (table 7.2). Associated with these differences in rates of oxygen consumption were striking differences in the percentage contribution to total body mass made by different organs (Hulbert and Else, 1989) (table 7.2). Whereas *A. vitticeps* had a higher percentage of mass due to skeleton, the most metabolically active tissues (in terms of oxygen consumed per gram)—brain, liver, kidney, and heart—represented only 3.7% of mass in the reptile but 6.2% of mass in the mammal. Although representing a minor fraction of

Table 7.2. Comparisons of Mammals and Reptiles of Comparable Mass and Body Temperature: the Rat (*Rattus norvegicus*) and the Bearded Dragon (*Amphibolurus vitticeps*)

	A. vitticeps	Rat	Statistical significance
I. BODY COMPOSITION[1]			
Body mass (g)	304	310	NS
% Body mass of major organs			
Brain	0.13	0.69	$P < .01$
Liver	2.84	4.21	$P < .01$
Kidney	0.41	0.89	$P < .01$
Heart	0.29	0.40	$P < .01$
Stomach	1.12	0.49	$P < .01$
Intestines	1.51	2.04	$P < .02$
Lung	0.81	0.68	NS
Reproductive	0.66	1.37	NS
Skin + fur	21.21	20.0	NS
Skeletal muscle	34.58	42.82	$P < .01$
Skeleton + other	36.42	25.94	$P < .01$
II. PROTEIN CONTENTS OF TISSUES (mg protein g tissue^{-1})[1]			
Liver	90	165	$P < .01$
Kidney	91	126	$P < .01$
Brain	53	105	$P < .01$
Heart	85	114	$P < .01$
Lung	60	90	$P < .01$
Skeletal muscle	81	120	$P < .02$
III. PHOSPHOLIPID FATTY ACID (FA) COMPOSITION OF LIVER[1]			
Phospholipid content (mg g tissue^{-1})	0.53	0.86	$P < .05$
Selected polyunsaturated fatty acids (mol %)			
20:4	13.7	30.6	$P < .001$
22:6	1.5	4.3	$P < .05$
% Unsaturated FA	61.1	53.7	$P < .005$
Unsaturation index: (mol% × double bonds)	155	185	$P < .01$
IV. TISSUE CYTOCHROME C OXIDASE ACTIVITY (nmol O_2 mg protein^{-1} min^{-1})[1]			
Liver	14.3	37.0	$P < .01$
Kidney	19.9	30.6	$P < .01$
Brain	12.2	16.9	$P < .05$
Heart	21.1	29.6	$P < .01$
Lung	2.5	9.4	$P < .01$
Skeletal muscle	6.7	15.6	$P < .01$
V. OXYGEN CONSUMPTION BY WHOLE ORGANISM AND HEPATOCYTES[2]			
Whole organism:			
Standard metabolic rate (ml O_2 h^{-1} g^{-1})	0.109	0.779	
Hepatocyte respiration rate (nmol O min^{-1} mg protein^{-1})	2.6	10.7	

[1]Data from Hulbert and Else (1989).
[2]Data from Brand et al. (1991).

body mass in a mammal, these four tissues may account for approximately 70% of basal metabolic rate (BMR) (Hulbert and Else, 1990). Liver alone may account for 20% of BMR in the rat (Brand et al., 1991). Therefore, a substantial fraction of the difference in whole body basal oxygen consumption rate between reptiles and mammals of similar mass and core temperature may be due to differences in the relative amounts of the most metabolically active tissues.

Differences in percentage contribution of highly metabolically active tissues to body mass fail to provide a complete picture of the physiologically important differences between homologous organs in reptiles and mammals, however. In addition to differences in relative contribution to mass, tissues of reptiles and mammals also differ significantly in a number of compositional properties, including protein and phospholipid content (table 7.2). Of major importance are differences between reptiles and mammals in the total volume of mitochondria per unit mass of tissue and the total amount of mitochondrial membrane surface area integrated over all organs. Because by far the largest fraction of oxygen consumed by the cell is due to mitochondrial activity (estimates put this fraction at 85–90% in rat liver [Couture and Hulbert, 1995]), any increase in mitochondrial respiration per unit mass could lead to a large increase in the preexponential a term.

In a comparison involving several species of mammals and reptiles that varied by about 100-fold in body mass, Else and Hulbert (1985) demonstrated that there is an approximately 60% higher fraction of cellular volume occupied by mitochondria in homologous organs of similar-sized mammals relative to reptiles. In addition, there may be a slight increase in the amount of internal mitochondrial membrane area per unit volume of mitochondria, although this difference seems of minor importance in explaining the higher mass-specific metabolic rates of mammals. When the effects of increased organ size and higher mitochondrial concentrations in mammals are summed together, it is found that the total amount of membrane surface area in similar-sized mammals and reptiles differs by approximately four-

fold. Differences in cytochrome-c oxidase activity of several organs reflect the differences in mitochondrial density, although the maximal difference in cytochrome-c oxidase is slightly under threefold (table 7.2). Thus, much of the difference in the preexponential a term may be due to different quantities of mitochondrial membrane, that is, to different amounts of enzymes for aerobic generation of ATP.

Mitochondria of reptiles and mammals differ in proton permeability

To appreciate more fully what these differences in mitochondrial membrane area mean in terms of heat-generating potential, it is important to consider a phenomenon discussed earlier in the context of thermogenesis by BAT: the generation of heat by "wasting" energy through uncoupled proton flux through the inner mitochondrial membrane. A substantial fraction of proton flux through the inner mitochondrial membrane is not coupled to synthesis of ATP even under normal conditions, i.e., in the absence of a need for high levels of thermogenesis. This fraction is estimated to be as high as 20–30% of oxygen consumption in mitochondria of rat liver and muscle under resting conditions (Nobes et al., 1989; reviewed in Ricquier and Bouillaud, 2000). Any means for enhancing this flux could, as already shown for BAT, lead to substantially greater heat production. It is conceivable, therefore, that a major "invention" made at the time of the origin of endothermy was an increase in the futile cycle of proton flux, as expressed on the basis of flux per unit surface area of inner mitochondrial membrane. That is, the increase in total heat generation from the proton futile cycling would not be a consequence of simply more mitochondrial surface area, but a result of a change in flux per unit membrane area times the increase in total area.

Substantial differences in the amounts of heat generated by the proton futile cycle seem likely to distinguish mitochondria of reptiles and mammals (Brand et al., 1991). Leakiness of the inner mitochondrial membrane, expressed as flux per unit area, was four- to fivefold higher in the rat relative to *A. vitticeps*

(Brand et al., 1991). The basis of the increased leakiness to protons in the inner mitochondrial membranes of mammals is not well understood, although potential mechanisms are apparent. In light of recent advances in the study of uncoupling proteins, as discussed in the context of BAT, it is plausible that one or more isoforms of UCP may be up-regulated in mitochondria of mammals to enhance the uncoupled flux of protons across the inner mitochondrial membrane. Because only a very small percentage of proton flux through the inner mitochondrial membrane is thought to occur through the lipid bilayer itself, independently of protein channels, the roles for UCPs could be substantial. In turn, the conductivity of proton channels like UCPs could be influenced by the composition of the bilayer. Comparisons of the phospholipid compositions of mitochondrial membranes from the rat and *A. vitticeps* revealed that the percentage of acyl chains represented by omega-3 fatty acids like the long-chain, polyunsaturate docosahexanoic acid ($C_{22:6}$) was seven times higher in the rat (Brand et al., 1991). The significance of high levels of long-chain omega-3 fatty acids is conjectured to lie in their abilities to disorder the middle portion of the bilayer. Brand et al. (1991) calculated that in the middle region (roughly, the central 30%) of the mitochondrial membranes of rats, there are approximately seven to eight times more double bonds than in the membranes of *A. vitticeps*. Energy barriers to diffusion and to the movement of membrane-spanning proteins are greatest near the center of membranes, so decreasing order in this region could have strong effects on rates of diffusion and on the conformational mobility of ion-conducting protein channels due to lowered viscotropic effects. Thus, increased disorder of the central portion of the bilayer may enhance proton conductivity through the lipid bilayer of the membrane or allow a higher conductance for membrane-spanning protein channels such as UCPs or nonspecific cation channels.

The higher leakiness to protons noted in the inner mitochondrial membranes of the rat relative to *A. vitticeps* has a parallel in the effects of thyroid hormones on respiration. Increased

levels of thyroid hormones lead to increased rates of respiration and mitochondrial proton leakage, and also to alterations in the fatty acid composition of mitochondrial membranes (Hafner et al., 1988, 1989; Brand et al., 1991). The thermogenic response to thyroid hormones may, then, mirror in important ways the changes that occurred evolutionarily when mammalian endothermic homeothermy first arose.

In summary, the total quantity of mitochondrial membrane surface area and the per unit area flux of protons through futile cycle channels are higher in mammals than in reptiles of similar body size. These differences in the quantitative and qualitative properties of mitochondria seem capable of accounting for much of the difference in mass-specific metabolic rate between mammals and reptiles; that is, they may provide a mechanistic account for the observed four- to fivefold difference in the *a* term in the allometric equation, $M = aW^{0.75}$.

Allometry of respiration rates in mammals: size-related "leakiness" of mitochondrial inner membranes

Surface-to-volume relationships render the task of keeping warm a much more difficult challenge for small than for large mammals. Therefore, other things (e.g., insulation, blood flow, and microhabitat) being equal, a small mammal would benefit from having a relatively high capacity for heat generation per unit body mass. That such a higher capacity exists for smaller mammals is apparent from the allometric scaling equation for respiration rate. Even though the higher mass-specific respiration rates of small mammals cannot be a consequence of selection for thermogenesis—recall that allometric scaling is also observed in ectothermic species—there is no question but that the higher heat-generating capacity of a gram of tissue of a small mammal is a powerful contributor to the organism's ability to maintain systemic endothermic homeothermy. Likewise, the low mass-specific respiration rates of very large mammals are important for preventing overheating of the body core. If an elephant had a mass-specific metabolic rate as high as that of a shrew, water might boil from the surface of the large mammal (for an excellent discussion of scaling relationships, see Schmidt-Nielsen, 1984). Allometric scaling of respiration rate thus can be viewed as offering an important "fringe benefit" or exaptation to mammals in terms of regulation of body temperature, even though the factors that are ultimate causes of metabolic scaling do not involve adaptation to temperature.

The mechanisms available for elevating mass-specific metabolic rate in small mammals, or for decreasing this rate in mammals with large body mass, involve the same types of "raw material" used to fabricate endothermic homeothermy in ancestral mammals. As in the comparisons between reptiles and mammals discussed above, differences in mass-specific metabolic rate among different-sized mammals are correlated with variation in activities of mitochondrial enzymes associated with aerobic generation of ATP (Emmett and Hochachka, 1981). Scaling of activities of aerobically poised enzymes shows allometry similar to that of whole organism respiration rate. However, similar allometric scaling patterns of aerobically poised enzymes are also found in ectotherms like fishes, which is another indication that metabolic scaling per se is not due to thermogenesis (Somero and Childress, 1980). In addition to size-related variation in concentrations of mitochondrial enzymes, changes in proton leakiness also may contribute importantly to the oxygen consumption rates of different-sized mammals. Porter et al. (1996) compared proton leakage rates of mitochondria isolated from liver tissue of nine species of mammals that varied in body mass by approximately 17,000-fold (horse to mouse). The proton leakage rate showed a significant allometric variation, increasing by about fivefold between the largest and smallest species (figure 7.34).

To determine the basis for this regular variation in rate of proton leakage, several characteristics of the mitochondria were measured, including inner membrane surface area per unit of matrix volume and fatty acid composition of mitochondrial membrane phospholipids. The largest share (about 70%) of the variation in proton flux rate appears to be due to differ-

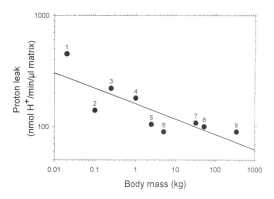

Figure 7.34. Allometric relationship of mitochondrial proton leak and body mass. Proton leak measured at a potential of 170 mV is expressed per unit volume (μl) of mitochondrial matrix. Numbers refer to the following species: (1) mouse, (2) hamster, (3) rat, (4) ferret, (5) Dutch rabbit, (6) New Zealand rabbit, (7) sheep, (8) pig, and (9) horse. (Figure modified after Porter et al. 1996.)

ences in membrane surface area (cm^2 per μl of matrix), which decreased regularly with increasing body size. The remaining difference in proton leakiness is proposed to be due to differences in membrane composition. In common with the differences found between mitochondrial membranes of *A. vitticeps* and the rat, a large and regular variation was observed between small and large mammals in the percentage contribution of omega-3 fatty acids to the total fatty pool of membrane phospholipids (figure 7.35). The percentage contribution of docosahexanoic acid ($C_{22:6}$) showed an allometric scaling with a mass-specific exponent (-0.276) similar to the exponent characterizing mass-specific respiration rate in mammals. Whether the correlation between content of omega-3 fatty acids like docosahexanoic acid and mass-specific respiration rate is causal remains to be determined. However, as discussed above in the context of a role for omega-3 fatty acids in the development of endothermy, a major role of long-chain polyunsaturated fatty acids on the order of the central region of the bilayer could be the modulation of rates of proton flux. And, as also considered in the context of reptilian versus mammalian systems, changes in levels and activities of uncoupling proteins could play central roles in

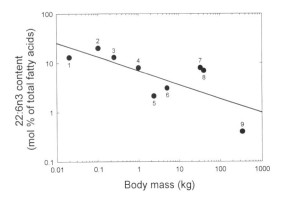

Figure 7.35. Variation in phospholipid composition of mitochondrial membranes in relation to body mass. The mole percent of 22:6 (*n*-3) fatty acids in the identified fatty acid pool of mitochondrial membrane phospholipids is plotted against body mass of nine mammals (see legend to figure 7.34 for identification of species). (Figure modified after Porter et al., 1996.)

modulating proton leakiness in different-sized mammals. Study of size-dependence of UCP concentration and activity is clearly warranted in order to define more fully the mechanisms underlying increased futile cycling of protons in mammalian mitochondria.

Cycling—futile or otherwise—of sodium and potassium ions

It was seen in the analysis of heater organ function in fishes that a substantial amount of heat can be generated through futile cycles involving operation of ATP-dependent Ca^{2+} pumps. Futile cycles involving other types of ions may play vital roles in thermogenesis in higher vertebrates. Because of the ubiquitous occurrence of the Na^+-K^+-ATPase in plasma membranes and the likelihood that this single enzyme may account for approximately 5–10% of BMR (Couture and Hulbert, 1995), there has been considerable interest in the possible role that cycling of Na^+ and K^+ might play in thermogenesis (Hulbert and Else, 1990). If the sodium pump were to function as the energy-utilizing part of an ion futile cycle, *all* cells of the body could play a role in thermogenesis.

As in the case of proton flux across the inner mitochondrial membrane, there appear to be differences in Na^+-K^+-ATPase activity between endotherms and ectotherms. Furthermore, within mammals as a single group, there is variation in activity of this enzyme in relation to body mass. Comparisons of ectotherms and endotherms suggest that a several-fold higher level of heat production due to activity of the sodium pump occurs in mammals. In a comparison of *A. vitticeps* and the rat, the estimated cost of operating the Na^+-K^+-ATPase was from 3.6-fold (brain) to 6.7-fold (liver) higher in the mammal (Else and Hulbert, 1987). Correlated with this difference in estimated costs of sodium pump activity were differences in the rates of passive efflux of K^+ and passive influx of Na^+ in liver cells (figure 7.36). The costs of maintaining transmembrane gradients in concentrations of Na^+ and K^+ are reflected in differences in sodium pump-dependent oxygen consumption. When ouabain, an inhibitor of the sodium pump, was used in studies of oxygen consumption by liver slices, a strong correlation was observed between sodium-dependent oxygen uptake and rate of sodium influx (figure 7.37; Hulbert and Else, 1990). In a broader comparison of mammals with a wide spectrum of ectotherms (representatives of reptiles, amphibians, fishes, and crustaceans), it was found that the energy demands for transporting Na^+ and K^+ were consistently much higher in mammalian cells: activities of the Na^+-K^+-ATPase were threefold, sixfold, 4.5-fold, and twofold higher in liver, skeletal muscle, brain, and kidney, respectively of mammals relative to ectotherms (Else et al., 1996).

The mechanism(s) responsible for setting higher Na^+-K^+-ATPase activities in cells of mammals may involve enzymes with higher specific activities rather than higher concentrations of enzymes with the same turnover numbers (k_{cat}) (Else et al., 1996). Using radiolabeled ouabain to quantify the numbers of Na^+-K^+-ATPase molecules in plasma membranes, no consistent differences between mammals and ectotherms could be detected. However, when Na^+-K^+-ATPase activity was measured on a per enzyme molecule basis, the specific activities of the enzymes from mammals were several-fold

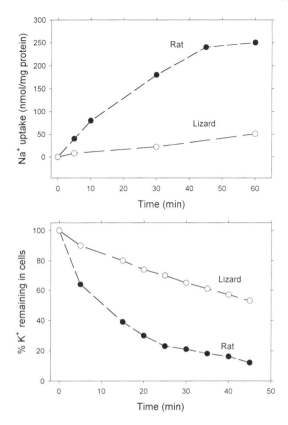

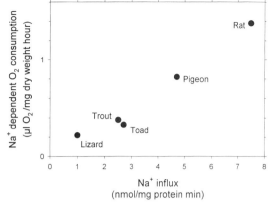

Figure 7.37. The relationship between passive Na^+ permeability of isolated liver cells from five species of vertebrates and Na^+-dependent oxygen consumption. (Figure modified after Hulbert and Else, 1990.)

Figure 7.36. Passive influx of Na^+ (upper panel) and passive efflux of K^+ (lower panel) in liver slices of the rat and a reptile (*Amphibolurus vitticeps*). Measurements were made in the presence of ouabain, an inhibitor of the sodium pump (Na^+-K^+-ATPase), at 37°C. Passive fluxes are higher in the "leakier" membranes of the mammal. (Data from Else and Hulbert, 1987.)

Is elevated activity of the Na^+-K^+-ATPase in mammals strictly an increased futile cycle activity?

In considering Ca^{2+} cycling in heater organs of fishes and proton flux through UCP1 channels in BAT, there seems to be little basis for doubting that these high ionic flux rates are representative of true futile cycles. Thus, in both cases no net work is accomplished and production of heat appears to be the sole function of these activities. A different scenario may occur in the case of elevated Na^+-K^+-ATPase activities in plasma membranes of mammals. There are at least two reasons for questioning whether heat-generating futile cycle activity is the sole function of this enhanced transmembrane movement of Na^+ and K^+. One reason is based on a somewhat a priori analysis of the optimal evolutionary strategies for heat generation: because futile cycling of protons appears to be an extremely effective means for generating large amounts of heat, why should evolution favor development of a second mechanism that entails the more complex process of making and, then, splitting of ATP? Whereas this question clearly is not amenable to experimental test, it nonetheless does call into doubt a simple explanation for elevated Na^+-K^+-

higher. These higher specific activities could be due to at least two distinct types of change: alteration in the intrinsic properties (k_{cat}) of the Na^+-K^+-ATPase itself, or modulations of the enzyme's activity through changes in the lipid domain surrounding the enzyme. The occurrence in membranes of mammals of higher concentrations of omega-3 fatty acids like docosahexanoic acid suggests that the latter mechanism could play a role in modulating activity of the Na^+-K^+-ATPase, albeit this conjecture has not been tested.

ATPase activity that is based solely on futile cycling of sodium and potassium ions.

A second and empirically substantiated reason for questioning the exclusive role of futile cycling in selection for high activities of the Na^+-K^+-ATPase relates to the fact that the transmembrane movement of organic molecules into the cell commonly depends on the electrochemical gradient of sodium ions. Thus, increased activity of the sodium pump would support higher rates of transport for amino acids, sugars, and other organic molecules that are critical for both catabolic and anabolic processes. The finding that tissues of mammals, relative to those of similar-sized reptiles, contain approximately 50% more protein (table 7.2; Hulbert and Else, 1989) supports the conjecture that increased levels of Na^+-K^+-ATPase activity in plasma membranes of mammalian cells fulfill important functions in addition to thermogenesis. Thus, initial selection for elevated activities of the sodium pump in mammalian cells could as well have been due to demands for increasing flux of sugars and amino acids into the cell as for increasing the capacities of the cells to produce heat.

Allometry of potassium ion flux in mammals

The flux of potassium ions (μmol K^+ per g tissue per min) across the plasma membranes of liver cells of mammals of different total body mass exhibits negative allometry, as does mass-specific respiration rate (Couture and Hulbert, 1995; figure 7.38). The scaling coefficients of ion flux are slightly smaller than those for oxygen consumption rate, however (−0.14 and −0.21, respectively). Higher mass-specific K^+ flux rates are assumed to be correlated with higher influx rates for Na^+, such that higher rates of heat generation and sodium-mediated transport occur in cells of smaller mammals. Because rates of protein synthesis scale similarly to metabolic rate (Blaxter, 1989), the higher potential for amino acid transport in cells of small mammals would appear to allow amino acid uptake to keep pace with the protein synthetic activity.

The proximate cause of the putative higher level of sodium and potassium ion flux in cells of small mammals may include simple geometrical considerations. It is worth noting that the linear dimensions and, therefore, the volumes of homologous cells in large and small mammals are different (Berrill, 1955). Based on differences in linear dimensions, it can be calculated that a hepatocyte from a small mammal like a mouse may have a volume only one-eighth that of a hepatocyte from an elephant. Therefore, surface-to-volume relationships may account in large measure for any differences in plasma membrane sodium pump activity that may exist between small and large mammals: the larger the mammal, the lower the surface-to-volume ratio of its cells and, therefore, the lower the Na^+-K^+-ATPase activity per gram wet weight of tissue.

What initially drove selection for "mammal-like" physiological properties?

The high mass-specific rates of oxygen consumption, the high rates of proton flux across the inner mitochondrial membrane, and the elevated levels of flux of sodium and potassium ions across plasma membranes are hallmarks of what distinguishes mammals from lower vertebrates, the reptiles, amphibians, and fishes. The contemporary importance of these "mammal-like" physiological properties in thermogenesis should not blind us to the possibility that the origin of some, if not all, of these traits may have had little, if anything, to do with the advantages of systemic endothermic homeothermy.

A primary basis for this caveat is another key difference found between mammals, on the one hand, and lower vertebrates, on the other: mammals typically have much higher capacities for sustained aerobic locomotory performance than the ectothermic tetrapods, reptiles and amphibians (Bennett, 1978; Bennett and Ruben, 1979). Although reptiles may far outclass mammals of similar size and body temperature in capacities for rapid sprint locomotion powered by anaerobic glycolysis, mammals generally have much higher abilities to support long-term, moderate velocity locomotion powered largely by aerobic metabolism. Thus, the initial development of a high level of

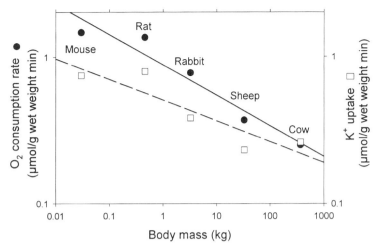

Figure 7.38. Allometry of oxygen consumption rates and potassium leakage rates for liver slices from five species of mammals that differ by four orders of magnitude in body mass. (Figure modified after Couture and Hulbert, 1995.)

aerobic capacity may have had more to do with predator–prey relationships than with the advantages of systemic endothermic homeothermy. However, in this scenario, as a high mass-specific respiration rate was being developed, the potential for systemic endothermic homeothermy arose as a potential side-benefit that came to assume major evolutionary significance once mechanisms for controlling the exchange of this metabolic heat with the environment were set in place.

If we examine in turn each of the major mechanisms used in mammals to support a high rate of heat production, we can generate a plausible scenario for adaptive value of the trait in question entirely within the context of increased potential for aerobic locomotory activity. The higher rates of flux of sodium and potassium ions through the plasma membrane can be viewed as supporting elevated rates of transport for substrates of energy metabolism and amino acids for protein synthesis. The higher protein concentrations of mammalian cells are hard to rationalize as "being there to enhance thermogenesis." Rather, the support of a high rate of protein turnover in mammals is seen to demand high rates of ATP turnover, as well as transport into the cells of substrates for catabolism and anabolism. The higher rates of proton futile cycling in mitochondria may

represent a "price that had to be paid" for the elevated rates of ATP synthesis in mammals. The fact that the higher rates of uncoupled flux of H^+ through the inner mitochondrial membranes of mammals appear to be a direct consequence of four- to fivefold larger areas of mitochondrial membrane surface per unit mass of tissue is consistent with the hypothesis that much of the increased uncoupled proton flux is a side-effect of more ATP production per unit mass of cell, rather than a specific adaptation for heat production. This is not to say, however, that modulation of proton flux, for instance through the involvement of UCPs, has not occurred to modify heat-generating capacity. The point is that the initial embellishment of ATP-generating capacity to support the energy demands of prolonged aerobic locomotory activity (and the energetically expensive enzymatic and contractile machinery on which this activity relies) may have been driven by fundamental ecological issues such as predator–prey relationships instead of thermogenesis.

The allometric variation in respiration rate, mitochondrial area, rates of uncoupled proton flux across the inner mitochondrial membrane, and plasma membrane sodium pump activity found in mammals appears consistent with selection for higher mass-specific rates of heat generation in small mammals. However, the

fact that the allometric scaling of aerobic metabolism is characterized by the same exponent in
ectotherms and endotherms refutes any hypothesis that proposes that the higher mass-specific
respiratory and transport activities in small
mammals reflect selection based primarily on
increased capacities for thermogenesis.

Although many uncertainties remain about
the ultimate and proximate causes of systemic
endothermic homeothermy in birds and mammals, work in this fascinating area has provided
a great number of important insights into major
issues in evolutionary and mechanistic physiology. Perhaps the most intriguing of these issues
are those involving the ways in which preexisting raw material has been exploited (exapted) to
allow the higher vertebrates to acquire their
unique abilities to govern their body temperatures and thereby attain substantial inde-
pendence from the vagaries of habitat
temperature. The importance of this ability is
shown very strikingly in the context of the
topic we next address: the dangers imposed by
ice formation in extra- and intracellular fluids.

THE FROZEN STATE: AVOIDANCE AND
TOLERANCE OF FREEZING

The Importance of Liquid Water and
the Dangers Posed by Ice

In previous sections of this chapter, as well as in
chapter 6, we have discussed several reasons
why liquid water is so critical for life. To briefly
review the salient points: (1) Water is essential
for driving the formation of the three-dimensional structures of macromolecules. These
structures, on which macromolecular function
depends, are encoded in a latent form in the
linear primary structures of proteins and nucleic
acids, but can be manifested only when liquid
water is present to foster hydrophobic interactions. (2) The assembly of bilayer membranes
from lipids and proteins likewise is driven in
large measure by hydrophobic effects. (3)
Water in the liquid state is a requirement for
most types of transport of materials between
organism and environment and between compartments within the organism. (4) Lastly, the

covalent chemistry of many metabolic transformations depends on liquid water, which may
serve as a reactant or product.

Much as liquid water is essential for life, frozen water, ice, is frequently lethal, especially if
ice formation occurs *within* the cell. Upon formation of ice, loss of liquid water may impair or
preclude the four basic water-related functions
listed above. In particular, the structures and
the activities of macromolecules and membranes may be severely damaged. In fact, the
harmful effects of ice formation are due to a
suite of physical and chemical effects. Physical
damage from ice crystals that form within a cell
can lead to rupture of membranes and the consequent dissipation of concentration gradients
between the cell and external fluids or between
membrane-bounded compartments within the
cell. Ice formation in the extracellular fluids
also can lead to damage to membranes as well
as to lethal dehydration of the cell, as water
moves down its concentration gradient from
the intracellular space to the now depleted
pool of liquid water in the extracellular space.
Dehydration of the cell not only deprives it of
water, but also leads to harmful and perhaps
lethal increases in the concentrations of inorganic ions, which remain behind in the cell.
Because the activities and structures of nucleic
acids and proteins are affected by the concentrations of ions in their milieu, dehydration is
expected to lead to perturbation of macromolecular structure and metabolic activity. It should
come as no surprise, therefore, that with rare
exceptions such as the fat body cells of certain
cold-tolerant insects (Lee et al., 1993b; Salt,
1962), ice formation within cells is lethal.

Freeze-Avoidance Strategies: Preventing
Formation and Growth of Ice Crystals

The threats posed by ice formation in the intracellular and extracellular fluids have favored
selection in diverse types of organisms for
mechanisms that either prevent the formation
of ice or minimize the potential for enlargement
of any small ice crystals that do form in the
internal fluids. These mechanisms are under
intense study, both because of their inherent
interest to evolutionary and ecological physiol-

ogists concerned with environmental tolerance relationships, and because of their potential in biomedical science for designing new strategies for the preservation of cells, tissues, organs, and whole organisms at low temperatures. Agricultural science is also focusing on freezing avoidance. For instance, there is an active effort to design frost-resistant plant species through bioengineering strategies. (Note: Agricultural science is also interested in the other side of the freeze-resistant/freeze-tolerant coin, by employing freeze-inducing bacteria whose outer membranes contain protein ice nucleators (PINs). Ingestion of these bacteria can cause crop-damaging insects to freeze [see Lee et al., 1993a].)

The wide diversity of organisms that have developed mechanisms allowing resistance to freezing may tend to belie the fact that only a few fundamental principles establish the potential adaptive routes that can be taken to prevent ice formation in biological fluids or to impede the growth of ice crystals that do form within the body. Our treatment of freezing resistance will focus on these core principles and illustrate numerous examples of evolutionary convergence on common solutions for solving the problems posed by threats of ice formation and ice growth.

Some Basic Physical Principles Related to Ice Formation and Ice Crystal Growth

To build an adequate foundation for understanding the different mechanisms used by organisms for preventing either the initial formation of ice crystals in biological fluids or the growth of existing crystals, some basic concepts and definitions need to be reviewed. Only by understanding some of the fundamental principles involved in the physics of ice formation and growth will it be possible to appreciate fully the problems posed by ice and the potential mechanisms by which organisms might avoid damage from freezing.

A central concept in the physics and chemistry of aqueous solutions involves what are termed *colligative relationships* or *colligative properties*. These are properties of solutions that depend only on the *number of solute particles* in a given volume of solution, not on the species of solutes that are present. Colligative properties comprise the freezing point, boiling point, vapor pressure, and osmotic pressure of the solution. For example, in a liter of water that contains a one molar solution of a nonelectrolyte such as glucose, the freezing point is $-1.86°C$ at one atmosphere pressure. A 0.5 M solution of a fully dissociated electrolyte such as NaCl will also have a freezing point of $-1.86°C$. Such solutions are termed 1 osmolar (1 Osm) solutions, and contain Avogadro's number (6.02×10^{23}) of solute particles. The fact that seawater is approximately 1 Osm in total concentration is an important point to recall at this juncture, because this central fact defines the problem faced by high-latitude marine teleost fishes, whose body fluids are only about 40% as concentrated as seawater.

Although colligative rules define the *thermodynamic* freezing point of a solution, the *kinetics* of freezing are such that rapid formation of ice does not necessarily occur at the instant temperature decreases to the point that freezing would be expected on the basis of the solution's osmolality. If initial *nucleation* of ice does not occur, aqueous solutions may *supercool* (*undercool*) by tens of degrees Celsius. Pure water may be supercooled to approximately $-40°C$, that is, by 40°C below its thermodynamic freezing point, as long as nucleation is avoided. At $-40°C$ the strengths of the hydrogen bonds between water molecules become great enough to induce *homogeneous nucleation*. At higher subzero temperatures, small nucleators such as dust particles may trigger ice formation, often at temperatures essentially identical to the thermodynamic freezing point. It would be predicted that biological fluids, which contain a wide variety of solutes and are bounded by surfaces, would tend to supercool much less than pure water. Many biological fluids in fact supercool by only about 0.1°C. In what may seem a paradoxical situation, the extracellular fluids of many freeze-tolerant organisms contain *ice-nucleating molecules* that function to prevent deep supercooling by triggering extracellular ice formation at relatively high temperatures (see "Freeze-Tolerance: Living with Internal Ice").

Another important physical concept in biological freezing relationships is *ice recrystallization*. This process involves a redistribution of ice crystal sizes in an ice-laden solution, such that some crystals grow in size while some shrink. The threat posed to cellular integrity from recrystallization arises from development of large crystals through joining together of smaller crystals. Organisms may be able to tolerate the presence of sufficiently small ice crystals in their body fluids, but if these crystals grow in size beyond a certain value, death may occur. For this reason, the study of mechanisms of freezing resistance includes not only adaptations for preventing the initial formation of ice in biological fluids, but also adaptations that limit the growth of any ice crystals that do form within the organism. Growth of individual crystals through addition of water molecules from the solution and growth due to recrystallization must be minimized.

Colligative defenses against ice formation

The simplest mechanism for preventing freezing, at least in terms of the physics involved, would seem to be to increase the concentrations of one or more solutes in the intra- and extracellular fluids to enable the freezing point to be depressed adequately to avoid ice formation. Colligative defenses are, in fact, very common as freeze avoidance adaptations in both terrestrial and aquatic organisms. As in the case of other mechanisms for preventing ice formation or for hindering crystal growth and recrystallization, a striking degree of convergent evolution is noted in the case of colligative defenses against freezing. A variety of taxa increase the concentrations of a relatively small set of low-molecular-mass organic solutes, for instance, glycerol, sorbitol, and trehalose, to reduce the freezing points of the cellular and extracellular fluids (Duman, 2001). Glycerol is often the major colligative antifreeze, notably in freeze-avoiding terrestrial arthropods such as insects. Although it may not be present at detectable levels in the hemolymph of summer-acclimatized insects, whose osmolality may be approximately 400–600 mOsmol kg^{-1}, glycerol concentrations in

winter-acclimatized specimens may reach 3–5 M (Karow, 1991). Polyols like glycerol not only enhance freezing avoidance through colligative effects, but also may lower the supercooling point of a solution by two to three times as much as the melting point is reduced. Thus, glycerol may confer much more protection because of its ability to enhance supercooling than it provides from strictly colligative effects on the equilibrium freezing/melting point. Glycerol-rich insects may supercool to approximately −60°C, the lowest temperature at which animals are known to remain unfrozen (Karow, 1991; Sømme, 1982). A 5 M solution of glycerol would be predicted to lower the freezing point by only 9.3°C (5 × −1.86°C), whereas an insect with this concentration of glycerol supercooled to −55°C (Ring, 1982). To enable such deep supercooling to occur, insects may eliminate ice nucleators from the body as winter approaches. For example, bacteria with ice-nucleating activities may be passed from the digestive system (Zachariassen, 1985, 1992).

One of the most surprising findings concerning the use of glycerol as a colligative antifreeze is that several teleost fishes from high-latitude waters in the northern hemisphere accumulate sufficient glycerol in winter to become iso-osmotic with seawater (Raymond, 1992, 1993). Teleost fishes are almost always strongly hypo-osmotic to seawater (chapter 6), and they would have to more than double the osmolality of their body fluids if they were to rely on colligative mechanisms for freezing avoidance. Nonetheless, several teleosts living in −1.9°C waters during winter, including species of smelt and greenling, accumulate glycerol to concentrations as high as approximately 0.4 M. Summer-acclimatized fish do not contain elevated levels of glycerol, indicating that glycerol production is regulated seasonally. This regulatory strategy makes sense in terms of energy relationships. Because the gills of these fishes are highly permeable to glycerol, the use of this molecule as a mechanism for avoiding freezing is likely to be quite energetically costly. A reduced carbon compound that could serve as a source of energy for synthesis of ATP or as a substrate for glycogen and lipid synthesis is lost to the environment. Perhaps because this mechanism for avoidance of freezing is so costly energetically, it appears to be restricted to a small subset of the teleost species that occur at high latitudes in freezing seawater.

In some Arctic and Antarctic bony fishes, the body fluids also contain relatively high concentrations of other classes of organic osmolytes, notably the metabolic dead-end compound trimethylamine-N-oxide (TMAO), which is a major osmolyte in cartilaginous fishes (chapter 6; Raymond, 1998; Raymond and DeVries, 1998). Trimethylamine-N-oxide is an especially interesting osmolyte to find at relatively high concentrations in fishes from high latitudes because it could play at least two quite different roles in adaptation to low temperature. First, its occurrence at high concentrations in both the intra- and extracellular compartments could lower the thermodynamic freezing points of all body fluids. Muscle concentrations of TMAO in some Antarctic notothenioids exceeded 140 mM, and blood concentrations ranged up to approximately 80 mM (Raymond and DeVries, 1998). Second, because methylammonium compounds like TMAO counteract perturbation of proteins by salt (chapter 6), TMAO could have favorable effects on proteins in these fishes, which contain atypically high concentrations of sodium and potassium ions. Temperate bony fishes typically contain approximately 170 mM concentrations of $Na^+ + K^+$, whereas some Antarctic notothenioids contain up to 220 mM concentrations of $Na^+ + K^+$ (Raymond, 1997).

Although colligative effects clearly play an important role in freeze-avoidance by high-latitude fishes, in the majority of these species a noncolligative type of mechanism involving macromolecular "antifreeze" compounds plays the central role in (i) preventing the formation of ice in the body fluids and, when ice crystal formation does occur, (ii) in inhibiting the potentially lethal processes of ice crystal growth and ice recrystallization.

Noncolligative defenses against ice formation: Antifreeze proteins and glycoproteins

Occurrence and defining properties of antifreeze proteins and antifreeze glycoproteins. One of the most interesting discoveries made in thermal biology during the last few decades of the twentieth century is that avoidance of freezing commonly is due to mechanisms that rely not on the colligative effects of small solutes, but on noncolligative effects that involve macromolecules, antifreeze proteins (AFPs) and glycoproteins (AFGPs). The discovery of macromolecular antifreezes in Antarctic notothenioid fishes by DeVries (1971, 1982) turned out to be only the proverbial tip of the iceberg. Subsequent to this discovery, various classes of macromolecular antifreezes have been found in a variety of other families of fishes, in terrestrial arthropods (insects, spiders, and mites), marine molluscs, plants, fungi, and bacteria (see Cheng, 1998; Duman, 2001; Duman and Olsen, 1993; Duman et al. 1993; Fletcher et al., 2001). All of these macromolecular antifreezes share certain properties in common. First, they are all polypeptides or proteins (biochemists have never agreed exactly when a polypeptide becomes large enough to merit being called a protein!). Certain of these antifreezes have carbohydrate moieties attached to threonine and serine residues, and therefore they are called antifreeze glycoproteins (AFGPs) (figure 7.39). When carbohydrate moieties are absent, the molecules are referred to simply as antifreeze proteins, AFPs. Second, all AFPs and AFGPs are characterized by an unusual effect on the freezing and melting points of ice crystals: solutions containing these antifreezes exhibit *thermal hysteresis*, which refers to the fact that the temperature at which an ice crystal grows in a solution containing the antifreeze (the *hysteric freezing point*) is lower than the temperature at which the crystal is observed to melt (thermodynamic freezing/melting point temperature of the solution). In other words, ice crystal growth appears to disobey colligative relationships.

It is important to examine the phenomenon of thermal hysteresis in some detail to appreciate how unusual the protein-based antifreezes

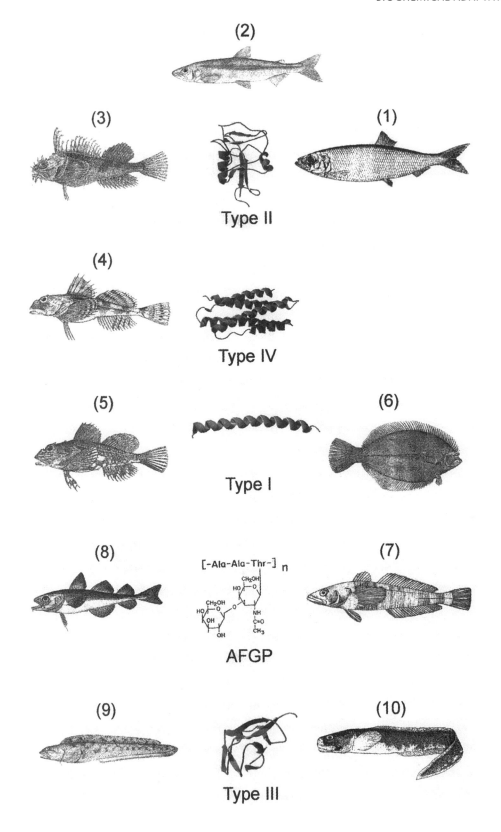

are in their function, and to gain an initial insight into the mechanism by which these antifreezes depress freezing points. It is also important to define carefully the concepts of "freezing point" and "melting point" as they are used in reference to macromolecular antifreezes, because the expression "freezing point" as used in analysis of AFPs and AFGPs is quite different from the freezing point discussed in the context of solutions that obey colligative rules. In typical freezing experiments with these antifreezes, a small ("seed") crystal of ice is formed in the device (e.g., a capillary tube) that contains the antifreeze solution (see Duman, 2001, and Fletcher et al., 2001, for discussions of the relevant methodologies). As the temperature of the solution is reduced, the investigator records the temperature at which growth of the small seed crystal is first evident. This temperature is defined as the "freezing point" of the AFP/AFGP-containing solution. In fact, this "freezing point" is really the temperature of *additional* freezing because ice is already present. In a solution containing solutes that obey colligative relationships, growth of a seed crystal would occur as soon as the temperature is reduced by approximately $0.01°C$–$0.02°C$. In other words, as predicted by colligative relationships, there should be no difference between the freezing and melting temperatures at equilibrium. In a solution containing a macromolecular antifreeze, however, the crystal may not increase in size until the solution is cooled by perhaps as much as $5°C$–$6°C$. The extent of cooling prior to crystal growth will depend on several factors, including the type of antifreeze present in the solution and its concentration, as discussed later. The size of the initial seed crystal will also influence the temperature of additional ice growth, with small crystals allowing greater depression of the freezing point (more thermal hysteresis) than large crystals (Duman, 2001). If, subsequent to freezing, the temperature of the solution is increased, melting of the ice does not occur at the "freezing point"—the temperature at which ice growth was observed—but only at a higher temperature. The ice melting temperature is, in fact, identical with the predicted thermodynamic (equilibrium) melting temperature set by colligative relationships. The amount of thermal hysteresis, then, is the difference between the equilibrium melting temperature of the solution and the temperature at which the ice crystal grew (a nonequilibrium freezing point). It has become common to refer to AFPs and AFGPs as *thermal hysteresis proteins* (THPs), to denote the common effect they have on ice crystal growth and disappearance. In the subsequent discussion, this generic acronym often will be used as a convenient shorthand when discussing properties common to all AFPs and AFGPs.

A third characteristic of THPs is their effect on the geometry of the new ice that forms in their presence (Raymond et al., 1986). Ice crystal growth is very different from that observed

Figure 7.39. The diversity of antifreeze proteins and antifreeze glycoproteins in marine fishes. Shown are the structures of four types of AFPs (I–IV) and the AFGP found in Antarctic notothenioids and Arctic cod. AFPs I–IV are shown as ribbon structures. The tripeptide repeat (–ala–ala–thr–) and carbohydrate moiety (galactosyl-*N*-acetylgalactosamine) of AFGPs illustrate the key element of AFGP structures in notothenioid and Arctic cod.

Type I AFPs are alanine-rich, amphipathic alpha helical proteins with characteristic repeat structures involving long stretches of alanines. Molecular masses of Type I AFPs are between 3.3 and 5 kDa. Like the AFGPs, Type I AFPs are extended molecules in which the polar side-chains are oriented along a common front. Type II AFPs are globular proteins with varied secondary structures. Type III AFPs are composed of small beta-strand elements and a single helix turn that gives the protein a flat-faced folded surface. Type IV AFP is conjectured to be a helix-bundle protein. (See Fletcher et al., 2001, for review.) Species: (1) Atlantic herring (*Clupea harengus harengus*), (2) American smelt (*Osmerus mordax*), (3) sea raven (*Hemitripterus americanus*), (4) longhorn sculpin (*Myoxocephalus octodecimspinosus*), (5) shorthorn sculpin (*Myoxocephalus scorpius*), (6) winter flounder (*Pleuronectes americanus*), (7) *Dissostichus mawsoni* (Antarctic notothenioid), (8) Arctic cod (*Boreogadus saida*), (9) ocean pout (zoarcid) (*Macrozoarces americanus*), (10) Antarctic zoarcid (*Lycodichthys dearborni*). (Figure modified after Fletcher et al., 2001.)

in solutions lacking THPs. When THPs are present, newly formed crystals are extremely elongated and needle-like, and they tend to grow rapidly. In normal ice, growth of the crystal typically occurs slowly, along flat planes, and needle-like spicules are uncommon.

A fourth characteristic of THPs that distinguishes them from solutes that are colligative in their effects on freezing points is that THPs are incorporated into the ice lattice (Raymond et al., 1986). As we will see when the mechanisms of THP activity are examined, the incorporation of THPs into ice crystals suggests that these molecules have a capacity to bind tightly to ice. Colligative solutes lack this ability and freeze out of solution, leading to the formation of ice that is composed of essentially pure water and pockets of concentrated solute that remain unfrozen down to very low temperatures. The pockets of dense brine found within sea ice are a manifestation of the freezing-out phenomenon.

A final defining characteristic of THPs is their ability to inhibit recrystallization. In the presence of THPs, small ice crystals tend not to aggregate into large crystals. As indicated above, inhibition of recrystallization may be an exceedingly important capacity in organisms facing the threat of freezing. Unless there is an absolute ability to prevent formation of ice in the body fluids, survival may depend on maintaining the ice crystals that do form at small enough sizes so they are not threatening to survival. Thus, even if THPs cannot completely prevent ice formation in body fluids, they nonetheless may fulfill an extremely important role as inhibitors of recrystallization.

Structures and evolutionary origins of fish AFPs and AFGPs. The origin and proliferation of AFPs and AFGPs is one of the more fascinating stories to have arisen in the broad field of molecular evolution during the past decade. The story is especially interesting because of its integrative nature: it weaves geological history, physiology, molecular genetics, protein biochemistry, and ice physics into a single narrative. This work also presents examples of how new functions can be generated from preexisting genes and proteins, and how a single type of gene or protein can be recruited by separate

evolutionary lineages to fabricate a new type of adaptation—*parallel convergence* in evolution (Fletcher et al., 2001). In essence, the emerging picture of the origins and evolutionary refinements of AFPs and AFGPs in fishes shows "how many ways the wheel can be reinvented" in evolution.

An appropriate starting point for developing this evolutionary story is to emphasize the diversity of types of THPs and the somewhat random way in which they are distributed among fishes. There are currently known to be four types of AFPs and one type of AFGP in marine fishes (figure 7.39). There is, however, no indication that any of the four types of AFPs are strongly linked to any particular evolutionary lineage. For example, there may be different types of AFPs in species as closely related as congeners. Thus, the shorthorn sculpin has a Type I AFP and its congener the longhorn sculpin has a Type IV AFP (figure 7.39). The variation in "who has what" among the AFP-containing fishes has implications for (i) the historical events that led to selection for THPs, (ii) the categories of genes and gene products that served as raw material for evolving THPs, and (iii) the molecular characteristics of THPs that underlie thermal hysteresis. We consider each of these themes of the story in turn.

The origins of AFPs and AFGPs appear to be relatively recent. In Antarctic notothenioid fishes, Chen et al. (1997a) conjecture that AFGPs arose between 5 and 14 million years ago, at the time that massive ice sheets began to form in the waters surrounding the Antarctic continent and water temperatures through most of the water column stabilized near $-1.86°C$ (see Eastman, 1993). An even more recent origin of THPs in northern fishes has been proposed (see Fletcher et al., 2001). As in the case of the Southern Ocean, where the separation of the Antarctic continent from lower latitude land masses approximately 30 million years ago led to circulation patterns that caused sea temperatures to fall dramatically, continental drift in the northern hemisphere led to changes in circulation that caused water temperatures in the Arctic Ocean to plummet. This rapid drop in sea temperature at high latitudes in the northern hemisphere may have started only 1–2 million years ago. At this time, many of the contemporary species found to contain THPs would have lacked these proteins. Clearly, the cooling that began 1–2 million years ago established a strong selective advantage for mechanisms conferring resistance to freezing, and many different species succeeded in developing these adaptations. It is the starting raw material and its subsequent exploitation that we now consider.

Where did the genetic raw material for AFPs and AFGPs originate, and how was this material modified to ensure effective THP function and the synthesis of adequate levels of THPs to allow freezing resistance? Although not all of the THPs found in fishes have had their genealogies mapped, it is now apparent that several types of ancestral genes provided raw material for THP evolution. In the case of the AFGPs of Antarctic notothenioids and Arctic cod (order Gadiformes), the tripeptide repeat, alanine–alanine–threonine, and the carbohydrates attached to the hydroxyls of the threonines (serines are present in some isoforms) are structural elements in common. The extremely similar protein sequences of these AFGPs, and the similar distribution of molecular masses among different isoforms, might suggest that the notothenioid and cod AFGPs originated from a common gene. In fact, this is not the case: the Antarctic and Arctic fishes have recruited different genes for their AFGPs (Chen et al., 1997a,b; Logsdon and Doolittle, 1997). Thus, the AFGPs provide an extremely interesting example of convergent evolution at the level of structure and function. The notothenioid AFGPs arose from a gene encoding pancreatic trypsinogen (figure 7.40; Chen et al., 1997a). What is notable about the origin of the notothenioid AFGP-encoding gene is that it arose from sections of the coding (exon) and the noncoding (intron) regions of the trypsinogen-encoding gene. A short region of the trypsinogen-encoding gene, which spanned the boundary between the first intron and the second exon, appears to have undergone extensive duplication and unequal crossing-over events to yield a gene that encodes a large polyprotein. In *Dissostichus mawsoni*, the AFGP gene sequenced by Chen et al. (1997a) had 41 tandemly repeated elements. Other AFGP genes may contain different numbers of repeats. The 5′ end of the original trypsinogen-encoding gene was retained in the AFGP-encoding gene. This 5′ region encodes a signal peptide that may be critical for secretion of AFGPs into the body fluids, much as the signal peptide attached to trypsinogen is needed for its secretion by the pancreas into the gut. Chen et al. (1997a) conjecture that the primordial AFGP in the notothenioids might have had as its function the prevention of ice formation in the intestine. Subsequently, AFGP synthesis may have been taken over by the liver, the primary, if not the sole site of AFGP synthesis in contemporary notothenioids. Antifreeze glycoproteins of notothenioids occur in at least eight size classes, with molecular masses from approximately 2.6 to 34 kDa (DeVries and Cheng, 1992; Duman et al., 1993).

The AFGPs of the Arctic cods such as *Boreogadus saida* arose from a different, and as yet unidentified gene (Chen et al., 1997b). Although the cod AFGP gene encodes a number of copies of the AFGP, as in the case of the notothenioid gene, the nucleotide sequences used to code for the –Ala–Ala–Thr– repeat, the intron–exon organizations of the genes, and the sites of proteolytic cleavage in the polyprotein differ between the two groups of fishes. The cod AFGPs are of much more recent origin; they may have appeared near the time of Arctic glaciation, approximately 1–2 million years ago.

The AFPs found in Arctic fishes also have a recent evolutionary origin. For the Type II AFPs, the genes from which the contemporary AFP-encoding genes arose are known (Fletcher et al., 2001). For the Type II AFPs of sea raven, herring, and smelt (figure 7.39), homologies in sequence and structure to the carbohydrate recognition domain of C-type lectins suggest that one or more lectin-encoding genes gave rise to the AFP-encoding genes. The phylogenies of these species make it extremely unlikely that the origin of an AFP-encoding gene occurred in a common ancestor. Rather, it is likely that Type II AFPs evolved from C-type lectin genes on several separate occasions. Thus, evolution of Type II AFPs represents *parallel*

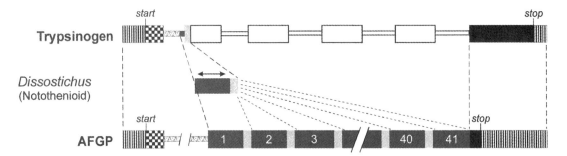

Figure 7.40. Structures of the genes encoding trypsinogen and the antifreeze glycoprotein (AFGP) of an Antarctic notothenioid (*Dissostichus mawsoni*). Thick boxes denote exons; thin box denote introns. Gene segments filled with vertical lines are untranslated (regions to the 5' of the start codon ("start") and at the 3' end of the genes). The gene segments filled with a checkered pattern are signal peptides. The AFGP gene of the Antarctic notothenioids is shown to have arisen from a highly duplicated portion of the trypsinogen gene that comprises part of the first intron and second exon. The double-headed arrow shown above the single AFGP-encoding segment in the middle of the figure denotes expansion of a sequence element present in the trypsinogen gene that has given rise to the canonical AFGP repeat unit. The AFGP-encoding sections of the gene are marked with numbers to indicate that the gene has 41 AFGP-encoding regions (dark shading). The lightly shaded regions joining the AFGP-encoding regions represent proteolytic sites. (Figure modified after Logsdon and Doolittle, 1997; based on data in Chen et al., 1997a,b.)

evolutionary convergence: in each case, a common type of gene was recruited and then modified, to generate a protein with thermal hysteresis properties. It should be appreciated that the convergence in evolution of Type II AFPs may be the result of recruitment of two or more genes from the large superfamily of genes encoding C-lectins. Thus, convergence in this scenario refers to recruitment from a gene family, and not necessarily to the recruitment of a single, common gene in all AFPII-containing lineages.

The parallel convergence noted in Type II AFPs has involved more than one molecular mechanism for effecting thermal hysteresis (reviewed by Fletcher et al., 2001). In the Type II AFPs of herring and smelt, thermal hysteresis is dependent on the presence of Ca^{2+} in the solution, a likely reflection of the fact that C-type lectins are calcium-dependent in their binding to sugars. However, unlike the AFPs of herring and smelt, the sea raven's Type II AFP does not require Ca^{2+} for ice-binding activity and thermal hysteresis. The sea raven AFP binds to ice through a different site on the protein from the Ca^{2+}-dependent site used in other Type II antifreezes. Therefore, the par-

allel convergence that is noted in the derivation of a common function (thermal hysteresis and ice binding) from a common genetic ancestor (genes encoding C-lectins) is not paired with exploitation of a common site on the lectin molecule for establishing antifreeze activity.

Type III AFPs have been identified only in eel pouts (zoarcids) (figure 7.39). These proteins contain most of the 20 amino acids, except for histidine and tryptophan. The Type III AFPs of Arctic and Antarctic zoarcids appear to be orthologous. This finding suggests that the Type III AFPs of zoarcids arose in a common ancestor of the contemporary polar species of this group. Because cooling of the Southern Ocean occurred many millions of years before the Arctic Ocean reached freezing temperatures, it appears probable that the ancestor of all AFP-containing zoarcids was a southern hemisphere species (Fletcher et al., 2001; Wang et al., 1995).

The THPs of organisms besides fishes are not as well characterized in terms of sequence or genetic origin (Duman, 2001). Insect THPs vary in mass from approximately 14 kDa to 20 kDa and have sequences with high percentages of polar amino acids (Duman et al., 1993).

Some insects have THPs with high cysteine contents, like those of the Type II AFPs of fishes. Most insects contain multiple variants of THP's, and these may function synergistically (see below). In certain vascular plants, for example, winter rye (*Secale cereale*), proteins that function in the context of pathogenesis have been recruited to serve as thermal hysteresis proteins (Hon et al., 1995; Yeh et al., 2000). These pathogenesis-related proteins include chitin-degrading enzymes, chitinases. Studies of chitinases of winter rye have shown that acclimation to low temperatures induces expression of unique forms of this enzyme that retain their abilities to hydrolyze chitin despite taking on a new function, that of a THP. This is the only case known in which a THP has retained its original physiological role. The chitinase THPs of winter rye are hypothesized to have arisen from duplicated chitinase genes. Following gene duplication, one chitinase-encoding gene is proposed to have acquired mutations that led (i) to a chitinase with the observed dual functions and (ii) to alterations in the gene's regulatory regions that allow the gene to be expressed only at low temperatures (Yeh et al., 2000). In many cases, the occurrence of THPs is indicated only indirectly: The presence of THPs is assumed because of thermal hysteresis activity that is abolished by treatment with proteases (see Duman and Olson, 1993).

Mechanism of action of THPs. Despite the diversity of sequences that exists among THPs of different taxa, it is very likely that a common physical mechanism of action is present, that accounts for all of the unusual behaviors of THP, from their capacity for generating thermal hysteresis to their integration into the ice lattice.

The mechanism of action of THPs is suggested by several of their properties. As mentioned above, the incorporation of THPs into the growing ice crystal suggests that a strong affinity exists between the ice surface and at least a part of the structure of all THP's. The precise elements of structure that are involved in ice binding by THPs remain to be characterized in most cases, although for some classes of THPs the likely mechanism

of ice binding is known. For the extended linear AFGPs, hydroxyl groups on the carbohydrate moieties appear to be critical for thermal hysteresis. Chemically modified AFGPs on which the carbohydrate moieties have been blocked or removed lose their unique properties as THPs and behave like normal (colligative) solutes. Despite lacking an AFGPs extended linear structure with a long front of ice-binding polar residues, the zoarcid Type III AFP binds effectively to ice because a very flat amphipathic surface is present on the molecule that permits formation of five hydrogen bonds between the AFP and ice (Jia et al., 1997). The spacing of the five hydrogen-bonding atoms of this AFP matches closely the spacing of O atoms on what is termed the prism face of the ice crystal. The residues interacting with ice appear to be highly stabilized in their three-dimensional orientations by interactions with other residues. Type III AFP thus may represent a case in which protein–ligand interaction does not entail a conformational change in the protein. Unlike enzymes, no catalytic vacuole needs to be formed by this ice-binding protein, and rigidity of the binding site rather than flexibility in this region may be essential for function. The flatness of the ice-binding surface, the orientation of the ice-binding residues, and the inflexibility of the geometry of the ice-binding region combine to favor strong interactions with ice and highly effective depression of the freezing point.

Despite the roles played by hydrogen bonding between THPs and ice, nonpolar groups also may play key roles in some THPs. There is evidence that hydrophobic faces on certain types of AFPs may be the ice-binding domains (Harding et al., 1999).

The diversity of THPs and the apparently wide range of sites on these proteins that are able to bind to ice is a reflection of the fact that the different planes of ice crystals are variable in their geometries, such that a number of targets are presented for THPs. Blockage of *any* plane on an ice crystal may suffice to keep it from growing or undergoing recrystallization, so that regardless of where or how a THP binds to ice, it can exert its freeze-avoiding influence.

A general model for THP function has been proposed, the *adsorption–inhibition model* (Raymond and DeVries, 1977), which applies regardless of the nature of the groups on the THP that bind to ice or the particular ice crystal plane at which binding takes place. The basic tenet of this model is quite simple: all types of THPs bind to the surface of ice and make growth of the ice crystal less energetically favorable (figure 7.41). Through binding to the surface of an ice crystal, the THPs force the crystal to grow along a path with a relatively high radius of curvature. Growth along a path with a high radius of curvature (compare the ice crystals in the upper left and right frames of figure 7.41) is less energetically favorable than growth along a relatively flat surface, due to what is termed the Kelvin Effect. In essence, the Kelvin Effect states that, when THPs are present, temperature must be reduced below the equilibrium melting/freezing point of THP-free ice, to allow water molecules to lose enough energy to join a highly curved growth surface.

Although the adsorption–inhibition mechanism may appear to make sense in terms of thermodynamic relationships, a reader versed in physical chemistry might question how the mechanism could work unless binding of the THP to the small ice crystal was irreversible. If the interaction between THP molecules and the ice crystal involved a freely reversible equilibrium—as is common in ligand-binding reactions that rely on noncovalent bonds—then there would likely be the opportunity for additional water molecules to add to the ice surface because the THP would not bind its ligand, the ice, 100% of the time. The way around this dilemma, as pointed out by Fletcher et al. (2001), appears to be based on the large sizes of THPs. Because each THP molecule possesses many ice binding elements, the probability that *all* of the THP–ice interactions would fail at once is remote and likely approaches zero. A useful analogy in this context involves the stabilization of structure of globular proteins. Each interaction between residues is weak, yet a global stability is achieved because of the improbability that adequate numbers of these interactions could

fail simultaneously and thus lead to denaturation—at least under normal physiological temperatures and pH values. Thermal hysteresis proteins likewise rely on large numbers of individually weak interactions to achieve their antifreeze activities.

It follows from the foregoing discussion that not all THPs are apt to be created equal in terms of their specific activities. As a general rule, there is a positive correlation between molecular mass of a particular type of THP and its capacity to depress the freezing point of a solution (support thermal hysteresis). Most THPs of fishes have similar specific activities (thermal hysteresis per mass of THP), despite the wide variation in structure among the teleost AFGPs and AFPs. However, the THPs of fishes are typically less potent in terms of specific activity than those of insects (Duman, 2001; Duman et al., 1993). Fish THPs, studied both in fish serum and in solutions of purified THPs, seldom generate more than $1.5°C$ of thermal hysteresis. In contrast, purified THPs of insects have thermal hysteresis activities almost twice as high, and when studied in unfractionated hemolymph, insect THPs may induce hysteresis as great as $8–9°C$. The disparity between the amounts of thermal hysteresis observed with purified THPs in vitro and with hemolymph suggests that factors in serum enhance the activities of THPs. Thus, the in-vivo functioning of THPs in insects may not be adequately simulated by simplified in-vitro experiments using only purified THPs.

At least two hemolymph constituents in insects are able to modify the efficacy of THPs. One factor operates on the principle that "bigger is better." The importance of presenting a large interacting surface to an ice crystal is perhaps most strikingly illustrated by insect THPs, whose activities are enhanced by a second component of the organism's cold weather strategy, protein ice nucleators (PINs) (Duman, 2001). The ice-nucleating functions of PINs will be discussed later, in the context of the complex strategies used by some insects to cope with freezing temperatures. In the present analysis, what is important to emphasize is that PINs are able to bind to multiple THP molecules and effectively create a massive THP with

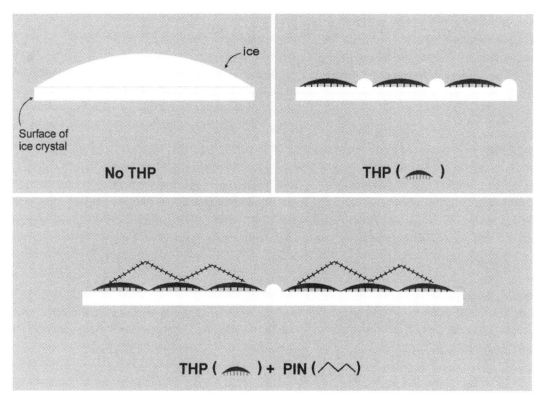

Figure 7.41. A model of the interactions between THP molecules and the surface of an ice crystal. (Upper left panel) In the absence of any THP, ice growth occurs with a low radius of curvature and thus is energetically favorable. (Upper right panel) The binding of THP molecules to the ice hinders addition of further water molecules from the solution because the higher radius of curvature of the growing ice crystal in the presence of THP molecules makes growth less energetically favorable (requires a lower temperature for crystal growth). The large size of the THP minimizes the probability that the THP will dissociate from the ice and allow the crystal to gain additional molecules of water. (Lower panel) The enhancement of THP function by an insect ice-nucleating protein (PIN) is shown. The PIN facilitates aggregation of THP molecules, thereby generating a larger sized antifreeze with enhanced ability to lower the hysteresis freezing temperature.

extraordinary ice-binding abilities (figure 7.41, lower panel).

A second set of components of hemolymph may also modify THP activity. Low-molecular-mass solutes like glycerol, sorbitol, citrate, and certain inorganic ions have been shown to enhance by up to sixfold (citrate) the abilities of insect THPs to support thermal hysteresis (Li et al., 1998). These enhancements of THPs activities were only observed at high concentrations of the solutes, 0.25 M to 1 M. Thus, glycerol and sorbitol are likely to be the only solutes tested (each gave a threefold enhancement) whose concentrations reach levels adequate to be physiologically relevant in this context.

The mechanism underlying the enhancing effect of these solutes could involve these solutes' stabilizing effects on proteins (chapter 6). For example, glycerol, a strong protein stabilizer, may favor aggregation of AFP monomers into large, more effective aggregates. Glycerol, then, may play a number of important roles in the over-wintering strategies of insects. It may confer adequate resistance to freezing through (i) colligative effects on the equilibrium freezing point, (ii) increases in supercooling ability, and (iii) enhancement of THP activity. Glycerol also may stabilize proteins and, through this effect, influence rates of enzymatic activity (see Glycerol and Other Stabilizing Solutes...").

A final point about the adsorption–inhibition model of THP function needs to be emphasized: this mechanism accounts for both the depressed freezing point of THP-containing solutions and the inhibition of recrystallization by THPs. Much lower concentrations of THPs appear to be sufficient for inhibiting recrystallization than are required to depress the freezing point, as manifested by the occurrence of thermal hysteresis (see Duman et al., 1993). Thus, in some species, the low concentrations of THPs that have been detected may function primarily as a means of preventing the formation of large ice crystals during freezing, rather than the prevention of freezing per se.

Thermal hysteresis protein efficacy differs among taxa: the issue of ultimate cause. The differences in molecular mass among THPs explain mechanistically a large fraction of the interspecific variation in thermal hysteresis activity. However, what is the ultimate cause, the selective basis, of the fact that THPs of fishes lack the high thermal hysteresis activity seen for THPs of insects, especially when the insect THPs are studied in hemolymph? The ultimate cause of the differences in potency between THPs of insects and fishes may be that fishes encounter much less threat from freezing than terrestrial insects. A teleost fish with a blood osmolality giving a colligatively determined freezing point of -0.6 to $-0.8°C$ will never experience water colder than $-1.86°C$, so it needs to reduce the freezing point of blood by only about $1°C$. In contrast, terrestrial insects may encounter winter temperatures below $-60°C$. It is possibly for this reason that selection has not led to even more potent THPs in fishes, and has led in insects not only to highly potent THPs, but also to a suite of other mechanisms for preventing freezing that are absent in fishes.

Polar fishes and cold-hardy beetles: contrasting scenarios for freeze-avoidance. With the information we now possess on the biochemistry, mechanism of action, and evolution of THPs,

it is appropriate to examine the functions of these molecules in a manner befitting an integrative ecological physiologist, to learn how the various mechanisms for freezing resistance play out in nature. We will see that differences in habitat thermal regime and phylogeny contribute to different scenarios in three types of animals whose freeze-avoidance relationships have been particularly well studied: Antarctic notothenioid fishes, Arctic fishes, and cold-hardy beetles.

The differences in specific activity of purified THPs from insects and teleost fishes, and the contrast between the specific activities of insect THPs when purified and when examined in whole serum, suggest that different strategies for freeze-avoidance may operate in marine teleosts and terrestrial insects. The contrast is most striking when the highly stenothermal Antarctic notothenioid fishes, which live continuously at near-freezing temperatures, are compared with (i) north temperate insects such as the beetle *Dendroides canadensis*, which encounters a wide range of temperatures during the annual seasonal cycle and must resist freezing down to deep subzero temperatures in winter, and (ii) Arctic fishes such as the winter flounder (*Pleuronectes americanus*), which experiences winter temperatures similar to those found year-round in the Antarctic, but temperatures well above freezing in other seasons.

Antarctic notothenioids. Consider first an Antarctic notothenioid living in McMurdo Sound, the southernmost region of the ocean. Throughout its life history, the fish has as stable a body temperature as an organism can have in any habitat. And, although this temperature is a low $-1.86°C$, it cannot get any lower (unless the fish freezes into the ice). To avoid freezing, the fish need only produce adequate amounts of THPs (AFGPs) to reduce the freezing point of its body fluids by just over $1.0°C$. In Antarctic notothenioids, unlike some Arctic fish, THPs appear to be synthesized only in the liver. From this site of synthesis, the THPs must be distributed to body fluids where the danger of ice formation occurs. These fluid spaces include, in addition to the blood, the interstitial, pericardial, peritoneal, and extradural fluids, and fluid within the intestine. In the last fluid space, low-molecular-mass AFGPs are predominant. Synthesis of high amounts of AFGPs is facilitated by high copy numbers of the genes that encode the AFGPs. In some northern fishes, families of 30 to 150 separate genes may encode AFPs in any given species (DeVries and Cheng, 1992). For AFGPs, the mechanism of enhancing gene dosage is different. In Arctic cod and Antarctic notothenioids, a single AFGP gene may contain multiple copies of the peptide-encoding region (Chen et al., 1997a,b; Hsaio et al., 1990). Proteolytic sites are found between the individual peptide-encoding regions, so that the polyprotein that is translated is hydrolyzed into dozens of individual AFGP molecules (figure 7.40). The proteolytic sites differ between AFGPs of Antarctic notothenioids and Arctic cod, with chymotrypsin sites occurring in the former and trypsin sites occurring in the latter (Fletcher et al., 2001). Expression of AFGP genes in Antarctic notothenioids is constitutive and continuous. Unlike high-latitude fishes from the northern hemisphere where the threat of freezing may be seasonal and THP synthesis may cease in summer, Antarctic notothenioids encounter the threat of freezing throughout their lives, and accordingly produce AFGPs continuously.

In Antarctic notothenioids, AFGPs likely perform both functions associated with THPs: prevention of ice crystal formation and enlargement, and inhibition of recrystallization. Antifreezes located near the body surface, for instance, in interstitial spaces among gill cells, may act as a peripheral defense and prevent inoculation of the cells and blood with ice. This peripheral defense may be especially important in cryopelagic species like *Pagothenia borchgrevinki*, which swims into the loose layer of ice crystals that lies beneath the solid sea ice. *Pagothenia borchgrevinki* has the highest concentrations of AFGPs of any notothenioid so far examined (DeVries and Cheng, 1992). The abundant small AFGPs in the intestinal fluids of notothenioids prevent freezing of this fluid when the fish ingests ice-laden seawater.

Despite the occurrence of AFGPs in Antarctic notothenioids at concentrations that would seem adequate to prevent formation of ice, there does in fact appear to be ice in the body fluids. The presence of ice is suggested by results of a novel heating experiment involving what is interpreted to be in-vivo melting of ice (DeVries and Cheng, 1992). When field-collected specimens of notothenioids were placed in hypersaline water and cooled to low temperatures, freezing was observed at $-2.7°C$. However, if the fish were first warmed to $0°C$, a temperature higher than they would experience during their lives, they then could be cooled to $-6°C$ before freezing took place. However, if the fish warmed to $0°C$ were then held at $-1.86°C$ for as little as one hour, they once again froze when temperature was reduced to $-2.7°C$. DeVries and Cheng interpret these results as providing evidence for existence of ice within the fishes. These ice crystals, whose location in the fish is not known, would trigger freezing near $-2.7°C$. However, if these crystals were removed by heating the fish, then the fish could be supercooled to a temperature about $4°C$ below its freezing point. Because notothenioids of McMurdo Sound never encounter temperatures above $-1.8°C$, the internal ice crystals would seem not to represent a threat to freezing, as long as the AFGPs keep the ice crystals small enough to prevent damage. However, because these fishes never have body temperatures high enough to melt ice, it seems probable that these small ice crystals could remain with these fishes throughout their lives, which may extend to approximately five decades. Ice crystals also may be present in northern fishes, as evidenced by anti-ice immunoglobulins, which have been detected in some freeze-resistant species (Verdier et al., 1996).

Arctic fishes—the winter flounder. Arctic fishes share many similarities in freezing avoidance strategies with Antarctic notothenioids, as just discussed. However, whereas notothenioids synthesize AFGPs constitutively, all of the Arctic fishes that produce AFGPs or AFPs exhibit seasonal patterns of synthesis. This is an energy-efficient strategy that avoids costly synthesis of THPs during warm seasons. Concentrations of THPs are strongly elevated at the onset of winter, and the degree to which THP concentrations are elevated reflects the severity of the threat of freezing. Mechanisms of THP synthesis differ among species, for instance in the kinetics of THP synthesis and the nature of post-translational processing of THPs, so no single model for regulation of THP concentrations fits all cases. The species for which most information on THP regulation is available is the winter flounder, in which a complex hierarchy of regulatory events links seasonal changes in the environment to production of plasma AFPs (figure 7.42; reviewed in Fletcher et al., 2001).

There are several major components to the regulatory cascade for controlling expression of AFP-encoding genes in winter flounder. The environmental factor that cues the need for THP production is photoperiod, not temperature. This makes sense because changes in day length are highly uniform year after year, whereas shifts in temperature are relatively unpredictable. For example, a warm autumn season might "fool" a fish that uses temperature as its cue for THP synthesis into postponing THP production; a sudden drop in temperature to freezing levels then could be lethal. In winter flounder, shortening of day length in fall elicits appearance of AFP mRNA in October, although plasma AFPs do not begin to accumulate until approximately one month later, when water temperatures usually have reached 4–6°C. It seems likely that turnover of AFP-mRNA is temperature dependent, such that the half-life of the message is extended significantly at low temperatures. Thus, although temperature is not the cue that controls transcription of the AFP-encoding gene, temperature does play an important role in determining message turnover and, thus, the timing of translation events.

The photoperiod signal regulating expression of AFP-encoding genes is processed in the central nervous system (CNS) (figure 7.42). A primary component in the regulatory cascade that follows photoperiod sensing is regulation of the production and release of growth hormone (GH) from the pituitary. In winter flounder no feeding or growth occurs in winter months, so down-regulation of GH synthesis in the pituitary by somatostatin is expected as day lengths

shorten. Hypophysectomy of summer-acclimatized fish results in induction of AFP synthesis, suggesting that production of GH by the pituitary plays an essential role in keeping AFP-encoding genes turned off.

It is not entirely clear how GH exerts its influences on AFP production, although some of the downstream effects of GH appear to involve influences on the concentrations or activity states of regulators of AFP gene transcription. Growth hormone levels may control synthesis of an insulin-like growth factor (IGF-1), which in turn may inhibit AFP gene enhancer (AEP) activity or inactivate a transcription factor termed CCAAT enhancer binding protein α (C/EBPα) through dephosphorylation. Both AEP and C/EBPα bind to an enhancer element located in the single intron of the AFP-encoding gene (Fletcher et al., 2001). Reduction in the amounts of GH binding to membrane receptors in liver cells is followed by (i) reductions in levels of IGF-1, (ii) concomitant activation of C/EBPα and AEP, and (iii) activation of transcription of the AFP-encoding genes.

The mRNA that is transcribed encodes a preproprotein. The pre-sequence is excised during translation, generating a proAFP protein having an accessible signal sequence that allows its secretion from the liver into the blood. There, the pro-sequence is removed to generate an active 37-residue AFP.

Disappearance of AFP mRNA in liver and AFP in plasma of winter flounder occurs in springtime as day length increases. During acclimatization to increasing day length, GH production rises, and the regulatory cascade shown on the left side of figure 7.42 leads to cessation of transcription and translation. Rising temperature may shorten the half-life of AFP-encoding message, leading to reduced translational activity for AFP.

Another major difference between certain Arctic fishes and Antarctic notothenioids is the occurrence of a second family of AFPs in the former fishes: skin AFPs. The discovery by Gong et al. (1996) that AFPs may exist within cells as well as in the extracellular fluids, and that the intracellular AFPs are encoded by a set of genes distinct from those encoding extra-

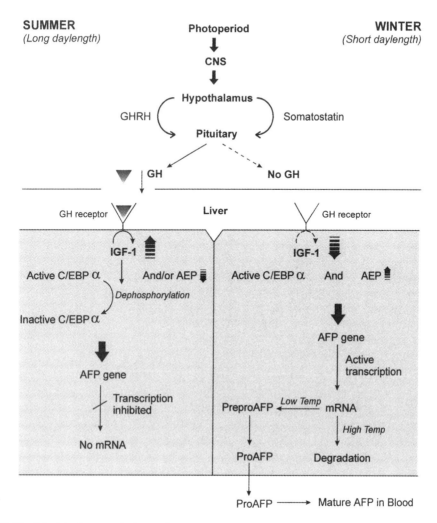

Figure 7.42. Model for regulation of AFP synthesis in winter flounder (*Pleuronectes americanus*). CNS: central nervous system; GHRH: growth hormone releasing hormone; GH: growth hormone; IGF-1: insulin-like growth factor-1; C/EBPα: CCAAT enhancer binding protein α; AEP: antifreeze enhancer-binding protein. See text for details. Arrows with striped tails denote up-regulation or down-regulation. (Figure modified after Fletcher et al., 2001.)

cellular AFPs, led to a paradigm shift in our thinking about freezing avoidance in fishes. In essence, the discovery of this second class of AFPs indicated that an important "peripheral defense" may be erected by Arctic fishes, one that would work to prevent inoculation of ice crystals into cells that come into contact with ice. Even though cell membranes do provide strong barriers to ice propagation, the thin, easily damaged epithelia found in structures such as the gill, in which only a single cell layer occurs between the blood and external

medium, makes ice propagation a concern. Skin AFPs thus could serve as a "peripheral defense" to prevent damaged cells from freezing, and to reduce the likelihood of propagation of ice from seawater into the blood. The skin AFPs are synthesized constitutively and manifest smaller seasonal changes in expression (approximately six- to ten fold variation) compared to plasma AFPs (500- to 700-fold change) (Fletcher et al., 2001). Skin-type AFPs also lack pro-sequences, consistent with their intracellular localization.

Arctic fishes exhibit variation in gene dosage and AFP expression levels that reflect the danger a given species or population faces from freezing. Winter flounder, which encounter substantial amounts of ice in their shallow habitat, possess 30–40 copies of liver-expressed AFP genes encoding plasma AFPs and synthesize high concentrations of AFP in winter (up to 10–15 mg ml^{-1}) (Scott et al., 1985). Yellowtail flounder (*Pleuronectes ferrugenia*) occur primarily in deeper water and face less danger from ice. This species produces less AFP (only 2–4 mg ml^{-1}) and contains only about one-third as many copies of the AFP-encoding genes (Scott et al., 1988). Differences in gene copy number and AFP titers also have been observed in intraspecific comparisons. Antifreeze protein concentrations in plasma of Newfoundland populations of ocean pout are 5–10 times higher than in southerly populations from New Brunswick (Fletcher et al., 1985), and gene copy number is also substantially lower in the southern populations (Hew et al., 1988). The differences noted among species and even among conspecifics in gene dosage and levels of AFP synthesis provide a striking example of how the quantity of a needed protein can be regulated in response to environmental demands.

Once synthesized, the THPs of fishes are not known to have their activities modulated by extrinsic factors. It is in the terrestrial arthropods where this additional level of regulation has been well described, and we now turn to an examination of the integrated nature of the response to threats of freezing in cold-hardy insects.

The cold-hardy beetle Dendroides canadensis. A very different scenario from those presented above can be sketched for a freeze-avoiding insect from the temperate zone, where the threat of freezing, while only seasonal, is much more severe than that faced by fishes from high latitudes. One of the best-studied freeze-avoiding insects is the beetle *Dendroides canadensis* (Duman, 2001; Duman et al., 1993). Compared to freeze-avoiding fishes, *D. canadensis* mounts a much more extensive freeze-avoidance response and

exploits a wider range of mechanisms in doing so.

Thermal hysteresis of hemolymph of *D. canadensis* increases approximately sixfold during autumn, in anticipation of the threat of freezing (Duman et al., 1993). Regulation of the levels and activities of THPs is complex. The cues utilized by insects to initiate synthesis of THPs, which occurs in the fat body cells, include temperature, photoperiod, and humidity. In *D. canadensis*, shortened photoperiod in autumn and lengthening photoperiod in spring are important in triggering and curtailing synthesis, respectively. As emphasized in the discussion of Arctic fishes, photoperiod is a far more reliable indicator of seasonal transitions than is temperature, so relying on photoperiod rather than exclusively on temperature (or thermoperiod) is a good regulatory strategy. Photoperiod-based regulation also permits anticipatory acclimatization of THP levels, such that freezing resistance can develop well before the threat of freezing ensues. Under field conditions, it is likely that photoperiod interacts with temperature and thermoperiod to control THP production (Horwath and Duman, 1986). A key mediator of the response is juvenile hormone, which has been shown to elevate production of THPs when applied to specimens of *D. canadensis* held under noninducing conditions (Xu et al., 1992). However, the beetle's response to juvenile hormone varies seasonally, as does the titer of juvenile hormone in the hemolymph. Summer specimens with low endogenous levels of the hormone did not induce THP synthesis even when dosed with juvenile hormone, whereas autumn-collected specimens showed a strong response.

The seasonal variation in thermal hysteresis found in *D. canadensis* is due to more than shifts in concentrations of THPs, however. Unlike the freezing-avoidance strategy of Antarctic and Arctic fishes, in which the amount of thermal hysteresis appears to be due strictly to the concentration of THPs in the body fluids, freeze-avoiding insects employ a complex set of mechanisms to achieve the high levels of thermal hysteresis found for hemolymph in winter-collected specimens.

Not only does acclimatization to falling temperatures lead to increases in levels of THPs, but in addition the milieu in which the THPs function is regulated to enhance their activities. In in-vitro experiments using purified THPs, glycerol, which occurs in substantial amounts in winter-acclimatized specimens, led to an approximately threefold increase in thermal hysteresis over control values (Li et al., 1998). Here, then, the activity of an important macromolecule is strongly influenced by the low-molecular-mass solutes in the milieu, a further illustration of the theme of macromolecular–micromolecular complementarity in adaptation. However, small solutes cannot fully explain the high levels of hysteresis found in hemolymph from winter specimens. Another key modulator of THP activity is an *endogenous THP-activator protein*, whose presence leads to a 3.64°C increase in thermal hysteresis (Wu and Duman, 1991). The THP-activator protein binds to THPs and is conjectured to exert its enhancement of thermal hysteresis through steric effects. A large ice-associated complex of THP molecules and THP-activators is proposed to block a relatively large area on an ice crystal, thereby significantly reducing the ability of water molecules to join the ice lattice (figure 7.41). A further enhancement of thermal hysteresis is a consequence of synergistic effects among the different classes of THPs present in the winter-acclimatized beetle (Wu and Duman, 1991). When studied in combination, the thermal hysteresis of the beetle THPs is much higher than the predicted sum of their effects noted in studies of separate THPs.

Another interesting effect noted in the freeze-avoidance strategy of *D. canadensis* involves the inactivation of an ice-nucleating agent. As discussed below in the context of freeze tolerance, ice-nucleating agents play important roles in controlling the temperatures at which ice formation first occurs. However, in freeze-avoiding species like *D. canadensis*, ice nucleator activity may need to be blocked if the insect is to be able to cool to deep subzero temperatures. Surprisingly, the THP-activator protein is an ice nucleator, a PIN. However, when bound to THPs, this nucleating activity is lost (Duman, 2001; Duman et al., 1993; Wu and Duman, 1991). When its ice-nucleating activity is inhibited, the THP-activator protein does not jeopardize the deep supercooling that may be critical for survival of *D. canadensis* during periods of extreme cold.

How, then, do THPs and other constituents of the hemolymph such as glycerol work together to enable a cold-hardy insect like *D. canadensis* to avoid freezing in very cold winters? In view of the fact that habitat temperatures in winter may fall to −30 to −40°C in extremely cold years, it would seem unlikely that the 5–6°C of thermal hysteresis provided by the hemolymph would protect the beetle during extremes of cold. An important caveat given earlier must be raised again at this point. The amount of thermal hysteresis measured with the conventional protocol involving a seed ice crystal is dependent on the size of that crystal (Zachariassen and Husby, 1982). The smaller the crystal, the greater the amount of thermal hysteresis. This relationship is very important in the context of inoculative freezing through an insect's cuticle. The sizes of the pores in the cuticle are much smaller than the sizes of the ice crystals used to measure thermal hysteresis in vitro. Thus, existing values for thermal hysteresis may significantly underestimate the degree of protection against inoculative freezing that is provided by THPs (see Duman, 2001; Duman et al., 1993). The presence of THPs in the epidermal cells under the cuticles of insects suggests that a peripheral defense against freezing is important, as has been conjectured in the case of fishes that have AFPs in their skins (Fletcher et al., 2001).

Supercooling also plays an important role in the freeze-avoidance behavior of insects, and a number of means are used to enhance the supercooling ability during cold seasons. First, colligative antifreezes like glycerol may accumulate to high concentrations, up to 5–6 M in some species. In addition to their strictly colligative function in reducing the equilibrium freezing/melting point, solutes like glycerol may be highly effective enhancers of supercooling. They may depress the supercooling point by two to three times as much as they lower the freezing/melting point. A second important means for enhancing supercooling is to block the nucleating action of ice nucleators, as was discussed above for the THP-activator protein of *D. canadensis*. Third, ice nucleators may be physically eliminated from the organism at the onset of winter. Ice-nucleating bacteria may be eliminated from the gut, and endogenous ice nucleators may be removed from the hemolymph. An interesting example of the latter type of adaptation is found in the stag beetle, *Ceruchus piceus*. Overwintering larvae of this species remove from the hemolymph a lipoprotein that is a potent ice nucleator (Neven et al., 1986). This lipoprotein is involved in intertissue shuttling of lipids during the warm season when the animals are fully active metabolically. In winter, the larvae enter a state of metabolic depression, so the need for this lipid transport protein is reduced, if not eliminated altogether, and it can be removed to facilitate supercooling. When this nucleator is not present, larvae of this beetle can supercool below $-20°C$ even in the absence of THPs. (Note: this is not a record in terms of supercooling ability by insects. Ring [1982] has shown that some Arctic insects can supercool to temperatures near $-60°C$.)

Overwintering insects thus rely on a complex battery of adaptations to prevent ice formation and the growth of existing ice crystals. Some adaptations are behavioral: overwintering insects may select hibernacula that are dry and, therefore, less apt to contain ice crystals that can seed freezing of the body fluids. Physiological defenses often are critical, however. Thermal hysteresis proteins are likely to be of major importance in reducing propagation of ice into the body and inhibiting recrystallization processes leading to large, damaging ice crystals. Thermal hysteresis proteins may also bind to, and mask the activities of, certain ice-nucleating compounds. Through removal of ice nucleators and accumulation of colligative antifreezes like glycerol, the equilibrium freezing/melting point and the supercooling point may be substantially lowered. Supercooling ability is the trait that gives the most extremely freeze-avoiding insects their capacities to cope with deep cold.

Lastly, to return briefly to one of the central themes of this volume, when examining the scenario for freeze-avoidance in a cold-hardy insect like *D. canadensis*, it becomes clear why an integrative approach to the study of adaptation is so important. Failure to appreciate the complex interactions among different components of this system could lead to a major underestimation of the resistance of the organism to freezing and prevent a full mechanistic understanding of how thermal hysteresis is achieved. Likewise, facets of the freeze-avoidance phenomenon involving habitat choice, role of anatomical features like cuticle pore size, and the dependence of freeze sensitivity on photoperiod and thermoperiod, must be integrated into a study, if the in-situ freeze-avoidance relationships of the organism are to be adequately understood.

Freeze-Tolerance: Living with Internal Ice

When, where, and why can ice form in biological fluids without lethal consequences?

Freeze-avoidance has numerous benefits, especially in species like fishes for which retention of locomotory activity at even the lowest ambient temperatures is necessary. Freeze-tolerance is a common strategy, however, notably in the case of terrestrial species that encounter deep subzero temperatures such as those that characterize the polar regions for much of the year and temperate regions in winter. Thus, tolerance of the lowest temperatures found in the biosphere often involves periodic entry into states of suspended animation, in which water enters a solid, glass-like state and metabolic activity largely or fully ceases. Terrestrial habitats in the Antarctic provide striking illustrations of this mode of life. In Antarctica's dry valleys, for instance, life is found in the ice layer covering permanently ice-covered freshwater lakes and in quartz-containing rocks housing endolithic cyanobacteria. In both niches, metabolic activity is confined to restricted periods of time in summer during which adequate melting of ice occurs to allow photosynthetic and heterotrophic activities to take place (Priscu et al., 1999). During the remainder of the year, these organisms are "solid-state" creatures in which liquid water is absent and metabolic activity is negligible.

Freeze-tolerance is also noted in less extreme, cold temperate environments, in which certain species elect to become "solid-state" even when their neighbors mount successful freeze-avoidance strategies of the types just described for terrestrial insects like *D. canadensis*. In fact, even the latter species has been observed to rely on freeze-tolerance under extreme conditions. The adoption of freeze tolerance in winter is noted in a wide variety of animal taxa, including numerous arthropods and even a few lower vertebrates, the freeze-tolerant frogs and reptiles (see Storey, 1990, for review). Plants, too, may spend much of the winter in a "solid-state" condition (Griffith and Antikainen, 1996).

To understand the nature of freeze-tolerance, it is critical to look carefully at (i) the nature of the solid-state water that forms, (ii) where this solid-state water can be generated without lethal effects, and (iii) how the formation of true ice, which is but one of water's potential solid states, is regulated to minimize damage from freezing. As we would predict from the earlier analysis of the types of damage caused by formation of ice in biological fluids, each of these three variables is critical for the development of a successful ability to withstand freezing.

Water at subzero temperatures can occur as what we commonly know as "ice" or as a "vitrified" form of solid-state water. Both forms of solid-state water have a high degree of organization among the water molecules. However, unlike ice, vitrified water does not manifest the expansion of volume that characterizes the formation of ice. Thus, unlike ice, vitrified water does not pose the threat of physical disruption of the cell as would result, for example, from structure-piercing spicules that can destroy the integrities of membranes. Furthermore, solutes are not frozen-out of vitrified water as they are from ice, so the threat of osmotic disturbance is less. For organisms that withstand intracellular solid-state water, it is vitrified water, not conventional ice, which almost invariably forms during cold stress.

A different picture emerges when formation of solid-state water in extracellular spaces is examined. Here, ice formation commonly occurs. Because extracellular fluids lack the complex membrane systems found within the cell, the potential for physical disruption of structures is much less than in cells. The tolerance of extracellular protein systems to increased solute concentration may also be greater than those of typical intracellular proteins, whose coordinated enzymatic functions generally are very sensitive to solute composition and concentration (chapter 6).

The requirements that must be met to gain the ability to tolerate freezing include the following: (1) The formation of true ice is restricted to the extracellular spaces. (2) The formation of ice in the extracellular fluids is not accompanied by extreme dehydration of the cells. (3) Rates of ice crystal formation and the sizes of ice crystals that are generated in the extracellular fluids are held at nonlethal values. (4) Any solid-state water that forms within cells is vitrified water, not true ice. To meet these requirements, freeze-tolerant organisms employ a variety of mechanisms to control the sites, rates, and sizes of ice crystal formation.

Controlling the rate of ice formation. Unlike the situation that obtains for freeze-avoiding species, freeze-tolerant species do not benefit from a capacity to deeply supercool. The danger that arises with deep supercooling is that, once ice formation does ensue, it leads to a rapid freezing of much of the organism's water. In freeze-tolerant species, slow, controlled freezing is often vital for survival. To achieve controlled formation of ice in the extracellular spaces, many freeze-tolerant organisms accumulate ice-nucleating agents, and often increase the concentrations of these substances with the onset of cold weather (Duman, 2001). These agents typically are proteins (PINs) that trigger ice formation at relatively high temperatures, thus minimizing supercooling. In the absence of PINs, supercooling may occur down to $-60°C$, whereas in the presence of PINs, supercooling generally is limited to $-6°$C to $-10°C$ (Duman, 2001). At these high freezing temperatures, initial freezing may incorporate only a small fraction of the extracellular water into ice crystals, leaving behind a more concentrated solution that remains liquid. In a deeply supercooled solution, a much larger fraction of the water would quickly form ice.

The levels of PINs found in the hemolymph of insects vary between freeze-avoiding and freeze-tolerant species and, especially in the former species, concentrations vary seasonally. Freeze-avoiding species generally reduce the ice-nucleating potential in their fluids, whereas freeze-tolerant species retain a substantial ice-nucleating capacity year-round. One of the ice nucleators that has been substantially characterized is a lipoprotein ice nucleator (LPIN) present in freeze-tolerant larvae of the cranefly (*Tipula trivittata*) (Neven et al., 1989). This 800 kDa LPIN is 45% protein, 51% lipid, and 4% carbohydrate. It functions in both lipid transport and ice nucleation. The ice-nucleating activity of the LPIN appears to depend on the hydroxyl groups of the phosphatidylinositol molecules, which may largely coat its surface, and on the protein itself. Although the complete structures of the two protein components of the LPIN have not been characterized, the proteins appear to share epitopes with bacterial ice nucleators. Both the insect LPIN and bacterial nucleators require lipids for activity. Aggregation of many LPIN molecules is needed for nucleating activity to occur. The aggregation process is postulated to bring the –OH groups of the phosphatidylinositol molecules into an orientation that allows favorable interaction with water. As mentioned earlier, freeze-avoiding species reduce levels of LPIN in winter (Duman, 2001). Because insects may become metabolically inactive in winter, the need for lipid transport is reduced, and LPIN concentrations thus can be lowered without posing problems for metabolic supply lines.

Freeze-tolerant insects and plants have been found to contain substantial concentrations of AFP's, a phenomenon that may appear paradoxical. However, THPs present in the extracellular fluids may contribute importantly to freeze-tolerance by inhibiting recrystallization, thus keeping the ice crystals that do form in the extracellular space small enough to prevent physical damage. Purified AFPs from a plant, the bittersweet nightshade (*Solarum dulcamara*), when added to a medium in which protoplasts (cells from which the cell wall has been removed) were frozen, conferred cryoprotection to the cells (see Duman, 2001).

Glycerol and other stabilizing solutes may have several distinct physiological effects at low temperatures. At numerous points in this volume we have shown how the effects of a particular type of biochemical change are not restricted to what may appear to be the primary physiological "problem" that the adaptation seems to intended to resolve. Instead, a given type of biochemical change may influence diverse aspects of an organism's physiology. For instance, the elevated concentrations of TMAO found in blood and organs of Antarctic fishes may serve to lower freezing points and to stabilize proteins in the face of the high concentrations of inorganic ions found in these species. Furthermore, because TMAO favors protein aggregation (chapter 6), it would be interesting to determine whether the concentrations of TMAO found in Antarctic notothenioids are sufficient to favor assembly of aggregates of AFGPs on the surface of ice crystals, leading to enhancement of antifreeze activity, in analogy with the effects of PINs on insect THPs.

Another potential effect of protein stabilizing solutes merits consideration in the context of freeze-avoiding and freeze-tolerant species that accumulate high concentrations of these compounds. As mentioned earlier, accumulation of polyols like glycerol may serve a number of physiological functions, whether or not these solutes prevent formation of solid-state water. One potentially significant effect of elevated glycerol concentrations arises from the enhanced stability of protein structure that is likely to result when glycerol concentrations are increased during the winter. Interactions between decreases in temperature and rising glycerol concentrations might work synergistically to slow down metabolic rates in the cold, for the reason given below.

The potential for a protein-stabilizing solute like glycerol to influence metabolic rates stems principally from the fact that stabilizing solutes may raise the energy barriers for the conformational changes that accompany catalysis. Earlier in this chapter we discussed how variations in k_{cat} among orthologs of A_4-LDH arise from amino acid substitutions that change the energy costs of catalytic conformational changes. Much as intrinsic differences in conformational mobility among orthologs alter k_{cat}, so can extrinsic factors such as organic osmolytes that modify protein stability. The combined effects of intrinsic and extrinsic factors on A_4-LDH function are illustrated in figure 7.43. Here, orthologs of A_4-LDH from a warm-temperate fish (*Gillichthys mirabilis*) and an Antarctic fish (*Parachaenichthys charcoti*) are contrasted in terms of how their activities are inhibited by glycerol. For both orthologs, increasing concentrations of glycerol inhibit pyruvate reduction to lactate. These inhibitory effects are greater at reduced temperatures: compare the inhibition curves for the ortholog of *Parachaenichthys* at 0°C (inset) and 20°C

(main figure). Therefore, for a species that builds up glycerol during acclimatization to low temperature, the resulting inhibition of enzymatic activity could lead to large Q_{10} values for enzymatic reactions. For species that remain inactive at low temperatures, the resulting large-scale decreases in metabolism as temperature falls and glycerol levels rise could spare metabolic substrates for subsequent periods of activity at higher temperatures. Enzymes are known to function in the frozen state, so the inhibitory influences of glycerol could be important whether or not solid-state water forms in the cell. In view of the similarity of the effects of protein stabilizers on different types of proteins and the importance of conformational changes in catalysis, the results shown in figure 7.43 for A_4-LDH orthologs of two fishes are likely to provide a general indication of how combinations of glycerol and low temperature would affect any type of enzymatic reaction whose rate-limiting step involves a conformational change, regardless of species.

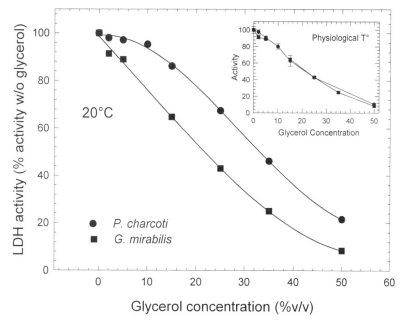

Figure 7.43. Effects of glycerol concentration and temperature on activities of A_4-LDH from an Antarctic notothenioid (*Parachaenichthys charcoti*) and a warm-temperate goby fish (*Gillichthys mirabilis*). Inset: the effects of glycerol concentration on the two orthologs at physiological temperatures of the species, 0°C for *P. charcoti* and 20°C for *G. mirabilis*. (Modified after Fields et al., 2001.)

Although the effects of a given type of solute tend to be qualitatively the same for orthologs of a particular protein, the quantitative effects of protein-stabilizing solutes may vary among species in accord with their adaptation temperatures. Note how the effects of glycerol vary among orthologs of A_4-LDH. The ortholog of *G. mirabilis* is more inhibited than the ortholog of *P. charcoti* at a common temperature of measurement. However, at the physiological temperatures of *G. mirabilis* and *P. charcoti*, approximately 20°C and 0°C, respectively, identical levels of inhibition by glycerol occurred (figure 7.43 inset). This similarity in effects of glycerol is consistent with conservation at physiological temperatures of flexibility in the "moving parts" of the enzyme that undergo catalytic conformational changes.

This digression into solute–temperature interactions on proteins serves as a further illustration of the need to examine macromolecular–micromolecular interactions to obtain a holistic picture of physiological adaptation.

THERMAL OPTIMA AND THERMAL TOLERANCE LIMITS

Developing a Physiological Perspective on the Effects of Global Climate Change

At the beginning of this chapter we emphasized how frequently biogeographic patterning correlates with gradients in environmental temperature. This temperature-related patterning in species' distributions serves as a strong indication of the pervasiveness of temperature effects on the biochemical structures and processes of organisms. Indeed, as we analyzed the effects of temperature on diverse biochemical components of cells we learned how sensitive each is to alterations in temperature, and how finely tuned each system is to the particular range of temperatures in which it must work. The detailed analysis of thermal relationships of contemporary organisms given in this chapter not only provides a picture of how organisms from all domains of life are adapted to their current habitats, but also can serve as a basis

for making predictions about the effects of global climate change on the biosphere. In this penultimate section of the chapter, we discuss some of the key issues that are entailed in developing predictions about the effects of global warming. This analysis will help to review and solidify some of the important points developed earlier in this chapter and will enable a physiological and biochemical foundation to be built for discussions of the biological consequences of global climate change.

Our focus on this broad, important, and controversial topic involves issues that fall under six interrelated headings:

(1) *Thermal optima*: Can we validly define thermal optima for physiological systems? If so, what are these thermal optima, and how much change in temperature is adequate to create a suboptimal state of function? Do all physiological systems of a species display similar thermal optima?

(2) *Mechanisms establishing thermal tolerance*: What mechanisms set the upper and lower thermal tolerance limits for organisms? Can we identify "weak links" in the physiological chain that are responsible for establishing upper and lower thermal tolerance limits? Are all links "weak"?

(3) *Thermal limits and current habitat temperatures*: How close do organisms live to the edge of their thermal tolerance limits? Do some species live closer to the edge than others? Are generalizations possible about groups of organisms that appear particularly threatened by global warming?

(4) *Potential for acclimatization*: To what extent can increases in temperature be compensated through phenotypic alterations—acclimatizations? Do some species have more acclimatization potential than other species?

(5) *Genetically based adaptations*: When is genetic change needed to allow an organism to succeed (or even survive) in a changing environment? How much genetic change is required to adaptively modify a protein or a gene regulatory process?

(6) *Compromises*: Does acquisition of heat tolerance reduce tolerance of cold, and vice versa? What limits exist to eurythermy?

Thermal optima: At what temperatures do physiological systems work best?

We treat this initial question only briefly because it represents a central theme that has appeared repeatedly in this chapter. In each context in which optimal thermal ranges were discussed, it was seen that temperature-sensitive properties of enzymes, membranes, and other cellular components have highly conserved values among differently thermally adapted species at their normal physiological temperatures. While it may seem circular to define these values as "optimal," we believe that this is an appropriate and logical step to take. Indeed, the extent to which conserved values for enzyme–ligand binding, membrane physical state, protein charge state (via alphastat pH regulation), and other physiological systems are observed among differently adapted taxa indicates that these are the states of the systems at which physiological function is best maintained. Adaptation leads to conservation of these optimal character states, a statement that indicates the highly conservative nature of biochemical and molecular adaptation—the "unity in diversity" that we have stressed at many junctures.

As emphasized earlier in this chapter, this definition of what is "optimal" does not refer to a Panglossian "best of all possible worlds" situation. Rather, "optimal" is to be taken as an adjective that denotes the ubiquitously conserved values for diverse physiological systems that have evolved within the constraints imposed by the sets of molecules and the physical laws governing their behavior on which life as we know it is based. Perhaps what we observe is a "best of all compromises" situation, which arises from the potentials and constraints afforded by biochemistry. The repeated observation that adaptation by species belonging to each of the three domains of life follows a similar course and employs the same raw material illustrates both the opportunities and constraints faced in adaptation.

It was emphasized at several points that optimization of traits commonly involves trade-offs or compromises, in the sense that it would be possible, in theory, to do a better job in designing any particular trait, but that success on one front often entails an unacceptable cost on another. One example of such trade-offs concerns the balance between stability and activity of enzymes: selection (or laboratory genetic engineering) can lead to extremely stable and long-lived enzymes, but these achievements commonly carry with them the cost of poor rates of function or poor binding ability. A similar relationship is seen in cases where metabolic down-regulation is accompanied by greatly enhanced protein stability (longer half-lives) but vastly reduced protein function. In metabolically quiescent cysts of the brine shrimp *Artemia*, for example, the half-life of cytochrome-c oxidase is enormously increased, but mitochondrial ATP generation is drastically reduced (Hand and Hardewig, 1996; Hofmann and Hand, 1990). Trade-offs are also evident in the case of membranes. Plasma membranes could be designed to greatly restrict loss of molecules from the cell, but these same membranes might perform poorly as regulators of transport or as a milieu for protein function. The fact that the optimal character states we might envision for a trait that evolves in a world unfettered by compromises are not found in nature shows how often trade-offs are made in the development of optimal traits.

To answer the question given in the heading to this section, then, we again provide what may appear to be a circular answer: physiological systems work best over the temperature ranges where the conserved values for the system can be maintained. As temperatures begin to climb or fall outside of this thermal range, we can speak of the phenomenon of *physiological denaturation*. The adjective "physiological" denotes that the system in question is not ceasing to function, but rather its properties are no longer optimal. For example, ligand-binding properties of a protein may become either too weak or too strong for optimal protein function. The protein itself is not denatured in the conventional sense of having lost activity through unfolding of its tertiary structure or loss of subunit association, but the physiological system is nonetheless impaired.

The amount of change in temperature that is sufficient to establish suboptimal status for a physiological system depends on a number of factors, including how temperature-sensitive the function in question is and how close the organism is living to its upper thermal limits. At one extreme, a eurythermal species living near the middle of its thermal tolerance range may be able to withstand a large increase or decrease in body temperature and yet maintain the properties of its physiological systems within the range of optimal values. For example, K_m values of enzymes from eurythermal species may be relatively unaffected by temperature compared to those for stenothermal species (see figure 7.7; Baldwin, 1971; Coppes and Somero, 1990). However, for any species, whether eurythermal or stenothermal, temperature increases that occur near the upper limits of the thermal tolerance range can quickly displace the values for the system into a suboptimal range. For example, the rapid increases in K_m that occur at above-optimal temperatures for a species are similar in both stenotherms and eurytherms. Thus, for species that are living close to their upper thermal tolerance limits, biochemical systems may be close to the edge of their optimal ranges. Increases in temperature of only a few degrees Celsius may be adequate to significantly impair function, that is, to cause physiological denaturation. Parallel arguments apply in the case of stress from low temperatures.

What are the biochemical and molecular determinants of thermal tolerance limits?

Can one identify weak links in the physiological chain that would appear to play dominant roles in setting thermal tolerance limits? In view of the fact that physiological systems maintain optimal functional states only over a finite range of temperatures, it seems likely that all systems are, to a greater or lesser degree, likely to play a role in setting thermal tolerance limits. However, although all links in the physiological chain are apt to be weak because of inherent thermal sensitivities, some links may be weaker than others. Cellular membranes have frequently been singled out as the strongest candidate for the "weakest link" in heat tolerance (see the review by Bowler and Manning, 1994). Thermal disruption of the physical states

of membranes, which may lead to alterations in permeability, enzymatic activity, and capacities for exo- and endocytosis, have been discussed as significant aspects of thermal perturbation. The fact that membranes so commonly show adaptive changes (homeoviscous and homeophasic adaptations) is an indication of how sensitive their properties are to alterations in temperature. Among the properties of membranes that appear most sensitive is synaptic transmission. As the study of Cossins et al. (1977) (figure 7.25) showed, acclimatory changes in the physical properties of synaptosomes were closely correlated with a number of behavioral changes that would affect survival.

Antarctic notothenioid fishes, the most cold-adapted and stenothermal vertebrates, offer a striking example of the potential for synaptic malfunction to lead to heat death (figure 7.44). As mentioned earlier, notothenioid fishes from McMurdo Sound cannot survive at temperatures above 4°C, even after prolonged warm acclimation at this temperature (Hofmann et al., 2000; Somero and DeVries, 1967; Somero et al., 1998). When placed into water with a temperature near 10°C, the fish quickly lose equilibrium; engage in short, uncoordinated bouts of swimming; and die within one to two hours. Two lines of biochemical evidence support the hypothesis that synaptic failure contributes to heat death. First, the rate at which quanta of the transmitter acetylcholine (ACh) are released at synapses rises rapidly as temperature is increased above approximately 8°C (figure 7.44, upper panel; Macdonald et al., 1988). Release of ACh becomes maximal between 12°C and 14°C, and then rapidly falls off at higher temperatures. Second, the enzyme responsible for degrading ACh, acetylcholine esterase (AChE), exhibits a highly temperature-dependent K_m^{ACh}, notably in the case of the enzyme from the Antarctic fish *Pagothenia borchgrevinki*, the species used in the studies of temperature effects on synaptic release of ACh (figure 7.44, lower panel; Baldwin, 1971). As temperatures rise above the physiological tolerance range for *P. borchgrevinki*, the affinity of AChE for ACh decreases very rapidly. Thus, as large quantities of transmitter are released into the synaptic cleft, the enzyme responsible

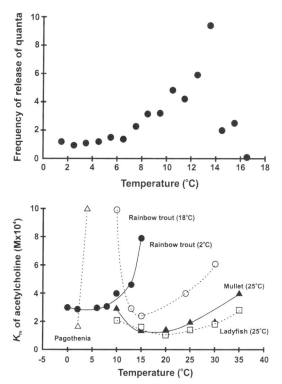

Figure 7.44. Effects of temperature on release of quanta of acetylcholine (ACh) at the neuromuscular junction of the extraocular nerve of the Antarctic fish *Pagothenia borchgrevinki* (upper panel: data from Macdonald et al., 1988), and on binding of acetylcholine to acetylcholine esterases of several marine fishes (lower panel: data from Baldwin, 1971.)

upswings in K_m^{ACh} found at low temperatures suggest that cold death, like heat death, may result from failures in synaptic events.

How do thermal tolerance limits compare to habitat (body) temperatures?

Although there is abundant evidence that species adapted to different temperatures differ in lethal temperatures, relatively few studies have examined the relationship between adaptation temperature and upper lethal temperature in a systematic and phylogenetically rigorous manner. Lethal temperature determinations seldom are done with a common methodology in different studies. Several variables can affect the values for upper lethal temperature that are obtained in laboratory studies. These variables include rate of heating, duration of exposure to a high temperature, and acclimatization or acclimation history of the specimens. Moreover, for species like many sessile intertidal invertebrates, death from exposure to high temperature may be a complex function of direct thermal effects on physiological processes and stresses arising from desiccation and hypoxia. Simulating or controlling these complex processes in the laboratory is difficult and seldom has been attempted in thermal tolerance studies.

Lessons from studies of intertidal organisms: porcelain crabs, snails, and mussels. With these caveats in mind, we turn to some examples of lethal temperature relationships that strongly suggest that some species are living close to their thermal limits and that capacities for extending these limits to higher temperatures through acclimatization may vary among species. We examine sets of congeneric species that are vertically distributed between the subtidal and intertidal zones. Congeners found in the intertidal may experience extremes of thermal stress, whereas their subtidal relatives may face relatively stable and nonthreatening thermal conditions. The differences in thermal sensitivities of physiological processes of congeners with different vertical distribution patterns offer excellent examples of how physiologically adap-

for degrading the transmitter loses its ability to bind its substrate. Effects of this sort could be instrumental in setting the thermal tolerance limits for neural function and, thus, for the whole organism. Note that acclimatory differences are found when AChEs of warm- and cold-acclimated rainbow trout are compared (Baldwin and Hochachka, 1970). The enzyme found in 18°C-acclimated trout differs from that in the 2°C-acclimated specimens in that it rapidly loses ACh binding ability as temperature is decreased below approximately 15°C. It is not known whether the differences in kinetics found between AChEs of warm- and cold-acclimated trout reflect different isoforms of the enzyme or differences in the lipids surrounding the protein. Whatever the underlying mechanisms, the rapid tations may influence species' distributions over small and large spatial scales.

Figure 7.45 shows the thermal tolerance limits (LT_{50}) for 19 species of porcelain crabs (genus *Petrolisthes*) from diverse temperate, subtropical, and tropical habitats. These congeners also differ in their vertical positions along the subtidal to high intertidal gradient (Stillman and Somero, 2000). Due to these differences in latitudinal and vertical distribution, the species encounter maximal habitat temperatures ranging from approximately 14°C to 43°C. When the upper lethal temperatures of the species are compared to their maximal habitat temperatures, there is a strong positive correlation between these two variables, a correlation that is retained when the effects of phylogeny are removed from the data using phylogenetically independent contrasts analysis (chapter 1; see Stillman and Somero, 2000). A striking feature of this interspecific pattern is that the difference between maximal habitat temperature and LT_{50} decreases with rising adaptation temperature. Thus, the most warm-adapted species, those with the highest LT_{50}'s, are also the species living closest to their thermal maxima. Several of these warm-adapted species encounter potentially lethal temperatures in their habitats. Species found in cooler habitats may encounter

maximal habitat temperatures that are as much as 10–12°C below the LT50.

The differences between warm- and cold-adapted porcelain crabs in terms of the threats posed by increasing habitat temperatures extend to their abilities to warm-acclimate (Stillman and Somero, 2000). Two relatively cold-adapted subtidal species, *P. eriomerus* and *P. manimaculis*, were able to increase their LT_{50} by 4°C when acclimated to higher temperature (18°C). In contrast, the intertidal, warm-adapted species, *P. cinctipes*, increased its LT_{50} by only half this amount. It would appear then that species of porcelain crabs currently living near the edge of their thermal tolerance ranges have substantially lower potentials for increasing their tolerance of high temperatures through acclimatization than do colder-adapted species.

Studies done with porcelain crabs also allow us to examine some of the physiological systems that may fail at or near lethal temperatures. In these comparisons the primary emphasis will be on two species, *P. cinctipes* and *P. eriomerus*, that occur at common latitudes but have different vertical distributions. *Petrolisthes cinctipes* occurs in the low- to mid-intertidal zone, where habitat temperatures as high as 33°C have been recorded during midday low tides on warm summer days. In its largely subtidal habitat, *Petrolisthes eriomerus* is much less frequently emersed and habitat temperatures seldom exceed 16°C, even in summer (Stillman and Somero, 1996). The LT_{50} temperatures of *P. cinctipes* and *P. eriomerus* are 32.3°C and 27.5°C, respectively (figure 7.45). Studies of the effects of temperature on rates of oxygen consumption by these two species revealed that *P. eriomerus* ceases to respire between 25°C and 30°C, whereas *P. cinctipes* continues to respire at 30°C. Heart function of the two species also responded differently to temperature (figure 7.46). The rate of the heart beat of *P. eriomerus* dropped precipitously above 26.6°C, the "break" temperature of the Arrhenius plot of log heart rate versus temperature. In the case of *P. cinctipes*, the ABT did not occur until 31.5°C. These ABT data illustrate two important points. First, the lower occurring, more cold-adapted species, *P. eriomerus*,

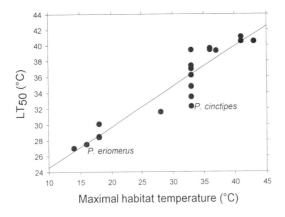

Figure 7.45. Thermal tolerance relationships of porcelain crabs. Relationship of habitat temperature to upper lethal temperature for 19 congeners of *Petrolisthes*. (Figure modified after Stillman and Somero, 2000.)

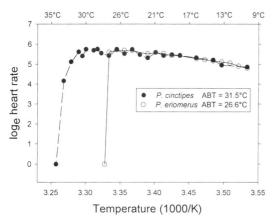

Figure 7.46. Effects of temperature on heart rate for two congeners of *Petrolisthes*. Data are presented as an Arrhenius plot to illustrate the sharp decline in heart rate (Arrhenius break temperature, ABT) that occurs at high temperatures. (Figure modified after Stillman and Somero, 1996.)

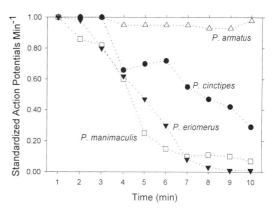

Figure 7.47. Effect of incubation at 30°C on the rate of action potential generation by a mechano-receptor nerve bundle for four congeners of *Petrolisthes*. (Unpublished data of J. Knape and G.N. Somero.)

cannot maintain heart function at the high temperatures experienced by its more warm-adapted congener. The different vertical distributions of these two species thus seem governed in part by physiological differences. Second, and of relevance to questions about the proximity of body temperatures to thermal limits, the heart of *P. cinctipes* loses function at temperatures very close to the maximal habitat temperatures the species encounters.

In keeping with the observations shown in figures 7.25 and 7.44, which support the hypothesis that neural activity is particularly sensitive to high temperatures, the effect of temperature on rates of action potential generation by nerves of differently adapted congeners of *Petrolisthes* shows large differences (figure 7.47). At a measurement temperature of 30°C, the rate of action potential generation by a mechanoreceptor nerve bundle of a warm-adapted porcelain crab, *P. armatus*, which occurs intertidally in the Gulf of California and encounters temperatures at least as high as 40°C, was stable over the 10 min period of measurement. In contrast, nerve preparations from *P. cinctipes* showed an approximately two-thirds reduction in rate of firing, and nerves from two temperate zone subtidal species, *P.*

eriomerus and *P. manimaculis*, essentially ceased to fire by the end of the 10 min period.

Studies of other sets of congeneric intertidal and subtidal invertebrates support the conjecture that some species currently live close to their upper thermal tolerance limits. When discussing the heat-shock response, we focused on snails of the widely occurring genus *Tegula*, to illustrate how differences among species in important characteristics of the heat-shock response—temperatures at which induction of hsp's occur, temperatures of maximal synthesis of hsp's, and rates of activation of the heat-shock response—varied adaptively among species from different latitudes and tidal heights. Another important lesson from the studies of *Tegula* congeners is the finding that lethal temperatures closely match the temperatures at which protein synthesis is curtailed. Thus, the ability to synthesize proteins may be another physiological trait that helps to establish upper thermal tolerance limits. An intertidal species like *T. funebralis* may encounter temperatures during low tides that come close to the upper thermal limits for protein synthesis. Subtidal congeners of *Tegula* fail to make proteins at temperatures commonly tolerated by higher occurring, more warm-adapted species like *T. funebralis*.

High temperatures may restrict organisms from certain habitats for reasons other than the short-term lethal effects discussed above. Studies of the heat-shock response in congeners of *Tegula* and mussels of the genus *Mytilus* (*Mytilus trossulus* and *Mytilus galloprovincialis*) (Hofmann and Somero, 1996b) suggest that high temperatures that are not lethal in the short term may nonetheless limit vertical distributions of organisms because of heat-caused increases in the amount of energy needed to repair thermal damage to proteins. These types of energy budget influences of high temperature, while not leading to rapid heat death, may yet play important roles in biogeographic patterning and in establishing the responses of organisms to global warming. It may prove to be too costly to persist in a warmer habitat, even if the increased temperatures of the habitat are not immediately lethal.

Another category of thermal effect on distribution patterns involves temperature-dependent rates of predation. Sanford (1999) demonstrated that predation by the sea star *Pisaster ochraceus* on *Mytilus californianus* was remarkably temperature-dependent. When water temperatures increased from approximately 8–9°C to 11–12°C, rates of predation by *Pisaster* increased severalfold. A rapid clearing of mussel beds by *P. ochraceus* occurred if warm temperatures persisted.

These varied effects of relatively small—in the range of a few degrees Celsius—changes in temperature on intertidal invertebrates show how dramatically global warming might affect these communities. There is in fact growing evidence that the effects of global warming are already altering diverse intertidal and terrestrial ecosystems (Hughes, 2000). Barry et al. (1995) showed that over the previous seven decades there had been a decrease in abundance of cold-adapted northern-occurring species and an increase in abundance of warm-adapted southern-occurring species in intertidal habitats of Monterey Bay in central California (see Sagarin et al., 1999, for an extended analysis of this phenomenon). Roemmich and McGowan (1995) showed that warming of the surface coastal waters along central and southern California was associated with a 60% reduction in zooplankton abundance, a change that was attributed in large measure to reduced

upwelling due to thermal stratification of the water column. Indeed, changes in oceanic circulation caused by elevated sea temperatures have the potential for causing major perturbation of the marine biota (Fields et al., 1993). In terrestrial communities, the biogeographic ranges of ectothermic species, for instance, butterflies, have shifted northwards and been truncated at lower latitudes (Hughes, 2000; Parmesan et al., 1999). Certain bird species in the United Kingdom have shown northwards range extensions (Thomas and Lennon, 1999). Although these correlations between shifts in ambient temperature and biogeographic patterning do not per se allow strong conclusions to be drawn about causation, the physiological effects of temperature examined throughout this chapter are certainly consistent with the hypothesis that the projected amounts of global warming likely to take place during this century (recent estimates by the Intergovernmental Panel on Climate Change (IPCC) predict between a 1.5 and 6°C increase) are apt to have pervasive effects on ecosystems through direct and indirect effects on physiological systems.

Thermal Limits: Lessons from Laboratory Evolution

Many of the central questions that were considered in the above discussion of thermal limits of naturally occurring populations have begun to be addressed in what are termed "laboratory evolution" studies. In these experiments, species with short generation times are "evolved" at different absolute temperatures and over different ranges of temperature to address such questions as: (i) How rapidly does adaptation to temperature occur, in terms of changing *thermal optima* and the *breadth of the thermal niche*? Is adaptation to high temperature faster than adaptation to low temperature? (ii) Do changes in thermal optima for performance necessarily correlate with changes in the breadth of the thermal niche? (iii) Does acquisition of increased tolerance of high temperature lead to reduced tolerance of lower temperature, and vice versa? These are basic questions about thermal relationships, and questions that may be difficult to address using the comparative method in studies of natural populations. Thus, studies of laboratory evolution, in which adaptive changes can be induced in relatively rapid time frames, stand to contribute importantly to the study of evolutionary adaptation to temperature.

Studies of *Escherichia coli* are yielding insights concerning several of the issues raised above (Bennett and Lenski, 1993, 1996; Bennett et al., 1990, 1992; for review, see Mongold et al., 1996). Use of *E. coli* for studies of this sort demonstrates the wisdom of following the August Krogh Principle (chapter 1). This species has a rapid generation time and is well understood in terms of genome sequence and physiology. Moreover, *E. coli* is a eurythermal bacterium that can be grown—or "evolved"—at a wide range of temperatures. Bennett, Lenski, and their colleagues have evolved strains of *E. coli* for many thousands of generations, providing sufficient time for mutations to occur at most, if not all, gene loci.

Before discussing some of the salient discoveries that have resulted from studies of laboratory evolution of *E. coli*, it is appropriate to sound some cautionary notes about the limitations of this type of evolutionary experimentation (see Mongold et al., 1996). The starting bacterial strains used in the studies were genetically homogeneous, and because the bacteria reproduced asexually, any new genetic potentials had to arise de novo by mutation. Thus there was an absence of the types of genetic recombination that take place in sexually reproducing animals and plants that occur in large populations that possess extensive genetic polymorphism. In this important sense, the bacteria used in these studies cannot serve as a paradigm for evolution in outcrossing eukaryotic species. (For a highly stimulating analysis of the differences between adaptive evolution in bacteria and eukaryotes, the review of Levin and Bergstrom [2000] is highly recommended.) Furthermore, in view of the major roles played in bacterial evolution by horizontal transmission of genes and accessory elements (plasmids, prophages, transposons, and integrons (genetic factors that are involved in the acquisition and control of expression of genes acquired by bacteria from external sources)), the absence of

opportunity for horizontal transfer of novel genetic information in these studies possibly erected large barriers to the extent to which adaptive change could occur (see below). Despite these limitations, however, studies of *E. coli* have yielded novel insights into issues related to evolution of thermal niches.

In several sets of experiments, populations were evolved for 2,000 generations at four constant temperatures: 20°C (a temperature slightly above the temperature at which cell division slows to a halt), 32°C, 37°C (close to the normal habitat temperature of this intestinal symbiont), and 42°C (a temperature within 1–2°C of the upper lethal temperature). An additional group was grown in a fluctuating thermal environment in which a daily shift between 32°C and 42°C occurred. Significant changes in thermal optima for performance and breadth of thermal niche occurred within 2,000 generations. The rate of evolution was higher when bacteria were evolved at high temperatures (e.g., 42°C), than at lower temperatures (e.g., 20°C). The mechanistic bases of these differences in rate of evolution are not understood, but it does appear that the differences in rate are not simply a consequence of temperature-dependent rates of mutation (Mongold et al., 1996).

The temperature range over which fitness changed relative to the control group (the founder population) reflected adaptation temperature (figure 7.48). In these comparisons, the evolved and control populations were compared in terms of their Malthusian (absolute) fitness, quantified as the slope of the natural logarithm of population density regressed over time. Only a slight difference from the common ancestor was observed in the cultures grown at 37°C. For cultures held at the lowest temperature (20°C), there was enhanced competitive ability at lower temperatures, but reduced fitness relative to the common ancestor above 30°C. The 32°C group also showed higher fitness relative to the ancestral population at lower temperatures (25–35°C). The populations evolved at the highest fixed temperature, 42°C, showed enhanced fitness at this higher temperature. The group that evolved under fluctuating temperatures (daily change between 32°C and 42°C) showed enhanced fitness at both high

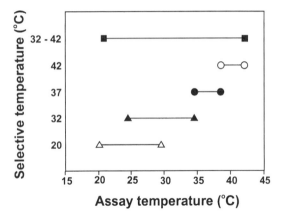

Figure 7.48. Consequences of laboratory evolution of *E. coli* for 2,000 generations at four fixed temperatures (20°C, 32°C, 37°C, and 42°C) and fluctuating temperatures (daily shifts between 32°C and 42°C). The solid lines connecting the symbols indicate the range of temperatures over which the mean fitness of each group was significantly elevated compared to the common ancestor (Anc). (Figure modified after Mongold et al., 1996.)

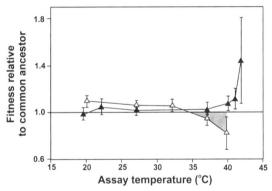

Figure 7.49. Mean fitness relative to a common ancestor of *E. coli* populations evolved at 20°C (open symbols) or 42°C (filled symbols). Error bars represent 95% confidence intervals ($n = 6$). (Figure modified after Mongold et al., 1996.)

and low temperatures, including temperatures several degrees lower than the minimal growth temperature. This group thus became thermal generalists, whereas the populations maintained at the constant temperatures can be viewed as thermal specialists.

The extent to which trade-offs occurred during adaptation to low (20°C) and high (42°C) temperatures is shown in more detail in figure 7.49. The 42°C-evolved group showed no loss of fitness at low temperatures relative to the common ancestor, even though it gained superior fitness at higher temperatures. In contrast, the 20°C-evolved population showed a significant trade-off in fitness: it lost relative fitness at higher temperatures during acquisition of superior fitness at lower temperatures.

Striking differences were observed between evolution of performance (fitness relative to common ancestor) (figures 7.48 and 7.49) and evolution of the breadth of the thermal niche, defined as the range of temperatures over which a given genotype was able to grow (reproduce) quickly enough to maintain a constant population size (figure 7.50). Only in the case of the population that was evolved at 20°C was there a

significant change in the thermal niche: a decrease in both upper and lower thermal limits occurred.

As Mangold and coauthors state in their review of this work, these studies involving asexually reproducing organisms originating from a common ancestor cannot be taken as

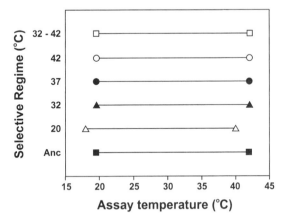

Figure 7.50. Thermal niche of the common ancestor (Anc) and five evolved populations of *E. coli*. The solid lines indicate the range of temperatures over which the different lines of bacteria were capable of maintaining a constant population density (able to offset the daily serial dilution). Only in the case of the 20°C population has the ancestral thermal niche been altered. (Figure modified after Mongold et al., 1996.)

paradigmatic for temperature adaptation in a broad sense. It remains to be determined how closely the results of these laboratory evolution studies simulate what occurs in nature for sexually reproducing species that carry high levels of genetic variation. Nonetheless, these laboratory studies are making important contributions to the study of evolution of thermal tolerance and thermal optima. In certain cases the results support conclusions from comparative studies of differently adapted species or conspecifics. One common conclusion is that increases or decreases in temperature of only a few degrees Celsius are sufficient to favor selection for temperature adaptive differences in physiology. This conclusion fits well with earlier discussions in this chapter, for instance, the issue of threshold effects on evolution of protein systems, and supports the arguments we have developed concerning the potential effects of global warming. Seemingly slight—perhaps only 1–2°C— increases in temperature are enough to "hurt."

The ability of bacteria evolved at high temperatures to retain good function at low temperatures whereas high-temperature function was impaired in cold-evolved bacteria mirrors the effects of temperature on enzyme-ligand binding abilities. As shown in figure 7.7, the K_m versus temperature relationships for enzymes from species adapted to high temperatures remain relatively flat as temperature is reduced, suggesting that these enzymes may continue to bind ligands well if temperature falls. Conversely, cold-adapted enzymes fail to retain good binding abilities as temperature is raised above the physiological thermal range. In a certain sense, enzymes appear to be more pre-adapted for function at lower temperatures than at higher temperatures, a trend consistent with the shifts in thermal tolerance observed in laboratory evolution studies.

An additional conclusion from the laboratory evolution studies, one that bears on the issue of acquisition of increased tolerance of high temperatures, is that *E. coli* showed no propensity to become an extremophile, despite many thousands of generations of "encouragement" to become more heat-adapted. One interpretation of the apparent inability of *E. coli* to increase its heat tolerance is that it lacks sets of genes on which extremely thermophilic (hyperthermophilic) species depend, for instance, genes encoding biosynthetic pathways for membrane-spanning lipids. Acquiring novel biosynthetic pathways is likely to be a vastly slower evolutionary process than the alteration of thermal optima of proteins already encoded in the genome. As discussed earlier in this chapter, a single amino acid substitution may suffice to alter the thermal optimum of a protein. Thus, as few as several thousand amino acid substitutions might be sufficient to increase the thermal stabilities and temperatures for optimal binding and catalysis of a bacterium's full suite of proteins. However, generating new *types* of genes that code for the novel biochemical systems that are needed to support a large increase in heat tolerance represents a vastly more complex and time-demanding challenge. It may be that the ability of bacteria to make major evolutionary "jumps" depends much more strongly on the many mechanisms allowing horizontal gene transfer than on accumulation of point mutations in the organism's existing set of genes (Levin and Bergstrom, 2000).

SOME FINAL THOUGHTS

The study of thermal relationships in different taxa has revealed the pervasive influence that temperature has on life. Temperature affects the structures of all large biomolecules—proteins, nucleic acids, lipids, and ensembles of these molecules. Because of this, a vast amount of fine-tuning of the properties of the "molecules of life" has occurred during evolution, to enable these essential molecules to carry out their tasks and retain their native structures at temperatures ranging from 60–80°C below zero up to at least 113°C. The fact that organisms are capable of carrying out highly similar metabolic reactions and information transfers (DNA to RNA to protein) over this wide a range of temperatures is not a reflection of insensitivity to temperature, but rather a testimony to the pervasiveness and success of adaptational processes. We have tried to define the most important of these processes, showing how common sets of raw material have been shaped by evolution to allow organisms to thrive in an enormous array of thermal conditions.

This analysis of adaptation to temperature also has revealed the complementary roles played by large and small molecules. Although most analyses of molecular evolution tend to focus exclusively on genes and proteins, a full understanding of adaptation can only be developed by examining the ways in which the "micromolecular" constituents of cells (see chapter 6) are modified qualitatively and quantitatively to provide an appropriate milieu for macromolecular structure and function. Low-molecular-mass organic solutes play critical roles in stabilizing macromolecules in the face of heat and cold stress and in modulating their activities, for instance, by improving the efficacy of insect THPs in preventing growth of ice crystals. Temperature-dependent regulation of proton activity is essential for retention of optimal function of proteins and membranes. The complex interplay among molecules and ions of all sizes emphasizes a point stressed in the introductory chapter: to understand a physiological system in its true complexity, an integrative perspective must be used.

Another major theme introduced in chapter 1 is illustrated especially well by the study of adaptation to temperature, and we end this chapter—and this volume—with a reiteration of this theme. The large amount of information that is available on adaptation to temperature in taxa from all three domains of life—the Eukarya, Bacteria, and Archaea—provides not only an extraordinary amount of fine detail on this critical aspect of evolution, but also an opportunity to develop general principles of adaptation that are common to all forms of life. Again and again, we found that common sets of raw material were exploited by diverse species to generate adaptations that are fundamentally conservative in nature. By discerning the traits or character states of organisms that are universally conserved in the face of environmental challenge, we can develop a profound sense of "what really matters" in the design of biological systems. What emerges from such an analysis is an illustration of a central tenet of comparative physiology that has been an over-arching theme of this volume: through the study of organismal diversity and adaptation, we may gain an unusually clear perspective on the underlying unity of living systems.

REFERENCES

Abad-Zapatero, C., J.P. Griffith, J.L. Sussman, and M.G. Rossmann (1987). Refined crystal structure of dogfish M_4 apo-lactate dehydrogenase. *J. Mol. Biol.* 198: 445–467.

Ali, A., S. Bharadwaj, R. O'Carroll, and N. Ovsenek (1998). Hsp90 interacts with and regulates the activity of heat shock factor 1 in *Xenopus* oocytes. *Mol. Cell. Biol.* 18: 4949–4960.

Anfinsen, C.B. (1973). Principles that govern the folding of protein chains. *Science* 8: 223–230.

Austin, J.H., F.W. Sunderman, and J.B. Camack (1927). The electrolyte composition and the pH of serum of a poikilothermous animal at different temperatures. *J. Biol. Chem.* 72: 677–685.

Bai, Y., T.R. Sosnick, L. Mayne, and S.W. Englander (1996). Protein-folding intermediates: Native-state hydrogen-exchange. *Science* 269: 192–197.

Bailey, A.J. (1968). The nature of collagen. In: *Comprehensive Biochemistry*, pp. 297–423, ed. M. Florkin and E.H. Stotz. Amsterdam: Elsevier.

Baldwin, J. (1971). Adaptation of enzymes to temperature: acetylcholinesterases in the central nervous system of fishes. *Comp. Biochem. Physiol.* 40: 181–187.

Baldwin, J., and P.W. Hochachka (1970). Functional significance of isoenzymes in thermal acclimatization: acetylcholinesterases from trout brain. *Biochem. J.* 116: 883–887.

Barnes, B.M. (1989). Freeze avoidance in a mammal: Body temperatures below 0°C in an Arctic hibernator. *Science* 244: 1593–1595.

Barry, J.P., C.H. Baxter, R.D. Sagarin, and S.E. Gilman (1995). Climate-related, long-term faunal changes in a California rocky intertidal community. *Science* 267: 672–675.

Behan-Martin, M., K. Bowler, G. Jones, and A.R. Cossins (1993). A near perfect temperature adaptation of bilayer order in vertebrate brain membranes. *Biochim. Biophys. Acta* 1151: 216–222.

Bennett, A.F. (1978). Activity metabolism of the lower vertebrates. *Annu. Rev. Physiol.* 40: 447–469.

Bennett, A.F., and R.E. Lenski (1993). Evolutionary adaptation to temperature. II. Thermal niches of experimental lines of *Escherichia coli. Evolution* 47: 1–12.

Bennett, A.F., and R.E. Lenski (1996). Evolutionary adaptation to temperature. V. Adaptive mechanisms and correlated responses in experimental lines of *Escherichia coli. Evolution* 50: 493–503.

Bennett, A.F., and R.A. Ruben (1979). Endothermy and activity in vertebrates. *Science* 206: 649–654.

Bennett, A.F., K.M. Dao, and R.E. Lenski (1990). Rapid evolution in response to high temperature selection. *Nature* 346: 79–81.

Bennett, A.F., R.E. Lenski, and J.E. Mittler (1992). Evolutionary adaptation to temperature. I. Fitness responses of *Escherichia coli* to changes in its thermal environment. *Evolution* 46: 16–30.

Berrill, N.J. (1955). Analysis of development. In: *The Determination of Size*, pp. 619–630, ed. B.H. Willier, P.A. Weiss, and V. Hamburger. Philadelphia: W.B. Saunders.

Blaxter, K. (1989). *Energy Metabolism in Animals and Man.* Cambridge: Cambridge University Press.

Block, B.A. (1987). Billfish brain and eye heater: A new look at nonshivering heat production. *News Physiol. Sci.* 2: 208–213.

Block, B.A. (1991). Endothermy in fish: thermogenesis, ecology and evolution. In: *Biochemistry and Molecular Biology of Fishes.* Vol. 1. pp. 269–311, ed. P.W. Hochachka and T. Mommsen. London: Elsevier.

Block, B.A. (1994). Thermogenesis in muscle. *Annu. Rev. Physiol.* 56: 535–577.

Bock, P.E., and C. Frieden (1974). pH-induced cold lability of rabbit skeletal muscle phosphofructokinase. *Biochemistry* 13: 4191–4196.

Bosch, T.C.G., S.M. Krylow, H.R. Bode, and R.E. Steele (1988). Thermotolerance and synthesis of heat-shock proteins: These responses are present in *Hydra attenuata* but absent in *Hydra oligactis. Proc. Natl. Acad. Sci. USA* 85: 7927–7931.

Bowler, K. and R. Manning (1994). Membranes as the critical targets in cellular heat injury and resistance adaptation. In: *Temperature Adaptation of Biological Membranes*, ed. A.R. Cossins, pp. 185–203. London: Portland Press.

Boyer, B.B., and B.M. Barnes (1999). Molecular and metabolic aspects of mammalian hibernation. *BioScience* 49: 713–724.

Brand, M.D., P. Couture, P.L. Else, K.W. Withers, and A.J. Hulbert (1991). Evolution of energy metabolism. *Biochem. J.* 275: 81–86.

Busa, W.B. and R. Nuccitelli (1984). Metabolic regulation *via* intracellular pH. *Am. J. Physiol.* *(Regulatory, Integrative Comp. Physiol. 15)* 246: R409–R438.

Cameron, J.N. (1989). Acid-base homeostasis: past and present perspectives. *Physiol. Zool.* 62: 845–865.

Carey, C. and J.R. Hazel (1989). Diurnal variation in membrane lipid composition of Sonoran desert teleosts. *J. Exp. Biol.* 147: 375–391.

Carey, F. (1990). Further observations on the biology of the swordfish. In: *Planning for the Future of Billfishes*, pp. 103–122, ed. R.H. Stroud. Savannah, Ga.: National Coalition for Marine Conservation.

Cary, S.C., T. Shank, and J. Stein (1998). Worms bask in extreme temperatures. *Nature* 391: 545–546.

Chaffee, R.R.J., and J.C. Roberts (1971). Temperature acclimation in birds and mammals. *Annu. Rev. Physiol.* 33: 155–202.

Chapelle, S., G. Brichon, and G. Zwingelstein (1982). Effect of environmental temperature on the incorporation of ^{3}H-ethanolamine into the phospholipids of the tissues of the crab *Carcinus meanas. J. Exp. Zool.* 224: 289–297.

Chen, L., A.L. DeVries, and C.-H. C. Cheng (1997a). Evolution of antifreeze glycoprotein gene from a trypsinogen gene in Antarctic notothenioid fish. *Proc. Natl. Acad. Sci. USA* 94: 3811–3816.

Chen, L., A.L. DeVries, and C.-H. C. Cheng (1997b). Convergent evolution of antifreeze glycoproteins in Antarctic notothenioid fish and Arctic cod. *Proc. Natl. Acad. Sci. USA* 94: 3817–3822.

Cheng, C.-H.C. (1998). Evolution of the diverse antifreeze proteins. *Curr. Opin. Genet. Dev.* 8: 715–720.

Ciulla, R.A., S. Burggraf, K.O. Stetter, and M.F. Roberts (1994). Occurrence and role of di-*myo*-inositol-1–1′-phosphate in *Methanococcus igneus. Appl. Environ. Microbiol.* 60: 3660–3664.

Clarke, A. (1991). What is cold adaptation and how should we measure it? *Amer. Zool.* 31: 81–92.

Clarke, M.R. (1979). The head of the sperm whale. *Sci. Amer.* 240: 128–141.

Cocca, E., M. Ratnayake-Lecamwasam, S.A. Parker, L. Camardella, M. Ciaramella, G. di Prisco, and H.W. Detrich (1995). Genomic remnants of α-globin genes in the hemoglobinless Antarctic icefishes. *Proc. Natl. Acad. Sci. USA* 92: 1817–1821.

Coppes, Z.L., and G.N. Somero (1990). Temperature-adaptive differences between the M_4-lactate dehydrogenases of stenothermal and eurythermal Sciaenid fishes. *J. Exp. Zool.* 254: 127–131.

Cossins, A.R., and K. Bowler (1987). *Temperature Biology of Animals.* London: Chapman and Hall.

Cossins, A.R., and J.A.C. Lee (1985). The adaptation of membrane structure and lipid composition to cold. In: *Circulation, Respiration, and Metabolism: Current Comparative Approaches*, pp. 543–552, ed. R. Gilles. Berlin: Springer-Verlag.

Cossins, A.R., M.J. Friedlander, and C.L. Prosser (1977). Correlations between behavioural temperature adaptations by goldfish and the viscosity and fatty acid composition of their synaptic membranes. *J. Comp. Physiol.* 120: 109–121.

Cossins, A.R., K. Bowler, and C.L. Prosser (1981). Homeoviscous adaptation and its effects upon membrane-bound enzymes. *J. Therm. Biol.* 6: 183–187.

Couture, P. and A.J. Hulbert (1995). Relationship between body mass, tissue metabolic rate, and sodium pump activity in mammalian liver and kidney. *Am. J. Physiol.* 268 (*Regulatory Integrative Comp. Physiol.* 37): R641–R650.

Craig, E.A., and C.A. Gross (1991). Is hsp70 the cellular thermometer? *Trends Biochem. Sci.* 16: 135–140.

Crowe, J.H., and L.M. Crowe (1992). Membrane integrity in anhydrobiotic organisms: toward a mechanism for stabilizing dry cells. In: *Water and Life*, pp. 87–103, ed. G.N. Somero, C.B. Osmond, and C.L. Bolis. Berlin: Springer-Verlag.

Cullen, K.E., and K.D. Sarge (1997). Characterization of hypothermic-induced cellular stress response in mouse tissues. *J. Biol. Chem.* 272: 1742–1746.

Dahlhoff, E., and G.N. Somero (1993a). Kinetic and structural adaptations of cytoplasmic malate dehydrogenases of eastern Pacific abalones (genus *Haliotis*) from different thermal habitats: biochemical correlates of biogeographical patterning. *J. Exp. Biol.* 185: 137–150.

Dahlhoff, E., and G.N. Somero (1993b). Effects of temperature on mitochondria from abalone (genus *Haliotis*): adaptive plasticity and its limits. *J. Exp. Biol.* 185: 151–168.

Dahlhoff, E., J. O'Brien, G.N. Somero, and R.D. Vetter (1991). Temperature effects on mitochondria from hydrothermal vent invertebrates: evidence for adaptation to elevated and variable habitat temperatures. *Physiol. Zool.* 1490–1508.

Davis, B.D. (1958). On the importance of being ionized. *Arch. Biochem. Biophys.* 78: 497–509.

Denborough, M. (1998). Malignant hyperthermia. *Lancet* 352: 1131–1136.

Deng, H., J. Zheng, A. Clarke, J.J. Holbrook, R. Callender, and J.W. Burgner II (1994). Source of catalysis in the lactate dehydrogenase system. Ground-state interactions in the enzyme-substrate complex. *Biochemistry* 33: 2297–2305.

DeVries, A.L. (1971). Glycoproteins as biological antifreeze agents in Antarctic fishes. *Science* 172: 152–155.

DeVries, A.L. (1982). Biological antifreeze agents in coldwater fishes. *Comp. Biochem. Physiol.* 73: 627–640.

DeVries, A.L., and C.-H.C. Cheng (1992). The role of antifreeze glycopeptides and peptides in the survival of cold-water fishes. In: *Water and Life*, pp. 301–315, ed. G.N. Somero, C.B. Osmond, and C.L. Bolis. Berlin: Springer-Verlag.

Dietz, T.J., and G.N. Somero (1993). Species- and tissue-specific synthesis patterns for heat-shock proteins HSP70 and HSP90 in several marine teleost fishes. *Physiol. Zool.* 66: 863–880.

Duman, J.G. (2001). Antifreeze and ice nucleator proteins in terrestrial arthropods. *Annu. Rev. Physiol.* 63: 327–357.

Duman, J.G., and T.M. Olsen (1993). Thermal hysteresis protein activity in bacteria, fungi, and phylogenetically diverse plants. *Cryobiology* 30: 322–328.

Duman, J.G., D-W. Wu, T. M. Olsen, M. Urrutia and D. Tursman (1993). Thermal-hysteresis proteins. *Adv. Low-Temp. Biol.* 2: 131–182.

Dumonteil, E., H. Barre, and G. Meissner (1995). Expression of sarcoplasmic reticulum Ca^{2+} transport proteins in cold-acclimating ducklings. *Am. J. Physiol. (Cell Physiol.)* 269: C955–C960.

Dunn, C.R., H.M Wilks, D.J. Halsall, T. Atkinson, A.R. Clarke, H. Muirhead, and J.J. Holbrook (1991). Design and synthesis of new enzymes based on the lactate dehydrogenase framework. *Phil. Trans. R. Soc. Lond. B* 332: 177–184.

Eastman, J.T. (1993). *Antarctic Fish Biology: Evolution in a Unique Environment.* San Diego: Academic Press.

Echtay, K.S., E. Winkler, and M. Klingenberg (2000). Coenzyme Q is an obligatory cofactor for uncoupling protein function. *Nature* 408: 609–613.

Ellis, R.J. (1996a). The "bio" in biochemistry: Protein folding inside and outside the cell. *Science* 272: 1448–1449.

Ellis, R.J. (1996b). *The Chaperonins.* San Diego: Academic Press.

Ellis, R.J., and S.M. van der Vies (1991). Molecular chaperones. *Annu. Rev. Biochem.* 60: 321–347.

Else, P.L., and A.J. Hulbert (1985). An allometric comparison of the mitochondria of mammalian and reptilian tissues: The implications for the evolution of endothermy. *J. Comp. Physiol.* B. 156: 3–11.

Else, P.L., and A.J. Hulbert (1987). Evolution of mammalian endothermic metabolism: "leaky" membranes as a source of heat. *Am. J. Physiol.* 253 (*Regulatory Integrative Comp. Physiol.* 22): R1–R7.

Else, P.L., D.J. Windmill, and V. Markus (1996). Molecular activity of sodium pumps in endotherms and ectotherms. *Am. J. Physiol.* 271 (*Regulatory Integrative Comp. Physiol.* 40): R1287–1294.

Emmett, B., and P.W. Hochachka (1981). Scaling of oxidative and glycolytic enzymes in the shrew. *Resp. Physiol.* 45: 261–267.

Farkas, T. and R. Roy (1989). Temperature mediated restructuring of phosphatidylethanolamines in livers of freshwater fishes. *Comp. Biochem. Physiol.* B 93: 217–222.

Feder, M. (1999). Organismal, ecological, and evolutionary aspects of heat-shock proteins and the stress response: established conclusions and unresolved issues. *Amer. Zool.* 39: 857–864.

Feder, M.E., and G.E. Hofmann (1999). Heat-shock proteins, molecular chaperones and the stress response: Evolutionary and ecological physiology. *Annu. Rev. Physiol.* 61: 243–282.

Feige, U., R.I. Morimoto, I. Yahara, and B.S. Polla (1996). *Stress Inducible Cellular Responses.* Basel: Birkhäuer.

Feller, G. and C. Gerday (1997). Psychrophilic enzymes: molecular basis of cold adaptation. *Cell. Mol. Life. Sci.* (1997) 830–841.

Fields, P.A., and G.N. Somero (1997). Amino acid sequence differences cannot fully explain interspecific variation in thermal sensitivities of gobiid fish A_4-lactate dehydrogenases (A_4-LDHs). *J. Exp. Biol.* 200: 1839–1850.

Fields, P.A., and G.N. Somero (1998). Hot spots in cold adaptation: Localized increases in conformational flexibility in lactate dehydrogenase A_4 orthologs of Antarctic notothenioid fishes. *Proc. Natl. Acad. Sci. USA.* 95: 11476–11481.

Fields, P.A., J.B. Graham, R.H. Rosenblatt, and G.N. Somero (1993). Effects of expected global climate change on marine faunas. *Trends Ecol. Evol.* 8: 361–367.

Fields, P.A., B.D. Wahlstrand, and G.N. Somero (2001). Intrinsic vs. extrinsic stabilization of enzymes: the interaction of solutes and temperature on A_4-lactate dehydrogenase orthologs from warm- and cold-adapted marine fishes. *Eur. J. Biochem.* 268: 4497–4505.

Fletcher, G.L., C.L. Hew, X. Li, K. Haya, and M.H. Kao (1985). Year-round presence of high levels of plasma antifreeze proteins in a temperate fish, ocean pout (*Macrozoarces americanus*). *Can. J. Zool.* 63: 488–493.

Fletcher, G.L., C.L. Hew, and P.L. Davies (2001). Antifreeze proteins of teleost fishes. *Annu. Rev. Physiol.* 63: 359–390.

Fleury, C., M. Neverova, S. Collins, S. Raimbault, O. Champigny, C. Levi-Meyrueis, Bouillaud, F., M. Seldin, R. Surwitt, D. Ricquier, and C. Warden (1997). Uncoupling protein-2: a novel gene linked to obesity and hyperinsulinemia. *Nature Genetics* 15: 269–272.

Frank, C.L. (1991). Adaptation for hibernation in the depot fats of a ground squirrel (*Spermophilus beldingi*). *Can. J. Zool.* 69: 2702–2711.

Frank, C.L. (1992). The influence of dietary fatty acids on hibernation by golden-mantled ground squirrels (*Spermophilus lateralis*). *Physiol. Zool.* 65: 906–920.

Fujii, D.K., and A.J. Fulco (1977). Biosynthesis of unsaturated fatty acids by bacilli—hyperinduction of desaturase synthesis. *J. Biol. Chem.* 252: 3660–3670.

Fujii, J., K. Otsu, F. Zorzato, S.D. Leon, V.K. Khanna, et al. (1991). Identification of a mutation in porcine ryanodine receptor associated with malignant hyperthermia. *Science* 253: 448–451.

Gates, R.D., and P.J. Edmunds (1999). The physiological mechanisms of acclimatization in tropical reef corals. *Amer. Zool.* 39: 30–43.

Gehring, W.J., and R. Wehner (1995). Heat shock protein synthesis and thermotolerance in *Cataglyphis*, an ant from the Sahara desert. *Proc. Natl. Acad. Sci. USA* 92: 2992–2998.

Geiser, F., B.T. Firth, and R.S. Seymour (1992). Polyunsaturated dietary lipids lower the selected body temperature of a lizard. *J. Comp. Physiol.* B. 162: 1–4.

Gellner, K., G. Praetzel, and T.C. Bosch (1992). Cloning and expression of a heat-inducible hsp70 gene in two species of *Hydra* which differ in their stress response. *Eur. J. Biochem.* 210: 683–691.

Gerstein, M. and C. Chothia (1991). Analysis of protein loop closure. Two types of hinges produce one motion in lactate dehydrogenase. *J. Mol. Biol.* 220: 133–149.

Gibbs, A.G. (1998). The role of lipid physical properties in lipid barriers. *Amer. Zool.* 38: 268–279.

Giver, L., A. Gershenson, P.-O. Freskgard, and F.H. Arnold (1998). Directed evolution of a thermostable esterase. *Proc. Natl. Acad. Sci. USA* 95: 12809–12813.

Gong, A., K.V. Ewart, Z. Hu, G.L. Fletcher, and C.L. Hew (1996). Skin antifreeze protein genes of the winter flounder, *Pleuronectes americanus*, encode distinct and active polypeptides without the secretory signal and prosequences. *J. Biol. Chem.* 271: 4106–4112.

Gracey, A.Y., J. Logue, P.E. Tiku, and A.R. Cossins (1996). Adaptation of biological membranes to temperature: biophysical perspectives and molecular mechanisms. *Soc. Exp. Biol. Sem. Ser., Animals and Temperature: Phenotypic and Evolutionary Adaptation*, 59: 1–21, ed. I.A. Johnston and A.F. Bennett. Cambridge: Cambridge University Press.

Graumann, P.L., and M.A. Marahiel (1998). A superfamily of proteins that contain the cold-shock domain. *Trends Biochem. Sci.* 23: 286–290.

Graves, J.E., and G.N. Somero (1982). Electrophoretic and functional enzymic evolution in four species of eastern Pacific barracudas from different thermal environments. *Evolution* 36: 97–106.

Griffith, M., and M. Antikainen (1996). Extracellular ice formation in freezing-tolerant plants. *Adv. Low-Temp. Biol.* 3: 107–139.

Hadley, N.F. (1981). Cuticular lipids of terrestrial plants and arthropods: A comparison of their structure, composition, and waterproofing function. *Biol. Rev.* 56: 23–47.

Hafner, R.P., C.D. Nobes, A.D. McGown, and M.D. Brand (1988). Altered relationship between protonmotive force and respiration rate in non-phosphorylating liver mitochondria isolated from rats of different thyroid hormone status. *Eur. J. Biochem.* 178: 511–518.

Hafner, R.P., M.J. Leake, and M.D. Brand (1989). Hypothyroidism in rats decreases mitochondrial inner membrane cation permeability. *FEBS Lett.* 248: 175–178.

Hand, S.C., and J.F. Carpenter (1986). pH-induced metabolic transitions in *Artemia* embryos mediated by a novel hysteretic trehalase. *Science* 232: 1535–1537.

Hand, S.C., and I. Hardewig (1996). Downregulation of cellular metabolism during environmental stress: Mechanisms and implications. *Annu. Rev. Physiol.* 58: 539–563.

Hand, S.C. and G.N. Somero (1983). Phosphofructokinase of the hibernator *Citellus beecheyi*: Temperature and pH regulation of activity via influences on the tetramer-dimer equilibrium. *Physiol. Zool.* 56: 380–388.

Haney, P.J., J.H. Badger, G.L. Buldak, C.I. Reich, C.R. Woese, and G.J. Olsen (1999). Thermal adaptation analyzed by comparison of protein sequences from mesophilic and extremely thermophilic *Methanococcus* species. *Proc. Natl. Acad. Sci. USA*. 96: 3578–3583.

Harding, M.M., L.G. Ward, and A.D.J. Haymet (1999). Type I 'antifreeze' proteins: Structure-activity studies and mechanisms of ice growth inhibition. *Eur. J. Biochem.* 264: 653–665.

Hartl, F.U. (1996). Molecular chaperones in cellular protein folding. *Nature* 293: 311–314.

Hazel, J.R. (1988). Homeoviscous adaptation in animal cell membranes. In: *Advances in Membrane Fluidity. Physiological Regulation of Membrane Fluidity*, pp. 149–188, ed. R.C. Aloia, C.C. Curtain, and L.M. Gordon. New York: Liss.

Hazel, J.R. (1990). Adaptation to temperature: phospholipid synthesis in hepatocytes of rainbow trout. *Am. J. Physiol.* 258 (*Regulatory Integrative Comp. Physiol.* 27): R1495–R1501.

Hazel, J.R. (1995). Thermal adaptation in biological membranes—is homeoviscous adaptation the explanation? *Annu. Rev. Physiol.* 57: 19–42.

Hazel, J.R., and R. Carpenter (1985). Rapid changes in the phospholipid composition of gill membranes during thermal acclimation of the rainbow trout, *Salmo gairdneri*. *J. Comp. Physiol. B.* 155: 597–602.

Hazel, J.R., and S.R. Landrey (1988). Timecourse of thermal acclimation in plasma membranes of trout kidney. 1. Headgroup composition. *Am. J. Physiol.* 255 (*Regulatory Integrative Comp. Physiol.* 24): R622–R634.

Hazel, J.R., and R.C. Livermore (1990). Fatty-acyl coenzyme A pool in liver of rainbow trout (*Salmo gairdneri*): effects of temperature acclimation. *Physiol. Zool.* 256: 31–37.

Hazel, J.R., and C.L. Prosser (1974). Molecular mechanisms of temperature compensation in poikilotherms. *Physiol. Rev.* 54: 620–677.

Hazel, J.R., and E.E. Williams (1990). The role of alterations in membrane lipid composition in enabling physiological adaptation of organisms to their physical environment. *Prog. Lipid Res.* 29: 167–227.

Hazel, J.R., S.J. McKinley, and E.E. Williams (1992). Thermal adaptation in biological membranes: interacting effects of temperature and pH. *J. Comp. Physiol. B.* 162: 593–601.

Henriques, V., and C. Hansen (1901). Vergleichende Untersuchungen über die chemische

Zusammensetzung des thierischen Fettes. *Skand. Arch. Physiol.* 11: 151–165.

Hensel, R., and H. Konig (1988). Thermoadaptation of methanogenic bacteria by intracellular ion concentration. *FEMS Microbiol. Lett.* 49: 75–79.

Hernández, G., F.E. Jenny, Jr., M.W.W. Adams, and D.M. LeMaster (2000). Millisecond time scale conformational flexibility in a hyperthermophile protein at ambient temperature. *Proc. Natl. Acad. Sci. USA.* 97: 3166–3170.

Hersko, A. and A. Ciechanover (1992). The ubiquitin system for protein degradation. *Annu. Rev. Biochem.* 61: 761–807.

Hew, C.L., N.C. Wang, S. Joshi, G.L. Fletcher, G.K. Scott, P.H. Hayes, B. Buettner, and P.L. Davies (1988). Multiple genes provide the basis for antifreeze protein diversity and dosage in the ocean pout, *Macrozoarces americanus. J. Biol. Chem.* 263: 12049–12055.

Hilser, V.J., D. Dowdy, T.G. Oas, and E. Freire (1998). The structural distribution of cooperative interactions in proteins: Analysis of the native state ensemble. *Proc. Natl. Acad. Sci. USA* 95: 9903–9908.

Himms-Hagen, J. (1990). Brown adipose tissue thermogenesis: interdisciplinary studies. *FASEB J.* 4: 2890–2898.

Hirata, F., and J. Axelrod (1980). Phospholipid methylation and biological signal transmission. *Science* 209: 1082–1090.

Hochachka, P.W., and G.N. Somero (1984). *Biochemical Adaptation.* Princeton: Princeton University Press.

Hofmann, G.E. and S.C. Hand (1990). Arrest of cytochrome c oxidase synthesis coordinated with catabolic arrest in dormant *Artemia* embryos. *Am. J. Physiol. (Integrative, Regulatory Comp. Physiol. 27)* 258: R1184–1191.

Hofmann, G.E., and G.N. Somero (1995). Evidence for protein damage at environmental temperatures: seasonal changes in levels of ubiquitin conjugates and hsp70 in the intertidal mussel *Mytilus trossulus. J. Exp. Biol.* 198: 1509–1518.

Hofmann, G.E., and G.N. Somero (1996a). Protein ubiquitination and stress protein synthesis in *Mytilus trossulus* occurs during recovery from tidal emersion. *Mol. Mar. Biol. Biotech.* 5: 175–184.

Hofmann, G.E., and G.N. Somero (1996b). Interspecific variation in thermal denaturation of proteins in the congeneric mussels *Mytilus trossulus* and *M. galloprovincialis*: evidence from the heat-shock response and protein ubiquitination. *Mar. Biol.* 126: 65–75.

Hofmann, G.E., B.A. Buckley, S. Airaksinen, J.E. Keen, and G.N. Somero (2000). Heat-shock protein expression is absent in the Antarctic fish *Trematomus bernacchii* (Family Nototheniidae). *J. Exp. Biol.* 203: 2331–2339.

Holeton, G.F. (1974). Metabolic cold adaptation of polar fish: Fact or artefact. *Physiol. Zool.* 47: 137–152.

Holland, L.Z., M. McFall-Ngai, and G.N. Somero (1997). Evolution of lactate dehydrogenase-A homologs of barracuda fishes (genus *Sphyraena*) from different thermal environments: Differences in kinetic properties and thermal stability are due to amino acid substitutions outside the active site. *Biochemistry* 36: 3207–3215.

Hon, W.-C., M. Griffith, A. Mlynarz, Y.C. Kwok, and D.S.C. Yang (1995). Antifreeze proteins in winter rye are similar to pathogenesis-related proteins. *Plant Physiol.* 109: 879–889.

Horikoshi, K., and W.D. Grant (1998). *Extremophiles: Microbial Life in Extreme Environments.* New York: Wiley-Liss.

Horwath, K.L., and J.G. Duman (1986). Thermoperiodic involvement in antifreeze protein production in the cold hardy beetle *Dendroides canadensis*: Implications for photoperiodic time measurement. *J. Insect Physiol.* 32: 799–806.

Hottinger, T., T. Boller, and A. Wiemken (1987). Rapid changes of heat and desiccation tolerance correlated with changes of trehalose content in *Saccharomyces cerevisiae* cells subjected to temperature shifts. *FEBS Lett.* 220: 113–115.

Hsaio, K.C., C.H. Cheng, I.E. Fernandes, H.W. Detrich, and A.L. DeVries (1990). An antifreeze glycopeptide gene from the Antarctic cod *Notothenia coriiceps neglecta* encodes a polyprotein of high peptide copy numbers. *Proc. Natl. Acad. Sci. USA* 94: 3811–3816.

Huey, R.B, and D. Berrigan (1996). Testing evolutionary hypotheses of acclimation. In: *Animals and Temperature: Phenotypic and Evolutionary Adaptation*, pp. 205–237, ed. I.A. Johnston and A.F. Bennett. Cambridge: Cambridge University Press.

Hughes, L. (2000). Biological consequences of global warming: is the signal already apparent? *Trends Ecol. Evol.* 15: 56–61.

Hulbert, A.J., and P.L. Else (1989). Evolution of mammalian endothermic metabolism: mitochondrial activity and cell composition. *Am. J. Physiol.* 256 (*Regulatory Integrative Comp. Physiol.* 25): R63–R69.

Hulbert, A.J., and P.L. Else (1990). The cellular basis of endothermic metabolism: A role for "leaky" membranes? *News Physiol. Sci.* 5: 25–28.

Hulbert, A.J., and P.L. Else (2000). Mechanisms underlying the cost of living in animals. *Annu. Rev. Physiol.* 62: 207–235.

Jaenicke, R. (1991). Protein stability and molecular adaptation to extreme conditions. *Eur. J. Biochem.* 202: 715–728.

Jaenicke, R. (2000). Do ultrastable proteins from hyperthermophiles have high or low conformational rigidity? *Proc. Natl. Acad. Sci. USA* 97: 2962–2964.

Jia, A.,C.I. DeLuca, H. Chao, and P.L. Davies (1997). Structural basis for the binding of a globular antifreeze protein to ice. *Nature* 384: 285–288.

Jiang, W., Y. Hou, and M. Inouye (1997). CspA, the major cold-shock protein of *Escherichia coli*, is an RNA chaperone. *J. Biol. Chem.* 272: 196–202.

Johnston, E.A., H.E. Guderley, C.E. Franklin, T. Crockford, and C. Kamunde (1994). Are mitochondria subject to evolutionary temperature adaptation? *J. Exp. Biol.* 195: 293–306.

Jones, P.G., M. Mitta, Y. Kim, W. Jiang, and M. Inouye (1996). Cold-shock induced a major ribosomal-associated protein that unwinds double-stranded RNA in *Escherichia coli*. *Proc. Natl. Acad. Sci. USA* 93: 76–80.

Kandror, O., and A.L. Goldberg (1997). Trigger factor is induced upon cold shock and enhances viability of *Escherichia coli* at low temperatures. *Proc. Natl. Acad. Sci.* 94: 4978–4981.

Karow, A.M. (1991). Chemical cryoprotection of metazoan cells. *BioScience* 41: 155–160.

Kawall, H.G., J.J. Torres, B.D. Sidell, and G.N. Somero (2001). Metabolic cold adaptation in Antarctic fishes: evidence from enzymatic activities of brain. *Mar. Biol.*, in press.

Ko, R., L. Tombras Smith, and G.M. Smith (1994). Glycine betaine confers enhanced osmotolerance and cryotolerance on *Listeria monocytogenes*. *J. Bacteriol.* 176: 426–431.

Krebs, R.A. and M.E. Feder (1997). Deleterious consequences of hsp70 overexpression in *Drosophila melanogaster* larvae. *Cell Stress Chaperones* 2: 60–71.

Laloi, M., M. Klein, J. Riesmeier, B. Müller-Röber, C. Fleury, F. Bouillaud, and D. Ricquier (1997). A plant cold-induced uncoupling protein. *Nature* 389: 135–136.

Langworthy, T.A., and J.L. Pond (1986). Membranes and lipids of thermophiles. In: *Thermophiles: General, Molecular, and Applied Microbiology.* 107–135, ed. T.D. Brock. New York: Wiley.

Lee, R.E. Jr., M.R. Lee, and J.M. Strong-Gunderson (1993a). Insect cold-hardiness and ice nucleating active microorganisms including their potential use for biological control. *J. Insect. Physiol.* 39: 1–12.

Lee, R.E., J.J. McGrath, R.T. Morason, and R.M. Taddeo (1993b). Survival of intracellular freezing, lipid coalescence and osmotic fragility in fat body cells of the freeze-tolerant gall fly *Eurosta solidaginis*. *J. Insect Physiol.* 39: 445–450.

Levin, B.R., and C.T. Bergstrom (2000). Bacteria are different: Observations, interpretations, speculations, and opinions about the mechanisms of adaptive evolution in prokaryotes. *Proc. Natl. Acad. Sci. USA* 97: 6981–6985.

Li, N., C.A. Andorfer, and J.G. Duman (1998). Enhancement of insect antifreeze protein activity by solutes with low molecular mass. *J. Exp. Biol.* 201: 2243–2251.

Lin, J.J., T.H. Yang, B. Wahlstrand, P.A. Fields, and G.N. Somero (2001). Phylogenetic relationships and biochemical properties of the duplicated cytosolic and mitochondrial isoforms of malate dehydrogenase from a teleost fish, *Sphyraena idiastes.* *J. Mol. Evol.*, in press.

Lindquist, S. (1986). The heat-shock response. *Annu. Rev. Biochem.* 55: 1151–1192.

Litman, B., and D. Mitchell (1996). A role for phospholipid polyunsaturation in modulating membrane protein function. *Lipids* S193–S197.

Liu, A.Y.C, H.J. Bian, L.E. Huang, and Y.K. Lee (1994). Transient cold-shock induces the heat-shock response upon recovery at 37 degrees C in human cells. *J. Biol. Chem.* 269: 14768–14775.

Liu, Y., M. Merrow, J.J. Loros, and J.C. Dunlap (1998). How temperature changes reset a circadian oscillator. *Science* 281: 825–829.

Logsdon, J.M. Jr., and W.F. Doolittle (1997). Origin of antifreeze protein genes: A cool tale in molecular evolution. *Proc. Natl. Acad. Sci. USA* 94: 3485–3487.

Logue, J.A., A.L. DeVries, E. Fodor, and A.R. Cossins (2000). Lipid compositional correlates of temperature-adaptive interspecific differences in membrane physical structure. *J. Exp. Biol.* 203: 2105–2115.

Louw, G.N., and M.K. Seely (1982). *Ecology of Desert Organisms*, London: Longman.

Low, P.S., and G.N. Somero (1976). Adaptation of muscle pyruvate kinases to environmental temperatures and pressure. *J. Exp. Zool.* 198: 1–12.

Low, P.S., J.L. Bada, and G.N. Somero (1973). Temperature adaptation of enzymes: roles of the free energy, the enthalpy, and the entropy of activation. *Proc. Natl. Acad. Sci. USA* 70: 430–432.

Lowell, B.B. (1996). Slimming with a leaner enzyme. *Nature* 382: 585–586.

Lowell, B.B., and B.M. Spiegelman (2000). Towards a molecular understanding of adaptive thermogenesis. *Nature* 404: 652–660.

Macdonald, A.G. (1984). The effects of pressure on the molecular structure and physiological functions of cell membranes. *Phil. Trans. R. Soc. Ser. B* 304: 47–68.

Macdonald, J.A., J.C. Montgomery, and R.M.G. Wells (1988). The physiology of McMurdo Sound fishes: current New Zealand research. *Comp. Biochem. Physiol. B.* 90: 567–578.

Malan, A., and E. Mioskowski (1988). pH-temperature interactions on protein function and hibernation: GDP binding to brown adipose tissue mitochondria. *J. Comp. Physiol. B.* 158: 487–493.

Martin, D.D., R.A. Ciulla, and M.F. Roberts (1999). Osmoadaptation in Archaea. *Appl. Environ. Microbiol.* 65: 1815–1825.

Matthews, B.W., H. Nicholson, and W.J. Becktel (1987). Enhanced protein thermostability from site-directed mutations that decrease the entropy of unfolding. *Proc. Natl. Acad. Sci. USA* 84: 6663–6667.

Mayr, E. (1982). *The Growth of Biological Thought.* Cambridge: Belknap-Harvard.

McArthur, M.D., C.C. Hanstock, A. Malan, L.C. Wang, and P.S. Allen (1990). Skeletal muscle pH dynamics during arousal from hibernation measured by ^{31}P NMR spectroscopy. *J. Comp. Physiol. B* 160: 339–347.

McElhaney, R.N. (1984). The structure and function of the *Acholeplasma laidlawii* membrane. *Biochim. Biophys. Acta* 779: 1–42.

McFall-Ngai, M., and J. Horwitz (1990). A comparative study of the thermal stability of the vertebrate eye lens: Antarctic fish to the desert iguana. *Exp. Eye Res.* 50: 703–709.

Mongold, J.A., A.F. Bennett, and R.E. Lenski (1996). Experimental investigations of evolutionary adaptation to temperature. In: *Animals and Temperature: Phenotypic and Evolutionary Adaptation*, pp. 239–264, ed. I.A. Johnston and A.F. Bennett. Cambridge: Cambridge University Press.

Morimoto, R.I. (1998). Regulation of the heat-shock transcriptional response: Cross talk between a family of heat-shock factors, molecular chaperones, and negative regulators. *Genes Devel.* 12: 3788–3796.

Morimoto, R.I., and M. G. Santoro (1998). Stress-inducible responses and heat shock proteins: New pharmacologic targets for cytoprotection. *Nature Biotech.* 16: 833–838.

Morita, M.T., Y. Tanaka, T.S. Kodama, Y. Kyogoku, H. Yanagi, and T. Yura (1999). Translational induction of heat-shock transcription by factor sigma^{32}: evidence for a built-in RNA thermosensor. *Genes Devel.* 13: 655–665.

Neelands, P.J., and M.T. Clandinin (1983). Diet fat influences liver plasma-membrane lipid composition and glucagon-stimulated adenylate cyclase activity. *Biochem. J.* 212: 573–583.

Neven, L.G., J.G. Duman, J.M. Beals, and F.J. Castellino (1986). Over-wintering adaptations of the stag beetle, *Ceruchus piceus*: removal of ice nucleators in winter to promote supercooling. *J. Comp. Physiol. B.* 156: 707–716.

Neven, L.G., J.G. Duman, M.G. Low, L.C. Sehl, and F.J. Castellino (1989). Purification and characterization of an insect hemolymph lipoprotein ice nucleator: evidence for the importance of phosphatidylinositol and apolipoprotein in the ice nucleator activity. *J. Comp. Physiol.* 159: 71–82.

Nobes, C.D., P.L. Lakin-thomas, and M.D. Brand (1989). The contribution of ATP turnover by the Na^+/K^+-ATPase to the rate of respiration of hepatocytes. Effects of thyroid status and fatty acids. *Biochim. Biophys. Acta* 976: 241–245.

O'Brien, J.E., E. Dahlhoff, and G.N. Somero (1991). Thermal resistance of mitochondrial respiration: hydrophobic interactions of membrane proteins may limit mitochondrial thermal resistance. *Physiol. Zool.* 64: 1509–1526.

Ourisson, G., M. Rohmer, and K. Poralla (1987). Prokaryotic hopanoids and other polyterpenoid sterol surrogates. *Annu. Rev. Microbiol.* 41: 301–333.

Padrón, D. M.E. Bizeau, and J.R. Hazel (2000). Is fluid-phase endocytosis conserved in hepatocytes of species acclimated and adapted to different temperatures? *Am J. Physiol. (Regulatory Integrative Comp. Physiol.)* 278: R529–R536.

Parmesan, C., N. Ryrholm, C. Stefanescu, J.K. Hill, C.D. Thomas, H. Descimon, B. Huntley, L. Kaila, J. Kullberg, T. Tammaru, W.J. Tennent, J.A. Thomas, and M. Warren (1999). Poleward shifts in geographical ranges of butterfly species associated with regional warming. *Nature* 399: 579–583.

Parsell, D.A. and S. Lindquist (1993). The function of heat-shock proteins in stress tolerance: Degradation and reactivation of damaged proteins. *Annu. Rev. Genet.* 27: 437–496.

Parsell, D.A., J. Taulien, and S. Lindquist (1993). The role of heat-shock proteins in thermotolerance. *Phil. Trans. Roy. Soc. Lond. B.* 339: 279–285.

Petersen, N.S., P. Young and V. Burton (1990). Heat-shock messenger RNA accumulation during recovery from cold shock in *Drosophila melanogaster. Insect Biochem.* 20: 679–684.

Pilon, M., and R. Schekman (1999). Protein translocation: how hsp70 pulls it off. *Cell* 97: 679–682.

Place, A.R., and D.A. Powers (1979). Genetic variation and relative catalytic efficiencies: lactate dehydrogenase-B allozymes of *Fundulus heteroclitus. Proc. Natl. Acad. Sci. USA* 76: 2354–2358.

Place, A.R., and D.A. Powers (1984). Purification and characterization of the lactate dehydrogenase (LDH-B$_4$) allozymes of *Fundulus heteroclitus. J. Biol. Chem.* 259: 1309–1318.

Poralla, K., T. Hartner, and E. Kannenberg (1984). Effect of temperature and pH on the hopanoid content of *Bacillus acidocaldarius. FEMS Microbiol. Lett.* 113: 107–110.

Porter, R.K., A.J. Hulbert, and M.D. Brand (1996). Allometry of mitochondrial proton leak: influence of membrane surface area and fatty acid composition. *Am. J. Physiol.* 271 (*Regulatory Integrative Comp. Physiol.* 40): R1550–R1560.

Powers, D.A. (1987). A multidisciplinary approach to the study of genetic variation within species. In: *New Directions in Ecological Physiology*, pp. 102–134, ed. M.E. Feder, A.F. Bennett, W.W. Burggren, and R.B. Huey. Cambridge: Cambridge University Press.

Powers, D.A., M. Smith, I. Gonzalez-Villasenor, L. DiMichelle, D. Crawford et al., (1993). A multidisciplinary approach to the selectionist/neutralist controversy using the model teleost *Fundulus heteroclitus.* In: *Oxford Surveys in Evolutionary Biology*, ed. D. Futuyma and J. Antonovics, 9: 43–107. Oxford: Oxford University Press.

Priscu, J.C., E.E. Adams, W.B. Lyons, M.A. Voytek, D.W. Mogk, R.L. Brown, C.P. McKay, C.D. Takacs, K.A. Welch, C.F. Wolk, J.D. Kirshtein, and R. Avci (1999). Geomicrobiology of subglacial ice above Lake Vostok, Antarctica. *Science* 286: 2141–2144.

Rahn, H., R.B. Reeves, and B.H. Howell (1975). Hydrogen ion regulation, temperature, and evolution. *Amer. Rev. Respir. Dis.* 112: 165–172.

Raskin, I., A. Ehmann, W.R. Melander, B.J.D. Meeuse (1987). Salicylic acid: A natural inducer of heat production in *Arum* lilies. *Science* 237: 1601–1602.

Raymond, J.A. (1992). Glycerol is a colligative antifreeze in some northern fishes. *J. Exp. Zool.* 262: 347–352.

Raymond, J.A. (1993). Glycerol and water balance in a near-isosmotic teleost, winter-acclimatized rainbow smelt. *Can. J. Zool.* 71: 1849–1854.

Raymond, J.A. (1997). Responses of marine fishes to freezing temperatures: a new look at colligative mechanisms. In: *Advances in Molecular and Cell Biology*, pp. 33–55, ed. J.S. Willis. Greenwich, Conn.: JAI.

Raymond, J.A. (1998). Trimethylamine oxide and urea synthesis in rainbow smelt and some other northern fishes. *Physiol. Zool.* 71: 515–523.

Raymond, J.A., and A.L. DeVries (1977). Adsorption inhibition as a mechanism of freezing resistance in polar fishes. *Proc. Natl. Acad. Sci. USA* 74: 2589–2593.

Raymond, J.A., and A.L. DeVries (1998). Elevated concentrations and synthetic pathways of trimethylamine oxide and urea in some teleost fishes of McMurdo Sound, Antarctica. *Fish. Physiol. Biochem.* 18: 387–398.

Raymond, J.A., P.W. Wilson, and A.L. DeVries (1986). Inhibition of growth on nonbasal planes in ice by fish antifreeze. *Proc. Natl. Acad. Sci. USA.* 86: 881–885.

Raynard, R.S. and A.R. Cossins (1991). Homeoviscous adaptation and thermal compensation of sodium pump of trout erythrocytes. *Am. J. Physiol.* 260 (*Regulatory Integrative Comp. Physiol.* 29): R916–R924.

Reeves, R.B. (1977). The interaction of body temperature and acid-base balance in ectothermic vertebrates. *Annu. Rev. Physiol.* 39: 559–586.

Ricquier, D., and F. Bouillaud (2000). The uncoupling protein homologues: UCP1, UCP2, UCP3, StUCP and AtUCP. *Biochem. J.* 345: 161–179.

Ring, J.A. (1982). Freezing-tolerant insects with low supercooling points. *Comp. Biochem. Physiol.* 73: 605–612.

Ritossa, F. (1962). A new puffing pattern induced by heat-shock and DNP in *Drosophila. Experientia* 18: 571–573.

Roberts, S.J., M.S. Lowery, and G.N. Somero (1988). Regulation of binding of phosphofructokinase to myofibrils in the red and white muscle of the barred sand bass, *Paralabrax nebulifer* (Serranidae). *J. Exp. Biol.* 137: 13–27.

Robertson, J.C., and J.R. Hazel (1995). Cholesterol content of trout plasma membranes varies with acclimation temperature. *Am. J. Physiol.* 269 (*Regulatory Integrative Comp. Physiol.* 38): R1113–R1117.

Robertson, J.C., and J.R. Hazel (1997). Membrane constraints to physiological function at different temperatures: does cholesterol stabilize membranes at elevated temperatures? *Soc. Exp. Biol. Sem. Ser., Global Warming: Implications for Freshwater and Marine Fish* 61: 25–49, ed. C.M. Wood and D.G. McDonald.

Robertson, J.C., and J.R. Hazel (1999). Influence of temperature and membrane lipid composition on the osmotic water permeability of teleost gills. *Physiol. Biochem. Zool.* 72: 623–632.

Robin, E.D. (1962). Relationship between temperature and plasma pH and carbon dioxide tension in the turtle. *Nature* 195: 249–251.

Roemmich, D., and J. McGowan (1995). Climatic warming and the decline of zooplankton in the California Current. *Science* 267: 1324–1326.

Rudolph, A., J. Crowe, and L. Crowe (1986). Effects of three stabilizing agents—proline, betaine and trehalose on membrane phospholipids. *Arch. Biochem. Biophys.* 245: 134–143.

Sagarin, R.D., J.P. Barry, S.E. Gilman, and C.H. Baxter (1999). Climate-related changes in an intertidal community over short and long time scales. *Ecol. Monogr.* 69: 465–490.

Salotra, P., D.K. Singh, K.P, Seal, N. Krishna, H. Jaffe, and R. Bhatnagar (1995). Expression of DnaK and GroEL homologs in *Leuconostoc mesenteriodes* in response to heat-shock, cold-shock or chemical stress. *FEMS Microbiol. Lettr.* 131: 57–62.

Salt, R.W. (1962). Intracellular freezing in insects. *Nature* 193: 1207–1208.

Sanford, E. (1999). Regulation of keystone predation by small changes in ocean temperature. *Science* 283: 2095–2097.

Schmid, S.R. and P. Linder (1992). D-E-A-D protein family of putative RNA helicases. *Mol. Microbiol.* 6: 283–292.

Schmidt-Nielsen, K. (1984). *Scaling: Why is Animal Size so Important?* Cambridge: Cambridge University Press.

Schulte, P.M., H.C. Glemet, A.A. Fiebig, and D.A. Powers (2000). Adaptive variation in lactate dehydrogenase-B gene expression: Role of a stress-responsive regulatory element. *Proc. Natl. Acad. Sci. USA* 97: 6597–6602.

Scott, G.K., C.L. Hew, and P.L. Davies (1985). Antifreeze protein genes are tandemly linked and clustered in the genome of the winter flounder. *Proc. Natl. Acad. Sci. USA* 82: 2613–2617.

Scott, G.K., P.L. Davies, H.H. Kao, and G.L. Fletcher (1988). Differential amplification of antifreeze protein genes in the pleuronectinae. *J. Mol. Evol.* 27: 29–35.

Seymour, R.S, and P. Schultze-Motel (1996). Thermoregulating lotus flowers. *Nature* 383: 305.

Sharp, V.A., B.E. Brown, and D. Miller (1997). Heat shock protein (hsp70) expression in the tropical reef coral *Goniopora djiboutiensis. J. Therm. Biol.*: 22: 11–19.

Shoichet, B.K., W.A. Baase, R. Kuroki, and B.W. Matthews (1995). A relationship between protein stability and protein function. *Proc. Natl. Acad. Sci. USA* 92: 452–456.

Sidell, B.D. (1977). Turnover of cytochrome c in skeletal muscle of green sunfish (*Lepomis cyanellus,* R.) during thermal acclimation. *J. Exp. Zool.* 199: 233–250.

Sidell, B.D., M.E. Vayda, D.J. Small, T.J. Moylan, R.L. Londraville, M.L. Yuan, K.J. Rodnick, Z.A. Eppley, and L. Costello (1997). Variable expression of myoglobin among the hemoglobinless Antarctic icefishes. *Proc. Natl. Acad. Sci. USA* 94: 3420–3524.

Simons, K. and E. Ikonen (2000). How cells handle cholesterol. *Science* 290: 1721–1726.

Sinensky, M. (1974). Homeoviscous adaptation—a homeostatic process that regulates the viscosity of membrane lipids in *Escherichia coli. Proc. Natl. Acad. Sci. USA* 71: 522–525.

Sinensky, M., F. Pinkerton, E. Sutherland, and F.R. Simon (1979). Rate limitation of (Na^+-K^+) ATPase by membrane acyl chain ordering. *Proc. Natl. Acad. Sci. USA* 76: 4893–4897.

Singer, M.A., and S. Lindquist (1998a). Thermotolerance in *Saccharomyces cerevisiae*: the Yin and Yang of trehalose. *Trends Biotech.* 16: 460–468.

Singer, M.A., and S. Lindquist (1998b). Multiple effects of trehalose on protein folding in vitro and in vivo. *Mol. Cell.* 1: 639–648.

Somero, G.N. (1986). Protons, osmolytes, and fitness of the internal milieu for protein function. *Am. J. Physiol.* 252 (*Regulatory Integrative and Comp. Physiol. 20)*: R197–R213.

Somero, G.N. (1995). Proteins and temperature. *Annu. Rev. Physiol.* 57: 43–68.

Somero, G.N. (1997). Temperature relationships: from molecules to biogeography. *Handbook of Physiology. Section 13. Comparative Physiology,* Vol. II, pp. 1391–1444, ed. W.H. Dantzler. Oxford: Oxford University Press.

Somero, G.N., and J.J. Childress (1980). A violation of the metabolism-size scaling paradigm: activities of glycolytic enzymes in muscle increase in larger size fishes. *Physiol. Zool.* 53: 322–337.

Somero, G.N., and A.L. DeVries (1967). Temperature tolerance of some Antarctic fishes. *Science* 156: 257–258.

Somero, G.N., and J.F. Siebenaller (1979). Inefficient lactate dehydrogenases of deep-sea fishes. *Nature* 282: 100–102.

Somero, G.N., A.C. Giese, and D.E. Wohlschlag (1968). Cold adaptation of the Antarctic fish *Trematomus bernacchii*. *Comp. Biochem. Physiol.* 26: 223–233.

Somero, G.N., P.A. Fields, G.E. Hofmann, R.B. Weinstein, and H. Kawall (1998). Cold adaptation and stenothermy in Antarctic notothenioid fishes: What has been gained and what has been lost? In: *Fishes of Antarctica. A Biological Overview*, pp. 97–109, ed. G. di Prisco, E. Pisano, and A. Clarke. Milan: Springer.

Sømme, L. (1982). Supercooling and winter survival in terrestrial arthropods. *Comp. Biochem. Physiol.* 73A, 519–543.

Stillman, J.H., and G.N. Somero (1996). Adaptation to temperature stress and aerial exposure in congeneric species of intertidal porcelain crabs (genus *Petrolisthes*): correlation of physiology, biochemistry and morphology with vertical distribution. *J. Exp. Biol.*, 199: 1845–1855.

Stillman, J.H., and G.N. Somero (2000). A comparative analysis of the upper thermal tolerance limits of Eastern Pacific porcelain crabs (genus *Petrolisthes*): influences of latitude, vertical zonation, acclimation and phylogeny. *Physiol. Biochem. Zool.* 73: 200–208.

Stillman, J.H., and G.N. Somero (2001). A comparative analysis of the evolutionary patterning and mechanistic bases of LDH thermal stability in porcelain crabs, genus *Petrolisthes*. *J. Exp. Biol.*, 204: 767–776.

Storey, K.B. (1990). Life in a frozen state: adaptive strategies for natural freeze tolerance in amphibians and reptiles. *Am. J. Physiol. (Regulatory Integrative Comp. Physiol. 27)* 258: R559–R568.

Storz, G. (1999). An RNA thermometer. *Genes Devel.* 13: 633–636.

Streyer, L. (1988). *Biochemistry*, third edition. New York: W.H. Freeman.

Suarez, R.K. (1998). Oxygen and the upper limits to animal design and performance. *J. Exp. Biol.* 201: 1065–1072.

Thomas, C.D. and J.J. Lennon (1999). Birds extend their ranges northwards. *Nature* 399: 213.

Tissières, A. H.K. Mitchell, and U.M. Tracy (1974). Protein synthesis in salivary glands of *Drosophila melanogaster*: Relation to chromosome puffs. *J. Mol. Biol.* 84: 389–398.

Tomanek, L., and G.N. Somero (1999). Evolutionary and acclimation-induced variation in the heat shock responses of congeneric marine snails (genus *Tegula*) from different thermal habitats: Implications for limits of thermotolerance and biogeography. *J. Exp. Biol.* 202: 2925–2936.

Tomanek, L., and G.N. Somero (2000). Time course and magnitude of synthesis of heat-shock proteins in congeneric marine snails (genus *Tegula*) from different tidal heights. *Physiol. Biochem. Zool.* 73: 249–256.

Tsvetkova, N.M., and P.J. Quinn (1994). Compatible solutes modulate membrane lipid phase behaviour. In: *Temperature Adaptation of Biological Membranes*, pp. 49–61, ed. A.R. Cossins. London: Portland Press.

Verdier, J.-M., K.V. Ewart, M. Griffith, and C.L. Hew (1996). An immune response to ice crystals in North Atlantic fishes. *Eur. J. Biochem.* 241: 740–743.

Wang, X., A.L. DeVries, C.-H. C. Cheng (1995). Genomic basis for antifreeze peptide heterogeneity and abundance in an Antarctic eel pout: Gene structures and organization. *Mol. Mar. Biol. Biotech.* 4: 135–147.

Watt, W.B., and A.M. Dean (2001). Molecular-functional studies of adaptive genetic variation in prokaryotes and eukaryotes. *Annu. Rev. Genet.* 34: 593–622.

Weinstein, R.B., and G.N. Somero (1998). Effects of temperature on mitochondrial function in the Antarctic fish *Trematomus bernacchii*. *J. Comp. Physiol. B.* 168: 190–196.

Williams, E.E. (1998). Membrane lipids: What membrane physical properties are conserved during physiochemically induced membrane restructuring? *Amer. Zool.* 38: 280–290.

Wodtke, E. (1981). Temperature adaptation of biological membranes. Compensation of the molar activity of cytochrome C oxidase in the mitochondrial enregy-transducing membrane during thermal acclimation. *Biochim. Biophys. Acta* 640: 710–720.

Wu, L., and J.G. Duman (1991). Activation of antifreeze proteins from the beetle *Dendroides canadensis*. *J. Comp. Physiol.* 161: 279–283.

Xu, L., J.G. Duman, W.G. Goodman, and D.W. Wu (1992). A role for juvenile hormone in the induction of antifreeze protein production by the fat body in the beetle *Tenebrio molitor*. *Comp. Biochem. Physiol.* 101B: 105–109.

Yancey, P.H., and G.N. Somero (1978). Temperature dependence of intracellular pH: its role in the conservation of pyruvate apparent K_m values of vertebrate lactate dehydrogenases. *J. Comp. Physiol.* 125B: 129–134.

Yang, T.-H., and G. N. Somero (1993). Effects of feeding and food deprivation on oxygen consumption, muscle protein concentration and activities of energy metabolism enzymes in muscle and brain of shallow-living (*Scorpaena guttata*) and deep-living (*Sebastolobus alascanus*) scorpaenid fishes. *J. Exp. Biol.* 181: 213–232.

Yeh, S., B.A. Moffatt, M. Griffith, F. Xiong, D.S.C. Yang, S.B. Wiseman, F. Sarhan, J. Danyluk, Y.Q. Xue, C.L. Hew, A. Doherty-Kirby, and G. Lajoie (2000). Chitinase genes responsive to cold encode antifreeze proteins in winter cereals. *Plant Physiol.* 124: 1251–1263.

Yocum, G.D., K.H. Joplin, and D.L. Denlinger 1991). Expression of heat-shock proteins in response to high and low temperature extremes in diapausing pharate larvae of the gypsy moth, *Lymantria dispar. Arch. Insect Biochem. Physiol.* 18: 239–250.

Zachariassen, K.E. (1985). Physiology of cold tolerance in insects. *Physiol. Rev.* 65: 799–832.

Zachariassen, K.E. (1992). Ice nucleating agents in cold-hardy insects. In *Water and Life*, pp. 261–281, ed. G.N. Somero, B. Osmond, and L. Bolis. Berlin: Springer-Verlag.

Zachariassen, K.E., and J.A. Husby (1982). Antifreeze effect of thermal hysteresis agents protects highly supercooled insects. *Nature* 298: 865–867.

Zhong, M., A. Orosz, and C. Wu (1998). Direct sensing of heat and oxidation by *Drosophila* heat shock transcription factor. *Mol. Cell.* 2: 101–108.

Zimmermann, C. and G. Hubold (1998). Respiration and activity of Arctic and Antarctic fish with different modes of life: A multivariate analysis of experimental data. In: *Fishes of Antarctica. A Biological Overview*, pp. 163–174, ed. G. di Prisco, E. Pisano, and A. Clarke. Milan: Springer.

Index

acceptor control. *See also* metabolic
control models
and [ADP], 57–63
acclimation
definition of, 13, 187
acclimatization
definition of, 13, 187
acetylcholine
hypoxic receptor down regulation,
126–127
in O_2 signal transduction, 180
acetylcholinesterase (AChE)
hypoxic receptor down regulation,
126–127
isozymes in temperature
acclimation, 430–431
actin. *See also* unconventional myosins
in cellular scaffolding, 276–277
in *Drosophila* flight muscle, 69
and glycolytic metabolon, 350
in intracellular movement, 68–69
in osmosensing mechanisms, 267
activated substrates, 274
activation energy (E_a)
definition of, 296
in enzymatic reactions, 296,
in temperature adaptation of
enzymes, 314–315
activation enthalpy ($\Delta H^{\ddagger}$)
definition of, 314
in temperature adaptation of
enzymes, 314–315
activation entropy ($\Delta S^{\ddagger}$)
definition of, 314
in temperature adaptation of
enzymes, 314–315
activation free energy ($\Delta G^{\ddagger}$)
definition of, 314
in metabolic control, 59, 62, 63
relation to k_{cat}, 314–315
in temperature adaptation of
enzymes, 314–315
acyl chain composition. *See also*
homeophasic adaptation;
homeoviscous adaptation;
membranes
acyl chain reshuffling, 371
and proton leak, 28–32
adaptation. *See also* acclimation;
acclimatization; aptation;
exaptation
philosophical issues with, 4–9
process of, 4–14
adaptational physiology
definition of, 9
history of, 9–13
adenosine diphosphate (ADP)
in allometry, 33

in BMR, 28
in coupling ATPases with aerobic
glycolysis, 55, 58
in coupling CPK with aerobic
glycolysis, 52, 194–197
in CPK function, 58–63, 165
in glycolytic control, 52, 58–63,
194–197
and metabolic control, 52, 58–63,
194–197
in respiratory control, 52, 58–63,
194–197
adenosine monophosphate (AMP)
in glycolytic control, 62
adenosine triphosphate (ATP)
as chemical fuel, 3, 20
coupling functions, 20, 27–32
and energy conservation, 20–24
in energy turnover, 27–32, 122,
124–125
yields in metabolism, 20–24, 50, 52,
120–125, 194–197
adenyl cyclase
in signal transduction, 135, 140
in thermogenesis in BAT, 385
adenylates. *See* adenosine
disphosphate; adenosine
monophosphate; adenosine
triphosphate; aerobic metabolism;
anaerobic metabolism
adsorption–inhibition model of
antifreeze action, 416. *See also*
antifreeze proteins and antifreeze
glycoproteins
aerobic–anaerobic transition. *See also*
hypoxia responses
and diving metabolism, 158
and induction of genes for glycolytic
enzymes, 130
and the Pasteur effect, 124
aerobic metabolism
and control coefficients in athletes,
201–204
during diving, 158–163, 165–166
in endothermic homeothermy,
382–390
and evolution of endothermic
homeothermy, 404–406
in human hypoxia tolerance,
188–203
and metabolic compensation to
temperature, 303–305
and metabolic regulation, 56–70,
201–204
pathways of, 22–24
properties of, 27–56
and training responses, 74–79
and tuna endothermy, 87–93, 393

alanopine
as an anaerobic end product, 21,
120, 122
dehydrogenase, 21, 120, 122
aldolase (ALD)
in evolutionary up-regulation of
glycolysis, 80–84
expression of, 80–86
functional properties of, 59–62
and glycolysis, 21
induction during hypoxia, 130–136
algebraic additivity in solute effects
on cellular proliferation, 241–242
concentration ratios giving effect,
238–242
on enzymes, 238–240
urea–methylammonium effects,
238–242
allometry. *See also* scaling
and BMR 32–34, 36–39
equation for, 32, 397
fractal model of, 34, 36–37
and insect flight muscle, 32
and maximum metabolism, 36–39
multiple contributors model, 37–39
and P/O ratios, 30
of potassium ion flux, 404
and proton leak, 32, 401
of respiration in mammals, 400
and tissue/organ metabolism, 27
allosterism, 62, 109
allozymes
definition of, 205–206
roles in temperature adaptation 304
alpha-imidazole (α_{imid}). *See* histidine,
pH
alphastat regulation. *See* pH
altitude
acute and acclimation responses,
187–194
and adaptable traits, 194–207
and ADP affinity adjustments,
194–195
and brain metabolism, 194–195
and conservative traits, 194
and enzyme adjustments, 195, 198,
199, 201
and genotypes, 204–207
and heart metabolism, 195–197
hemoglobin adaptations to,
108–113, 200
and human evolution, 207–212
and the lactate paradox 189–192
and metabolic regulation, 194–197,
201–204
and oxygen sensing, 197–200
and phenotypes, 200–204
amino acid metabolism